Gluten-Free Diet

Gluten-Free Diet

Special Issue Editor

Luca Elli

MDPI • Basel • Beijing • Wuhan • Barcelona • Belgrade

Special Issue Editor
Luca Elli
Fondazione IRCCS Ca Granda Ospedale Maggiore Policlinico
Italy

Editorial Office
MDPI
St. Alban-Anlage 66
4052 Basel, Switzerland

This is a reprint of articles from the Special Issue published online in the open access journal *Nutrients* (ISSN 2072-6643) from 2018 to 2019 (available at: https://www.mdpi.com/journal/nutrients/special_issues/gluten_free_diet)

For citation purposes, cite each article independently as indicated on the article page online and as indicated below:

LastName, A.A.; LastName, B.B.; LastName, C.C. Article Title. *Journal Name* **Year**, *Article Number*, Page Range.

ISBN 978-3-03897-736-0 (Pbk)
ISBN 978-3-03897-737-7 (PDF)

Contents

About the Special Issue Editor

Luca Elli, MD received his degree in Medicine at the University of Milano and in 2004 became a specialist in Gastroenterology and Endoscopy. Again at the University of Milano, he received his PhD in Gastroenterological sciences. Throughout his career, Luca Elli has dealt with celiac disease, acquiring an important clinical and scientific experience. He is the author of more than 100 articles published in international journals. Moreover, during the last few years, Luca Elli has become an expert in small bowel endoscopy both videocapsule and double balloon enteroscopy, which has successfully been applied in the management of celiac disease. In fact, he is the head of the Center for Prevention and Diagnosis of Celiac Disease, Fondazione IRCCS Ca' Granda Opsedale Maggiore Policlinico, Milano, Italy.

nutrients

MDPI

Editorial

Gluten Rhapsody

Luca Elli * and Beatrice Marinoni

Center for the Prevention and Diagnosis of Coeliac Disease, Division of Gastroenterology and Endoscopy, Fondazione IRCCS Ca' Granda Ospedale Maggiore Policlinico, Milan 20122, Italy; beatrice.marinoni@unimi.it
* Correspondence: luca.elli@policlinico.mi.it

Received: 3 March 2019; Accepted: 5 March 2019; Published: 11 March 2019

Keywords: gluten; gluten-free diet; coeliac disease; non-celiac gluten sensitivity; non-coeliac wheat sensitivity; gliadin; microbiota

---

For decades, gluten-free dieting (GFD) has been accepted as the only therapeutic approach to coeliac disease (CD) and, more recently, for non-coeliac gluten sensitivity (NCGS), a term to refer to the so-called gluten-related disorders (GRD) [1].

GFD has become popular among the general population for its supposed beneficial effects on human health [2]. GFD is also the most frequently suggested dietary regimen in irritable bowel syndrome (IBS) [3].

In fact, there are several concerns and misconceptions regarding GFD, which deserve special attention. For such a reason, this Special Issue on "Gluten-Free Diet" comprises 23 peer-reviewed papers, reporting on the most recent evidence and topics about GFD. In particular, the impact of GFD on human health and quality of life; the emerging evidence of its beneficial effects in IBS; and the difficult problems of compliance, costs, and availability of GF food are discussed.

Several sources of evidence support the notion that, despite its remarkable effectiveness in remitting the vast majority of GRD symptoms, GFD comes with both a social and financial burden. Gluten-free foods are still less available and more expensive than their gluten-containing versions [4], thus causing patients social and psychological consequences in securing good quality of life and compliance with the advised dietary regimen.

As Joelson AM et al. have shown, the prevalence of depression among the sufferers of coeliac disease (CD) is high and depressive symptoms may mask the relationship between symptoms and inadvertent gluten exposure, and thus make it more difficult to detect any lack of adherence to GFD [5]. With a systematic review and meta-analysis, Busby at al. have confirmed that gluten elimination may well represent an effective treatment strategy for mood disorders for individuals with GRD [6].

As permanent adherence to GFD is difficult, with repeated transgression and frequent contaminations, a reliable tool to assess compliance is currently advocated [7]. In their review, Rodrigo L. et al. establish that the determination of the immunogenic gluten peptides in isolated samples of faeces or urine has proven useful for assessing adherence to GFD [8].

In the opinion of some authors, several factors contribute to greater adherence to GFD; that is, good knowledge of the disease and its treatment, high level of education, high economic status, female sex, young age, high self-esteem, good grades at school, good availability and labelling of products, good contact with a doctor and a dietitian, and finally membership of the Coeliac Society [9–12]. Conversely, the factors responsible for not adhering to GFD are poor taste of gluten-free products, high price and poor availability, being adolescent, the absence of immediate symptoms following the intake of small amounts of gluten, and low awareness of the disease [9,11,12].

From a study conducted by Czaja-Bulsa et al., it has emerged that GFD adherence has improved over the last ten years, thanks to the popularity gained by GFD and GF food becoming more available [13].

Further evidence, recently accepted, shows that in spite of improvements in food formulation over the last few years, GF foods still present with a reduced nutritional profile when compared with gluten-containing products, with higher lipid and trans-fat content; lower level of proteins; and lower degree of fortification with micronutrients, especially Ca, Fe, Mg, and Zn [14]. Similarly, Wiech et al. have shown that CD children adhering to GFD for a year showed a higher increase in weight and body mass index (BMI) when compared with healthy controls, suggesting a tendency towards metabolic syndrome [15]. However, there is growing evidence supporting the protective effect of GFD on bone metabolism [16] and the possible prevention of diabetes through GFD [17].

In preparing this Special Issue, GFD and fermentable oligo/di/monosaccharides and polyols (FODMAP) as dietary therapies in individuals with IBS was an issue that the Editors found to be important [18]. In a study evaluating the intake of foods containing fermentable oligo/di/monosaccharides and polyols (FODMAP) in CD patients, Roncoroni et al. confirmed that the prevalence of IBS-type symptoms among CD patients is higher than in the general population. Moreover, they demonstrated that CD patients consume a diet high on FODMAP, which is a factor that possibly induces gastrointestinal symptoms in treated CD patients [19,20]. Moreover, in the first RCT DB intervention controlled study, the same researchers showed that CD patients on GFD, but with persisting functional gastrointestinal symptoms, had a positive response to a diet low on FODMAP. Thus, GFD associated with a low-FODMAP content is beneficial, as a support therapy, for a group of CD patients with persistent gastrointestinal symptoms [21].

A number of questions still remain unanswered; namely, the modifications by GFD of the gut microbiota in different populations [22,23]; the effects of gluten intake on both gastric and gallbladder motility [24]; and the persistent motor disorders in CD patients, despite GFD, which can be explained by low-grade mucosal inflammation [25].

Several open issues regarding GFD also remain, such as, most importantly, the ingestion threshold for the amount of gluten considered tolerable has not been defined yet. Furthermore, the appropriateness of a lifelong indication to GFD, particularly for patients with sub-clinical and potential CD (i.e., not confirmed by histology), is still a matter of debate [26], especially on consideration of the impact on patients' quality of life posed by a restrictive gluten-free diet [27]. Finally, in a study on the immunogenic potential of α-gliadins in Triticale, Ruiz-Carnicer et al. demonstrated that by substituting a natural amino acid to the most immunogenic fraction of gluten (DQ2.5-glia-a 1, DQ2.5-glia-a2, and DQ2.5-glia-a3), the toxicity of three T-cell epitopes was eliminated, while the technological properties of commercial wheat were maintained [28]. These results may offer the opportunity to generate wheat varieties with a reduced CD immunogenicity not safe for consumption by patients, but that might help to prevent the onset of CD in people that carry genetic risk factors.

In conclusion, we would like to acknowledge all the authors for their valuable contributions and the reviewers for their constructive comments. Special thanks are owed to the publishing team of *Nutrients* for their professional assistance in the development of this Special Issue.

Funding: This research received no external funding

Conflicts of Interest: Luca Elli is a member of special dietary foods manufacturer Dr. Schär's Advisory Board.

References

1. Elli, L.; Villalta, D.; Roncoroni, L.; Barisani, D.; Ferrero, S.; Pellegrini, N.; Bardella, M.T.; Valiante, F.; Tomba, C.; Carroccio, A.; et al. Nomenclature and diagnosis of gluten-related disorders: A position statement by the Italian Association of Hospital Gastroenterologists and Endoscopists (AIGO). *Dig. Liver Dis.* **2017**, *49*, 138–146. [CrossRef] [PubMed]
2. Kim, H.S.; Patel, K.G.; Orosz, E.; Kothari, N.; Demyen, M.F.; Pyrsopoulos, N.; Ahlawat, S.K. Time Trends in the Prevalence of Celiac Disease and Gluten-Free Diet in the US Population: Results from the National Health and Nutrition Examination Surveys 2009–2014. *JAMA Intern. Med.* **2016**, *176*, 1716–1717. [CrossRef]

3. Catassi, C.; Alaedini, A.; Bojarski, C.; Bonaz, B.; Bouma, G.; Carroccio, A.; Castillejo, G.; De Magistris, L.; Dieterich, W.; Di Liberto, D.; et al. The Overlapping Area of Non-Celiac Gluten Sensitivity (NCGS) and Wheat-Sensitive Irritable Bowel Syndrome (IBS): An Update. *Nutrients* **2017**, *9*, 1268. [CrossRef] [PubMed]
4. Allen, B.; Orfila, C. The Availability and Nutritional Adequacy of Gluten-Free Bread and Pasta. *Nutrients* **2018**, *10*, 1370. [CrossRef] [PubMed]
5. Joelson, A.M.; Geller, M.G.; Zylberberg, H.M.; Green, P.H.R.; Lebwohl, B. The Effect of Depressive Symptoms on the Association between Gluten-Free Diet Adherence and Symptoms in Celiac Disease: Analysis of a Patient Powered Research Network. *Nutrients* **2018**, *10*, 538. [CrossRef] [PubMed]
6. Busby, E.; Bold, J.; Fellows, L.; Rostami, K. Mood Disorders and Gluten: It's Not All in Your Mind! A Systematic Review with Meta-Analysis. *Nutrients* **2018**, *10*, 1708. [CrossRef] [PubMed]
7. Syage, J.A.; Kelly, C.P.; Dickason, M.A.; Ramirez, A.C.; Leon, F.; Dominguez, R.; Sealey-Voyksner, J.A. Determination of gluten consumption in celiac disease patients on a gluten-free diet. *Am. J. Clin. Nutr.* **2018**, *107*, 201–207. [CrossRef] [PubMed]
8. Rodrigo, L.; Perez-Martinez, I.; Lauret-Brana, E.; Suarez-Gonzalez, A. Descriptive Study of the Different Tools Used to Evaluate the Adherence to a Gluten-Free Diet in Celiac Disease Patients. *Nutrients* **2018**, *10*, 1777. [CrossRef] [PubMed]
9. Freeman, H.J. Dietary compliance in celiac disease. *World J. Gastroenterol.* **2017**, *23*, 2635–2639. [CrossRef] [PubMed]
10. Silvester, J.A.; Weiten, D.; Graff, L.A.; Walker, J.R.; Duerksen, D.R. Is it gluten-free? Relationship between self-reported gluten-free diet adherence and knowledge of gluten content of foods. *Nutrition* **2016**, *32*, 777–783. [CrossRef] [PubMed]
11. Greco, L.; Mayer, M.; Ciccarelli, G.; Troncone, R.; Auricchio, S. Compliance to a gluten-free diet in adolescents, or "what do 300 coeliac adolescents eat every day?". *Ital. J. Gastroenterol. Hepatol.* **1997**, *29*, 305–310. [PubMed]
12. Kurppa, K.; Lauronen, O.; Collin, P.; Ukkola, A.; Laurila, K.; Huhtala, H.; Maki, M.; Kaukinen, K. Factors associated with dietary adherence in celiac disease: A nationwide study. *Digestion* **2012**, *86*, 309–314. [CrossRef] [PubMed]
13. Czaja-Bulsa, G.; Bulsa, M. Adherence to Gluten-Free Diet in Children with Celiac Disease. *Nutrients* **2018**, *10*, 1424. [CrossRef] [PubMed]
14. Rybicka, I. The Handbook of Minerals on a Gluten-Free Diet. *Nutrients* **2018**, *10*, 1683. [CrossRef] [PubMed]
15. Wiech, P.; Chmiel, Z.; Bazalinski, D.; Salacinska, I.; Bartosiewicz, A.; Mazur, A.; Korczowski, B.; Binkowska-Bury, M.; Dabrowski, M. The Relationship between Body Composition and a Gluten Free Diet in Children with Celiac Disease. *Nutrients* **2018**, *10*, 1817. [CrossRef] [PubMed]
16. Tovoli, F.; Negrini, G.; Sansone, V.; Faggiano, C.; Catenaro, T.; Bolondi, L.; Granito, A. Celiac Disease Diagnosed through Screening Programs in At-Risk Adults Is Not Associated with Worse Adherence to the Gluten-Free Diet and Might Protect from Osteopenia/Osteoporosis. *Nutrients* **2018**, *10*, 1940. [CrossRef] [PubMed]
17. Haupt-Jorgensen, M.; Holm, L.J.; Josefsen, K.; Buschard, K. Possible Prevention of Diabetes with a Gluten-Free Diet. *Nutrients* **2018**, *10*, 1746. [CrossRef] [PubMed]
18. Rej, A.; Sanders, D.S. Gluten-Free Diet and Its 'Cousins' in Irritable Bowel Syndrome. *Nutrients* **2018**, *10*, 1727. [CrossRef] [PubMed]
19. Sainsbury, A.; Sanders, D.S.; Ford, A.C. Prevalence of irritable bowel syndrome-type symptoms in patients with celiac disease: A meta-analysis. *Clin. Gastroenterol. Hepatol.* **2013**, *11*, 359–365. [CrossRef] [PubMed]
20. Roncoroni, L.; Elli, L.; Doneda, L.; Bascunan, K.A.; Vecchi, M.; Morreale, F.; Scricciolo, A.; Lombardo, V.; Pellegrini, N. A Retrospective Study on Dietary FODMAP Intake in Celiac Patients Following a Gluten-Free Diet. *Nutrients* **2018**, *10*, 1769. [CrossRef] [PubMed]
21. Roncoroni, L.; Bascunan, K.A.; Doneda, L.; Scricciolo, A.; Lombardo, V.; Branchi, F.; Ferretti, F.; Dell'Osso, B.; Montanari, V.; Bardella, M.T.; et al. A Low FODMAP Gluten-Free Diet Improves Functional Gastrointestinal Disorders and Overall Mental Health of Celiac Disease Patients: A Randomized Controlled Trial. *Nutrients* **2018**, *10*, 1023. [CrossRef] [PubMed]
22. Garcia-Mazcorro, J.F.; Noratto, G.; Remes-Troche, J.M. The Effect of Gluten-Free Diet on Health and the Gut Microbiota Cannot Be Extrapolated from One Population to Others. *Nutrients* **2018**, *10*, 1421. [CrossRef] [PubMed]

23. Garcia-Mazcorro, J.F.; Rivera-Gutierrez, X.; Cobos-Quevedo, O.J.; Grube-Pagola, P.; Meixueiro-Daza, A.; Hernandez-Flores, K.; Cabrera-Jorge, F.J.; Vivanco-Cid, H.; Dowd, S.E.; Remes-Troche, J.M. First Insights into the Gut Microbiota of Mexican Patients with Celiac Disease and Non-Celiac Gluten Sensitivity. *Nutrients* **2018**, *10*, 1641. [CrossRef] [PubMed]
24. Massironi, S.; Branchi, F.; Fraquelli, M.; Baccarin, A.; Somalvico, F.; Ferretti, F.; Conte, D.; Elli, L. Effects of a Gluten-Containing Meal on Gastric Emptying and Gallbladder Contraction. *Nutrients* **2018**, *10*, 910. [CrossRef] [PubMed]
25. Usai-Satta, P.; Oppia, F.; Lai, M.; Cabras, F. Motility Disorders in Celiac Disease and Non-Celiac Gluten Sensitivity: The Impact of a Gluten-Free Diet. *Nutrients* **2018**, *10*, 1705. [CrossRef] [PubMed]
26. Norsa, L.; Branchi, F.; Bravo, M.; Ferretti, F.; Roncoroni, L.; Somalvico, F.; Conte, D.; Bardella, M.T.; Fabiano, S.; Barigelletti, G.; et al. Celiac Disease 30 Years After Diagnosis: Struggling with Gluten-free Adherence or Gaining Gluten Tolerance? *J. Pediatr. Gastroenterol. Nutr.* **2018**, *67*, 361–366. [CrossRef] [PubMed]
27. Itzlinger, A.; Branchi, F.; Elli, L.; Schumann, M. Gluten-Free Diet in Celiac Disease-Forever and for All? *Nutrients* **2018**, *10*, 1796. [CrossRef] [PubMed]
28. Ruiz-Carnicer, A.; Comino, I.; Segura, V.; Ozuna, C.V.; Moreno, M.L.; Lopez-Casado, M.A.; Torres, M.I.; Barro, F.; Sousa, C. Celiac Immunogenic Potential of alpha-Gliadin Epitope Variants from Triticum and Aegilops Species. *Nutrients* **2019**, *11*, 220. [CrossRef] [PubMed]

nutrients

Article

The Effect of Depressive Symptoms on the Association between Gluten-Free Diet Adherence and Symptoms in Celiac Disease: Analysis of a Patient Powered Research Network

Andrew M. Joelson [1], Marilyn G. Geller [2], Haley M. Zylberberg [3], Peter H. R. Green [3] and Benjamin Lebwohl [3,4,*]

1. Department of Internal Medicine, New York Presbyterian Hospital, New York, NY 10032, USA; amj9033@nyp.org
2. Celiac Disease Foundation, Woodland Hills, CA 91364, USA; marilyn.geller@celiac.org
3. Celiac Disease Center, Department of Medicine, Columbia University Medical Center, 180 Fort Washington Avenue, Suite 936, New York, NY 10032, USA; hmz2105@columbia.edu (H.M.Z.); pg11@cumc.columbia.edu (P.H.R.G.)
4. Deartment of Epidemiology, Mailman School of Public Health, Columbia University Medical Center, New York, NY 10032, USA

* Correspondence: BL114@columbia.edu; Tel.: +1-212-305-5590

Received: 8 March 2018; Accepted: 23 April 2018; Published: 26 April 2018

Abstract: Background: The prevalence of depression in celiac disease (CD) is high, and patients are often burdened socially and financially by a gluten-free diet. However, the relationship between depression, somatic symptoms and dietary adherence in CD is complex and poorly understood. We used a patient powered research network (iCureCeliac®) to explore the effect that depression has on patients' symptomatic response to a gluten-free diet (GFD). Methods: We identified patients with biopsy-diagnosed celiac disease who answered questions pertaining to symptoms (Celiac Symptom Index (CSI)), GFD adherence (Celiac Dietary Adherence Test (CDAT)), and a 5-point, scaled question regarding depressive symptoms relating to patients' celiac disease. We then measured the correlation between symptoms and adherence (CSI vs. CDAT) in patients with depression versus those without depression. We also tested for interaction of depression with regard to the association with symptoms using a multiple linear regression model. Results: Among 519 patients, 86% were female and the mean age was 40.9 years. 46% of patients indicated that they felt "somewhat," "quite a bit," or "very much" depressed because of their disorder. There was a moderate correlation between worsened celiac symptoms and poorer GFD adherence ($r = 0.6$, $p < 0.0001$). In those with a positive depression screen, there was a moderate correlation between worsening symptoms and worsening dietary adherence ($r = 0.5$, $p < 0.0001$) whereas in those without depression, the correlation was stronger ($r = 0.64$, $p < 0.0001$). We performed a linear regression analysis, which suggests that the relationship between CSI and CDAT is modified by depression. Conclusions: In patients with depressive symptoms related to their disorder, correlation between adherence and symptoms was weaker than those without depressive symptoms. This finding was confirmed with a linear regression analysis, showing that depressive symptoms may modify the effect of a GFD on celiac symptoms. Depressive symptoms may therefore mask the relationship between inadvertent gluten exposure and symptoms. Additional longitudinal and prospective studies are needed to further explore this potentially important finding.

Keywords: Celiac Disease; depression; gluten-free diet; dietary adherence

1. Introduction

Celiac Disease (CD) is an autoimmune disorder that, by recent estimates, affects roughly 0.7% of the United States population [1]. The disease is caused by gut mucosal immune activation against gluten, a protein component of wheat, rye, and barley [2]. The clinical manifestations are numerous and often differ between adults and children. While potential new therapies are being studied, the only current treatment is strict avoidance of gluten in the diet [3]; a treatment that for many is expensive, socially isolating, and can result in anxiety about accidental ingestion [3].

There are many well-described neuropsychiatric manifestations of CD. Many studies have examined the association between CD and depression [4–12], anxiety [7,10], bipolar disorder [10], and schizophrenia [3,6]. The prevalence of depression in CD has been reported as anywhere between 6% and 57% [13], and a 2011 meta-analysis showed that depression is more common in CD than the general population [5]. However, other studies have demonstrated that the prevalence of depression in CD is the same as in the general population [14] and in other cohorts that suffer from chronic illness [5,15]. Many pathophysiologic mechanisms behind the CD-depression association have been postulated and studied including regional cerebral hypoperfusion [12], comorbid autoimmune thyroid disease [11], and decreased levels of cerebrospinal fluid monoamines in celiac patients, which improve with a gluten-free diet (GFD) [16,17]. The GFD can be expensive, burdensome, and socially isolating [3]. It is therefore conceivable that adhering to such a diet may be associated with worsening of affective symptoms. However, one cross-sectional study demonstrated an association between less severe depression scores and being on a gluten-free diet for more than five years [8] and another longitudinal study found improvements in quality of life after one year of treatment of a GFD, with less improvement in those who adhered poorly [18]. Simsek et al. (2015) identified improved depression scores in pediatric patients adherent to a GFD [19] as did Borghini et al. [20] in adult patients, where another study suggested improvement in anxiety only, with no change in depressive symptoms after one year of a GFD [21]. Furthermore, depressed patients who suffer from chronic illnesses have been found to be less compliant with treatment than non-depressed individuals [22]. A recent meta-analysis examined 8 cross-sectional studies and concluded that an association between poorer GFD adherence and self-reported depressive symptoms is likely [23]. Another study followed 66 patients, randomized to receive or not receive psychological support and found reduced depression scores and better adherence to their diet at six months in patients receiving psychological support [24]. This suggests that a relationship may exist between depressive symptoms and GFD adherence; however, the common use of self-reported depression and dietary adherence scales challenges the study of the topic. Furthermore, many of these studies do not specifically examine symptoms of CD. As many common CD symptoms may mimic those of depression, this remains a challenging relationship to evaluate scientifically.

In order to involve patients in clinical research, the Patient-Centered Outcomes Research Institute (PCORI) created the National Patient-Centered Clinical Research Network. As an outcome of this initiative, the Celiac Disease Foundation created iCureCeliac®, a patient-governed forum for clinical research. We implemented this tool to study the effect of self-reported depressive symptoms as relating to CD on the association between CD symptoms and adherence to a GFD. We hypothesized that the presence of depressive symptoms modifies the symptomatic response to a GFD.

2. Patients and Methods

We performed a cross-sectional analysis of pre-existing study data, utilizing the research questionnaire from iCureCeliac® a patient-powered research network. Beginning in January 2016, the questionnaire was posted on the Celiac Disease Foundation website and reminders were periodically emailed to newsletter subscribers. Patients had the option to enter as much or as little data as they desired on an entirely voluntary basis with no financial incentive offered.

2.1. Inclusion Criteria

At the time of data analysis, the iCureCeliac® questionnaire included data from 1724 individuals, with gluten-related disorders that included CD, non-celiac gluten sensitivity, dermatitis herpetiformis, wheat allergy, and self-diagnosed gluten-related disorder. We included patients of all ages who indicated in the questionnaire a diagnosis of CD, diagnosed at any age by endoscopy and biopsy and who answered the questions that applied to our study between the inception of the patient-powered research network on 30 January 2016 and 25 August 2016. A parent or legal guardian completed responses for children. Although per ACG and AGA guidelines [25,26], a diagnosis of CD is made using a combination of serology and a confirmatory biopsy of the small bowel to diagnose CD in patients with typical signs and symptoms, we assumed that biopsy-proven diagnoses were made in patients with symptoms and serology suggestive of celiac disease.

2.2. Data Collection

We collected basic demographic information including age, sex, education level, time to diagnosis from symptom onset, and degree of adherence to a gluten-free diet. We extracted data from one question asking patients about depression as it relates to their gluten-related disorder, phrased as follows: "I feel depressed because of my gluten-related disorder". Five responses were offered ranging from "not at all" to "very much". We considered the responses "somewhat", "quite a bit", and "very much" to indicate the presence of depressive symptoms, whereas "not at all" and "a little bit" to indicate the absence of depressive symptoms. A smaller subset of patients responded to the PROMIS (Patient Reported Outcomes Measurement Information System) Depression instrument. PROMIS is a set of validated, self-reported measures that evaluate various physical, psychological and social symptoms designed for use in adult and pediatric populations for research. The PROMIS Depression instruments include a complete 28-item assessment, as well as 4-, 6-, and 8-question short forms. Upon completion of the questionnaire, a raw score is generated, which corresponds to a T-score (based on a conversion table provided) with an instrument-specific range (41.0 to 79.4 for the 4-question short form used in the iCureCeliac® questionnaire). The T score is compared to the population mean with standard errors provided.

We also extracted data from questions administered to questionnaire respondents relating to symptoms and dietary adherence, which comprised most of the Celiac Symptom Index (CSI) and Celiac Dietary Adherence Test (CDAT) questions outlined by Leffler et al. [27,28]. The CSI and CDAT are clinically oriented, easily administered, questionnaires with 16 and 7-items, respectively. The CSI performed well as a surrogate measure of disease activity [27] and the CDAT was shown to perform better than tissue transglutaminase titers for evaluating dietary adherence [28].

2.3. Data Analysis

The iCureCeliac® questionnaire asked fifteen of the sixteen questions included in the CSI (missing question: "How much physical pain have you had during the last 4 weeks"?) and five out of the seven questions included in the CDAT (missing scaled questions: "I do not consider myself a failure" and "Before I do something, I carefully consider the consequences"). As not all of the CSI and CDAT questions were included in the initial iCureCeliac® questionnaire, the instruments are incomplete. We therefore analyzed these responses out of a total of 75 and 25 possible points, respectively (compared with 80 and 35, respectively). Higher CSI scores correlate with more severe symptoms and higher CDAT scores correlate with poorer dietary adherence, as described by Leffler et al. [27,28].

We calculated correlation coefficients with 95% confidence intervals between: (1) adherence to a GFD (CDAT) and CD symptoms (CSI); (2) depression and CD symptoms (CSI); and (3) depression and adherence to a GFD (CDAT). We then stratified patients based on the presence of depressive symptoms so as to determine whether these symptoms modify the association between adherence to a GFD and CD symptoms. To formally test for interaction, we constructed a multiple linear regression model with CSI score as the outcome, and CDAT score, the presence of depression, and the interaction term (depression*CDAT) as the dependent variables.

As a means of validating our chosen screening question for depressive symptoms, we calculated a correlation coefficient to compare our question to the 4-item PROMIS depression score in the smaller subset of respondents who completed both sets of questions regarding depression. For all PROMIS Depression instruments, a T-score of 50 is equivalent to the mean of the general population with a standard deviation of 10. The 4-item depression short form has been validated against the Center for Epidemiologic Studies Depression Scale [29]. For the purpose of this study, patients with a raw score greater than or equal to 11 (corresponding to a T score of, $\geq$60.5 or 1 SD above the mean of the general population) were considered to have a positive depression screen.

We used the guidelines set forth by Evans [30] for interpretation of correlation coefficient values.

We used SAS version 9.4 (SAS Institute Inc. 2013, Cary, NC, USA) to calculate Pearson correlation coefficients for the variables listed above. Although the study was designed after data collection, our hypothesis was developed prior to data analysis. Informed consent was obtained from each patient prior to completion of the survey. This study conforms to the ethical guidelines set forth by the 1975 declaration of Helsinki and was approved by the Institutional Review Board of Columbia University Medical Center on 22 September 2016.

3. Results

We identified 519 patients with biopsy-diagnosed CD who met criteria for inclusion in our study. The characteristics of our study population are displayed in Table 1. The participants were predominantly female (86%). The mean age was 40.9 years (standard deviation (SD) $\pm$ 16.7), 26 patients were aged 16 years or less, 92% of our study population self-reported their race as white and 65% had completed at least one year of college-level education. Feeling depressed was reported by 46% of respondents ("very much" by 6.7%, "quite a bit" by 12.5%, and "somewhat" by 26.8%). The mean ($\pm$SD) CDAT score was 12.81 ($\pm$2.53, out of a 25-point scale, IQR = 16) and the mean ($\pm$SD) CSI score was 36.1 ($\pm$11.2 out of a 75-point scale, IQR = 11).

Depression had a weak correlation with worse symptoms (r = 0.35, 95% CI 0.26–0.43, p < 0.0001) and a weaker correlation with GFD adherence (r = 0.25, 95% CI 0.16–032, p < 0.0001). There was a moderate correlation between worse symptoms and poorer GFD adherence (r = 0.60, 95% CI 0.53–0.66, p < 0.0001).

In patients with a positive depression screen, there was a moderate correlation between worsening symptoms and worsening dietary adherence (r = 0.50, 95% CI 0.37–0.60, p < 0.0001) whereas in those without depression, the correlation was still moderate, although stronger (r = 0.64, 95% CI 0.55–0.71, p < 0.0001). When patients <16 years of age were removed from the analysis (n = 370), the results were unchanged. The difference in CSI vs. CDAT scores in depressed vs. non-depressed patients is shown in Figure 1. When formally testing for interaction (n = 392), the beta coefficient for CDAT*depression was −0.935 (95% CI −1.65–−0.22, p = 0.0109), suggesting that the relationship between CSI and CDAT is modified by depression.

137 patients answered the 4-item PROMIS Depression instrument. Using a cutoff of one standard deviation above the mean, 24 patients (17.5%) met criteria for depression (T score $\geq$ 11) and 113 (82.5%) were not depressed (T score $\leq$ 10). The mean PROMIS raw score was 6.9 (SD $\pm$ 3.6) corresponding to a T score of 53.9 (SE 2.4). 91 patients (66.4%) scored below the mean and 46 (33.6%) patients scored above the mean. Our chosen depression screening question correlated moderately (r = 0.48, p < 0.0001) with the PROMIS score. Furthermore, in the same subset of patients, we found a similarly moderate correlation between symptoms and adherence in depressed patients (r = 0.46, p = 0.03) and moderate, although stronger correlation in patients who were not depressed (r = 0.57, p < 0.0001).

Table 1. Patient characteristics of our study population. As the questionnaire was voluntary, some questions are missing responses from all 519 participants.

Characteristic		Study Population (n = 519)
Gender		
Male		74 (14%)
Female		445 (86%)
Age (mean ± SD)		40.9 (±16.7)
Race/Ethnicity (n = 509)		
Black/African American		3 (0.6%)
Latino/Hispanic		8 (1.6%)
White		469 (92.1%)
Other (including more than 1)		29 (5.7%)
Highest education level (n = 207)		
Less than a college degree		60 (29%)
College degree or equivalent		85 (41.1%)
Master's degree or degree beyond Bachelor's degree		49 (23.7%)
Doctorate degree		13 (6.3%)
Currently working (n = 209)		
Yes		149 (71.3%)
No—on disability		5 (2.4%)
No—retired		24 (11.5%)
No—other		24 (11.5%)
Degree of Strict Gluten Free Diet Adherence (n = 516)		
Always		453 (87.3%)
Often		51 (9.8%)
Sometimes		9 (1.7%)
Rarely		2 (0.4%)
Never		1 (0.2%)
Skipped/Missing		3 (0.6%)
Length of time from symptom onset to Celiac Disease diagnosis		
<5 years		356 (68.6%)
5–15 years		67 (12.9%)
>15 years		38 (7.3%)
Don't Know/missing		58 (11.2%)
Depressed (n = 519)		
Yes	Very Much	35 (6.7%)
	Quite A bit	65 (12.5%)
	Somewhat	139 (26.8%)
No	A little bit	157 (30.3%)
	Not at all	125 (23.7%)
Celiac Dietary Adherence Test (n = 519)		
Mean (±SD)		12.8 (±2.5)
First Quartile		3
Median		13
Third Quartile		14
Interquartile Range		11
Celiac Symptom Index (n = 392)		
Mean (±SD)		36.1 (±11.2)
First Quartile		27
Median		36
Third Quartile		43
Interquartile Range		16

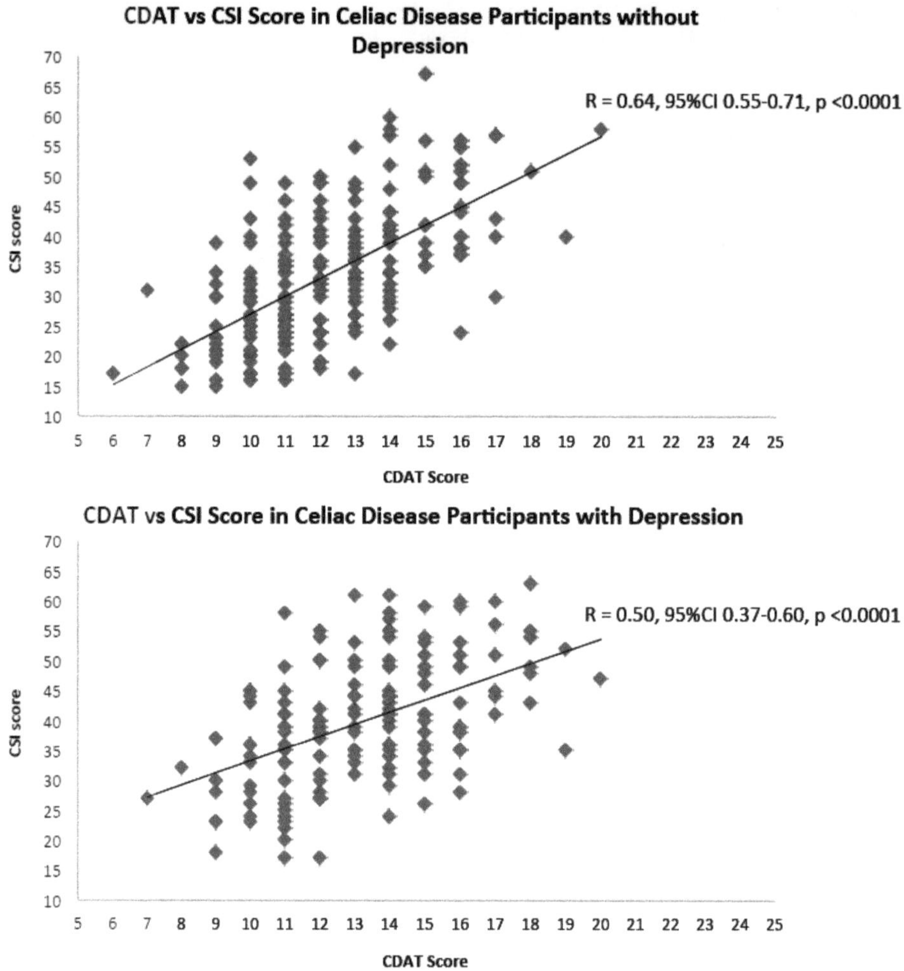

Figure 1. Celiac Dietary Adherence Test vs. Celiac Symptom Index Scores in patients with depressive symptoms versus those without depressive symptoms.

4. Discussion

In this cross-sectional study of 519 patients with biopsy-diagnosed CD, we found that self-reported depressive symptoms were common, occurring in 46% of the respondents. We also found that the relationship between CD symptoms and adherence to a GFD may be attenuated based on the presence of depressive symptoms related to having celiac disease. In those without depressive symptoms, the correlation between symptoms and dietary adherence was moderate, although stronger than in those with a positive depression screen. This was further supported by our regression analysis demonstrating significant interaction of depression on the relationship between GFD adherence and CD symptoms. These results suggest that the presence of depressive symptoms may attenuate the relationship between adherence to a GFD and symptoms of CD as those with depression may have less symptomatic relief from better adherence to a GFD than those without depressive symptoms.

We also found a weak correlation between higher levels of depression (based on our screening question) and poor dietary adherence. The association between adherence to a GFD and depression was further evaluated in a recent meta-analysis, which found a likely association between poor GFD adherence and worsened depressive symptoms. Furthermore, Addolorato et al. demonstrated that CD patients who received six months of psychological counseling had better adherence to their diets and lower rates of depression [24]. The weak correlation found in our study does not support the relationship between poor dietary adherence and depression described by others [23]. Rather, our results suggest that depression affects the relationship between adherence to a GFD and CD symptoms. One possible, reason for this effect modification is that patients with depression may have their symptoms driven or exacerbated by factors other than gluten exposure, which may manifest physically. However, there are many other potential causes of symptoms in CD including functional bowel disorders, inadvertent gluten exposure, and concomitant food intolerances. The relationship between celiac symptoms and depressive symptoms is complex and identifying which symptoms are attributable to each process can be challenging for clinicians.

This study has a number of limitations, some of which are inherent to its retrospective, self-reported and observational nature. The study was compiled from a voluntary questionnaire in a patient-powered research network. Although there was no financial incentive to complete the questionnaire, the study population represents a self-selected cohort of patients, who may be more aware of their illnesses and therefore may be more adherent to a GFD than the general CD population. This is supported by the high percentage (87%) of patients reporting they "always" adhere to a GFD. Furthermore, the majority of our research cohort was comprised of white, highly educated females. Unfortunately, the initial questionnaire did not contain all of the questions that make up the CSI and the CDAT, so each of these instruments is incomplete. However, for the purpose of our study, the trend (higher CDAT scores representing worse dietary adherence and higher CSI scores representing more symptomatic patients) was sufficient to evaluate our research question. Moreover, we feel that the correlation of higher CD symptom scores (worse symptoms) with poorer dietary adherence suggests validity, despite the abbreviated indices available.

Another limitation was in our utilization of a single question to screen patients for depression. Our screening question demonstrated moderate correlation with the validated 4-item PROMIS Depression instrument. However the PROMIS questions were completed by only a small subset of participants, which may lead to selection for more depressed patients. By PROMIS criteria, the prevalence of depression in our study was 17.5%. In contrast, using our 1-item screening question, depressive symptoms in our study were more common, with nearly half of respondents (46%) reporting that they felt at least "somewhat" depressed with regards to their disease. This difference may be due to the use of the chosen depression screening question which may signify the emotional reaction to having CD as opposed to clinical depression. Addolorato et al. [21] demonstrated a 57% prevalence of depression in their study, but others have shown the prevalence of active depressive symptoms in CD patients to be lower [4]. The prevalence of depression found in our study should therefore be interpreted with caution, as it may represent a self-selecting, more symptomatic population. Furthermore, these results represent self-reported data at a point in time, and not diagnoses made by health care professionals.

5. Conclusions

In conclusion, our analysis of data provided through a CD patient-powered research network, suggests that depression may modify the relationship between adherence to a GFD and the presence of symptoms in CD. In patients who screened positive for depressive symptoms, the correlation between CD symptoms and response to a GFD was attenuated. These findings support that screening for depression should be considered in patients with CD, as those with depression may have less improvement in symptoms despite better adherence to the diet than those without depression. The study of this topic remains a challenge due to a lack of longitudinal and prospective studies. The relationship between dietary adherence and depression remains complex and the direction of the association remains unclear [23]. As suggested previously, patients receiving psychological counseling may show better adherence to a GFD [24], but further prospective and randomized studies are needed to explore whether or not treatment for depression improves how patients respond symptomatically to a GFD. Ideally, future studies will encompass more diverse groups that represent the true CD population in the United States with validated measures of depression to further substantiate these findings. Our study also provides demonstrable evidence of the value of patient-powered research networks in the ongoing study of celiac disease.

Author Contributions: Andrew M. Joelson researched the study and wrote and submitted the manuscript. Marilyn G. Geller assisted with questionnaire data acquisition. Haley M. Zylberberg assisted with statistical analysis. Peter H. R. Green and Benjamin Lebwohl assisted with study planning and revisions.

Acknowledgments: Special thanks to Marilyn G. Geller for her assistance with the iCureCeliac questionnaire, Haley M. Zylberberg for her assistance with data analysis, Peter H. R. Green and Benjamin Lebwohl for their guidance and oversight. The iCureCeliac Patient Powered Research Network is funded by an Engagement Award from the Patient-Centered Outcomes Research Institute (Award #1306-04899).

Conflicts of Interest: The authors declare no conflicts of interest.

References

1. Rubio-Tapia, A.; Ludvigsson, J.F.; Brantner, T.L.; Murray, J.A.; Everhart, J.E. The prevalence of celiac disease in the United States. *Am. J. Gastroenterol.* **2012**, *107*, 1538–1544. [CrossRef] [PubMed]
2. Green, P.H.; Cellier, C. Celiac disease. *N. Engl. J. Med.* **2007**, *357*, 1731–1743. [CrossRef] [PubMed]
3. Lebwohl, B.; Ludvigsson, J.F.; Green, P.H. Celiac disease and non-celiac gluten sensitivity. *BMJ* **2015**, *351*, h4347. [CrossRef] [PubMed]
4. Ludvigsson, J.F.; Reutfors, J.; Osby, U.; Ekbom, A.; Montgomery, S.M. Coeliac disease and risk of mood disorders—A general population-based cohort study. *J. Affect. Disord.* **2007**, *99*, 117–126. [CrossRef] [PubMed]
5. Smith, D.F.; Gerdes, L.U. Meta-analysis on anxiety and depression in adult celiac disease. *Acta Psychiatr. Scand.* **2012**, *125*, 189–193. [CrossRef] [PubMed]
6. Jackson, J.R.; Eaton, W.W.; Cascella, N.G.; Fasano, A.; Kelly, D.L. Neurologic and psychiatric manifestations of celiac disease and gluten sensitivity. *Psychiatr. Q.* **2012**, *83*, 91–102. [CrossRef] [PubMed]
7. Zingone, F.; Swift, G.L.; Card, T.R.; Sanders, D.S.; Ludvigsson, J.F.; Bai, J.C. Psychological morbidity of celiac disease: A review of the literature. *United Eur. Gastroenterol. J.* **2015**, *3*, 136–145. [CrossRef] [PubMed]
8. Van Hees, N.J.; Van der Does, W.; Giltay, E.J. Coeliac disease, diet adherence and depressive symptoms. *J. Psychosom. Res.* **2013**, *74*, 155–160. [CrossRef] [PubMed]
9. Addolorato, G.; Stefanini, G.F.; Capristo, E.; Caputo, F.; Gasbarrini, A.; Gasbarrini, G. Anxiety and depression in adult untreated celiac subjects and in patients affected by inflammatory bowel disease: A personality "trait" or a reactive illness? *Hepatogastroenterology* **1996**, *43*, 1513–1517. [PubMed]
10. Carta, M.G.; Conti, A.; Lecca, F.; Sancassiani, F.; Cossu, G.; Carruxi, R.; Boccone, A.; Cadoni, M.; Pisanu, A.; Francesca, M.; et al. The Burden of Depressive and Bipolar Disorders in Celiac Disease. *Clin. Pract. Epidemiol. Ment. Health* **2015**, *11*, 180–185. [CrossRef] [PubMed]
11. Carta, M.G.; Hardoy, M.C.; Boi, M.F.; Mariotti, S.; Carpiniello, B.; Usai, P. Association between panic disorder, major depressive disorder and celiac disease: A possible role of thyroid autoimmunity. *J. Psychosom. Res.* **2002**, *53*, 789–793. [CrossRef]
12. Addolorato, G.; Di Giuda, D.; De Rossi, G.; Valenza, V.; Domenicali, M.; Caputo, F.; Gasbarrini, A.; Capristo, E.; Gasbarrini, G. Regional cerebral hypoperfusion in patients with celiac disease. *Am. J. Med.* **2004**, *116*, 312–317. [CrossRef] [PubMed]
13. Garud, S.; Leffler, D.; Dennis, M.; Edwards-George, J.; Saryan, D.; Sheth, S.; Schuppan, D.; Jamma, S.; Kelly, C.P. Interaction between psychiatric and autoimmune disorders in coeliac disease patients in the Northeastern United States. *Aliment. Pharmacol. Ther.* **2009**, *29*, 898–905. [CrossRef] [PubMed]
14. Häuser, W.; Janke, K.H.; Klump, B.; Gregor, M.; Hinz, A. Anxiety and depression in adult patients with celiac disease on a gluten-free diet. *World J. Gastroenterol.* **2010**, *16*, 2780–2787. [CrossRef] [PubMed]
15. Fera, T.; Cascio, B.; Angelini, G.; Martini, S.; Guidetti, C.S. Affective disorders and quality of life in adult coeliac disease patients on a gluten-free diet. *Eur. J. Gastroenterol. Hepatol.* **2003**, *15*, 1287–1292. [CrossRef] [PubMed]

16. Hernanz, A.; Polanco, I. Plasma precursor amino acids of central nervous system monoamines in children with coeliac disease. *Gut* **1991**, *32*, 1478–1481. [CrossRef] [PubMed]
17. Hallert, C.; Sedvall, G. Improvement in central monoamine metabolism in adult coeliac patients starting a gluten-free diet. *Psychol. Med.* **1983**, *13*, 267–271. [CrossRef] [PubMed]
18. Nachman, F.; del Campo, M.P.; González, A.; Corzo, L.; Vázquez, H.; Sfoggia, C.; Smecuol, E.; Sánchez, M.I.; Niveloni, S.; Sugai, E.; et al. Long-term deterioration of quality of life in adult patients with celiac disease is associated with treatment noncompliance. *Dig. Liver Dis.* **2010**, *42*, 685–691. [CrossRef] [PubMed]
19. Simsek, S.; Baysoy, G.; Gencoglan, S.; Uluca, U. Effects of Gluten-Free Diet on Quality of Life and Depression in Children with Celiac Disease. *J. Pediatr. Gastroenterol. Nutr.* **2015**, *61*, 303–306. [CrossRef] [PubMed]
20. Borghini, R.; Di Tola, M.; Salvi, E.; Isonne, C.; Puzzono, M.; Marino, M.; Donato, G.; Picarelli, A. Impact of gluten-free diet on quality of life in celiac patients. *Acta Gastroenterol. Belg.* **2016**, *79*, 447–453. [PubMed]
21. Addolorato, G.; Capristo, E.; Ghittoni, G.; Valeri, C.; Mascianà, R.; Ancona, C.; Gasbarrini, G. Anxiety but not depression decreases in coeliac patients after one-year gluten-free diet: A longitudinal study. *Scand. J. Gastroenterol.* **2001**, *36*, 502–506. [CrossRef] [PubMed]
22. DiMatteo, M.R.; Lepper, H.S.; Croghan, T.W. Depression is a risk factor for noncompliance with medical treatment: Meta-analysis of the effects of anxiety and depression on patient adherence. *Arch. Intern. Med.* **2000**, *160*, 2101–2107. [CrossRef] [PubMed]
23. Sainsbury, K.; Marques, M.M. The relationship between gluten free diet adherence and depressive symptoms in adults with coeliac disease: A systematic review with meta-analysis. *Appetite* **2018**, *120*, 578–588. [CrossRef] [PubMed]
24. Addolorato, G.; De Lorenzi, G.; Abenavoli, L.; Leggio, L.; Capristo, E.; Gasbarrini, G. Psychological support counselling improves gluten-free diet compliance in coeliac patients with affective disorders. *Aliment. Pharmacol. Ther.* **2004**, *20*, 777–782. [CrossRef] [PubMed]
25. Rubio-Tapia, A.; Hill, I.D.; Kelly, C.P.; Calderwood, A.H.; Murray, J.A.; American College of Gastroenterology. ACG clinical guidelines: Diagnosis and management of celiac disease. *Am. J. Gastroenterol.* **2013**, *108*, 656–676. [CrossRef] [PubMed]
26. Rostom, A.; Murray, J.A.; Kagnoff, M.F. American Gastroenterological Association (AGA) Institute technical review on the diagnosis and management of celiac disease. *Gastroenterology* **2006**, *131*, 1981–2002. [CrossRef] [PubMed]
27. Leffler, D.A.; Dennis, M.; Edwards George, J.; Jamma, S.; Cook, E.F.; Schuppan, D.; Kelly, C.P. A validated disease-specific symptom index for adults with celiac disease. *Clin. Gastroenterol. Hepatol.* **2009**, *7*, 1328–1334. [CrossRef] [PubMed]
28. Leffler, D.A.; Dennis, M.; Edwards George, J.B.; Jamma, S.; Magge, S.; Cook, E.F.; Schuppan, D.; Kelly, C.P. A simple validated gluten-free diet adherence survey for adults with celiac disease. *Clin. Gastroenterol. Hepatol.* **2009**, *7*, 530–536. [CrossRef] [PubMed]
29. Pilkonis, P.A.; Yu, L.; Dodds, N.E.; Johnston, K.L.; Maihoefer, C.C.; Lawrence, S.M. Validation of the depression item bank from the Patient-Reported Outcomes Measurement Information System (PROMIS) in a three-month observational study. *J. Psychiatr. Res.* **2014**, *56*, 112–119. [CrossRef] [PubMed]
30. Evans, J.D. *Straightforward Statistics for the Behavioral Sciences*; Brooks/Cole Pub. Co.: Pacific Grove, CA, USA, 1996.

nutrients

MDPI

Article

Effects of a Gluten-Containing Meal on Gastric Emptying and Gallbladder Contraction

Sara Massironi [1,*], Federica Branchi [1,2], Mirella Fraquelli [1], Alessandra Baccarin [1,2], Francesco Somalvico [3], Francesca Ferretti [1,2], Dario Conte [1,2] and Luca Elli [1,4]

1 Gastroenterology and Endoscopy Unit, Fondazione IRCCS Ca' Granda Ospedale Maggiore Policlinico, 20122 Milan, Italy; federica.branchi@gmail.com (F.B.); mfraquelli@yahoo.it (M.F.); alessandra85.baccarin@gmail.com (A.B.); francesca.ferretti01@gmail.com (F.F.); dario.conte@unimi.it (D.C.); luca.elli@policlinico.mi.it (L.E.)

2 Department of Pathophysiology and Transplantation, Università degli Studi di Milano, 20122 Milan, Italy

3 Alphasearch, 20100 Milan, Italy; alphasearch@tin.it

4 Center for the Prevention and Diagnosis of Celiac Disease, Fondazione IRCCS Ca' Granda Ospedale Maggiore Policlinico, 20122 Milan, Italy

* Correspondence: sara.massironi@policlinico.mi.it; Tel.: +39-02-55033445

Received: 28 May 2018; Accepted: 12 July 2018; Published: 16 July 2018

Abstract: The ingestion of gluten has been associated with gastrointestinal symptoms even in the absence of detectable immune responses. Little is known about the pathophysiological effects of gluten on the upper gastrointestinal tract. We aimed to assess whether the ingestion of gluten leads to an impairment of the physiological mechanisms of gastric emptying, gallbladder contraction and relaxation. A total of 17 healthy subjects underwent ultrasound evaluation of gastric emptying dynamics and gallbladder contractions at baseline and every 30 min after a standard gluten-containing and gluten-free meal (250 kcal, 70% carbohydrates). The pattern of gastric emptying was similar after a standard meal with or without gluten, but differed in terms of the peak of the antral filling curve, which was wider (mean area 5.69, median 4.70, range 3.71-9.27 cm^2 vs. mean 4.89, median 4.57, 2.27-10.22 cm^2, $p = 0.023$) after the gluten-containing meal. The pattern of gallbladder contractions was different after the gluten-free meal ($p < 0.05$), with higher gallbladder volumes in the late refilling phases. The results of this study show that gluten ingestion exerts objective effects on gastric and gallbladder motility. Although the underlying pathophysiological mechanism remains unknown, these results could account for some of the gluten-related symptoms reported by patients with celiac disease and non-celiac gluten sensitivity.

Keywords: gluten; gastric emptying; cholecyst; celiac disease; non celiac gluten sensitivity

1. Introduction

The ingestion of gluten-containing food has reportedly been involved in the development of a broad range of symptoms. Gluten is a structural protein found in wheat, barley and rye, composed of two main fractions, gliadins and glutenins [1]. In celiac disease (CD), the dietary intake of gluten leads to the intestinal exposure to gluten-derived peptides. This exposure triggers a T-cell mediated autoimmune reaction eventually leading to villous atrophy and malabsorption [2]. In wheat allergy (WA), an adverse IgE-mediated immune reaction develops against proteins contained in wheat (i.e., alpha-amylase/trypsin inhibitor, lipid transfer protein, gliadins, glutenins) with different clinical presentations [3]. However, recent data have suggested that the consumption of gluten-containing food can cause gastrointestinal symptoms even in the absence of detectable immune responses or signs of inflammation [4–6], which prompted the definition of a new class of gluten-related disorders, the non-celiac sensitivity (NCGS) or non-celiac wheat sensitivity. NCGS describes a spectrum of gastrointestinal and extra-intestinal symptoms occurring shortly after the dietary exposure to gluten and resolving when a gluten-free diet (GFD) has started [7–9]. Interestingly, GFD has shown benefits in terms of reduction of gastrointestinal symptoms when tested in a population with already known gastrointestinal disorders, such as inflammatory bowel disease or irritable bowel syndrome [10,11]. In spite of the growing evidence on the potential direct effects of gluten or related wheat-derived proteins on the gastrointestinal and immune system [12–15], there is still little data concerning the pathophysiological effects of gluten on the upper gastrointestinal tract. It is known that patients with CD tend to have higher fasting gallbladder volumes and slower gastric emptying before starting on GFD, possibly because of impaired levels of somatostatin and cholecystokinin [16,17]. However, these alterations of the upper gastrointestinal dynamics were considered more as a consequence of small bowel mucosal damage than a direct effect of gluten on the gastrointestinal system mediated by innate or adaptive immune response.

One can conjecture that, in subjects with disorders belonging to the spectrum of functional gastrointestinal disorders, as well as in those with a diagnosis of NCGS, the ingestion of gluten exerts a direct effect on gastrointestinal dynamics: this would explain the onset of symptoms following gluten-containing meals. Recent data have suggested that gluten may trigger a rapid innate immune response after ingestion also in subjects not affected by CD [15]. Magnetic resonance studies have showed that the ingestion of wholemeal bread results in delayed gastric emptying and reduced postprandial small bowel waters compared to a rice meal [18]. However, no significant effect on gastric emptying and small bowel and colonic distension was observed in a subsequent study investigating the effect of bread with different ingredients, including different gluten contents [19]. Ultrasound is a non-invasive, readily available technique that can be successfully applied in the setting of gastrointestinal dynamics [17,20]. To date, only a small-scale study has investigated, with the aid of ultrasound, the effect of gluten intake on healthy volunteers: it has shown no differences in gastric and gallbladder emptying in healthy volunteers after a gluten-containing vs. gluten-free meal [21]. With these premises, the aim of this study was to evaluate the effect of a gluten-containing meal on gastric emptying and gallbladder (GB) contraction and relaxation, as compared to a gluten-free isocaloric meal, in order to collect more data on the relationship between dietary intake of gluten and gastrointestinal dynamics.

2. Materials and Methods

2.1. Study Population

Between June 2014 and June 2015, 17 healthy volunteers were enrolled at the academic Gastroenterology and Endoscopy Unit, Fondazione IRCCS Ca' Granda, Ospedale Maggiore Policlinico, Milan (Italy). The criteria for excluding the enrolment as healthy volunteers were: the presence of clinically relevant diseases (especially as concerns CD, food allergies and gastrointestinal diseases including functional gastrointestinal disorders), on-going pregnancy, active smoking habits. The absence of CD was proven by means of serological testing of tissue transglutaminase antibodies (TTG). All the subjects gave their written informed consent to the study, which was approved by the local ethics committee (n. 1491/2014). Basal clinical history data were collected and a physical examination was carried out for every subject. Anthropometric parameters (weight, height) were collected and the body mass index (BMI) was computed for each individual, using the standard formula: weight (kg)/height^2 (m^2).

2.2. Ultrasound Study of Gastric and Gallbladder Dynamics

The primary outcomes of the study were the assessment of changes in the gastric antrum size, in the dynamics of gastric emptying and of gallbladder contraction. All the subjects underwent the ultrasound evaluation of gastric and gallbladder dynamics twice: after a standard normocaloric balanced gluten-free meal and an isocaloric gluten-containing meal. Each subject received each meal in fasting conditions and after at least 72 h on a normocaloric balanced gluten-free diet.

2.3. Meal Administration

The composition of the administered meals was as follows:

a. gluten-free meal—a standard fatty meal consisting of cooked egg albumen (110 g), two slices of toasted gluten-free bread (rice, millet and quinoa flour basis) (50 g), strawberry jam (20 g), water (120 mL). The meal contained 250 kcal, of which 70% from carbohydrates.
b. gluten-containing meal—an isocaloric meal differing only as regards the type of bread, which was gluten-containing (wheat flour basis).

2.4. Ultrasonographic Evaluation

Gastric emptying and gallbladder motility were evaluated by real-time ultrasound examination with a Philips iU22 system (Philips Ultrasound, Bothell, WA, USA), equipped with a multi-frequency convex transducer (C5-2, 5-2MHz). The gastric antral area was measured three times and the mean values of the two diameters were used to calculate the area, assuming an elliptical shape, by means of the formula: $\pi AB/4$, where A is the longitudinal diameter and B the anteroposterior diameter as measured at the cross-section of the gastric antrum, corresponding to the sagittal plane passing through the superior mesenteric vein, according to Bolondi et al. [20]. The basal antral measurements were taken after overnight fasting (basal time, 0 min). After having the standard meal, all the subjects underwent US measurements every 30 min until complete gastric emptying. Gastric emptying was considered ended when the antral area returned to basal values and remained then unchanged for at least 30 min. The gallbladder volume was calculated by the ellipsoid formula: $\pi AxBxC/6$ as previously described by Dodds et al. [22], where A is the longitudinal, B the transverse and C the antero-posterior diameter. Gallbladder measurements were taken at time 0 and every 30 min after the standard meal, until the refilling occurred after an initial contraction. Also for the gallbladder three different measurements were taken in rapid sequence and the mean values were used. The gallbladder residual volume (mL) was the smallest volume measured at the completion of the meal-induced emptying. The in-percent difference between the basal volume and the residual volume represented the gallbladder ejection volume (mL) (GB EF%). All the examinations were obtained and evaluated in real time by two expert operators (SM and AB) blinded as regards the type of meal received by the participants. At the end of the observation time, all subjects were asked to fill in a questionnaire regarding the onset of common dyspeptic symptoms after each meal, i.e., upper abdominal pain or discomfort, nausea, vomiting, fullness, bloating, early satiety and belching, as well as their intensity measured by means of visual analogic scales ranging from 0 to 10.

2.5. Statistical Analysis

This study was designed as a pilot study and a sample size estimation was not considered possible as this preliminary stage. Demographic and clinical data were expressed as medians and ranges or means and SD, unless stated otherwise. The difference in mean gastric antral area variations after the two meals was evaluated by means of ANOVA or Friedman's model. The areas under the curve were calculated for both the gastric emptying and gallbladder contraction dynamics and the differences were analyzed with the paired *t*-test or the Wilcoxon matched-pairs signed rank test. The presence of any association between the onset of symptoms and variation in the gastric antral area or other US parameters was evaluated by means of Pearson's correlation test. All the data were tested for a normal distribution using the Kolmogoroff–Smirnoff test. Statistical analysis was performed with the software package SPSS v. 19 (IBM SPSS Statistics, rel. 2010, Armonk, NY, USA: IBM Corp). A two-tailed p value < 0.05 was considered statistically significant.

3. Results

The study population consisted of 17 subjects, 11 females and six males, with a median age of 30.5 years (range 25–41) and a median BMI of 20.8 Kg/m^2 (range 17.7–29.9). No participant had relevant concomitant conditions nor drug intake, nor alcohol consumption (defined as more than 1 alcoholic unit per day). Only one participant was a smoker (five cigarettes a day).

After the gluten-containing meal, the postprandial filling peak was significantly wider than after the gluten-free meal (median antral area 4.70 cm^2, range 3.71–9.27 vs. 4.57 cm^2, range 2.27–10.22, $p = 0.025$, Figure 1). Also the mean difference between the basal antral area and the antral filling curve peak was significantly higher after the gluten-containing meal (3.02 $\pm$ 1.74 cm^2 vs. 1.89 $\pm$ 1.68 cm^2, $p = 0.01$). Overall, gastric emptying dynamics were similar for both types of meals (Figure 2) and the time-to-peak of the antral filling curve was not significantly different between the two meals (mean 45.9 $\pm$ 30.2 min after the gluten-containing meal vs. 52.9 $\pm$ 34.4 min after the gluten-free meal, $p = 0.47$). Regarding gastric emptying, the emptying time was slightly longer after the gluten-containing meal than after the gluten-free meal, although this finding was not statistically significant (mean 222.35 $\pm$ 81.5 min vs. 202 $\pm$ 64.97 min, $p = 0.37$). The results are summarized in Table 1. Age, sex and BMI did not correlate with the gastric filling curve nor did they with the time-to-peak and the gastric emptying time.

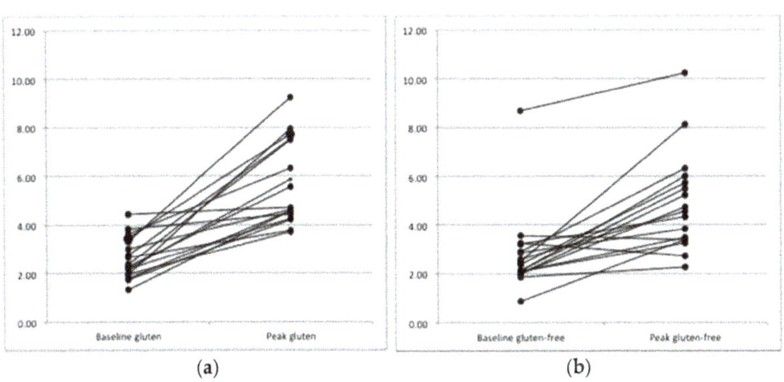

Figure 1. Changes in the gastric antral area at peak of the 17 healthy volunteers after gluten-containing (**a**) and gluten-free meals (**b**); $p = 0.01$. y-curve: area, cm^2.

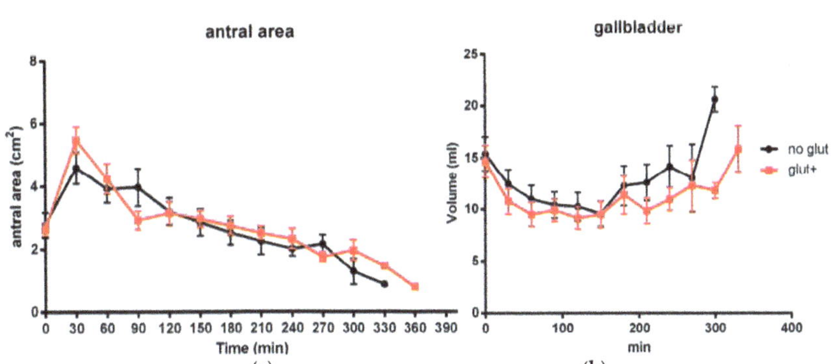

Figure 2. Detailed gastric filling and emptying patterns (**a**) and gallbladder contraction (**b**) after the two meals. Data are shown as mean (standard deviation).

Table 1. Parameters of the gastric dynamics after gluten-containing and gluten-free meals.

Parameters	Gluten-Containing Meal	Gluten-Free Meal	*p*
Gastric filling peak area in cm^2, median (range)	4.70 (3.71–9.27)	4.57 (2.27–10.22)	0.023
Difference peak-basal area in cm^2, median (range)	3.02 ± 1.74	1.89 ± 1.68	0.01
Time to peak mins, mean (SD)	45.9 ± 30.2	52.9 ± 34.4	0.47
Gastric emptying time mins, mean (SD)	222.4 (81.5)	202 (65.0)	0.37

SD: standard deviation.

The gallbladder contraction patterns were different between the gluten-containing and the gluten-free meal aftermaths (area under the curve, AUC: 3.711 vs. 3.630, $p = 0.001$), with higher gallbladder volumes being observed especially in the late refilling phases ($p = 0.039$ at 240 min, <0.01 at 300 min). The gallbladder ejection fraction did not differ between the two meals. The fasting gallbladder volume did not correlate with age, sex, BMI nor with the basal antral area (Table 2). Interestingly, no subject reported the onset of gastrointestinal symptoms after either meal.

Table 2. Parameters of the gallbladder dynamics after gluten-containing and gluten-free meals.

Parameters	Gluten-Containing Meal	Gluten-Free Meal	*p*
GB basal volume mL, mean (SD)	14.7 (6.5)	15.4 (6.8)	0.76
Gallbladder ejection fraction %, mean (SD)	44.4 (28.1)	44.2 (28.1)	0.9
GB volume at 240 min mL, median (range)	10.8 (5.2–13.4)	14.3 (12.1–21.2)	0.039
Pattern of GB contraction mL*min, AUC	3711	3630	0.001

GB: gallbladder; AUC: area under the curve.

4. Discussion

The results of our study show that the ingestion of a gluten-containing meal may cause specific effects on the upper gastrointestinal dynamics irrespective of the presence of a gluten-related disorder. In the group of healthy volunteers we examined, small but significant differences were observed in both the gastric filling and gallbladder contraction dynamics. Regarding gastric filling and emptying dynamics, a significantly wider antral area was observed after a gluten-containing meal than after the isocaloric gluten-free meal, although the filling and emptying times and the general dynamic pattern were not altered by the different composition of meals. The gallbladder contraction after the two meals did not vary significantly as regards the entity of the contraction, but after the gluten-containing meal a longer contraction time was observed, with a significantly longer time required to return to the basal fasting volume.

In patients with known gastrointestinal disorders, the ingestion of gluten-containing food exerts upper gastrointestinal symptoms which are to date not commonly explained from a pathophysiological point of view (in the case of NCGS) or only partially explained by the immune response to gluten (in the case of celiac disease). Thus, this study was performed in order to objectively analyze the presence of differences in gastric and/or gallbladder motility according to the content of gluten in a meal, irrespective of the onset of symptoms on healthy subjects. The differences we observed, though not dramatic, appear to confirm the hypothesis that the ingestion of gluten may exert a direct effect on the gastrointestinal tract and thus cause symptoms through a pathogenetic mechanism other than those associated with the development of celiac disease.

In fact, gluten, or gluten-related peptides, can reportedly elicit several reactions when they are in contact with the gut and in particular with immune cells [15,23,24]. The alteration of gut permeability, as a consequence of a direct effect of gluten-derived peptides or through the triggering of an immediate innate immune response, has been studied in both animal models and human subjects with the aim of explaining the pathogenesis of both celiac disease and NCGS [23,24]. Moreover, the increase in the secretion of hormones, such as insulin, links to the exposure to gliadin peptides in animal models and in vitro [25]. A direct link between gluten and the secretion of gastrointestinal hormones has not been demonstrated at a molecular level; however, one can suppose that the interaction between gluten-derived peptides and immune cells in the intestinal mucosa and submucosa might also directly influence the secretion of these hormones and thus the dynamics of gastric emptying and gallbladder contractions [17,26]. This is in line with the observation of an impaired gallbladder motility in patients with celiac disease in relation to a reduced secretion of enteric hormones and/or decreased gallbladder sensitivity to them. In particular, untreated celiac patients, when compared to controls, have showed low levels of postprandial cholecystokinin and increased fasting somatostatin levels [17]. Moreover, a gastric emptying time longer than in controls has been observed in untreated celiac patients, along with the concomitant increase in plasma neurotensin levels [26].

Other mechanisms that possibly explain our observations, particularly the potential role of proteins other than gluten on the gastric and gallbladder motility are: the increased gastric filling observed at ultrasound after the gluten-containing meal which is possibly a consequence of other wheat components, such as amylase-tripsin inhibitors (ATI) [13] or fructans, which have been linked to the development of gastrointestinal symptoms in both patients with NCGS and irritable bowel syndrome [27–29]. However, this study is limited since the exact content of ATI and fructans in our meals was not calculated. Further data would be useful to directly compare the effect of ATI, fructans and gluten on the upper gastrointestinal dynamics.

As for the limitations of our study, first of all the small sample size may have led to less precision of the estimates; further studies will have to be designed in order to overcome this limit. Moreover, the group of participants was not entirely balanced as it included more women (11/17, 65%). However, considering the cross-over design of the study, every patient acted as their own control, which helps reduce biases. Finally, the investigation of gastric and gallbladder dynamics by means of ultrasound is not the standard methodology for the diagnosis of altered gastric emptying, although it is easy and non-invasive and has already been evaluated in previous studies [17,20–22].

It is worth noting that none of our healthy subjects reported the onset of gastrointestinal symptoms after the meals, irrespective of the actual changes on gastric volume or gallbladder dynamics observed. It is known that in subjects with functional gastrointestinal disorders, alterations in visceral motility or distension considered within "normal" range are associated with the onset of symptom [30]. One can hypothesize that in patients reporting symptoms after having a gluten-containing meal, the alterations caused by the meal would be perceived differently, thus corroborating the hypothesis of an enhanced visceral sensitivity in patients with the irritable bowel syndrome spectrum [30]. Of course, numerous other factors could impact symptoms and responses in patients, including innate immune reactions, size of the meals, so that the specific role of gluten still has to be clarified. In order to prove this speculative hypothesis, further studies should investigate the effects of meals with different gluten content on patients with IBS or NCGS.

5. Conclusions

In conclusion, the results of our study support the hypothesis of a direct effect of gluten intake on both gastric and gallbladder motility, especially regarding the dynamics of gastric filling and the gallbladder contraction pattern. Although the underlying pathophysiological mechanism is still unknown, these observations could, if substantiated by further studies on patients, explain some of the gluten-related symptoms reported by patients with NCGS and other gastrointestinal disorders, who are improving through GFD.

Author Contributions: Conceptualization, S.M., F.B. and L.E.; Methodology, S.M. and F.B.; Validation, S.M. and L.E.; Formal Analysis, M.F. and F.S.; Investigation, S.M., A.B. and F.F.; Data Curation, S.M. and A.B.; Writing-Original Draft Preparation, F.B.; Writing: Review and Editing, M.F. and D.C.; Visualization, S.M. and F.B.; Supervision, D.C. and L.E.; Project Administration, S.M.

Funding: This research received no external funding.

Conflicts of Interest: The authors declare no conflict of interest.

References

1. Shewry, P.R.; Halford, N.G.; Belton, P.S.; Tatham, A.S. The structure and properties of gluten: An elastic protein from wheat grain. *Philos. Trans. R. Soc. Lond. B Biol. Sci.* **2002**, *357*, 133–142. [CrossRef] [PubMed]
2. Rubio-Tapia, A.; Murray, J.A. Celiac disease. *Curr. Opin. Gastroenterol.* **2010**, *26*, 116–122. [CrossRef] [PubMed]
3. Ludvigsson, J.F.; Leffler, D.A.; Bai, J.C.; Biagi, F.; Fasano, A.; Green, P.H.; Hadjivassiliou, M.; Kaukinen, K.; Kelly, C.P.; Leonard, J.N.; et al. The Oslo definitions for coeliac disease and related terms. *Gut* **2013**, *62*, 43–52. [CrossRef] [PubMed]
4. Elli, L.; Tomba, C.; Branchi, F.; Roncoroni, L.; Lombardo, V.; Bardella, M.T.; Ferretti, F.; Conte, D.; Valiante, F.; Fini, L.; et al. Evidence for the Presence of Non-Celiac Gluten Sensitivity in Patients with Functional Gastrointestinal Symptoms: Results from a Multicenter Randomized Double-Blind Placebo-Controlled Gluten Challenge. *Nutrients* **2016**, *8*, 84. [CrossRef] [PubMed]
5. Biesiekierski, J.R.; Newnham, E.D.; Irving, P.M.; Barrett, J.S.; Haines, M.; Doecke, J.D.; Shepherd, S.J.; Muir, J.G.; Gibson, P.R. Gluten causes gastrointestinal symptoms in subjects without celiac disease: A double-blind randomized placebo-controlled trial. *Am. J. Gastroenterol.* **2011**, *106*, 508–514. [CrossRef] [PubMed]
6. Di Sabatino, A.; Volta, U.; Salvatore, C.; Biancheri, P.; Caio, G.; De Giorgio, R.; Di Stefano, M.; Corazza, G.R. Small amounts of gluten in subjects with suspected nonceliac gluten sensitivity: A. randomized, double-blind, placebo-controlled, cross-over trial. *Clin. Gastroenterol. Hepatol.* **2015**, *13*, 1604–1612. [CrossRef] [PubMed]
7. Carroccio, A.; Rini, G.; Mansueto, P. Non-celiac wheat sensitivity is a more appropriate label than non-celiac gluten sensitivity. *Gastroenterology* **2014**, *146*, 320–321. [CrossRef] [PubMed]
8. Sapone, A.; Bai, J.C.; Ciacci, C.; Dolinsek, J.; Green, P.H.; Hadjivassiliou, M.; Kaukinen, K.; Rostami, K.; Sanders, D.S.; Schumann, M.; et al. Spectrum of gluten-related disorders: Consensus on new nomenclature and classification. *BMC Med.* **2012**, *10*, 13. [CrossRef] [PubMed]
9. Verdu, E.F.; Armstrong, D.; Murray, J.A. Between celiac disease and irritable bowel syndrome: The "no man's land" of gluten sensitivity. *Am. J. Gastroenterol.* **2009**, *104*, 1587–1594. [CrossRef] [PubMed]
10. Aziz, I.; Branchi, F.; Pearson, K.; Priest, J.; Sanders, D.S. A study evaluating the bidirectional relationship between inflammatory bowel disease and self-reported non-celiac gluten sensitivity. *Inflamm. Bowel Dis.* **2015**, *21*, 847–853. [CrossRef] [PubMed]
11. Aziz, I.; Trott, N.; Briggs, R.; North, J.R.; Hadjivassiliou, M.; Sanders, D.S. Efficacy of a gluten-free diet in subjects with irritable bowel syndrome-diarrhea unaware of their HLA-DQ2/8 genotype. *Clin. Gastroenterol. Hepatol.* **2016**, *14*, 696–703. [CrossRef] [PubMed]
12. Doherty, M.; Barry, R.E. Gluten-induced mucosal changes in subjects without overt small-bowel disease. *Lancet* **1981**, *1*, 517–520. [CrossRef]
13. Junker, Y.; Zeissig, S.; Kim, S.J.; Barisani, D.; Wieser, H.; Leffler, D.A.; Zevallos, V.; Libermann, T.A.; Dillon, S.; Freitag, T.L.; et al. Wheat amylase trypsin inhibitors drive intestinal inflammation via activation of toll-like receptor 4. *J. Exp. Med.* **2012**, *209*, 2395–2408. [CrossRef] [PubMed]
14. Palová-Jelínková, L.; Rozková, D.; Pecharová, B.; Bártová, J.; Sedivá, A.; Tlaskalová-Hogenová, H.; Spísek, R.; Tucková, L. Gliadin fragments induce phenotypic and functional maturation of human dendritic cells. *J. Immunol.* **2005**, *175*, 7038–7045. [CrossRef] [PubMed]

15. Brottveit, M.; Beitnes, A.C.; Tollefsen, S.; Bratlie, J.E.; Jahnsen, F.L.; Johansen, F.E.; Sollid, L.M.; Lundin, K.E. Mucosal cytokine response after short-term gluten challenge in celiac disease and non-celiac gluten sensitivity. *Am. J. Gastroenterol.* **2013**, *108*, 842–850. [CrossRef] [PubMed]
16. Marciani, L.; Coleman, N.S.; Dunlop, S.P.; Singh, G.; Marsden, C.A.; Holmes, G.K.; Spiller, R.C.; Gowland, P.A. Gallbladder contraction, gastric emptying and antral motility: Single visit assessment of upper GI function in untreated celiac disease using echo-planar MRI. *J. Magn. Reson. Imaging* **2005**, *22*, 634–638. [CrossRef] [PubMed]
17. Fraquelli, M.; Bardella, M.T.; Peracchi, M.; Cesana, B.M.; Bianchi, P.A.; Conte, D. Gallbladder emptying and somatostatin and cholecystokinin plasma levels in celiac disease. *Am. J. Gastroenterol.* **1999**, *94*, 1866–1870. [CrossRef] [PubMed]
18. Marciani, L.; Pritchard, S.E.; Hellier-Woods, C.; Costigan, C.; Hoad, C.L.; Gowland, P.A.; Spiller, R.C. Delayed gastric emptying and reduced postprandial small bowel water content of equicaloric whole meal bread versus rice meals in healthy subjects: Novel MRI insights. *Eur. J. Clin. Nutr.* **2013**, *67*, 754–758. [CrossRef] [PubMed]
19. Coletta, M.; Gates, F.K.; Marciani, L.; Shiwani, H.; Major, G.; Hoad, C.L.; Chaddock, G.; Gowland, P.A.; Spiller, R.C. Effect of bread gluten content on gastrointestinal function: A crossover MRI study on healthy humans. *Br. J. Nutr.* **2016**, *115*, 55–61. [CrossRef] [PubMed]
20. Bolondi, L.; Bortolotti, M.; Santi, V.; Calletti, T.; Gaiani, S.; Labò, G. Measurement of gastric emptying time by real-time ultrasonography. *Gastroenterology* **1985**, *89*, 752–759. [CrossRef]
21. Di Stefano, M.; Carnevale Maffè, G.; Bergonzi, M.; Mengoli, C.; Formagnana, P.; Di Sabatino, A.; Corazza, G.R. The effect of gluten on intestinal fermentation, gastric and gallbladder emptying in healthy volunteers. *Dig. Liver Dis.* **2015**, *47*, 751–756. [CrossRef] [PubMed]
22. Dodds, W.J.; Groh, W.J.; Darweesh, R.M.; Lawson, T.L.; Kishk, S.M.; Kern, M.K. Sonographic measurement of gallbladder volume. *Am. J. Roentgenol.* **1985**, *145*, 1009–1011. [CrossRef] [PubMed]
23. Sapone, A.; Lammers, K.M.; Casolaro, V.; Cammarota, M.; Giuliano, M.T.; De Rosa, M.; Stefanile, R.; Mazzarella, G.; Tolone, C.; Russo, M.I.; et al. Divergence of gut permeability and mucosal immune gene expression in two gluten-associated conditions: Celiac disease and gluten sensitivity. *BMC Med.* **2011**, *9*, 23. [CrossRef] [PubMed]
24. Sapone, A.; Lammers, K.M.; Mazzarella, G.; Mikhailenko, I.; Cartenì, M.; Casolaro, V.; Fasano, A. Differential mucosal IL-17 expression in two gliadin-induced disorders: Gluten sensitivity and the autoimmune enteropathy celiac disease. *Int. Arch. Allergy Immunol.* **2010**, *152*, 75–80. [CrossRef] [PubMed]
25. Larsen, J.; Dall, M.; Antvorskov, J.C.; Weile, C.; Engkilde, K.; Josefsen, K.; Buschard, K. Dietary gluten increases natural killer cell cytotoxicity and cytokine secretion. *Eur. J. Immunol.* **2014**, *44*, 3056–3067. [CrossRef] [PubMed]
26. Bardella, M.T.; Fraquelli, M.; Peracchi, M.; Cesana, B.M.; Bianchi, P.A.; Conte, D. Gastric emptying and plasma neurotensin levels in untreated celiac patients. *Scand. J. Gastroenterol.* **2000**, *35*, 269–273. [PubMed]
27. Biesiekierski, J.R.; Peters, S.L.; Newnham, E.D.; Rosella, O.; Muir, J.G.; Gibson, P.R. No effects of gluten in patients with self-reported non-celiac gluten sensitivity after dietary reduction of fermentable, poorly absorbed, short-chain carbohydrates. *Gastroenterology* **2013**, *145*, 320–328. [CrossRef] [PubMed]
28. Mansueto, P.; Seidita, A.; D'Alcamo, A.; Carroccio, A. Role of FODMAPs in patients with irritable bowel syndrome. *Nutr. Clin. Pract.* **2015**, *30*, 665–682. [CrossRef] [PubMed]
29. Halmos, E.P.; Power, V.A.; Shepherd, S.J.; Gibson, P.R.; Muir, J.G. A diet low in FODMAPs reduces symptoms of irritable bowel syndrome. *Gastroenterology* **2014**, *146*, 67–75. [CrossRef] [PubMed]
30. Drossman, D.A.; Hasler, W.L. Rome IV-functional GI disorders: Disorders of gut-brain interaction. *Gastroenterology* **2016**, *150*, 1257–1261. [CrossRef] [PubMed]

nutrients

MDPI

Article

A Low FODMAP Gluten-Free Diet Improves Functional Gastrointestinal Disorders and Overall Mental Health of Celiac Disease Patients: A Randomized Controlled Trial

Leda Roncoroni [1,2,*,†], Karla A. Bascuñán [1,3,†], Luisa Doneda [2], Alice Scricciolo [1], Vincenza Lombardo [1], Federica Branchi [1], Francesca Ferretti [1], Bernardo Dell'Osso [4,5,6], Valeria Montanari [1], Maria Teresa Bardella [1] and Luca Elli [1]

1. Centre for the Prevention and Diagnosis of Celiac Disease/Division of Gastroenterology and Endoscopy, Fondazione IRCCS Ca' Granda Ospedale Maggiore Policlinico, 20122 Milan, Italy; kbascunan@med.uchile.cl (K.A.B.); scricciolo.alice@gmail.com (A.S.); vicky.l@hotmail.it (V.L.); federica.branchi@gmail.com (F.B.); francesca.ferretti01@gmail.com (F.F.); montanari.valeria8@gmail.com (V.M.); mariateresa.bardella@yahoo.com (M.T.B.); luca.elli@policlinico.mi.it (L.E.)
2. Department of Biomedical, Surgical and Dental Sciences, University of Milano, 20100 Milan, Italy; luisa.doneda@unimi.it
3. Department of Nutrition, University of Chile, 8380453 Santiago, Chile
4. Department of Pathophysiology and Transplantation, Università degli Studi di Milano, Fondazione IRCCS Ca' Granda, Ospedale Maggiore Policlinico, 20100 Milan, Italy; bernardo.dellosso@unimi.it
5. Department of Psychiatry and Behavioral Sciences, Bipolar Disorders Clinic, Stanford University, Stanford, CA 94305-5723, USA
6. CRC "Aldo Ravelli" for Neuro-technology & Experimental Brain Therapeutics, University of Milan, 20100 Milan, Italy

* Correspondence: leda.roncoroni@unimi.it; Tel.: +39-025-503-3384

† These authors have contributed equally to this work.

Received: 3 July 2018; Accepted: 1 August 2018; Published: 4 August 2018

Abstract: A subset of patients with celiac disease (CD) on a gluten-free diet (GFD) reported the persistence of functional gastrointestinal disorders. Foods containing fermentable, oligosaccharides, disaccharides, monosaccharides, and polyols (FODMAP) can trigger a broad range of gastrointestinal symptoms in sensitive individuals. We evaluated the effects of a low FODMAP diet (LFD) on gastrointestinal and psychological symptomatology in CD patients. A total of 50 celiac patients on GFDs and with persistence of gastrointestinal symptoms were included. The patients were randomly allocated to one of two dietary groups—one on a low FODMAP GFD (LF-GFD, $n = 25$) and the other on a regular GFD (R-GFD, $n = 25$)—for 21 days. Psychological symptomatology and quality of life were evaluated by the Symptom Checklist-90-R (SCL-90) and the Short Form (36) Health Survey (SF-36) questionnaires, respectively. Gastrointestinal symptomatology and general well-being were evaluated by visual analogue scale (VAS) scores. After 21 days, 21 and 23 patients completed the dietary treatment on LF-GFD and R-GFD, respectively. A reduced global SCL-90 index ($p < 0.0003$) was found in the LF-GFD group but not in the R-GFD one. However, the SF-36 scores did not differ between groups after treatment. The VAS for abdominal pain was much lower, and the VAS for fecal consistency enhanced after treatment in the LF-GFD group. General well-being increased in both groups but with a much higher improvement in the LF-GFD ($p = 0.03$). A short-term LFD regimen helps to improve the psychological health and gastrointestinal symptomatology with enhanced well-being of CD patients with persisting functional gastrointestinal symptomatology. The long-term clinical effects of LFD in particular subgroups of CD patients need further evaluation.

Keywords: gluten-free diet; gastrointestinal symptoms; quality of life

1. Introduction

Celiac disease (CD) is an autoimmune multisystem disorder triggered by gluten ingestion [1,2]. CD affects genetically susceptible individuals who are known to possess the Human Leukocyte Antigen HLA DQ2 (90%–95%) or the HLA DQ8 (5%–10%) haplotypes [3]. CD symptomatology is mainly gastrointestinal with patients usually reporting diarrhea, bloating, abdominal pain, and weight loss [2]. Extra-intestinal symptoms can be also frequent [4].

A gluten-free diet (GFD) is the current treatment for CD [5]. In this dietary treatment, foods containing gluten, which is a protein found in grains, such as wheat, barley, rye, and triticale, are excluded. Gluten induces small intestine inflammation, and a GFD helps to counteract the clinical signs/symptoms and to prevent complications [6]. Although this treatment is highly successful, following a strict GFD poses great difficulty to patients in their family, social, and working contexts, thus deteriorating their quality of life [7] and causing psychological distress [8].

It is not uncommon that patients on GFDs report symptoms resembling those of irritable bowel syndrome (IBS), which is a frequent condition in clinical practice. Reportedly, around 20–23% of treated CD patients fulfill the Rome III criteria for IBS and also suffer from various functional gastrointestinal symptoms, further affecting their quality of life [9]. In fact, a meta-analysis has shown that IBS-like symptoms are common in CD patients (the pooled prevalence of IBS symptoms in treated CD patients was 38%), concluding that higher levels of adherence to a GFD are possibly associated with some reduction in symptomatology [10]; however, the authors also highlighted that in some patients, IBS-like symptoms persist even after following a strict GFD.

Functional gastrointestinal disorders are characterized by recurrent or current gastrointestinal symptoms that have no identifiable structural or biochemical basis. The most common functional gastrointestinal disorder is IBS [11]. The variety of clinical manifestations has limited the effective treatment of these syndromes, and most treatments to date only alleviate the primary manifestation. A novel option for IBS treatment, which is currently generating great excitement, is the dietary regimen with reduced amounts of fermentable, oligosaccharides, disaccharides, monosaccharides, and polyols (FODMAP) [12]. FODMAP are short-chain carbohydrates that are poorly absorbed in the small intestine and increase gas production and intestinal osmolarity because of their rapid fermentation and osmotic action [13–15]. Foods containing FODMAP can trigger gastrointestinal symptoms in sensitive individuals [13,16].

A low FODMAP diet (LFD) appears to be associated with the reduction of IBS symptoms [17]. A very recent meta-analysis found evidence for the short-term efficacy and safety of LFD for patients with IBS, but the long-term effects are still under investigation [18]. Recently, LFD has been evaluated in patients with inflammatory bowel disease, showing improved symptomatology after treatment [19]. From a clinical point of view, CD and IBS may coexist [20]. However, it is more likely that the inflammatory process occurring in CD does not revert completely in some patients on GFD, and similar low-grade inflammation can be present both in patients with CD and IBS [9,21]. To date there are no reports showing the potential effect of LFD on gastrointestinal symptomatology for patients with CD; thus, we have evaluated the role of LFD on treated CD patients with the persistence of functional gastrointestinal disorders. In addition, given the frequent manifestation of psychopathological and behavioral abnormalities in CD patients undergoing dietary changes, their overall psychological distress and disability were also assessed. In particular, we hypothesized that patients being administered LFD would show improved conditions in terms of gastrointestinal and psychopathological symptoms compared with patients on regular-GFD (R-GFD).

2. Materials and Methods

This was a randomized double-blind intervention-controlled study, previously registered at ClinicalTrials.gov (ref. no. IDNCT02946827). All the authors had access to the study data and reviewed and approved the final version of the manuscript. The patients were recruited at the Center for Prevention and Diagnosis of Celiac Disease of Fondazione IRCCS Ca' Granda Ospedale Maggiore Policlinico in Milan (Italy). The University of Milan's Institutional Review Board reviewed and approved the study protocol according to the Helsinki Declaration, the Project Identification Code of the Ethics Committee Approval of our study: 744_2015bis, the protocol was approved by the Ethics Committee of Milano Area B (date 10.11.2015). All the patients gave and signed their informed consent prior to participation in this study.

Between December 2015 and December 2017, we studied patients with CD fulfilling the following inclusion criteria: adult age (between 18 and 60 years), treated with a GFD for at least one year, with negative plasma tissue transglutaminase values, with IBS-like symptoms and functional gastrointestinal disorders according to the Rome III criteria [22], and with a global well-being score assessed by a visual analogue scale (VAS) of <4. As exclusion criteria, we considered the following: low adherence to the GFD (as evaluated by the Celiac Dietary Adherence Test [23]), refractory CD (as evaluated through biopsy to assess the persistence of intestinal atrophy while on a GFD and by means of interview carried out by a trained nutritionist, who assessed patients' adherence to the diet), individual intolerance to disaccharides (as evaluated by hydrogen test (lactose and fructose), history of previous nutritionist evaluation or nutritional treatment for the dietary management of IBS, taking IBS pharmacological therapy, abdominal surgery, and type 2-diabetes.

CD was diagnosed according to positivity to the serological tests of endomysial antibodies and tissue transglutaminase antibodies and on the basis of histological abnormalities at duodenal biopsy according to the modified Marsh classification (following the European Society for Pediatric Gastroenterology and Nutrition criteria) [24]. The allocation ratio was 1:1, and the recruited patients ($n = 50$) were randomly allocated to either of two dietary treatments—a low FODMAP GFD (LF-GFD, $n = 25$) or a R-GFD (R-GFD, $n = 25$)—for a time length of 21 days. Before randomization (baseline) and at day 21, the patients underwent a physical examination, and biochemical and nutritional parameters were assessed. After the intervention period, 21 patients in the LF-GFD and 23 in the R-GFD group completed the protocol and were included for the analyses reported in this study. The primary outcome was change in the VAS score for general well-being after 21 days of intervention. Secondary outcomes were changes in the VAS score for gastrointestinal symptomatology and the Short Form (36) Health Survey (SF-36) and the Symptom Checklist-90-R (SCL-90) scores for quality of life and psychological symptomatology, respectively.

The sample size was calculated using G*Power v. 3.1.9.2 for Windows (Düsseldorf, Germany [25]) based on the difference in the reduction of overall IBS-like symptomatology of at least 50% after 21 days following a LFD or high-FODMAP diet in IBS patients, as reported by McIntosh et al. [26]. Considering an α-error 1% (two-tailed test) and a power of 90%, with a response of 72% after the LFD and 21% after the high-FODMAP diet, the estimated sample size was estimated in 22 patients per group, including an additional 20% of patients for potential losses during the follow-up. The random allocation sequence was planned by one of the researchers (L.R.), and the participants' enrollments were carried out by F.B., F.F., and L.E. Both the researchers (gastroenterologists and trained nutritionists) and the patients were blind after the assignment to each intervention group.

2.1. Clinical Evaluation

At the baseline and at the end of the intervention period, each patient underwent a clinical and nutritional evaluation (by two gastroenterologists and two trained nutritionists). Overall health and gastrointestinal and extra-gastrointestinal symptoms were assessed, and the gastrointestinal symptomatology was further classified.

2.2. Diets

The nutritional evaluation aimed at assessing anthropometrical parameters, nutritional status, and usual dietary patterns. After clinical evaluation, a personalized GFD adjusted to match energy and macronutrients and micronutrients daily requirements was indicated to each patient. This task was carried out by a trained nutritionist who was only in charge of performing this task, without involvement in patient management. In each dietary treatment, a structured 21-day dietary plan excluding all food gluten sources was indicated. The dietary plan included structured daily meals and specific foods/beverages and was explained in detail to each patient at the beginning of the study. After the initial explanation, the nutritionist was available to answer any doubts or issues strictly related to the dietary plan via e-mail or telephone. As all the patients received a structured dietary plan, both the R-GFD, as well as the LF-GFD, received a review of their current dietary habits, in addition to the change in FODMAP content in the LF-GFD group. The FODMAP content of the R-GFD and LF-GFD was a median (interquartile range) of 21.8 (18.5–22.5) and 3.7 (3.0–4.12) g/day, respectively, as previously described [27,28]. An example of the meals and foods used in both types of diets is shown in Table 1. The group with the LF-GFD received an in-depth GFD review, food education regarding GFD and LFD, and dietary counseling to initiate the modification of the FODMAP content towards the LFD. The patients in the R-GFD group received an in-depth GFD review together with food education regarding their diet. Compliance and doubts about the diet were checked 10 days later by means of a telephone call by the same nutritionist.

Table 1. Examples of the two different prescribed diets for a typical day [1].

Meal	LF-GFD (3.54 g/day FODMAP)	R-GFD (19.9 g/day FODMAP)
Breakfast	1 cup of tea 80 g of gluten free biscuits	1 glass of fresh orange juice 3 slices of gluten-free bread 3 teaspoons of honey
Morning snack	1 banana	1 apple
Lunch	130 g of gluten free pasta with zucchini 60 g of chicken 150 g of carrots	120 g of turkey thighs 200 g of cauliflowers
Afternoon snack	1 cup of blueberries	1 pear
Dinner	180 g of seafood 150 g of tomatoes	200 g of asparagus soup 70 g of fresh cheese 150 g of carrots
During the day	130 g of gluten free bread 6 tea spoons and half of virgin olive oil	160 g of gluten free bread 2 tea spoons of virgin olive oil

[1] Dietary data represent the typical diet for a patient with an approximate energy expenditure of 1800 kcal/day. FODMAP: Fermentable, oligosaccharides, disaccharides, monosaccharides, and polyols; R-GFD: regular gluten-free diet; and LF-GFD: low-FODMAP diet.

2.3. Psychological Symptoms and Quality of Life

The Symptom Checklist-90-R (SCL-90) questionnaire was used to evaluate a broad range of psychological problems and symptomatology [29]. The scale is composed of 90 questions and assesses the presence and severity of symptoms of mental distress regarding different symptomatic domains (somatization, obsessive-compulsive, interpersonal sensitivity, depression, anxiety, hostility, phobic anxiety, paranoid ideation, and psychotic). Each question is awarded a score on a five-point Likert scale with extremes from "not at all" (0 points) to "extremely" (4 points). In addition to the scores rating specific symptoms' intensities, a global severity index was calculated to estimate the assessment of the patient's psychopathological state and as an indicator of symptomatic severity and psychic distress.

The Short Form (36) Health Survey (SF-36) questionnaire evaluated the patients' quality of life. This is a 36-question-long instrument conceptually referring to eight health domains: physical activity (10 questions), role limitations due to physical health (4 questions), role limitations due to emotional state (3 questions), physical pain (2 questions), general health perception (5 questions), vitality (4 questions), social activities (2 questions), mental health (5 questions), and a single question on changes in the state of health [30]. The scores for each domain ranged between 0 and 100, where 100 represents the best possible perception of quality of life.

2.4. Gastrointestinal Symptoms

We used a series of 10-cm long visual analogue scales (VASs) referring to the level of satisfaction with their health status and the severity of specific symptoms (abdominal pain, satisfaction with stool consistency, bloating, postprandial fullness, early satiety, epigastric pain, and other symptoms). A further VAS evaluated satisfaction with general well-being (0 being extremely poor satisfaction and 10 very high satisfaction). These VASs were previously used by our group in a population with Non Celiac Gluten Sensitivity to evaluate gastrointestinal manifestations and general well-being [31]. The magnitude of change in gastrointestinal symptoms between the baseline and at the end of the 21-day-long intervention was assessed as follows: (a) comparing each VAS score at both time points, and (b) estimating the number of patients achieving a change in VAS score for general well-being higher than or equal to 50% from the baseline.

2.5. Statistical Analysis

The data were described as median ± Standard Deviation (SD) or median (inter-quartile range), depending on the parametric or non-parametric distribution of variables as assessed by graphical inspection and the Shapiro–Wilk test. All the patients who had fully completed the intervention period, were included in the analysis (per-protocol analysis). For SCL-90 and SF-36 scores, a within-group comparison at both time points (the baseline and day 21) and a between-group comparison at day 21 was conducted using an independent Student's *t*-test or the non-parametric Wilcoxon rank sum test, depending on the distribution of variables. For the main outcome, the VAS score for general well-being, with two-way Analysis of Variance (ANOVA) (factors 'treatment' and 'time') with one repeated measure ('time'), was used. The magnitude of change in the VAS score for the general well-being comparison between groups at day 21 was evaluated by Fisher's exact two-tailed test. A 5% significance level was used, and the software packages STATA® v. 13.1 (StataCorp LLC, College Station, TX, USA) and GraphPad Prism v. 6 (GraphPad Software, La Jolla, CA, USA) were used for analysis and figures processing.

3. Results

3.1. Patients

The participant flow is shown in Figure A1. The patients were middle-aged, mainly women, and within the normal weight range, according to mean body-mass index (Table 2). Regarding their clinical symptomatology at the baseline, 64% reported the presence of IBS-like symptoms, whereas 34% reported functional symptomatology (Table 2). Among the specific symptoms, diarrhea and constipation were the most frequently reported (34% and 32%, respectively) with lower frequencies of mixed and non-specified gastrointestinal symptoms (12% and 8%, respectively). At the baseline the LF-GFD and R-GFD groups were similar in relation to the presence of evaluated symptoms.

Table 2. Background and gastrointestinal symptoms at baseline [1].

Variable	Overall (n = 50)	R-GFD (n = 25)	LF-GFD (n = 25)	p value †
Age, years	41.1 ± 10.1	40.4 ± 10.1	41.9 ± 10.2	0.73
Gender, female (%)	44 (88)	25 (100)	22 (3 no data)	0.09
BMI, kg/m^2	22.5 ± 4.1	22.3 ± 3.6	22.1 ± 5.4	0.87
Diarrhea, n (%)	17 (34)	6 (6 no data)	11 (4 no data)	0.18
Constipation, n (%)	16 (32)	9 (7 no data)	7 (2 no data)	0.2
Mixed symptoms, n (%)	6 (12)	4 (10 no data)	2 (5 no data)	0.36
Non-specified, n (%)	4 (8)	3 (12 no data)	1 (9 no data)	0.29
Dyspepsia, n (%)	17 (34)	8 (5 no data)	9 (3 no data)	0.95

[1] Data shown as mean ± Standard Deviation (SD) for continuous variables and frequency and percentage for nominal variables. † p-value for comparison between groups using an independent t-test for continuous variables or Chi-square or Fisher's exact tests for nominal variables. BMI: body-mass index; R-GFD: regular gluten-free diet; and LF-GFD: low-FODMAP gluten-free diet.

3.2. Psychological Symptoms and Quality of Life

A consistent reduction in most SCL-90 scores was found in the LF-GFD group but not in the R-GFD group, with the global SCL-90 score being significantly reduced ($p < 0.0003$) compared with the R-GFD group at day 21 ($p < 0.04$, Table 3, and Figure S1 in the Supplementary Materials). With respect to specific sub-items of the SCL-90, there were no differences in the R-GFD group. However, in the LF-GFD group some significant changes were observed between the baseline and day 21 in relation to the majority (7 out of 9) of the psychopathological dimensions (Table 3).

Table 3. SCL-90 scores according to studied groups [1].

	R-GFD			LF-GFD			
	Baseline (n = 25)	21-day (n = 23)	p-Value within Group †	Baseline (n = 25)	21-day (n = 21)	p-Value within Group †	p-Value between Groups
Global index	1.61 ± 0.39	1.44 ± 0.29	0.13 ‡	1.49 ± 0.17	1.26 ± 0.18	0.0003	0.04
Somatization	1.87 (0.71)	1.50 (0.58)	0.13	1.83 (0.62)	1.45 (0.40)	0.01	0.43
Obsessive-compulsive	1.70 (1.0)	1.60 (0.70)	0.41	1.60 (0.50)	1.30 (0.60)	0.01	0.15
Interpersonal sensitivity	1.55 (0.66)	1.38 (0.65)	0.09	1.22 (0.44)	1.11 (0.44)	0.09	0.58
Depression	1.57 (0.73)	1.50 (0.73)	0.33	1.54 (0.46)	1.38 (0.46)	0.01	0.26
Anxiety	1.30 (0.65)	1.10 (0.51)	0.17	1.30 (0.40)	1.10 (0.15)	0.02	0.60
Hostility	1.42 (0.50)	1.42 (0.58)	0.75	1.33 (0.50)	1.16 (0.08)	0.01	0.11
Phobic anxiety	1.0 (0.14)	1.0 (0.14)	0.81	1.0 (0.14)	1.0 (0.0)	0.10	0.12
Paranoid ideation	1.66 (0.83)	1.16 (0.66)	0.22	1.33 (0.50)	1.0 (0.33)	0.01	0.20
Psychotic	1.20 (0.50)	1.10 (0.25)	0.13	1.20 (0.10)	1.0 (0.10)	0.03	0.26

[1] Data shown as mean ± SD or median (interquartile range) for non-parametrical variables. † p-value for comparison within groups using a non-parametric Wilcoxon rank sum test unless otherwise is indicated; ‡ independent t-test. R-GFD: regular gluten-free diet; LF-GFD: low-FODMAP gluten-free diet.

The results of the SF-36 scores are shown in Table 4. Overall, there were no differences in the SF-36 sub-scores both within and between groups through the intervention (Table 4 and Figure S2 in the Supplementary Materials). However, when evaluating the change percentage at day 21, a statistically significant improvement in health perception, as well as in the physical functioning scores was found in the LF-GFD compared with the R-GFD group (Figure 1).

Table 4. Short Form (36) Health Survey (SF-36) subscales and global score [1].

	R-GFD			LF-GFD			
	Baseline (n = 25)	**21-day (n = 23)**	***p*-value within Group** †	**Baseline (n = 25)**	**21-day (n = 21)**	***p*-value within Group** †	***p*-value between Groups**
Health perception	46.44 ± 29.62	52.0 ± 26.93	0.53	44.54 ± 24.25	53.27 ± 18.92	0.17	0.87
Physical functioning	95.0 (15.0)	100 (30)	0.94 ‡	95.0 (7.5)	95.0 (10.0)	0.25	0.91
Role physical	75.0 ± 34.6	81.3 ± 32.2	0.40 ‡	79.2 ± 28.2	87.5 ± 26.4	0.18	0.65
Role emotional	69.3 ± 35.9	77.1 ± 35.9	0.41 ‡	65.3 ± 37.4	81.8 ± 28.6	0.10	0.82
Bodily Pain	60.88 ± 23.90	64.93 ± 26.37	0.62	65.91 ± 19.29	72.77 ± 20.54	0.25	0.33
Mental health	63.91 ± 19.47	69.33 ± 14.78	0.33	62.38 ± 16.92	66.18 ± 13.89	0.40	0.51
Vitality	50.20 ± 18.14	59.66 ± 19.77	0.14	55.20 ± 14.02	57.27 ± 12.41	0.59	0.68
Social functioning	69.0 ± 22.27	78.33 ± 20.30	0.18	69.27 ± 18.78	76.13 ± 17.63	0.20	0.73
General health	53.25 ± 26.12	62.26 ± 25.28	0.29	57.47 ± 18.91	62.36 ± 17.08	0.36	0.98

[1] Data shown as mean ± SD or median (interquartile range) for non-parametrical variables. † p-value for comparison within groups using an independent t-test unless otherwise is indicated; ‡ non-parametric Wilcoxon rank sum test. R-GFD: regular gluten-free diet; LF-GFD: low-FODMAP gluten-free diet.

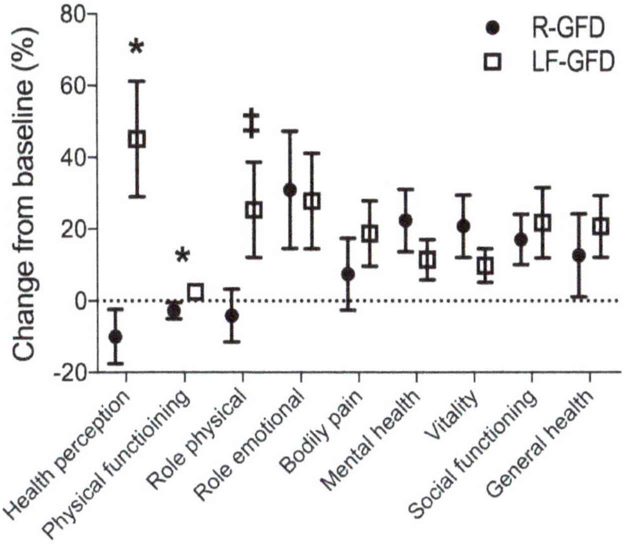

Figure 1. Change in the SF-36 questionnaire scores between the baseline and day 21 from intervention. Data shown as mean (symbol) ± SEM (upper and lower whiskers). For each sub-item, the difference between the values after intervention and the baseline was calculated and divided by the respective baseline value, expressed as a percentage, * $p < 0.05$; ‡ $p = 0.06$, for comparison between groups for each sub-item. R-GFD: regular gluten-free diet; and LF-GFD: low-FODMAP gluten-free diet.

3.3. *Gastrointestinal Symptoms*

A significant interaction was found with regard to the VAS score of abdominal pain with a significant decrease in the LF-GFD group versus the R-GFD group at day 21 ($p < 0.01$, Figure 2, and Figure S3 in the Supplementary Materials). The VAS score for satisfaction about fecal consistency showed a tendency for a higher increase in the LF-GFD group at day 21 ($p < 0.09$). Post-prandial fullness severity was lower in the LF-GFD group and decreased in both groups at day 21 ($p < 0.006$) but without significant interaction (Figure 2 and Figures S4 and S5 in the Supplementary Materials). No differences were found for non-specific functional gastrointestinal symptoms.

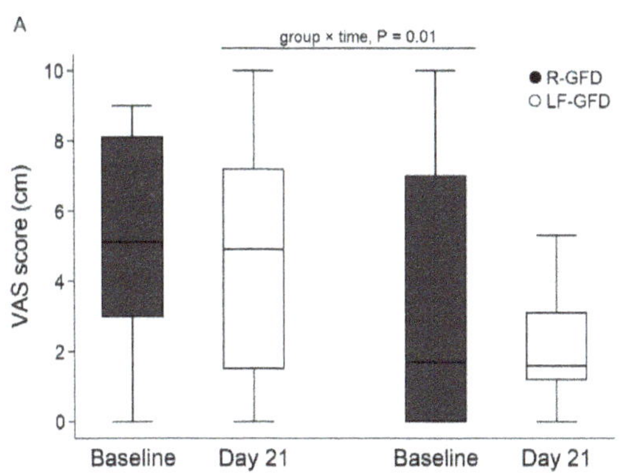

Figure 2. *Cont.*

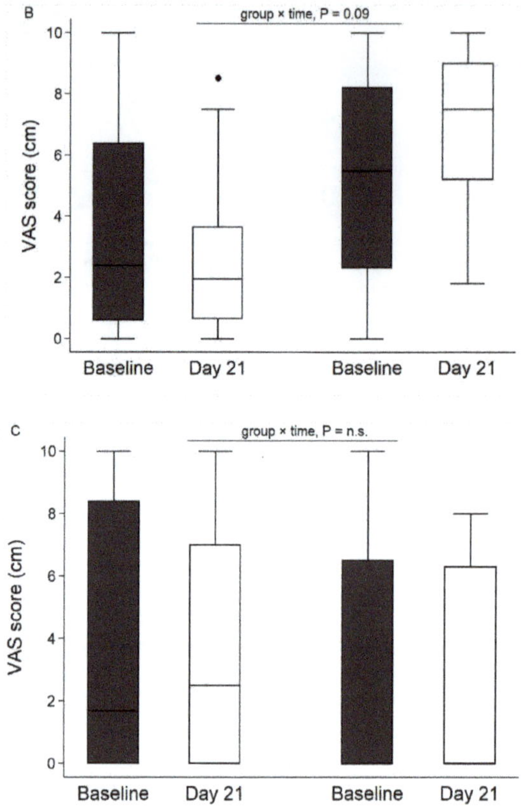

Figure 2. Visual analogue scale (VAS) score for gastrointestinal symptoms. VAS for abdominal pain (**A**), fecal consistency (**B**), and post-prandial fullness severity (**C**). In each plot, data is shown as median (line), inter-quartile range (box limits), and min/max (whiskers); Black dot in B) indicates an extreme value. R-GFD: regular gluten-free diet; LF-GFD: low-FODMAP gluten-free diet; and n.s.: non-significant.

The VAS score for satisfaction about general well-being was significantly enhanced in both groups. However, the improvement in well-being was greater in the LF-GFD group ($p < 0.01$, Figure 3). Consistently, the evaluation of the change in this VAS score of general well-being from the baseline revealed a greater change at day 21 in the LF-GFD group as compared with the R-GFD group (Figure 3).

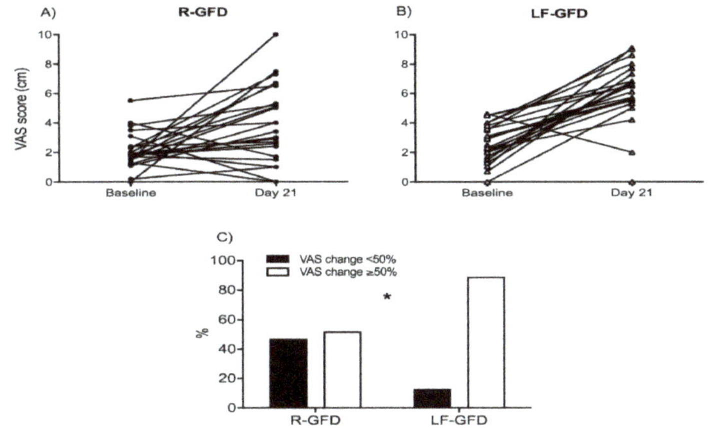

Figure 3. Change in the VAS of well-being between the baseline and day 21 from intervention. VAS score for overall well-being was evaluated at the baseline and at the end of the intervention period (day 21) for the R-GFD (**A**) and LF-GFD (**B**) groups; the magnitude of change in well-being perception (**C**) was calculated by estimating the number of patients (shown in percentage for each group) with a change in VAS score greater than or equal to 50% of the baseline value. Data are individual values at both time points. R-GFD: regular gluten-free diet; LF-GFD: low-FODMAP gluten-free diet; VAS: visual analogue scale. * $p = 0.03$ Fisher´s exact test.

4. Discussion

To our knowledge this is the first randomized double-blind intervention-controlled study that has investigated the effects of a LFD on patients with CD following GFDs but with persisting functional gastrointestinal symptoms. Our results showed a positive response to LFD, an improvement in psychological health scores—but only a limited change in quality of life—and a significant improvement in gastrointestinal symptoms with improved perception of well-being by the patients on the LFD.

Foods containing FODMAP can trigger IBS-like symptoms. These dietary compounds can trigger an increase in flatulence, diarrhea, and bloating that may lead to abdominal pain [13]. Our results suggest that LFD may improve persistent gastrointestinal symptomatology in those patients who undergo GFD and also successfully improve the psychological aspects already described in this group of patients [32]. After our intervention, the severity of gastrointestinal symptoms, such as abdominal pain and stool consistency, decreased when compared with the situation at the baseline and with the R-GFD group, along with improvement in the general well-being VAS. These results are in agreement with those reported by Halmos and colleagues, who showed that a low-FODMAP diet effectively reduced functional gastrointestinal symptoms in patients with IBS [17]. On the other hand, a study conducted on patients with inflammatory bowel disease has showed a positive response to LFD, thus suggesting that a reduction in FODMAP intake offers an efficacious strategy for those patients who present with concurrent functional gastrointestinal symptoms [33]. Although we were able to show an effect on symptomatology as measured by VAS in the LF-GFD group, we also observed that the patients receiving GFD reinforcement (our comparison group) did also show a decrease in symptomatology. This issue has already been addressed in Sainsbury and co-workers, [10], who emphasized that in-depth dietary revision as carried out by a trained nutritionist can improve any persistent symptomatology in CD patients. Nevertheless, our results have showed that such improvement was to a greater extent in the LF-GFD group.

Together with the improvements in IBS-like symptoms, we have also found that LF-GFD can overall improve the psychopathological symptoms as measured by a well-validated instrument. The relationship between psychological and psychiatric disturbances and CD is already well-established, significantly influencing the reduction of the quality of life and worsening the symptoms of affected patients [34]. The results related to the SCL-90 questionnaire have shown post-intervention differences in the LF-GFD group but none for the patients on the R-GFD. In the former group, in fact, we have observed a change in the vast majority of the dimensions as compared with the baseline, suggesting that the decrease in gastrointestinal symptoms may positively influence the improvement of a patient's overall psychopathological burden. These results are consistent with those reported by a previous study, in which patients with CD undertook GFDs and for whom a post-intervention change was observed, which determined a decrease in the score for anxiety but not for depression [32].

In another report some patients newly diagnosed with CD were evaluated in relation to the dimensions of SCL-90 and compared with a healthy control group: the scores for somatization, obsessive-compulsive, interpersonal sensitivity, depression, anxiety, and sleep were found to be higher in CD patients [8]. The use of SCL-90 in a population that suffers from gastrointestinal symptoms has been already evaluated in IBS patients, who exhibited significantly more distress compared with other groups. In addition, the patients with gastrointestinal symptoms as a group, compared with the healthy controls, were characterized by high levels of irritable depression and somatization [35]. From this perspective, the results from the present study, which shows a significant psychopathological improvement in CD patients on the LF-GFD versus the R-GFD, provide an important confirmation about the relationship between gastrointestinal and mental health in CD patients who undergo different types of diet. In particular, to our knowledge this present study offers the first report demonstrating a significant amelioration for CD patients of most SCL-90 items in the short-term (i.e., after 21 days) as a result of following a LF-GFD.

The quality-of-life perception, as assessed by means of the SF-36 questionnaire, has shown only minor differences between the studied groups: we could not establish for this group of celiac patients any significant improvement in this regard after the LFD. This finding is in discordance with what was previously reported. Previous data about our group of patients with non-celiac gluten sensitivity treated with GFDs, showed an improvement in the majority of the SF-36 scores after 7 days of treatment in a cross-over study, with both mental and physical components of the SF-36 questionnaire being significantly lower for patients positive to a gluten challenge [31]. Other authors have shown a quality-of-life improvement in patients with atypical and typical CD, compared with healthy controls after a one-year-long treatment, but only with differences in two items (general health and vitality) for subjects with typical CD [36].

Of note, even though we were not able to demonstrate any improvement in quality of life when comparing our study groups, when the percent change was evaluated for each of the items consulted, both health perception and physical functioning turned out higher in the LF-GFD group compared with the R-GFD group. Therefore, we could not rule out that the aforementioned mixed results possibly depended on the limited period of observation, with a longer follow-up period to be required in order to better assess the changes in quality of life for CD patients following the LF-GFD.

Among the strengths of our report there is the fact that it comes from the first randomized double-blind study performed on patients with CD and to evaluate the potential effects of a reduction in dietary FODMAP on overall health and gastrointestinal symptomatology. As a limitation, even if we could show significant improvement in clinical symptoms, our results were obtained only after a short period of time (i.e., limited to three weeks) and only on patients who had fully completed the intervention (92% and 84% in the R-GFD and LF-GFD groups, respectively).

In conclusion, our results show that nutritional intervention by a LFD can have beneficial effects for CD patients who are on a GFD but present with persisting functional gastrointestinal disorders, even without major changes in their quality-of-life perception. The same results also suggest that, for those patients with CD being treated with a GFD and experiencing IBS-like symptoms, a LFD can be indicated by a trained nutritionist, but its beneficial effects and long-term clinical effects for this group of selected CD patients need further investigation.

ClinicalTrials.gov, ref. no. DNCT02946827.

Supplementary Materials: The following are available online at www.mdpi.com/2072-6643/10/8/1023/s1, Figure S1: SCL-90 global index, Figure S2: SF-36 score for general health, Figure S3: VAS score for abdominal pain, Figure S4: VAS score for fecal consistency, Figure S5: VAS score for postprandial fullness severity.

Author Contributions: Conceptualization, L.R., K.A.B., and L.E.; Methodology, L.R., K.A.B., and L.E.; Investigation, L.R., A.S., V.L., F.B., F.F., and L.E.; Data Curation, L.R.; Formal analysis, L.R., K.A.B., and L.E.; Original Draft Preparation, L.R. and K.A.B.; Review and Editing of Manuscript, L.R., K.A.B., B.D.O., L.D., M.T.B., and L.E.; and Funding Acquisition, L.E.

Funding: This research was funded by Fondazione IRCCS Ca' Granda and received grants from Italy's Ministry of Health and Lombardy's Regional Government Authority (Ministero della Salute e Regione Lombardia, grant number 2011-02348234. The Article Processing Charge was funded by Fondazione IRCCS Ca' Granda Ospedale Maggiore Policlinico and Università degli Studi di Milano, Milan, Italy.

Conflicts of Interest: The authors declare no conflict of interest.

Appendix A

CONSORT

TRANSPARENT REPORTING of TRIALS

CONSORT 2010 Flow Diagram

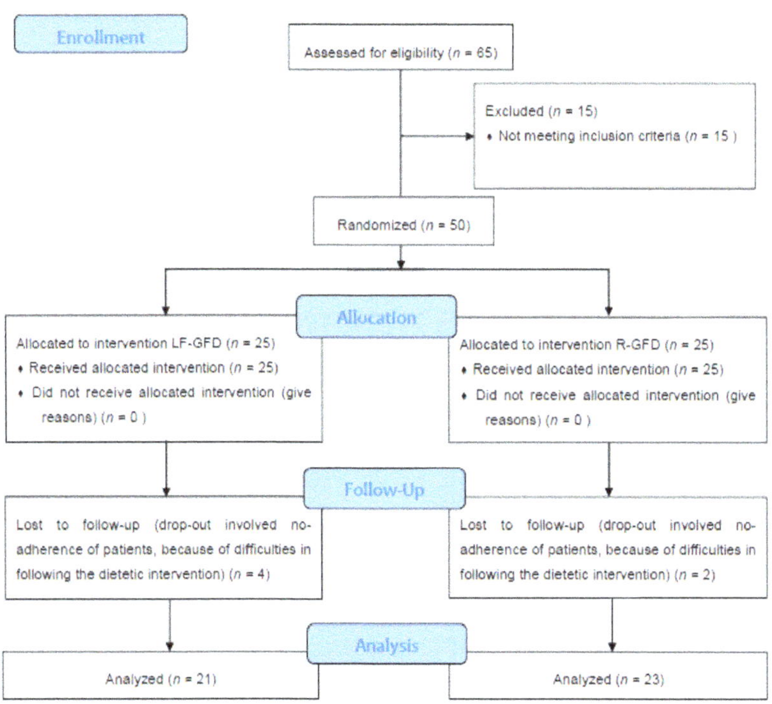

Figure A1. CONSORT Flow diagram.

References

1. De Re, V.; Magris, R.; Cannizzaro, R. New Insights into the Pathogenesis of Celiac Disease. *Front. Med.* **2017**, *4*. [CrossRef] [PubMed]
2. Lebwohl, B.; Sanders, D.S.; Green, P.H.R. Coeliac disease. *Lancet* **2017**. [CrossRef]
3. Karell, K.; Louka, A.S.; Moodie, S.J.; Ascher, H.; Clot, F.; Greco, L.; Ciclitira, P.J.; Sollid, L.M.; Partanen, J. HLA types in celiac disease patients not carrying the DQA1*05-DQB1*02 (DQ2) heterodimer: Results from the European genetics cluster on celiac disease. *Hum. Immunol.* **2003**, *64*, 469–477. [CrossRef]
4. Leffler, D.A.; Green, P.H.R.; Fasano, A. Extraintestinal manifestations of coeliac disease. *Nat. Rev. Gastroenterol. Hepatol.* **2015**, *12*, 561–571. [CrossRef] [PubMed]
5. Bascuñán, K.A.; Vespa, M.C.; Araya, M. Celiac disease: Understanding the gluten-free diet. *Eur. J. Nutr.* **2016**, 1–11. [CrossRef] [PubMed]
6. Francavilla, R.; Cristofori, F.; Stella, M.; Borrelli, G.; Naspi, G.; Castellaneta, S. Treatment of celiac disease: From gluten-free diet to novel therapies. *Minerva Pediatr.* **2014**, *66*, 501–516. [PubMed]
7. Hauser, W.; Stallmach, A.; Caspary, W.F.; Stein, J. Predictors of reduced health-related quality of life in adults with coeliac disease. *Aliment Pharmacol. Ther.* **2007**, *25*, 569–578. [CrossRef] [PubMed]
8. Passananti, V.; Siniscalchi, M.; Zingone, F.; Bucci, C.; Tortora, R.; Iovino, P.; Ciacci, C. Prevalence of eating disorders in adults with celiac disease. *Gastroenterol. Res. Pract.* **2013**, *2013*. [CrossRef] [PubMed]
9. O'Leary, C.; Wieneke, P.; Buckley, S.; O'Regan, P.; Cronin, C.C.; Quigley, E.M.M.; Shanahan, F. Celiac disease and irritable bowel-type symptoms. *Am. J. Gastroenterol.* **2002**, *97*, 1463–1467. [CrossRef] [PubMed]
10. Sainsbury, A.; Sanders, D.S.; Ford, A.C. Prevalence of irritable bowel syndrome-type symptoms in patients with celiac disease: A meta-analysis. *Clin. Gastroenterol. Hepatol.* **2013**, *11*, 359–365. [CrossRef] [PubMed]
11. Quigley, E.M.M. Prokinetics in the Management of Functional Gastrointestinal Disorders. *Curr. Gastroenterol. Rep.* **2017**, *19*, 53. [CrossRef] [PubMed]
12. Marsh, A.; Eslick, E.M.; Eslick, G.D. Does a diet low in FODMAPs reduce symptoms associated with functional gastrointestinal disorders? A comprehensive systematic review and meta-analysis. *Eur. J. Nutr.* **2016**, *55*, 897–906. [CrossRef] [PubMed]
13. Gibson, P.R.; Shepherd, S.J. Evidence-based dietary management of functional gastrointestinal symptoms: The FODMAP approach. *J. Gastroenterol. Hepatol.* **2010**, *25*, 252–258. [CrossRef] [PubMed]
14. De Roest, R.H.; Dobbs, B.R.; Chapman, B.A.; Batman, B.; O'Brien, L.A.; Leeper, J.A.; Hebblethwaite, C.R.; Gearry, R.B. The low FODMAP diet improves gastrointestinal symptoms in patients with irritable bowel syndrome: A prospective study. *Int. J. Clin. Pract.* **2013**, *67*, 895–903. [CrossRef] [PubMed]
15. Shepherd, S.J.; Parker, F.C.; Muir, J.G.; Gibson, P.R. Dietary Triggers of Abdominal Symptoms in Patients with Irritable Bowel Syndrome: Randomized Placebo-Controlled Evidence. *Clin. Gastroenterol. Hepatol.* **2008**, *6*, 765–771. [CrossRef] [PubMed]
16. Varjú, P.; Farkas, N.; Hegyi, P.; Garami, A.; Szabó, I.; Illés, A.; Solymár, M.; Vincze, Á.; Balaskó, M.; Pár, G.; et al. Low fermentable oligosaccharides, disaccharides, monosaccharides and polyols (FODMAP) diet improves symptoms in adults suffering from irritable bowel syndrome (IBS) compared to standard IBS diet: A meta-analysis of clinical studies. *PLoS ONE* **2017**, *12*. [CrossRef] [PubMed]
17. Halmos, E.P.; Power, V.A.; Shepherd, S.J.; Gibson, P.R.; Muir, J.G. A diet low in FODMAPs reduces symptoms of irritable bowel syndrome. *Gastroenterology* **2014**, *146*, 67–75. [CrossRef] [PubMed]
18. Schumann, D.; Klose, P.; Lauche, R.; Dobos, G.; Langhorst, J.; Cramer, H. Low fermentable, oligo-, di-, mono-saccharides and polyol diet in the treatment of irritable bowel syndrome: A systematic review and meta-analysis. *Nutrition* **2018**, *45*, 24–31. [CrossRef] [PubMed]
19. Pedersen, N.; Ankersen, D.V.; Felding, M.; Wachmann, H.; Végh, Z.; Molzen, L.; Burisch, J.; Andersen, J.R.; Munkholm, P. Low-FODMAP diet reduces irritable bowel symptoms in patients with inflammatory bowel disease. *World J. Gastroenterol.* **2017**, *23*, 3356–3366. [CrossRef] [PubMed]
20. Ball, A.J.; Hadjivassiliou, M.; Sanders, D.S. Is gluten sensitivity a no man's land or a fertile crescent for research. *Am. J. Gastroenterol.* **2010**, *105*, 222–223. [CrossRef] [PubMed]
21. El-Salhy, M. Irritable bowel syndrome: Diagnosis and pathogenesis. *World J. Gastroenterol.* **2012**, *18*, 5151–5163. [CrossRef] [PubMed]
22. Drossman, D.A.; Dumitrascu, D.L. Rome III: New standard for functional gastrointestinal disorders. *J. Gastrointest. Liver Dis.* **2006**, *15*, 237–241.

23. Leffler, D.A.; Dennis, M.; Edwards George, J.B.; Jamma, S.; Magge, S.; Cook, E.F.; Schuppan, D.; Kelly, C.P. A Simple Validated Gluten-Free Diet Adherence Survey for Adults with Celiac Disease. *Clin. Gastroenterol. Hepatol.* **2009**, *7*. [CrossRef] [PubMed]
24. Husby, S.; Koletzko, S.; Korponay-Szabo, I.R.; Mearin, M.L.; Phillips, A.; Shamir, R.; Troncone, R.; Giersiepen, K.; Branski, D.; Catassi, C.; et al. Nutrition European Society for Pediatric Gastroenterology, Hepatology, and Nutrition guidelines for the diagnosis of coeliac disease. *J. Pediatr. Gastroenterol. Nutr.* **2012**, *54*, 136–160. [CrossRef] [PubMed]
25. Faul, F.; Erdfelder, E.; Lang, A.-G.; Buchner, A. G*Power: A flexible statistical power analysis program for the social, behavioral, and biomedical sciences. *Behav. Res. Methods* **2007**, *39*, 175–191. [CrossRef] [PubMed]
26. McIntosh, K.; Reed, D.E.; Schneider, T.; Dang, F.; Keshteli, A.H.; De Palma, G.; Madsen, K.; Bercik, P.; Vanner, S. FODMAPs alter symptoms and the metabolome of patients with IBS: A randomised controlled trial. *Gut* **2017**, *66*, 1241–1251. [CrossRef] [PubMed]
27. Muir, J.G.; Rose, R.; Rosella, O.; Liels, K.; Barrett, J.S.; Shepherd, S.J.; Gibson, P.R. Measurement of short-chain carbohydrates in common Australian vegetables and fruits by high-performance liquid chromatography (HPLC). *J. Agric. Food Chem.* **2009**, *57*, 554–565. [CrossRef] [PubMed]
28. Biesiekierski, J.R.; Rosella, O.; Rose, R.; Liels, K.; Barrett, J.S.; Shepherd, S.J.; Gibson, P.R.; Muir, J.G. Quantification of fructans, galacto-oligosacharides and other short-chain carbohydrates in processed grains and cereals. *J. Hum. Nutr. Diet.* **2011**, *24*, 154–176. [CrossRef] [PubMed]
29. Derogatis, L.R. *Symptom Checklist-90-R (SCL-90-R): Administration, Scoring, and Procedures Manual*; NCS Pearson: Minneapolis, MN, USA, 1994.
30. Ware, J.J.; Sherbourne, C. The MOS 36-item short-form health survey (SF-36): I. Conceptual framework and item selection. *Med. Care* **1992**, *30*, 473–483. [CrossRef] [PubMed]
31. Elli, L.; Tomba, C.; Branchi, F.; Roncoroni, L.; Lombardo, V.; Bardella, M.T.; Ferretti, F.; Conte, D.; Valiante, F.; Fini, L.; et al. Evidence for the presence of non-celiac gluten sensitivity in patients with functional gastrointestinal symptoms: Results from a multicenter randomized double-blind placebo-controlled gluten challenge. *Nutrients* **2016**, *8*, 84. [CrossRef] [PubMed]
32. Addolorato, G.; Capristo, E.; Ghittoni, G.; Valeri, C.; Mascianà, R.; Ancona, C.; Gasbarrini, G. Anxiety but not depression decreases in coeliac patients after one-year gluten-free diet: A longitudinal study. *Scand. J. Gastroenterol.* **2001**, *36*, 502–506. [CrossRef] [PubMed]
33. Gearry, R.B.; Irving, P.M.; Barrett, J.S.; Nathan, D.M.; Shepherd, S.J.; Gibson, P.R. Reduction of dietary poorly absorbed short-chain carbohydrates (FODMAPs) improves abdominal symptoms in patients with inflammatory bowel disease-a pilot study. *J. Crohns Colitis* **2009**, *3*, 8–14. [CrossRef] [PubMed]
34. Cossu, G.; Carta, M.G.; Contu, F.; Mela, Q.; Demelia, L.; Elli, L.; Dell'Osso, B. Coeliac disease and psychiatric comorbidity: Epidemiology, pathophysiological mechanisms, quality-of-life, and gluten-free diet effects. *Int. Rev. Psychiatry* **2017**, *29*, 489–503. [CrossRef] [PubMed]
35. Kovács, Z.; Seres, G.; Kerékgyártó, O.; Czobor, P. Psychopathological symptom dimensions in patients with gastrointestinal disorders. *J. Clin Psychol Med Settings* **2010**, *17*, 378–386. [CrossRef] [PubMed]
36. Johnston, S.D.; Rodgers, C.; Watson, R.G.P. Quality of life in screen-detected and typical coeliac disease and the effect of excluding dietary gluten. *Eur. J. Gastroenterol. Hepatol.* **2004**, *16*, 1281–1286. [CrossRef] [PubMed]

nutrients

Correction

Correction: Roncoroni, L. et al. A Low FODMAP Gluten-Free Diet Improves Functional Gastrointestinal Disorders and Overall Mental Health of Celiac Disease Patients: A Randomized Controlled Trial. *Nutrients* 2018, *10*, 1023

Leda Roncoroni [1,2,*,†], Karla A. Bascuñán [1,3,†], Luisa Doneda [2], Alice Scricciolo [1], Vincenza Lombardo [1], Federica Branchi [1], Francesca Ferretti [1], Bernardo Dell'Osso [4,5,6], Valeria Montanari [1], Maria Teresa Bardella [1] and Luca Elli [1]

1 Centre for the Prevention and Diagnosis of Celiac Disease/Division of Gastroenterology and Endoscopy, Fondazione IRCCS Ca' Granda Ospedale Maggiore Policlinico, 20122 Milan, Italy; kbascunan@med.uchile.cl (K.A.B.); scricciolo.alice@gmail.com (A.S.); vicky.l@hotmail.it (V.L.); federica.branchi@gmail.com (F.B.); francesca.ferretti01@gmail.com (F.F.); montanari.valeria8@gmail.com (V.M.); mariateresa.bardella@yahoo.com (M.T.B.); luca.elli@policlinico.mi.it (L.E.)

2 Department of Biomedical, Surgical and Dental Sciences, University of Milano, 20100 Milan, Italy; luisa.doneda@unimi.it

3 Department of Nutrition, University of Chile, 8380453 Santiago, Chile

4 Department of Pathophysiology and Transplantation, Università degli Studi di Milano, Fondazione IRCCS Ca' Granda, Ospedale Maggiore Policlinico, 20100 Milan, Italy; bernardo.dellosso@unimi.it

5 Department of Psychiatry and Behavioral Sciences, Bipolar Disorders Clinic, Stanford University, Stanford, CA 94305-5723, USA

6 CRC "Aldo Ravelli" for Neuro-technology & Experimental Brain Therapeutics, University of Milan, 20100 Milan, Italy

* Correspondence: leda.roncoroni@unimi.it; Tel.: +39-025-503-3384

† These authors have contributed equally to this work.

Received: 4 February 2019; Accepted: 28 February 2019; Published: 6 March 2019

The authors have requested that the following changes be made to their paper [1].

In Table 2, page 6, the frequency (and percentage) of gastrointestinal symptoms are shown for each group (regular gluten-free diet (R-GFD) and low fermentable, oligosaccharides, disaccharides, monosaccharides, and polyols (FODMAP)—gluten free diet (LF-GFD)). Instead of showing the percentages for each group, "No data" was included in parentheses instead of the percentages corresponding to the frequency of symptoms in each group. The table should read as follows.

Table 2. Background and gastrointestinal symptoms at baseline [1].

Variable	Overall (n = 50)	R-GFD (n = 25)	LF-GFD (n = 25)	p Value †
Age, years	41.1 ± 10.1	40.4 ± 10.1	41.9 ± 10.2	0.73
Gender, female (%)	44 (88)	25 (100)	22 (88)	0.09
BMI, kg/m^2	22.5 ± 4.1	22.3 ± 3.6	22.1 ± 5.4	0.87
Diarrhea, n (%)	17 (34)	6 (24)	11 (44)	0.18
Constipation, n (%)	16 (32)	9 (36)	7 (28)	0.2
Mixed symptoms, n (%)	6 (12)	4 (16)	2 (8)	0.36
Non-specified, n (%)	4 (8)	3 (12)	1 (4)	0.29
Dyspepsia, n (%)	17 (34)	8 (32)	9 (36)	0.95

[1] Data shown as mean ± standard deviation (SD) for continuous variables and frequency and percentage for nominal variables. † p-value for comparison between groups using an independent t-test for continuous variables or Chi-square or Fisher's exact tests for nominal variables. BMI: body mass index; R-GFD: regular gluten-free diet; LF-GFD: low fermentable, oligosaccharides, disaccharides, monosaccharides, and polyols (FODMAP)—gluten free diet (LF-GFD).

In Figure 2, page 8, visual analogue scale scores for abdominal pain, fecal consistency, and post-prandial fullness severity are shown. Instead of stating only both times of assessment (at "baseline" and "day 21"), a duplicate in the writing of the x-axis legend was found. The figure should read as follows.

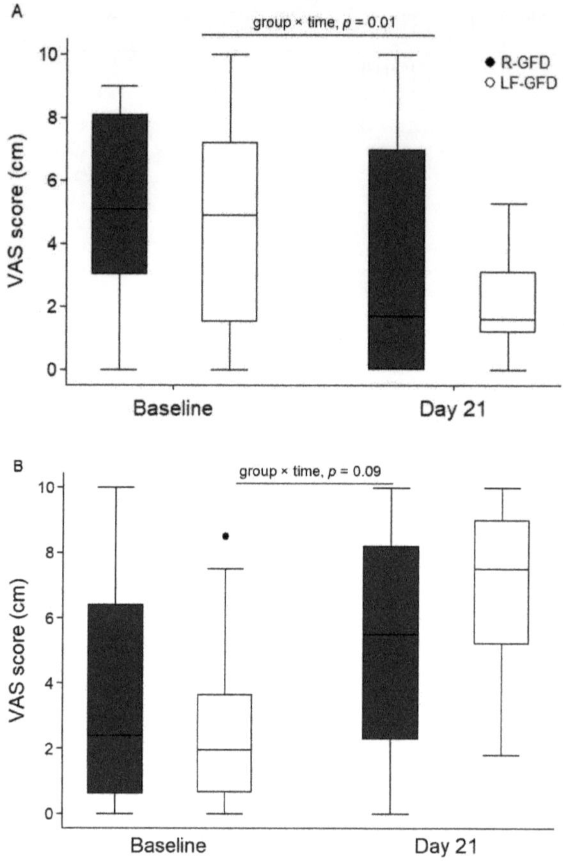

Figure 2. *Cont.*

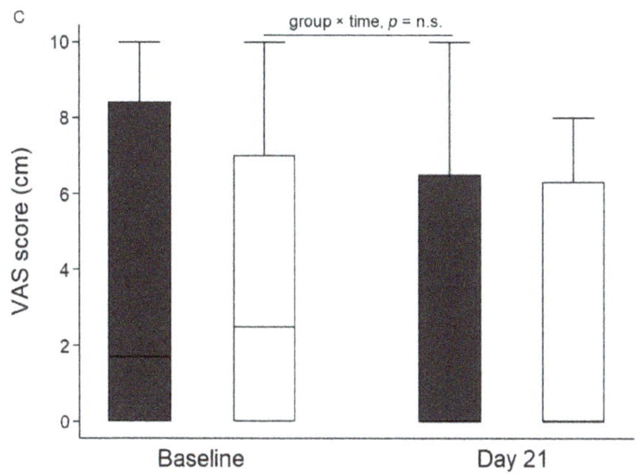

Figure 2. Visual analogue scale (VAS) score for gastrointestinal symptoms. VAS for abdominal pain (**A**), fecal consistency (**B**), and post-prandial fullness severity (**C**). In each plot, data is shown as median (line), inter-quartile range (box limits), and min/max (whiskers); R-GFD: regular gluten-free diet; LF-GFD: low-FODMAP gluten-free diet; n.s.: non-significant.

The authors apologize to the readers for any inconvenience caused by these changes. It is important to state that both corrections do not affect our study's results and involve no changes or modifications in the original data supporting our results. The original manuscript will remain online on the article webpage, with reference to this Correction.

Reference

1. Roncoroni, L.; Bascuñán, K.A.; Doneda, L.; Scricciolo, A.; Lombardo, V.; Branchi, F.; Ferretti, F.; Dell'osso, B.; Montanari, V.; Bardella, M.T.; et al. A low FODMAP gluten-free diet improves functional gastrointestinal disorders and overall mental health of celiac disease patients: A randomized controlled trial. *Nutrients* **2018**, *10*, 8. [CrossRef] [PubMed]

nutrients

MDPI

Article

Quality of Life of Celiac Patients in Brazil: Questionnaire Translation, Cultural Adaptation and Validation

Claudia B. Pratesi [1,2], Winfred Häuser [3], Rosa Harumi Uenishi [1,2], Nicole Selleski [1,2], Eduardo Yoshio Nakano [4], Lenora Gandolfi [1,2], Riccardo Pratesi [1,2] and Renata Puppin Zandonadi [5,*]

1 Interdisciplinary Laboratory of Biosciences and Celiac Disease Research Center, School of Medicine, University of Brasilia, 70910-900 Brasilia, DF, Brazil; claudiapratesi@hotmail.com (C.P.P.); rosa.uenishi@gmail.com (R.H.U.); selleskinicole@gmail.com (N.S.); lenoragandolfi1@gmail.com (L.G.); pratesiunb@gmail.com (R.P.)

2 Post-graduate Program in Health Sciences, School of Health Sciences, University of Brasilia, 70910-900 Brasilia, DF, Brazil

3 Department of Internal Medicine I, Klinikum Saarbrücken and Department of Psychosomatic Medicine and Psychotherapy, Technische Universität München, 80333 München, Germany; whaeuser@klinikum-saarbruecken.de

4 Department of Statistics, University of Brasilia, 70910-900 Brasilia, DF, Brazil; eynakano@gmail.com

5 Department of Nutrition, School of Health Sciences, University of Brasilia, 70910-900 Brasilia, DF, Brazil

* Correspondence: renatapz@yahoo.com.br; Tel.: +55-61-98103-3600

Received: 6 August 2018; Accepted: 22 August 2018; Published: 25 August 2018

Abstract: (1) Background: Celiac disease (CD) is a common autoimmune disorder. The manifestations of the disease and the obligatory life-long gluten-free diet (GFD) are associated with the impairment of patients' quality of life. Therefore, the present study aimed to translate, culturally adapt and validate a celiac disease quality of life (CD-QoL) questionnaire and apply it to a representative number of Brazilian CD patients. (2) Methods: A cross-cultural Brazilian-Portuguese version of the CD-QoL was developed according to revised international guidelines. The questionnaire was administered to 450 celiac patients. The reliability, reproducibility and validity were studied. (3) Results: The Brazilian CD-QoL questionnaire presents valid measures of reproducibility and internal consistency. Early diagnosis is related to higher scores of Brazilian CD-QoL social, sub- and total scale. There was a positive correlation between higher education level and higher QoL. Individuals with partners tend to have a better emotional subscale of QoL. CD-patients who follow a strict GFD have highest QoL scale values. Men scored higher than women on the CD-QoL. All results were statistically significant except for the gastrointestinal subscale. (4) Conclusions: Brazilian CD-QoL allows comparative research between different celiac populations in the world. QoL research will help in the development of effective strategies to improve Brazilian celiac patients' quality of life.

Keywords: Brazilian CD-QoL; quality of life; celiac disease; questionnaire

1. Introduction

Celiac disease (CD) is an autoimmune enteropathy that occurs in genetically susceptible individuals through the consumption of gluten and affects approximately 1% of the population worldwide [1,2]. Although there are asymptomatic patients, the disorder is generally characterized by the combination of gluten-dependent symptoms such as diarrhea, malabsorption, abdominal pain and weight loss. Extra-intestinal manifestations may also occur, such as arthralgia, osteoporosis, chronic fatigue, iron-deficiency anemia, depression and in some cases infertility and miscarriage [3,4].

Despite significant advances in understanding the physiopathology and treatment of celiac disease, the only available treatment continues to be a strict lifelong gluten-free diet (GFD) [5]. The dietary restrictions and the symptoms can significantly impact the patient's quality of life (QoL) [6–9].

The knowledge of the QoL is essential for the evaluation and implementation of measures that can reduce the physical, emotional and social burden on patients affected. In this context, the celiac disease quality of life (CD-QoL) questionnaire is a valuable tool to evaluate the difficulties faced by the celiac patient, regarding symptoms, GFD and social exclusion [6,7]. It is also essential to provide data to promote the improvement of public health policies and consequently, the wellbeing of CD patients.

Quality of life questionnaires specific for celiac patients have been validated and applied in Germany (original), Italy, Turkey and France [7–10]. However, none have been adapted, validated and performed to assess the QoL of Brazilian CD patients.

It is important to highlight that the prospect for celiac patients in Brazil is not optimal and therefore their QoL is impacted [11]. Although there has been an increase in the number of gluten-free products in Brazil, the market is still much smaller than that of conventional products. Finding gluten-free products with adequate taste and nutritional value at an affordable price is a challenge for celiac patients. Additionally, eating out becomes an even bigger challenge for celiac patients, due to lack of information about ingredients used and the risk of cross-contamination [12,13].

Therefore, the present study aimed to translate, culturally adapt, validate and apply a CD-QoL questionnaire to a representative sample of the Brazilian celiac population. We expect that the present study will allow future comparative research between different celiac populations. Potentially, this could also help health professionals and governmental institutions develop effective strategies to improve the quality of life of Brazilian celiac patients.

2. Materials and Methods

The study was developed in six steps: (i) translation, (ii) cultural adaptation, (iii) validation of the questionnaire, (iv) evaluation of the internal consistency and reproducibility of the QoL, (v) application of the questionnaire to Brazilian celiac patients and (vi) statistical analysis. The study was approved by the Health Sciences Ethics Committee, University of Brasilia, No. 69119317.3.0000.0030 and followed the guidelines established by the Declaration of Helsinki.

2.1. Questionnaire

This study followed the original version of the CD-QoL by Häuser et al. [7], which consists of 28 items divided into four areas (with seven items in each): (i) emotions (depressed, restless, relaxed, happy, physically fatigued, tearful); (ii) gastrointestinal symptoms (loose bowels, sudden urge for bowel movement, abdominal cramps, bloating, incomplete bowel evacuation, belching, nausea); (iii) concerns (being diagnosed too late, fear of medical examinations, afraid of cancer, lack of medical expertise, problems with health providers, inheritance of the disease to children); (iv) social (lack of understanding by colleagues, difficulties in recreation/sports, professional limitations, lack of understanding by family/friends, invitation/dinner, feeling of exclusion from others, sexual activities).

In the original questionnaire, responses were scored on a seven-point Likert scale in which "7" corresponds to the best function and "1" to the worst. The total CD-QoL score ranges from 49 to 196. The scores of each area range from 7 to 49, where a higher score indicates a better quality of life. All questions asked were based on the respondent's experience in the past two weeks to reduce memory bias. We chose the questionnaire designed by Häuser et al. [7] due to its capacity to evaluate attitudes and perceptions of celiac patients, covering physical, social and emotional aspects.

2.2. Translation, Cultural Adaptation and Validation

The translation and cultural adaptation of the instrument was done in three phases following an adaptation of the parameters established by the International Quality of Life Assessment (IQOLA) project methodology [14] and the Delphi method [15].

2.2.1. Translation and Retranslation

For the translation phase, two bilingual health professionals independently translated the CD-QoL questionnaire from English to Portuguese, emphasizing conceptual rather than literal translation. The English questionnaire was translated to a Brazilian Portuguese 7th-grade reading level to obtain a better understanding of the questions by the general population. After the first translation, both translators, along with two health professionals with extensive experience with CD, met to resolve any discrepancies and integrate both translations into a single version. A single version was retranslated from Brazilian Portuguese to English, by two different bilingual translators working independently from each other, to confirm its accuracy to the original questionnaire. Lastly, the four translators jointly checked the final questionnaire version for accuracy. An adapted and modified version of the Delphi method [15] was used for the validation process.

2.2.2. Cultural Adaptation, Semantic Evaluation and Validation (First Step)

The validation of an instrument consists of a methodological procedure to evaluate its quality, which is related to the capacity of the instrument to accurately measure what it is intended to measure [16]. Therefore, the validation of the questionnaire occurred in two different steps. In the first step, the cultural adaptation, semantic evaluation and content validation were analyzed by a panel composed of professionals and researchers recognized in their areas. The expert panel consensus helps to define the instrument items which should be maintained, revised, or excluded [17,18].

Twelve health professionals were contacted by email. They were invited to participate and assist with cultural adaptation and semantic evaluation of the questionnaire; ten agreed to participate. Following their consent, participants received an email with a link to the questionnaire in Brazilian Portuguese that was placed on SurveyMonkey® (San Mateo, CA, USA), an online survey platform. The online survey contained all 28 questions translated to Portuguese. The judges rated the questions on a five-point Likert Scale for clarity and, when applicable, made suggestions to improve the questionnaire regarding cultural adaptation, comprehension and clarity.

The mean grade for the evaluation of clarity and content validation of each item and semantic evaluation was calculated considering the answers provided by the experts. The degree of agreement among the experts for the assessment of importance and clarity of the items was evaluated through the Kendall (W) coefficient of concordance, which ranges from 0 to 1. High W-values ($W \geq 0.66$) indicate that the experts applied the same standards of evaluation as opposed to Low W-values, which suggest disagreement among the experts [16]. The criteria established for the approval of the item was a minimal of 80% of agreement between the experts (W-values ≥ 0.8) [12]. Items considered unclear were rewritten in a different manner and subject to further evaluation by the experts. Once the ten participants approved all questions, two bilingual translators met and compared the new Brazilian Portuguese version of the questionnaire to the original version in English. This phase ensured that the Brazilian Portuguese version of the questionnaire was of appropriate cultural relevance while maintaining its fidelity to the original version.

2.2.3. Pilot Test (Second Step)

In the pilot study, the new version of CD-QoL was applied to four celiac subjects that had been patients at the University of Brasilia Hospital (HUB) out-patient celiac clinic for over ten years. These patients rated the questions for reliability, clarity and ease of comprehension. Subsequently, a second evaluation was carried out a week later with four other longstanding celiac patients from the clinic. When the reliability, clarity and ease and of comprehension of each question achieved the score (80% of agreement) the step of internal consistency and reproducibility of the QoL was achieved.

2.2.4. Internal Consistency and Reproducibility of the Brazilian CD-QoL

The internal consistency and reproducibility of the Brazilian CD-QoL were evaluated using 18 celiac patients' (who did not participate in previous phases) responses. The celiac patients answered the Brazilian CD-QoL and after one week they were invited to answer the same questionnaire again. The Cronbach alpha measure evaluated the internal consistency of the QoL subscales. The test-retest reliability (reproducibility) of the questionnaire was verified using the Pearson correlation coefficient and the intra-class correlation coefficient (ICC).

2.3. Brazilian CD-QoL Application

The final step was to place the Brazilian Portuguese CD-QoL questionnaire on the SurveyMonkey® platform and apply it to a representative number of Brazilian celiac patients. The first page of the survey contained the consent form that included the established exclusion/inclusion criteria; where participants had to be 18 years of age or older and have been positively diagnosed by a physician for over a year. At that point, participants gave their consent to participate. Those that did not agree to participate were directed to a page thanking them for their time; while those that agreed, were directed to the first page of the survey containing ten social demographic questions. The third part of the survey consisted of applying the 28 translated and culturally adapted questions to Brazilian celiac patients.

2.4. Psychometric Evaluation, Validation and Statistics

The statistical analysis was carried out following the score proposed by the original study by Häuser et al. research [7] where a higher score indicates a higher quality of life. Questions left blank where substituted by a median value of the corresponding dimensions. The total score was calculated for each demographic and clinical dimension. If more than 25% of the questions were left blank the questionnaire was eliminated from the analysis.

The descriptive statistics (mean, median, standard deviation, floor effect and ceiling effect) of the subscales of the Celiac Disease Questionnaire (CDQ) were presented. Student's *t*-test and Variance Analysis (ANOVA) followed by Tukey post-hoc analysis was used to compare the values of the CDQ subscales with the variables of interest. All tests considered two-tailed hypotheses with a significance level of 5%. Confirmatory factor analysis was used to assess the factor validity. The Root Mean Square Error of Approximation (RMSEA) and the Chi-squared test of minimum discrepancy [19] evaluated the factor validity. The RMSEA ranges from 0 to 1, with smaller values indicating better model fit. A value of 0.06 or less is indicative of an acceptable model fit [20]. The statistical analyses were performed using IBM SPSS (Statistical Package for Social Sciences) version 22 (IBM SPSS Statistics for Windows, Version 22.0. IBM Corp, Armonk, NY, USA) and IBM SPSS AMOS (Analysis of Moment Structures) version 22 (Amos (Version 22.0), IBM SPSS, Chicago, IL, USA).

3. Results

3.1. Translation, Cultural Adaptation, Semantic Evaluation and Content Validation

The summary of stages of the Brazilian questionnaire process is displayed in Figure 1. The Brazilian CD-QoL (Supplementary Material S1) was constructed considering the translation/retranslation and suggestions made by the experts and celiac patients in the pilot test. After the translation/retranslation steps, the first stage of the content validation and the semantic evaluation was performed by judges and they decided to maintain all of the 28 questions with cultural and semantic adaptations since we opted to follow an existing CD-QoL questionnaire [7]. In total, three rounds of evaluations were necessary to obtain agreement among the experts for the content validation and semantic evaluation. After that, a pilot study with eight celiac patients was conducted. In the first round of the questionnaire, questions were considered adequate regarding reliability, clarity and easy comprehension.

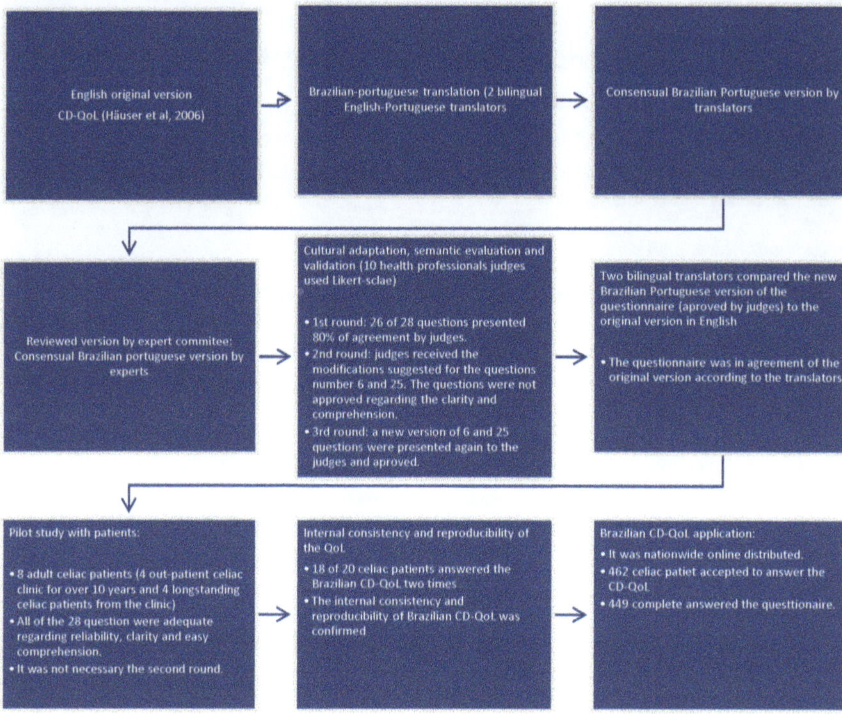

Figure 1. Process stages of the Brazilian celiac disease questionnaire of quality life (CD-QoL).

Internal Consistency, Construct Validity and Reproducibility of the Brazilian CD-QoL

The concordances of the answers (internal consistency) were verified by the Cronbach's alpha measure (Table 1). All four domains of the CD-QoL indicated good internal consistency (Cronbach's alpha > 0.7).

Table 1. Descriptive and internal consistency of the Brazilian CD-QoL.

	Mean (SD)	Median (IQR)	Range	Floor Effect (%)	Ceiling Effect (%)	Internal Consistency (Cronbach's Alpha)
Emotion	26.70 (9.55)	27 (20–34)	7–49	1.3%	0.2%	0.927
Social	31.15 (8.18)	32 (25–38)	10–48	0%	0%	0.703
Worries	27.25 (9.85)	27 (20–34)	7–49	0.4%	0.9%	0.832
Gastrointestinal	34.87 (8.61)	36 (29–41)	10–49	0%	2.4%	0.793
Total Score	119.79 (30.16)	120 (99–142)	51–181	0%	0%	0.925

SD—Standard deviation; IQR—Interquartile range. The factor/construct validity was examined by confirmatory factor analysis. The four domains (emotion, social, worries and gastrointestinal) presented a good fit in the confirmatory factor analysis (Root Mean Square Error of Approximation (RMSEA) = 0.016 and χ^2 = 309.04, df = 278, p = 0.097).

The test-retest reliability (reproducibility) of the questionnaire was verified using the paired t test, Pearson correlation coefficient and the intraclass correlation coefficient (Table 2). None of the four domains composing the final questionnaire showed significant divergence among the evaluators ($p > 0.05$ in the paired t test). The Pearson coefficient and Interclass correlation coefficient (ICC) are ideally more substantial and significant ($p < 0.05$). Therefore, the questionnaire presents proper measures of reproducibility.

Table 2. CD-QoL scale reproducibility (n = 18 participants).

	Score			Pearson Correlation		Intraclass Correlation Coefficient	
	Phase 1 Mean (SD)	**Phase 2 Mean (SD)**	p *	**Correlation**	p	**ICC**	p
Emotion	25.50 (10.16)	27.06 (10.08)	0.153	0.905	<0.001	0.947	<0.001
Social	33.00 (9.17)	34.67 (7.08)	0.224	0.769	<0.001	0.850	<0.001
Worries	30.06 (7.68)	31.17 (8.54)	0.291	0.863	<0.001	0.923	<0.001
Gastrointestinal	37.06 (6.91)	35.17 (6.23)	0.247	0.486	0.041	0.647	0.018
Total	125.61 (27.11)	128.06 (27.08)	0.531	0.821	<0.001	0.905	<0.001

* paired t-test. ICC: Interclass correlation coefficient. $p < 0.05$ is statistically significant.

3.2. CD-QoL Application

During the period from July to October of 2017, a link to the Brazilian CD-QoL was distributed nationwide by email to multiple Brazilian Celiac Associations (*Associação dos Celíacos do Brasil—Acelbra; and Federação Nacional das Associações de Celíacos do Brasil Fenacelbra*). Those associations either emailed the link to CD patients registered with them or published the link to the survey through social media that was subsequently shared by members. In addition to Brazilian Celiac Associations, dietitians and gastroenterologists were also asked to distribute the link to their CD patients. Therefore, we used a convenience sample to perform the present study.

A total of 462 participants from 18 out of 26 Brazilian States agreed to answer the questionnaire. The eight Brazilian States not represented were those with no Celiac Associations. Of the 462 questionnaires, 12 were excluded because they were not filled out. The remaining 450 questionnaires responses were analyzed. The questionnaire took an average of six minutes to be completed. Characteristics of the responders and their association with the CD-QoL subcategories are presented in Table 3.

We divided the marital status category into either *in a stable relationship* (married or with a live-in partner) or *not in a stable relationship* (those that are single, divorced, or widowed). We also divided the Gluten-Free Diet category into two. Only participants that answered "always" were considered to be on a GFD, those that responded, "almost always", "almost never"; "never" and "sometimes", were considered not to be on a GFD.

Participants over the age of 40 presented higher values on the scale (statistically significant only for the total scale and the social subscale). Early diagnosis is related to higher scores on the social, sub- and total scale. There was a positive correlation between higher education level and higher QoL.

Individuals with partners tend to have a better QoL emotional subscale score (represent higher values on the scale). Regarding other subscales, the marital aspect did not influence the QoL. Individuals that follow a strict GFD have higher QoL scale values (except for the worries subscale) and those who do not take antidepressants have a higher quality of life.

The men's scores for the CD-QoL were higher than the women's. All results were statistically significant except for the gastrointestinal subscale, where there is no significant difference between women and men ($p > 0.05$).

Table 3. Sub-scores of the CD-QoL scale subcategorized by sex, age, time of diagnosis, schooling, marital status and diet.

	Emotion	Social	Worries	Gastrointestinal	Total
	Mean (SD)	Mean (SD)	Mean (SD)	Mean (SD)	Mean (SD)
Gender *					
Women (n = 425)	26.42 (9.51)	30.08 (8.14)	26.80 (9.69)	34.75 (8.63)	118.55 (29.98)
Men (n = 25)	30.88 (9.03)	36.40 (6.57)	34.71 (9.96)	36.84 (8.33)	139.33 (25.95)
p	0.023	0.000	0.000	0.238	0.001
Age *					
39 and under (n = 271)	26.01 (9.13)	30.28 (7.93)	26.87 (9.64)	34.28 (8.45)	117.34 (28.98)
40 and over (n = 179)	27.74 (10.08)	32.48 (8.40)	27.82 (10.17)	35.77 (8.79)	123.52 (31.59)
p	0.065	0.006	0.032	0.074	0.036
Time of diagnosis *					
29 and under (n = 170)	25.27 (8.76)	29.97 (8.14)	26.75 (9.61)	33.99 (8.51)	115.72 (29.16)
30 and over (n = 273)	27.48 (9.92)	31.80 (8.20)	27.27 (9.93)	35.34 (8.67)	121.75 (30.58)
p	0.015	0.024	0.588	0.109	0.043
Educational level **					
Elementary (n = 26)	23.00 (10.92) [a]	28.44 (6.68) [a]	24.23 (10.78) [a]	29.42 (8.68) [a]	106.12 (30.32) [a]
High School (n = 116)	24.10 (9.60) [a,b]	29.29 (8.20) [a,b]	25.69 (9.69) [a,b]	32.69 (9.36) [a,b]	111.57 (30.21) [a,b]
College (n = 152)	27.32 (9.13) [b,c]	31.34 (8.06) [a,b]	27.29 (9.54) [a,b]	35.43 (8.22) [b,c]	121.01 (29.36) [b,c]
Graduate & Post-grad (n = 156)	28.65 (9.14) [c]	32.79 (8.16) [b]	28.88 (9.90) [b]	36.86 (7.67) [c]	127.01 (28.86) [c]
p	0.000	0.002	0.022	0.000	0.000
Marital status *					
With partners (n = 275)	27.51 (9.68)	31.69 (8.25)	27.30 (9.68)	35.36 (8.39)	121.78 (29.85)
Without partners (n = 175)	25.43 (9.22)	30.31 (8.02)	27.18 (10.14)	34.11 (8.91)	116.68 (30.47)
p	0.025	0.085	0.908	0.136	0.084
Gluten-free diet compliance *					
No (n = 51)	20.61 (9.37)	28.10 (7.43)	25.16 (10.97)	29.73 (8.71)	104.20 (30.00)
Yes (n = 399)	27.48 (9.30)	31.53 (8.20)	27.52 (9.68)	35.53 (8.38)	121.76 (29.64)
p	0.000	0.005	0.108	0.838	0.000
Antidepressant medicines *					
No (n = 371)	27.67 (9.37)	31.67 (7.98)	27.76 (9.78)	35.50 (8.49)	122.45 (29.63)
Yes (n = 79)	22.15 (9.09)	28.79 (8.72)	24.85 (9.90)	31.95 (8.63)	107.73 (29.81)
p	0.000	0.004	0.017	0.001	0.000

* Student t-test. ** Anova with Tukey post-hoc test. Groups with the same letters do not differ significantly. Different letters on the same column represent statistical differences.

4. Discussion

Health is defined as "a state of complete physical, mental and social well-being" [21]. According to the World Health Organization, to achieve optimal health, it is essential to comprehend the patient's perception of quality of life [22]. The Celiac Disease-specific Quality of Life Scale is an important and cost-effective tool to understand aspects related to the QoL of celiac patients. The scale helps us understand elements present in daily choices, management of mental and physical well-being as well as the social limitations imposed by this chronic disease due to the necessity for lifelong commitment [7,9].

When the quality of life assessment instrument is used in a variety of cultural settings, it is imperative to establish whether the same aspects of life are equally important to the group studied. Groups of people, particularly in different cultures, are likely to assign different levels of importance to various aspects of their life; therefore, cultural and semantic validation is crucial [23]. To the best of our knowledge, our study is the first characterization of the emotional, worries, gastrointestinal and social features related to the quality of life in CD Brazilian adults. In this context, we validated the first specific QoL instrument for CD patients in Brazilian Portuguese, based on the Hauser et al. [7] instrument.

The linguistic validation process (translation and retranslation) is recommended when the original instrument is developed in a language other than the target language and there is no translated and validated version in the target language [22]. Therefore, the first step of this study was to translate/retranslate the original version of CD-QoL to English/Portuguese/English. The translation was followed by the cross-cultural adaptation process that followed the guidelines predominant in the literature [24,25]. To acquire a reliable instrument, it is also vital to perform a semantic evaluation, which measures the comprehension of the instrument. This step ensures the instrument is clear and easy to understand [17]. The Brazilian Portuguese versions of the instrument demonstrate cultural and semantic adequacy and therefore represent the first Brazilian Portuguese version developed. A pilot study was conducted to evaluate the reliability and internal consistency of the instrument with celiac patients.

Reliability is an estimate of the instrument's ability to reproduce results provided that no change in the outcome has taken place [22]. In this study, it was measured with internal consistency and test-retest stability. The internal instrument consistency is an estimate of the extent to which the included items of a score correlate with each other. Cronbach's alpha coefficient was used for this estimate for all patients, in all domains of the CD-QoL at baseline [26]. Internal consistency was considered acceptable when Cronbach's alpha was 0.70 or higher [27]. None of the 28 items composing the final questionnaire showed significant divergence among the evaluators (>0.05 in the Cronbach alpha test) (Table 1). The 28-items of the CD-QoL show reliable internal consistency; therefore, the questionnaire presents good measures of reproducibility, which indicates that similar results under consistent conditions are reproducible.

Once validated, the instrument was sent nationwide to Brazilian celiac patients to evaluate their quality of life. Similar to the other studies of CD-QoL in different countries [7–9], most of the respondents in this study were female (95%). It was expected, since the CD prevalence is higher in female patients than male patients [1,3,28] and women tend to be more concerned about health and participate more often in health studies [29–32]. The study conducted by Ramirez-Cervantes et al. [33] also had more responses from female participants (75%) compared to male participants in Mexico. In Brazil, Castilhos et al. [32] conducted a study with celiac patients that were registered in the Southern Brazilian Celiac Association (ACELPAR), which also showed a low rate of male participation (6.8%). They attribute these findings to the low participation rate of men in the ACELPAR meetings where the questionnaires were administered and more broadly, to the low interest in their health when compared to women [32].

In the present study, women's scores for the CD-QoL were lower than men's scores, except for the gastrointestinal subscale. Studies have shown that CD women experience a lower level of quality of life than men [13,34–36]. Women also report more distress caused by daily life restrictions and perceive a higher burden with CD than men [35].

Individuals that follow a strict GFD have higher QoL scale values (except for subscale worries). The strict adherence to the GFD tends to enhance physical and physiological aspects. Despite the food restriction, social wellbeing aspects can also be achieved, since symptoms and other conditions related to CD tend to be improved with the treatment adherence [37]. In line with previous studies, we found that diet-compliant CD patients (with an internal LoC (locus of control)) had a better QoL than noncompliant patients [7,9,32,38–40]. According to Wagner et al. [38], the GFD compliance is essential for celiac patients to obtain optimal QoL. Psychological and educational support is also essential for patients that are having difficulty adhering to a GFD [32,38]. According to Castilhos et al. [32], most of the CD patients felt well informed, showed no declining trend and showed no constant worry about their food. They believed that these results are related to the information and support received by the celiac association (ACELPAR). These results reinforce the importance of information and support to improve the QoL of CD patients.

Other studies showed similar results to ours; Wagner et al. (Wagner et al., 2008 [38]) showed that better physical health, lower CD-associated burden and fewer social problems, were found in participants who had a longer period since being diagnosed, indicating the importance of the earliest possible diagnosis. Ramírez-Cervantes et al. [33] also concluded that, at the time of diagnosis, CD patients had a reduced quality of life, compared to those with a longer diagnosis period—likely due to better knowledge about the disease and acceptance of the lifestyle. In the study conducted by Castilhos et al. [32], patients newly diagnosed were compared with those who had the longer diagnosis. The study showed that patients that were longer diagnosed had better QoL, suggesting that the limitations imposed by disease and GFD influence the patients QoL. They also indicate that over the years, there is a better adaptation to the restrictions imposed by the treatment [32]. Another study of Brazilian CD patients showed that the longer the time since diagnosis, the lower the chances that these patients had positive serological tests, indicating a better comprehension and adherence to the treatment [11].

Several studies highlight the positive role families can play in providing support to patients when adopting a GFD, as well as the support in coping with CD [13,41,42]. This active support provided is likely the reason why those "with partner" under marital status scored higher in the emotional subscale CD-QoL.

Past research has demonstrated that a higher educational level significantly contributes to the patient's physical and social function, health perception and mental health. Low education amplifies the adverse effects of many chronic medical conditions due to lack of knowledge [43–46]. Our results, which corroborate the above findings, showed a positive correlation between higher education level and higher QoL. The education level tends to be associated with higher socioeconomic status [44]. A study suggests that income modulates both health-seeking behavior and access to health care [47], which is related to higher QoL.

A potential limitation to our study was selection bias created by the manner in which the survey was disseminated, that is, over the internet and with the use of email and social media. According to a census by the Brazilian Institute of Geography and Statistics (IBGE), approximately half of the Brazilian population 25 years of age and younger have less than eighth-grade education [48]. However, 56% of our respondents had a college degree or above, which is not representative of the Brazilian population. Consequently, there was also a selection bias regarding the socioeconomic level of the respondents, which is much higher than the national average.

5. Conclusions

There is growing interest in assessing the outcome of CD, given the chronic nature of the disease. The development of a self-administered Brazilian-Portuguese CD-QoL instrument that captures the perceptions and concerns of CD individuals is an important step forward in the care of these patients. The Brazilian-Portuguese CD-QoL questionnaire version presents good measures of reproducibility and internal consistency. In Brazil, the time since diagnosis, higher education level, strict adherence to GFD and male gender are related to the highest scores of CD-QoL. Knowledge of the quality of life is important to help implement effective strategies to improve Brazilian celiac patients' quality of life and for reducing the physical, emotional and social burden on them. Besides the Brazilian CD-QoL, an Italian, German, French and Turkish version of the CD-QoL have been published, which allows for comparative research between different celiac populations in the world.

Supplementary Materials: The following are available online at http://www.mdpi.com/2072-6643/10/9/1167/s1. Supplementary Material S1: Brazilian CD-QoL in Portuguese.

Author Contributions: Conceptualization, C.P.P., W.H., L.G., R.P. and R.P.Z.; Methodology, C.P.P., W.H., L.G., R.P. and R.P.Z.; Validation, C.P.P., W.H., N.S., E.Y.N., R.H.U., L.G., R.P. and R.P.Z.; Formal Analysis, C.P.P., L.G., R.P., E.Y.N. and R.P.Z.; Investigation, C.P.P., N.S., E.Y.N., R.H.U., L.G., R.P. and R.P.Z.; Resources, R.P., L.G.; Data Curation, R.P.; Writing-Original Draft Preparation, C.P.P., L.G., R.P. and R.P.Z.; Writing-Review & Editing, C.P.P., W.H., E.Y.N., L.G., R.P. and R.P.Z.; Visualization, C.P.P., W.H., E.Y.N., L.G., R.P. and R.P.Z.; Supervision, C.P.P., L.G., R.P. and R.P.Z.; Project Administration, C.P.P., L.G., R.P. and R.P.Z.

Funding: This research received no external funding.

Acknowledgments: I would like to thank Matthew Rogers, Marcelo Pratesi and Molly Glasby for all their editing help and for their love and patience throughout the research process.

Conflicts of Interest: The authors declare no conflict of interest.

References

1. Shamir, R.; Heyman, M.B.; Koning, F.; Wijimenga, C.; Gutierrez-Achury, J.; Catassi, C.; Gatti, S.; Fasano, A.; Discepolo, V.; Korponay-Szabó, I.R.; et al. Celiac Disease. *J. Pediatr. Gastroenterol. Nutr.* **2014**, *59*, S1. [CrossRef] [PubMed]
2. Schuppan, D.; Junker, Y.; Barisani, D. Celiac Disease: From Pathogenesis to Novel Therapies. *Gastroenterology* **2009**, *137*, 1912–1933. [CrossRef] [PubMed]
3. Barada, K.; Abu Daya, H.; Rostami, K.; Catassi, C. Celiac Disease in the Developing World. *Gastrointest. Endosc. Clin. N. Am.* **2012**, *22*, 773–796. [CrossRef] [PubMed]
4. Barker, J.M.; Liu, E. Celiac disease: Pathophysiology, clinical manifestations and associated autoimmune conditions. *Adv. Pediatr.* **2008**, *55*, 349–365. [CrossRef] [PubMed]
5. Kaukinen, K.; Lindfors, K.; Mäki, M. Advances in the treatment of coeliac disease: An immunopathogenic perspective. *Nat. Rev. Gastroenterol. Hepatol.* **2014**, *11*, 36–44. [CrossRef] [PubMed]
6. Zingone, F.; Iavarone, A.; Tortora, R.; Imperatore, N.; Pellegrini, L.; Russo, T.; Dorn, S.D.; Ciacci, C. The Italian translation of the Celiac Disease-specific Quality of Life Scale in celiac patients on gluten free diet. *Dig. Liver Dis.* **2013**, *45*, 115–118. [CrossRef] [PubMed]
7. Häuser, W.; Gold, J.; Stein, J.; Caspary, W.F.; Stallmach, A. Health-related quality of life in adult coeliac disease in Germany: Results of a national survey. *Eur. J. Gastroenterol. Hepatol.* **2006**, *18*, 747–754. [CrossRef] [PubMed]
8. Marchese, A.; Klersy, C.; Biagi, F.; Balduzzi, D.; Bianchi, P.I.; Trotta, L.; Vattiato, C.; Zilli, A.; Rademacher, J.; Andrealli, A.; et al. Quality of life in coeliac patients: Italian validation of a coeliac questionnaire. *Eur. J. Intern. Med.* **2013**, *24*, 87–91. [CrossRef] [PubMed]
9. Aksan, A.; Mercanlıgil, S.M.; Häuser, W.; Karaismailoğlu, E. Validation of the Turkish version of the Celiac Disease Questionnaire (CDQ). *Health Qual. Life Outcomes* **2015**, *13*, 82. [CrossRef] [PubMed]
10. Pouchot, J.; Despujol, C.; Malamut, G.; Ecosse, E.; Coste, J.; Cellier, C. Validation of a French version of the quality of life "Celiac Disease Questionnaire". *PLoS ONE* **2014**, *9*, e96346. [CrossRef] [PubMed]
11. Machado, J.; Gandolfi, L.; Coutinho De Almeida, F.; Malta Almeida, L.; Puppin Zandonadi, R.; Pratesi, R. Gluten-free dietary compliance in Brazilian celiac patients: Questionnaire versus serological test. *Nutr. Clin. Diet. Hosp.* **2013**, *33*, 46–49. [CrossRef]
12. Farage, P.; Puppin Zandonadi, R.; Cortez Ginani, V.; Gandolfi, L.; Pratesi, R.; de Medeiros Nóbrega, Y.K. Content Validation and Semantic Evaluation of a Check-List Elaborated for the Prevention of Gluten Cross-Contamination in Food Services. *Nutrients* **2017**, *9*, 36. [CrossRef] [PubMed]
13. Sverker, A.; Hensing, G.; Hallert, C. 'Controlled by food'—Lived experiences of coeliac disease. *J. Hum. Nutr. Diet.* **2005**, *18*, 171–180. [CrossRef] [PubMed]
14. Bullinger, M.; Alonso, J.; Apolone, G.; Leplège, A.; Sullivan, M.; Wood-Dauphinee, S.; Gandek, B.; Wagner, A.; Aaronson, N.; Bech, P.; et al. Translating health status questionnaires and evaluating their quality: The IQOLA Project approach. International Quality of Life Assessment. *J. Clin. Epidemiol.* **1998**, *51*, 913–923. [CrossRef]
15. Okoli, C.; Pawlowski, S.D. The Delphi method as a research tool: An example, design considerations and applications. *Inf. Manag.* **2004**, *42*, 15–29. [CrossRef]
16. De Lima, T.C.; Gallani, M.C.B.J.; de Freitas, M.I.P. Content validation of an instrument to characterize people over 50 years of age living with human immunodeficiency virus/acquired immunodeficiency syndrome. *Acta Paul. Enferm.* **2012**, *25*, 4–10. [CrossRef]
17. Conti, M.A.; Scagliusi, F.; Kawamura De Oliveira Queiroz, G.; Hearst, N.; Cordás, T.A. Cross-cultural adaptation: Translation and Portuguese language content validation of the Tripartite Influence Scale for body dissatisfaction. *Cad. Saude Publ.* **2010**, *26*, 503–513. [CrossRef]
18. Polit, D.F.; Beck, C.T. *Nursing Research: Principles and Methods*; Lippincott Williams & Wilkins: Philadelphia, PA, USA, 2004; ISBN 0781737338.
19. Kline, R.B. *Principles and Practice of Structural Equation Modeling*, 3rd ed.; The Guilford Press: New York, NY, USA, 2011; ISBN 978-1-60623-877-6.
20. Hu, L.; Bentler, P. Cutoff criteria for fit indices in covariance structure analysis: Conventional criteria versus new alternatives. *Struct. Equ. Model.* **1999**, *6*, 1–55. [CrossRef]
21. World Health Organization. *The Third Ten Years of the World Health Organization*, 1st ed.; WHO: Geneva, Switzerland, 2008; ISBN 978 92 4 156366 6.

22. Fagerdahl, A.-M.; Boström, L.; Ulfvarson, J.; Bergström, G.; Ottosson, C. Translation and validation of the wound-specific quality of life instrument Cardiff Wound Impact Schedule in a Swedish population. *Scand. J. Caring Sci.* **2014**, *28*, 398–404. [CrossRef] [PubMed]
23. Saxena, S.; Carlson, D.; Billington, R.; Orley, J. The WHO quality of life assessment instrument (WHOQOL-Bref): The importance of its items for cross-cultural research. *Qual. Life Res.* **2001**, *10*, 711–721. [CrossRef] [PubMed]
24. Guillemin, F.; Bombardier, C.; Beaton, D. Cross-cultural adaptation of health-related quality of life measures: Literature review and proposed guidelines. *J. Clin. Epidemiol.* **1993**, *46*, 1417–1432. [CrossRef]
25. Beaton, D.E.; Bombardier, C.; Guillemin, F.; Ferraz, M.B. Guidelines for the process of cross-cultural adaptation of self-report measures. *Spine* **2000**, *25*, 3186–3191. [CrossRef] [PubMed]
26. Streiner, D.L. Starting at the Beginning: An Introduction to Coefficient Alpha and Internal Consistency Starting at the Beginning: An Introduction to Coefficient Alpha and Internal Consistency. *J. Pers. Assess.* **2003**, *80*, 99–103. [CrossRef] [PubMed]
27. Streiner, D.L.; Norman, G.R. *Health Measurement Scales: A Practical Guide to Their Development and Use*; Oxford University Press: Oxford, UK, 2008; ISBN 9780199231881.
28. Mäki, M.; Collin, P. Coeliac disease. *Lancet* **1997**, *349*, 1755–1759. [CrossRef]
29. Davidson, D.J.; Freudenburg, W.R. Gender and Environmental Risk Concerns. *Environ. Behav.* **1996**, *28*, 302–339. [CrossRef]
30. Chen, M. Consumers' health and taste attitude in Taiwan. *Br. Food J.* **2013**, *115*, 526–540. [CrossRef]
31. Lee, A.R.; Wolf, R.; Contento, I.; Verdeli, H.; Green, P.H.R. Coeliac disease: The association between quality of life and social support network participation. *J. Hum. Nutr. Diet.* **2016**, *29*, 383–390. [CrossRef] [PubMed]
32. Castilhos, A.C.; Gonçalves, B.C.; Macedo e Silva, M.; Lanzoni, L.A.; Metzger, L.R.; Kotze, L.M.S.; Nisihara, R.M. Quality of life evaluation in celiac patients from Southern Brazil. *Arq. Gastroenterol.* **2015**, *52*, 171–175. [CrossRef] [PubMed]
33. Ramírez-Cervantes, K.L.; Remes-Troche, J.M.; del Pilar Milke-García, M.; Romero, V.; Uscanga, L.F. Characteristics and factors related to quality of life in Mexican Mestizo patients with celiac disease. *BMC Gastroenterol.* **2015**, *15*, 4. [CrossRef] [PubMed]
34. Hallert, C.; Grännö, C.; Hultén, S.; Midhagen, G.; Ström, M.; Svensson, H.; Valdimarsson, T. Living with coeliac disease: Controlled study of the burden of illness. *Scand. J. Gastroenterol.* **2002**, *37*, 39–42. [CrossRef] [PubMed]
35. Hallert, C.; Sandlund, O.; Broqvist, M. Perceptions of health-related quality of life of men and women living with coeliac disease. *Scand. J. Caring Sci.* **2003**, *17*, 301–307. [CrossRef] [PubMed]
36. Zarkadas, M.; Cranney, A.; Case, S.; Molloy, M.; Switzer, C.; Graham, I.D.; Butzner, J.D.; Rashid, M.; Warren, R.E.; Burrows, V. The impact of a gluten-free diet on adults with coeliac disease: Results of a national survey. *J. Hum. Nutr. Diet.* **2006**, *19*, 41–49. [CrossRef] [PubMed]
37. Bellini, A.; Zanchi, C.; Martelossi, S.; Di Leo, G.; Not, T.; Ventura, A. Compliance with the Gluten-Free Diet: The Role of Locus of Control in Celiac Disease. *J. Pediatr.* **2011**, *158*, 463–466. [CrossRef] [PubMed]
38. Wagner, G.; Berger, G.; Sinnreich, U.; Grylli, V.; Schober, E.; Huber, W.-D.; Karwautz, A. Quality of Life in Adolescents with Treated Coeliac Disease: Influence of Compliance and Age at Diagnosis. *J. Pediatr. Gastroenterol. Nutr.* **2008**, *47*, 555–561. [CrossRef] [PubMed]
39. Roma, E.; Roubani, A.; Kolia, E.; Panayiotou, J.; Zellos, A.; Syriopoulou, V.P. Dietary compliance and life style of children with coeliac disease. *J. Hum. Nutr. Diet.* **2010**, *23*, 176–182. [CrossRef] [PubMed]
40. Häuser, W.; Stallmach, A.; Caspary, W.F.; Stein, J. Predictors of reduced health-related quality of life in adults with coeliac disease. *Aliment. Pharmacol. Ther.* **2007**, *25*, 569–578. [CrossRef] [PubMed]
41. Jacobsson, L.R.; Friedrichsen, M.; Göransson, A.; Hallert, C. Impact of an Active Patient Education Program on Gastrointestinal Symptoms in Women With Celiac Disease Following a Gluten-Free Diet. *Gastroenterol. Nurs.* **2012**, *35*, 200–206. [CrossRef] [PubMed]
42. Taylor, E.; Dickson-Swift, V.; Anderson, K. Coeliac disease: The path to diagnosis and the reality of living with the disease. *J. Hum. Nutr. Diet.* **2013**, *26*, 340–348. [CrossRef] [PubMed]
43. Gazmararian, J.A.; Williams, M.V.; Peel, J.; Baker, D.W. Health literacy and knowledge of chronic disease. *Patient Educ. Couns.* **2003**, *51*, 267–275. [CrossRef]
44. Everson, S.A.; Maty, S.C.; Lynch, J.W.; Kaplan, G.A. Epidemiologic evidence for the relation between socioeconomic status and depression, obesity and diabetes. *J. Psychosom. Res.* **2002**, *53*, 891–895. [CrossRef]

45. Rojas-García, A.; Ruiz-Perez, I.; Rodríguez-Barranco, M.; Gonçalves Bradley, D.C.; Pastor-Moreno, G.; Ricci-Cabello, I. Healthcare interventions for depression in low socioeconomic status populations: A systematic review and meta-analysis. *Clin. Psychol. Rev.* **2015**, *38*, 65–78. [CrossRef] [PubMed]
46. Elovainio, M.; Pulkki-Råback, L.; Jokela, M.; Kivimäki, M.; Hintsanen, M.; Hintsa, T.; Viikari, J.; Raitakari, O.T.; Keltikangas-Järvinen, L. Socioeconomic status and the development of depressive symptoms from childhood to adulthood: A longitudinal analysis across 27 years of follow-up in the Young Finns study. *Soc. Sci. Med.* **2012**, *74*, 923–929. [CrossRef] [PubMed]
47. Mehra, S.; Leffler, D.A.; Pallav, K.; Tariq, S.; Shah, S.; Green, P.H.; Hansen, J.; Dennis, M.; Kelly, C.P. Socioeconomic Status Influences Celiac Disease Diagnosis. *Gastroenterology* **2011**, *140*, S-438. [CrossRef]
48. IBGE. *Pesquisas de Orçamentos Familiares*; Brasília, Brazil, 2010. Available online: https://biblioteca.ibge.gov.br/visualizacao/livros/liv50063.pdf (accessed on 3 June 2018).

nutrients

MDPI

Article

The Availability and Nutritional Adequacy of Gluten-Free Bread and Pasta

Beatrice Allen and Caroline Orfila *

School of Food Science and Nutrition, University of Leeds, Leeds LS2 9JT, UK; beatriceallen@hotmail.co.uk
* Correspondence: c.orfila@leeds.ac.uk; Tel.: +44-113-343-2966

Received: 23 August 2018; Accepted: 21 September 2018; Published: 25 September 2018

Abstract: Management of coeliac disease (CD) requires the removal of gluten from the diet. Evidence of the availability, cost, and nutritional adequacy of gluten-free (GF) bread and pasta products is limited. GF flours are exempt from UK legislation that requires micronutrient fortification of white wheat flour. This study surveyed the number and cost of bread and pasta products available and evaluated the back-of-pack nutritional information, the ingredient content, and the presence of fortification nutrients of GF bread and pasta, compared to standard gluten-containing equivalent products. Product information was collected from four supermarket websites. Standard products were significantly cheaper, with more products available than GF ($p < 0.05$). GF bread products were significantly higher in fat and fiber ($p < 0.05$). All GF products were lower in protein than standard products ($p < 0.01$). Only 5% of GF breads were fortified with all four mandatory fortification nutrients (calcium, iron, niacin, and nicotinic acid or nicotinamide), 28% of GF breads were fortified with calcium and iron only. This lack of fortification may increase the risk of micronutrient deficiency in coeliac sufferers. It is recommended that fortification legislation is extended to include all GF products, in addition to increased regulation of the nutritional content of GF foods.

Keywords: coeliac disease; celiac disease; gluten; gluten-free diet; fortification; micronutrient; cost

---

1. Introduction

Coeliac disease (CD) affects 1% of the population in Europe [1,2]. Gluten is a collection of storage proteins present in major cereals such as wheat, barley, and rye, which compromise the main components of common UK foods, bread and pasta [3]. When consumed, gluten proteins trigger an immune-mediated enteropathy, leading to intestinal damage in genetically pre-disposed individuals. Management of CD requires exclusion of dietary gluten, which proves a challenge for CD sufferers due to the presence of gluten in many food products [4]. Cereals and their products contribute important dietary nutrients, including high levels of protein, fiber and B vitamins such as niacin and thiamin. In addition, white wheat flour is fortified by law in the UK with calcium, iron, niacin, and thiamin. Thus, removal of wheat products from the diet may result in nutrient insufficiency in coeliac diets.

The manufacturing of gluten-free (GF) products is challenging, as gluten contributes vital structural, rheological, and organoleptic properties to bread and pasta [3]. Currently, no direct substitute for gluten is available and a combination of refined unfortified cereal flours (e.g., maize and rice), hydrocolloids (e.g., hydroxypropyl methylcellulose) and proteins (e.g., egg white) are used to make GF products, which are often unpalatable [5]. There is inadequate evidence on the impact these foods have on the health of consumers; however, studies have demonstrated a strong impact of a GF diet on diet-related quality of life, affecting in particular their ability to eat socially and outside the home [6].

In addition to a reduced nutritional profile of GF foods, consuming a GF diet (GFD) has financial and psychological effects on CD patients. The inability to purchase affordable food easily may result in CD patients experiencing higher levels of depression and increased psychological stress regarding food consumption, especially in social situations [7].

The UK National Diet and Nutrition Survey (NDNS) reported white bread was the most commonly consumed carbohydrate source, and pasta consumption is increasing [8]. If CD patients are directly exchanging standard products for GF equivalents, GF products need to be of a similar nutritional standard. Due to the high intakes of bread, UK manufacturers are required by the Bread and Flour Regulations (1998) to fortify bread flours with calcium, iron, niacin, and thiamin [9] to prevent micronutrient deficiencies in the population. The Science Advisory Committee on Nutrition advised in 2017 mandatory folic acid fortification of standard flour to prevent anencephaly and spina bifida in developing fetus [10], although currently no changes to legislation have been made. GF flours and bread are exempt from these regulations, the reasons for which are unclear.

It is generally considered that GF foods are less nutritionally adequate than standard products, although evidence is limited. Fry et al. (2018) observed higher levels of fat, sugar and salt in UK GF foods compared to standard foods, although the study focusses solely on front-of-pack macronutrient levels [11]. Thompson (1999) found only 9% of US GF bread products were fortified with thiamin, riboflavin, and niacin [12]. Thompson (2000) reported iron fortification in 23% of GF breads and no fortification in US GF pasta products [13]. Recent studies have demonstrated low intakes of micronutrients in coeliac diets [14–17], this may be of particular concern in children [17].

The Department for Environment Food & Rural Affairs (2013), supported by manufacturing industry representatives and public health officials, confirmed its retention of the existing fortification legislation. According to the review, fortification of foods is cheap, convenient for manufacturers and nutritionally beneficial for the general population. There is no apparent reason GF products are not included in fortification legislation. This lack of fortification of GF foods may increase the risk of micronutrient deficiency and have severe health consequences for CD patients and consumers who choose to avoid gluten. However, recent studies have shown that CD patients may accumulate heavy metals, due to higher metaloprotein expression in enterocytes [18] so any fortification strategy must be carefully considered.

This study aims to examine the availability, cost and nutritional composition of GF bread and pasta, specifically addressing the macronutrient content and micronutrient fortification of these foods.

2. Materials and Methods

This study was a cross-sectional survey of the availability, cost, ingredient labels and nutritional values of standard and GF products available to buy in the four major UK supermarkets through online retailer websites. Products selected for the GF data had a clear GF declaration or description on the packaging. For each available GF product, a standard gluten containing product of similar characteristics was selected e.g., a GF white roll matched with a standard white roll. The four product categories selected were white bread, brown bread, seeded bread and white pasta, to reflect common UK consumption habits. A list of products identified through the survey is available as supplementary material, and includes information on brand, cost, back-of-pack energy, macronutrient and salt content, and presence of fortification nutrients.

2.1. Data Collection

2.1.1. Search Strategy

To represent the majority of purchasing options available to UK consumers, the four biggest supermarkets were chosen; Tesco, Sainsbury's, ASDA and Morrisons. Collectively, these supermarkets had a 73.2% market penetration in the UK grocery market in 2015. High end supermarkets and specialist health shops, such as Waitrose and Holland & Barrett, were excluded from the study because of the higher price range of products and smaller numbers of stores, which may not be accessible to all coeliac consumers. Discount retailers such as Aldi and Lidl that display no product or nutritional information online were excluded from the study.

The data was collected between September 2017 and December 2017. The product name, the cost (£/100 g), the ingredient label and the nutritional information (per 100 g) were recorded. Values relating to micronutrient levels were recorded where available, although this was limited in many products. Branded products found in multiple supermarkets were recorded once in the study. Where the same products were available in multiple formats (e.g., branded bread at 400 g and 800 g), only one format was selected for the study.

Two search methods were used; typing in general product names (e.g., white bread) into the search bar function on the supermarket websites and secondly by selecting product categories, as defined by the supermarkets e.g., category: bread, sub-category: white bread. Both search methods returned relevant products; however, both relied on the efficiency of the website and the correct labelling of the products and food categories by the supermarkets. Using both methods of searching for products and cross-referencing the resulting products in each category allowed the relevant products to be made available to the study. This was necessary, as using the search bar often returned irrelevant products, or the category selection did not include all available GF products. Search terms for GF products included GF, coeliac and free-from, and was used in addition to selecting the GF product category on the supermarket websites.

2.1.2. Food Categories

Products included in the evaluation for bread included whole loaves, sliced loaves, rolls (and their regional names e.g., baps). Bread products not included in the evaluation were part-baked breads, bread flours, crackers, wraps, pittas, bagels, crumpets, English muffins, 50/50 bread (half white/half brown), and naan breads as these often did not have GF equivalents. Brown bread and seeded bread products were recorded separately owing to the impact that seeds may have on the nutritional content. The brown bread category included any bread that was labelled as wholemeal or brown. Any bread product with labelling such as grains, granary, malted or any labelling referring to a seed were categorized as "seeded" and included in the "seeded bread" data set.

Pasta products used for the standard products evaluation included dry white pasta. Nutrient values were recorded as to the dry weight to ensure that products were comparable. Standard pasta products not recorded in the review included wholemeal pasta, canned pasta, pasta ready meals, gnocchi, 50/50 pasta, and fresh pasta. GF pasta products selected were direct substitutes of white pasta, therefore products such as pea pasta or red lentil pasta were not included in the study, as they do not directly mimic standard white pasta characteristics. The list of all the products included in the survey can be found Table S1.

2.1.3. Nutritional Content

The back-of-pack nutritional information was recorded for each product, including energy (kJ) per 100 g, energy (kcal) per 100 g and the following nutrients recorded in g per 100 g; fat, saturated fat, carbohydrates, sugars, fiber, protein, salt. Other nutrients were recorded where the information was provided, including calcium (mg), folic acid (μg), iron (mg), niacin (mg), omega-3 fatty acids (g), riboflavin (mg) and thiamin (g). The mean value and standard deviation was calculated and a graphical representation was created. The percentage of the contribution to the Reference Nutrient Intake (RNI) per portion was calculated using the mean value for 100 g of bread and 75 g of pasta for standard and GF products. The nutrient content of all the products included is listed in Table S1.

2.1.4. Ingredient Labels

The ingredient label was recorded for each product and a detailed list of the individual ingredients was compiled. Ingredients that had the same origins, for example, rice flour, rice starch, rice flakes etc. were grouped together under an appropriate collective term, e.g., rice. The functions of the ingredient (e.g., preservative) and the general nutritional contribution (e.g., protein) were recorded. The total number of ingredients that occurred in each product was calculated, in addition to the mean number of ingredients for each product category. The percentage of standard and GF foods containing each ingredient was calculated. Word it Out (2018) online software was used to analyze the frequency in which ingredients were found on labels. The list of ingredients for all the products included in this survey can be found in Table S2 (standard products) and Table S3 (GF products).

2.1.5. Fortification of Products

The fortification count of GF products was established by examining each ingredient label for the following nutrients; calcium carbonate, iron, niacin, and thiamin. The mean nutrient content was calculated for products where values were given, and the resulting information used to calculate the contribution to the RNI. The estimated contribution to the RNI for the standard breads was calculated using the minimum fortification values for each micronutrient per 100 g of wheat flour (the Bread and Flour Regulations, 1998). The presence of fortification for each product in the survey was recorded in Table S1.

2.2. Calculations and Statistical Analysis

Microsoft Excel was used to calculate the mean values, standard deviation for this study and perform all statistical tests for this study. Mean and standard deviation for each product category were calculated, and their differences assessed using an f-test, followed by a *t*-test (two-tailed distribution and two-sample unequal variance (heteroscedastic) settings). Statistically significant differences between means were considered when $p < 0.05$.

3. Results

3.1. Availability of GF Bread and Pasta

GF breads and pasta were available from all four websites and each supermarket sold an own-brand GF range. Often the same brands e.g., Genius and Schar were available from all websites, thus the products available may be repetitive and indicate a low level of consumer choice.

As shown in Figure 1, there were significantly more standard products available than GF products across all categories. The mean number of standard products available ranged between 23 and 62, while the mean available GF products ranged between 4 and 11. There was a significant difference between the number of GF white breads available, compared to the standard ($p = 0.003$). The lower number of GF brown breads compared to the standard was significant ($p \leq 0.001$). This is indicative of the limited choice available for GF consumers. GF pasta had significantly lower numbers of products available than standard products ($p = 0.012$). There were 83%–88% fewer GF white and brown breads and pasta products available compared to standard products. There were 69% fewer GF seeded breads than the standard equivalent.

A total of 110 products was used in the cost and nutritional analysis section of this study. All the available GF products ($n = 49$) on the websites were used and compared to equivalent standard products ($n = 61$).

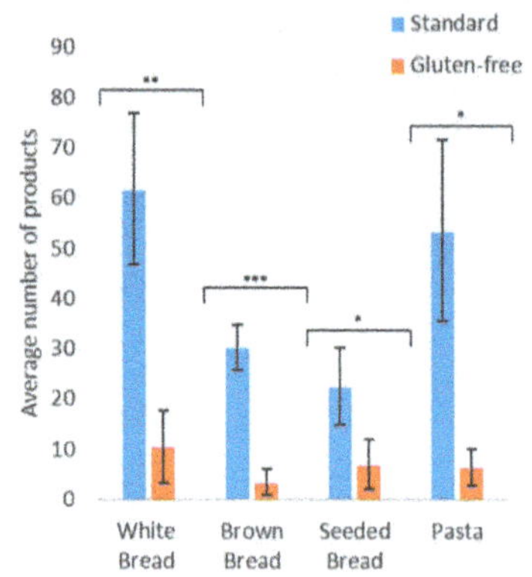

Figure 1. The average number of standard and gluten-free products available in four major UK supermarket websites. Key: * = $p < 0.05$, ** = $p < 0.01$, *** = $p < 0.001$.

3.2. Product Cost

The average cost of standard and GF products is shown in Figure 2. GF products were significantly more expensive across all four product categories than the standard equivalents. A highly significant difference was observed between the higher cost of GF pasta and standard pasta ($p = 0.004$). An extremely significant difference was observed in the cost of GF white and seeded breads compared to the standard equivalents ($p < 0.001$). When compared to standard products, an increase in the average cost of GF products was observed in white (+307%), brown (+314%) and seeded (+220%) breads. The cost of GF pasta increased by 70% compared to standard pasta.

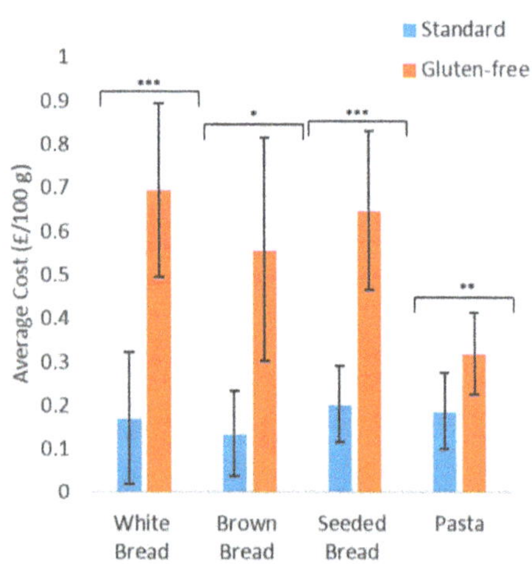

Figure 2. The average cost (£/100 g) of standard and gluten-free products available in four major UK supermarket websites. Key: * = $p < 0.05$, ** = $p < 0.01$, *** = $p < 0.001$.

3.3. Ingredient Labels and Nutritional Adequacy of Products

The total number of different ingredients used for GF bread was 98 and 44 for standard breads. A list of ingredients for all products in this survey can be found in Table S2 (standard products) and Table S3 (GF products). On average, eight different ingredients were used for GF pasta and one for standard pasta. The average number of ingredients used in standard bread products was 14 compared to 20 for GF bread. The higher number of ingredients was not associated with higher cost. The most common GF ingredients used are shown in Figure 3, with common ingredients being cereal flours, plant fibers and emulsifiers.

The nutrient content per portion of standard and GF products and their contribution to RNI is shown in Figure 4. The average total energy, saturated fat, and salt values (Figure 4A,C,H) were similar between standard and GF products. Carbohydrate values were significantly lower in GF white bread ($p = 0.004$); however, the carbohydrate values were similar and not statistically different for other product types (Figure 4D).

Standard products contained higher levels of sugar (Figure 4E) than GF products, significantly so in brown bread ($p = 0.041$) and pasta ($p = <0.001$). The RNI is the daily intake needed to satisfy the nutritional requirements of the majority (97.5%) of the population, as shown in Table 1. The sugar content in one portion of standard brown bread and pasta as a contribution to the RNI is 4% and 2% respectively (Table 1).

Table 1. Macronutrient and salt content of standard and gluten-free (GF) products per portion (100 g) and pasta (75 g) and the percentage contribution to reference nutrient intake (RNI).

Nutrition Attribute	RNI Value Per Day	Category	Standard Products		GF Products	
			Intake Per Portion	% Contribution to RNI	Intake Per Portion	% Contribution to RNI
Energy (kJ)	8400	White bread	1043	12	1016	12
		Brown bread	984	12	1035	12
		Seeded bread	1168	14	1113	13
		Pasta	1134	14	1117	13
Fat (g)	<70	White bread	3	4	5	7
		Brown bread	3	4	6	9
		Seeded bread	7	10	9	13
		Pasta	1	2	1	2
Saturates (g)	<20	White bread	1	3	0	2
		Brown bread	1	3	1	3
		Seeded bread	1	5	1	4
		Pasta	0	1	0	2
Carbohydrate (g)	260	White bread	46	18	42	16
		Brown bread	39	15	39	15
		Seeded bread	39	15	37	14
		Pasta	54	21	51	20
Sugars (g)	90	White bread	3	4	3	3
		Brown bread	3	4	2	2
		Seeded bread	4	4	2	3
		Pasta	2	2	0	0
Protein (g)	50	White bread	9	17	4	9
		Brown bread	10	21	8	16
		Seeded bread	11	22	6	12
		Pasta	9	18	5	9
Salt (g)	6	White bread	1	16	1	16
		Brown bread	1	15	1	15
		Seeded bread	1	15	1	15
		Pasta	0	1	0	1
Fiber (g)	30	White bread	3	9	7	22
		Brown bread	6	21	8	26
		Seeded bread	6	22	8	26
		Pasta	2	8	1	4

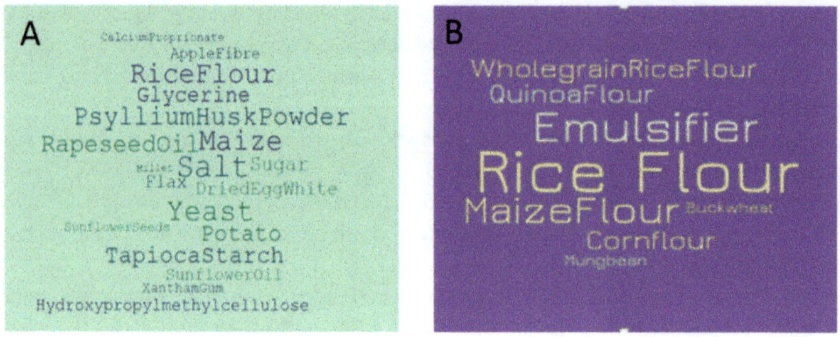

Figure 3. Key ingredients used in gluten-free (**A**) bread products and (**B**) pasta products. Ingredients frequently used in multiple products are indicated by larger font sizes. For a full list of ingredients, please refer to supplementary material.

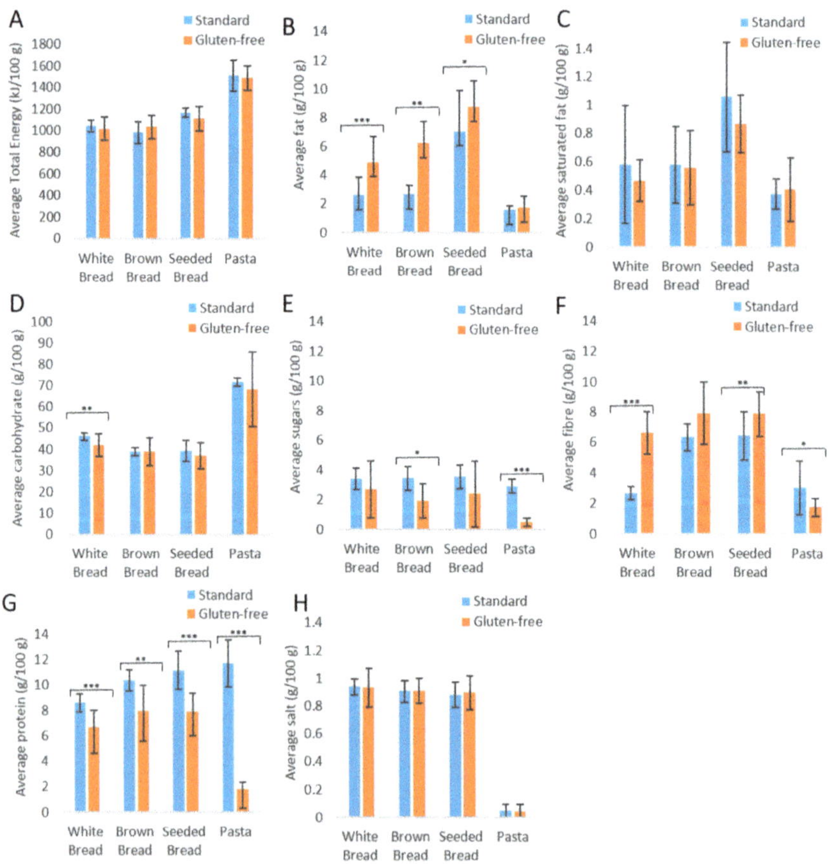

Figure 4. The average nutritional values of standard and gluten-free products for (**A**) total energy; (**B**) fat; (**C**) saturated fat; (**D**) carbohydrate; (**E**) sugars; (**F**) fiber; (**G**) protein; (**H**) salt. Key: * = $p < 0.05$, ** = $p < 0.01$, *** = $p < 0.001$.

Fiber was higher in all GF bread products (Figure 4F), significantly in white bread ($p \leq 0.001$) and seeded bread ($p = 0.008$). A portion of GF bread contributes 22%–26% of the fiber RNI, compared to standard breads providing 9%–21%. Standard white bread contained the lowest levels of fiber at 3 g per 100 g. The fiber content of GF pasta is significantly lower than standard pasta ($p = 0.039$), contributing 50% less fiber to the RNI than the standard, at 4% and 8% respectively.

As shown in Figure 4B, GF products contain significantly higher fat levels in white ($p \leq 0.001$), brown ($p = 0.006$) and seeded ($p = 0.038$) breads, with a minimal difference noted in pasta products. A portion of GF bread could contribute 7%–13% of the fat RNI, compared to standard products ranging between 4% and 10%.

Protein (Figure 4G) was significantly lower in all GF products, especially in white and brown breads ($p \leq 0.001$) and pasta ($p \leq 0.001$) when compared to standard products. All GF products contribute between 9%–16% of the RNI per portion, compared to standard products which contribute 17%–22% of the RNI.

3.4. Fortification of Bread and Pasta

All white bread is fortified with calcium carbonate, iron, niacin, and thiamin in accordance with UK law [19]. Standard brown (30%) and seeded (94.7%) breads contained fortified wheat flour although it is assumed that the use of wholemeal flour and seeds may increase the micronutrient content of these products. In total, 10% of standard bread products contained added folic acid.

Our analysis showed that only 28% of GF breads were fortified with calcium carbonate and iron, and only 5% of the total GF breads were fortified with all four fortification minerals, in addition to folic acid and riboflavin. Only two of the 14 GF manufacturers, Genius and Warburtons, fortified their products. None of the standard and GF pasta products surveyed was fortified.

Fortification of bread with nutrients contributes substantially to the RNI, especially that of calcium (23.5%) and thiamin (24%–30%) (Table 2). These results demonstrate that where fortification is present, a considerable percentage of the RNI can be achieved in one portion of bread. Most GF products on the market are not contributing to this intake.

Table 2. Reference nutrient intake (RNI) for calcium, iron, niacin and thiamin and the contribution of 100 g of standard bread.

Micronutrient	RNI (mg/day)		Contribution to RNI (%)	
	Male	Female	Male	Female
Calcium	1000	1000	23.5	23.5
Iron	8.7	14.8	19	11
Niacin	18	14	9	11
Thiamin	1	0.8	24	30

4. Discussion

The results of this study clearly show that CD sufferers are at risk of nutritional inadequacy owing to three main factors: (1) the low availability and high cost of commercial GF alternatives to bread and pasta; (2) the reduced nutritional quality of GF products compared to their equivalent gluten-containing staples; (3) the widespread lack of fortification.

4.1. Availability and Cost

These results demonstrate significantly lower numbers of GF products were available, compared to standard products. However, the true number of available products may be considerably lower, as the websites list GF products as sold throughout the country. It is likely that the actual number of in-store products will relate to the size of the supermarket and thus, in smaller supermarkets the number of GF products may be further restricted. This may considerably impact CD patients living in rural areas or those with access to only one supermarket. The limited number of products and potentially limited access to food may contribute to increased anxiety and depression surrounding food choice reported in CD patients [7]. However, global sales of GF food grew by 12.6% in 2016, with the market expected to increase [20]. This could be due to increased awareness of CD and a consumer perception that GF products are healthier. Despite the limited number of GF products currently available, the expansion of the GF product market can only contribute positively to coeliac food choice.

The results also showed that GF products are more expensive, in line with previous findings by Fry, Madden [11] which found GF products were on average 159% more expensive than the standard equivalents. Generally, standard bread loaves in the UK weigh 800 g, thus the average price of a standard white bread loaf is £1.35, compared to the higher GF cost of £5.52 of comparable weight.

The results of this study demonstrate that in addition to the limited number of products available to the consumer, the cost of GF products is significantly more expensive than standard products. The increased economic burden of CD and the reduced availability of products may increase the likelihood of some CD patients being unable to comply with a GFD.

4.2. Nutritional Profile According to Back-of-Pack Labelling

The results indicated that GF products tend to contain more fiber and fat, but less sugar and protein. The higher fiber content of GF breads may be attributed to the frequent use of plant fibers in GF products (Figure 3). Ingredients such as psyllium husk powder, cellulose polymers such as hydroxypropyl methylcellulose and apple fibers are commonly used to in GF manufacturing, as confirmed by the findings of Capriles and Areas [5]. The NDNS [21] reported that cereals and cereal products provide the largest source of dietary fiber, with only 9% of adults aged 19 to 64 years achieving the RNI of 30 g per day. CD patients following a GFD consume inadequate fiber levels, especially women, with intakes of 13.7 g per day [15] and 12 g per day [14] observed in UK dietary studies (fiber expressed as non-starch polysaccharides). There is limited scientific evidence of the effects these products have on the digestive system, but recently a study has shown that a subset of CD patients is sensitive to fermentable fibers [22]. Understanding these effects is important, especially as the digestive mechanism of CD patients may differ to that of the general population, as CD is an abnormal immune response to a food component.

Wild et al. found that CD patients following a GFD consumed significantly higher intakes of fat at 68.4 g per day and 93.2 g per day for women and men respectively, the latter exceeding the RNI of fat of <70 g per day [15]. These levels are higher than those observed by Kinsey et al. [14] who reported mean fat intakes of 59 g per day, which equates to 85% of the RNI for fat. Cereals account for a substantial 23% of UK protein intake [23]. Both studies found that coeliac protein consumption exceeded the RNI of 70 g per day with mean values of 74.1 g and 75 g of protein consumed per day, respectively. Therefore, while GF products are significantly lower in protein, this is unlikely to put CD sufferers at risk of protein deficiency. These results are supported by those of Fry et al. who compared the front-of-pack nutritional content of GF and standard products for example breads, cereals, pizza, and crackers [11]. Their study found that GF breads contained higher fat and fiber, and lower protein values than standard breads. Their study has several limitations, including the unexplained exclusion of GF products containing xanthan gum and egg white replacer, which are common in GF foods (Figure 3A). Although there is a statistically significant difference in the sugar content of GF and standard products, the small amount of sugar consumed per portion is unlikely to impact on consumer health.

Wild et al. reported lower intakes of micronutrients in CD patients when compared to the standard population, particularly iron, folate, and magnesium [15], although Kinsey et al. concluded adequate intakes of iron in the coeliac diet [14]. The study found that 47% of patients had been prescribed a calcium and vitamin D supplement. On average, patients who had not been prescribed with a calcium supplement consumed less than the RNI. Low calcium intakes are supported by the findings of Kinsey et al. who observed intakes of 866 mg per day [14]. This is below the specific coeliac RNI of

1000 mg per day, which is advised as an osteoporosis prevention measure. Further research into the micronutrient intake of CD patients is needed.

While bread and pasta are staples and major contributors to nutrient intake, other sources of nutrients need to be considered to assess nutrient intake in the CD population.

4.3. Fortification

GF products are currently excluded from fortification legislation, possibly because when the fortification legislation came into place, CD was relatively unknown. The Department for Environment Food & Rural Affairs [9] concluded in their review of the regulations that fortification is cheap, nutritionally beneficial for the population and convenient for manufacturers. The present study showed that fortification of bread contributes to nutrient intake, particularly of calcium (23.5% of RNI) and thiamin (24%–30% of RNI). We propose that the mandatory fortification of GF foods is necessary to provide equivalent nutrition to the healthy population. Fortification levels for GF foods must be carefully considered, taking into account CD pathophysiology, including potential accumulation of metals [18].

4.4. Limitations

This study represents a survey of GF bread and pasta products available in the four major British supermarkets, through online retailing. While this represents over 70% of the market penetration in the UK, we did not survey the remaining 30% of retailing places, including specialist shops selling GF foods. The survey only revealed 49 GF products (bread and pasta) available. While this is a small sample which limits the generalizability of the results, it does reflect the limited availability of GF products. We had to exclude some bread categories (such as crumpets, muffins, naan bread) because the GF version of these products could not be found in these supermarkets. The nutrient analysis was based on back-of-pack information. While this is an improvement compared to studies using front-of-pack information, chemical analysis of food should be applied to verify nutrient content, especially micronutrient content.

5. Conclusions

Despite improvements in the formulation and availability of GF in the last decade, GF foods are still less available and more expensive than gluten-containing versions. The macronutrient profile suggests that GF foods generally have adequate levels of fiber and sugar, but lower levels of protein and higher levels of fat, compared to their equivalent gluten-containing products. Very few GF foods were found to be fortified with micronutrients. As mandatory fortification of wheat flour is considered a successful health initiative for the general population, fortification should be extended to include GF products. Fortification of these products may reduce the risk of micronutrient deficiency and therefore deficiency-related diseases in CD patients.

Supplementary Materials: The following are available online at http://www.mdpi.com/2072-6643/10/10/1370/s1. Table S1: List of products identified in the survey with their back-of-pack nutrient information (energy, macronutrients, and salt values in g per 100 g) and fortification; Table S2: Ingredient list for standard bread and pasta products identified in the supermarket survey; Table S3: Ingredient list for gluten-free (GF) bread and pasta products identified in the supermarket survey.

Author Contributions: B.A. and C.O. contributed to the design of the research and the writing the manuscript. B.A. carried out data collection and analysis, C.O. supervised the project.

Conflicts of Interest: The authors declare no conflict of interest.

References

1. Coeliac U.K. How Common Is Coeliac Disease? About Coeliac Disease. 2018. Available online: https://www.coeliac.org.uk/coeliac-disease/about-coeliac-disease-and-dermatitis-herpetiformis/ (accessed on 23 September 2018).
2. Mustalahti, K.; Catassi, C.; Reunanen, A.; Fabiani, F.; Heier, M.; Millian, M.C.; Murry, L.; Metzger, M.H.; Gasparin, M.; Bravi, E.; et al. The prevalence of celiac disease in Europe: Results of a centralized, international mass screening project. *Ann. Med.* **2010**, *42*, 587–595. [CrossRef] [PubMed]
3. Wieser, H. Chemistry of gluten proteins. *Food Microbiol.* **2007**, *24*, 115–119. [CrossRef] [PubMed]
4. Ludvigsson, J.F.; Leffler, D.A.; Bai, J.C.; Biagi, F.; Fasano, A.; Green, P.H.R.; Hadjivassiliou, M.; Kaukinen, K.; Kelly, C.P.; Leonard, J.N.; et al. The Oslo definitions for coeliac disease and related terms. *Gut* **2013**, *62*, 43–52. [CrossRef] [PubMed]
5. Capriles, V.D.; Areas, J.A.G. Novel approaches in gluten-free breadmaking: Interface between food science, nutrition, and health. *Compr. Rev. Food Sci. Food* **2014**, *13*, 871–890. [CrossRef]
6. Black, J.L.; Orfila, C. Impact of coeliac disease on dietary habits and quality of life. *J. Hum. Nutr. Diet.* **2011**, *24*, 582–587. [CrossRef]
7. Van Hees, N.J.; Van der Does, W.; Giltay, E.J. Coeliac disease, diet adherence and depressive symptoms. *J. Psychosom. Res.* **2013**, *74*, 155–160. [CrossRef]
8. Whitton, C.; Nicholson, S.K.; Roberts, C.; Roberts, C.; Prynne, C.J.; Pot, G.K.; Olson, A.; Fitt, E.; Cole, D.; Teucher, B.; et al. National diet. and nutrition survey: UK food consumption and nutrient intakes from the first year of the rolling programme and comparisons with previous surveys. *Br. J. Nutr.* **2011**, *106*, 1899–1914. [CrossRef] [PubMed]
9. Department for Environment Food & Rural Affairs. *Bread and Flour Regulations 1998—A Summary of Responses to the Consultation and Government Reply*; F.R.A. Department for Environment: London, UK, 2013.
10. Wald, N.J.; Morris, J.K.; Blakemore, C. Public health failure in the prevention of neural tube defects: Time to abandon the tolerable upper intake level of folate. *Public Health Rev.* **2018**, *39*, 2. [CrossRef] [PubMed]
11. Fry, L.; Madden, A.M.; Fallaize, R. An investigation into the nutritional composition and cost of gluten-free versus regular food products in the UK. *J. Hum. Nutr. Diet.* **2018**, *31*, 108–120. [CrossRef] [PubMed]
12. Thompson, T. Thiamin, riboflavin, and niacin contents of the gluten-free diet: Is there cause for concern? *J. Am. Diet. Assoc.* **1999**, *99*, 858–862. [CrossRef]
13. Thompson, T. Folate, iron, and dietary fiber contents of the gluten-free diet. *J. Am. Diet. Assoc.* **2000**, *100*, 1389–1396. [CrossRef]
14. Kinsey, L.; Burden, S.T.; Bannerman, E. A dietary survey to determine if patients with coeliac disease are meeting current healthy eating guidelines and how their diet compares to that of the British general population. *Eur. J. Clin. Nutr.* **2008**, *62*, 1333–1342. [CrossRef] [PubMed]
15. Wild, D.; Robins, G.G.; Burley, V.J.; Howdle, P.D. Evidence of high sugar intake, and low fibre and mineral intake, in the gluten-free diet. *Aliment. Pharmacol. Ther.* **2010**, *32*, 573–581. [CrossRef] [PubMed]
16. Abenavoli, L.; Delibasic, M.; Peta, V.; Turkulov, V.; Lorenzo, A.D.; Medić-stojanosk, M. Nutritional profile of adult patients with celiac disease. *Eur. Rev. Med. Pharmacol. Sci.* **2015**, *19*, 4285–4292.
17. Ohlund, K.; Olsson, C.; Hernell, O.; Ohlund, I. Dietary shortcomings in children on a gluten-free diet. *J. Hum. Nutr. Diet.* **2010**, *23*, 294–300. [CrossRef] [PubMed]
18. Elli, L.; Pigatto, P.D.; Guzzi, G. Evaluation of Metals Exposure in Adults on a Gluten-Free Diet. *Clin. Gastroenterol. Hepatol.* **2018**, *16*, 152. [CrossRef] [PubMed]
19. The Bread and Flour Regulations. Schedule 1: Essential Ingredients in Flour in No. 141. 1998. Available online: http://www.legislation.gov.uk/uksi/1998/141/made (accessed on 23 September 2018).
20. Terazono, E. Healthy Appetites Drive Jump in Sales of Gluten-free Foods, in Financial Times. 2017. Available online: https://www.ft.com/content/4ec0f2f2-2c0a-11e7-9ec8-168383da43b7 (accessed on 23 September 2018).
21. National Diet and Nutrition Survey. Results of the National Diet and Nutrition Survey (NDNS) Rolling Programme for 2014 to 2015 and 2015 to 2016. 2018. Available online: http://www.mrc-ewl.cam.ac.uk/results-of-the-national-diet-and-nutrition-survey-ndns-rolling-programme-years-78-combined-2014-to-2015-and-2015-to-2016-are-now-published/ (accessed on 23 September 2018).

22. Roncoroni, L.; Bascuñán, K.; Doneda, L.; Scricciolo, A.; Lombardo, A.; Branchi, F.; Ferretti, F.; Dell'Osso, B.; Montanari, V.; Bardella, M.T. A low FODMAP gluten-free diet improves functional gastrointestinal disorders and overall mental health of celiac disease patients: A randomized controlled trial. *Nutrients* **2018**, *10*, 1023. [CrossRef] [PubMed]
23. Nutrients, Food and Ingredients: Protein. 2018. Available online: https://www.nutrition.org.uk/nutritionscience/nutrients-food-and-ingredients/protein.html?limit=1&start=1 (accessed on 23 September 2018).

nutrients

Article

Preparation of a Defined Gluten Hydrolysate for Diagnosis and Clinical Investigations of Wheat Hypersensitivities

Herbert Wieser † and Katharina A. Scherf *

Leibniz-Institute for Food Systems Biology at the Technical University of Munich, 85354 Freising, Germany; h.wieser2@gmx.de

* Correspondence: k.scherf.leibniz-lsb@tum.de; Tel.: +49-8161-712927

† Retired.

Received: 10 September 2018; Accepted: 25 September 2018; Published: 2 October 2018

Abstract: Gluten is the trigger for celiac disease (CD), non-celiac gluten/wheat sensitivity (NCGS), and wheat allergy. An oral food challenge is often needed for diagnosis, but there are no standardized gluten challenge materials with known composition available. To fill this gap, two materials, commercially available gluten and a food-grade gluten hydrolysate (pepgluten), were extensively characterized. Pepgluten was prepared from gluten by incubation with a pepsin dietary supplement and acetic acid at 37 °C for 120 min. The components of pepgluten were crude protein (707 mg/g), starch (104 mg/g), water (59 mg/g), fat (47 mg/g), dietary fiber (41 mg/g) and ash (11 mg/g). The protein/peptide fraction of pepgluten (1 g) contained equivalents derived from 369 mg gliadins and 196 mg glutenins, resulting in 565 mg total gluten equivalents, 25 mg albumins/globulins, 22 mg α-amylase/trypsin inhibitors and 48 mg pepsin capsule proteins. The slightly acidic, dough-like smell and bitter taste of pepgluten could be completely camouflaged in multivitamin juice with bitter lemon, grapefruit juice, or vegetable and fruit smoothies. Thus, pepgluten met the criteria for placebo-controlled challenges (active and placebo materials are identical regarding appearance, taste, smell, and texture) and is appropriate as a standard preparation for the oral food challenge and clinical investigations to study wheat hypersensitivities.

Keywords: celiac disease; diagnosis; gliadin; gluten; glutenin; non-celiac gluten sensitivity; oral food challenge; pepsin; wheat allergy

1. Introduction

Wheat hypersensitivities can be classified into celiac disease (CD) and related disorders (dermatitis herpetiformis Duhring and gluten ataxia), non-celiac gluten/wheat sensitivity (NCGS), non-IgE-mediated allergies and IgE-mediated allergies such as food allergy, skin allergy, respiratory allergy (e.g., baker's asthma), and wheat-dependent exercise-induced anaphylaxis (WDEIA) [1,2]. Additionally, a subgroup of individuals suffering from irritable bowel syndrome (IBS), especially diarrhea-predominant IBS, appears to be sensitive to wheat products and may profit from adhering to a gluten-free diet [3,4].

A wide variety of wheat proteins may trigger these hypersensitivities in susceptible individuals with a certain genetic predisposition (HLA-DQ2/8-positive) or sensitization. The causative factors in wheat are gluten (gliadins and glutenins, 70–80% of wheat proteins) and non-gluten proteins (albumins/globulins, 20–30% of wheat proteins). Classically, wheat proteins are subdivided according to extractability into albumins/globulins soluble in aqueous salt solution: gliadins are soluble in aqueous alcohols, and glutenins soluble in aqueous alcohols only after reduction of disulfide bonds [5]. Gluten comprises more than one hundred single proteins and serves as a source of nitrogen and amino acids for the wheat germ, whereas albumins/globulins mainly contain metabolic and protective proteins such as enzymes and enzyme inhibitors. Gluten proteins are hydrophobic, compact, and characterized by repetitive amino acid sequences rich in glutamine and proline, which makes them resistant to human gastrointestinal enzymes [6]. Based on amino acid sequence similarities, gliadins are subdivided into the gluten protein types ω5-, ω1,2-, α- and γ-gliadins and glutenins into glutenin-bound ωb-gliadins, high-molecular-weight (HMW) and low-molecular-weight (LMW) glutenin subunits (GS) [7]. While CD is caused by gluten only, wheat allergy occurs following sensitization with both gluten and non-gluten proteins. In the case of NCGS, α-amylase/trypsin-inhibitors (ATIs) belonging to non-gluten proteins have been identified as activators of innate immunity and adjuvant of several inflammatory reactions [8,9], but gluten proteins may be involved as well.

The differential diagnosis of wheat hypersensitivities is complex and requires a high level of clinical suspicion. Especially in inconclusive cases, open or single- or double-blinded oral challenge of the patients with the suspected triggering factor needs to be performed. A 14-day provocation test with gluten is necessary to achieve a clear diagnosis in CD patients who have already voluntarily adopted a gluten-free diet [10]. Stepwise challenges with half-logarithmic dose increments of wheat proteins at intervals of at least 20 min are needed to diagnose an immediate wheat allergy [11,12]. For WDEIA, gluten ingestion is combined with exercise or other cofactors [13]. The diagnosis of NCGS and diarrhea-predominant IBS is known to be especially difficult due to the lack of specific biomarkers and frequent placebo or nocebo effects [2,14,15]. Therefore, a double-blind, placebo-controlled food challenge is regarded as the gold standard to establish whether wheat is involved in symptom induction [16], although this is difficult to undertake in daily clinical practice [3].

A number of different materials, for example, wheat bread [17] or cookies [18], udon noodles [19], wheat-containing daily meals [4], and wheat gluten as is [13], as gastrosoluble capsules [16,20] or added to bakery products such as muffins [21] have been used for oral challenge. However, the amount and composition of wheat proteins used in these materials were often not determined or indicated. For example, commercial wheat gluten (vital gluten) has been frequently assumed to consist of 100% gluten proteins, but the protein content is typically only about 70–80% based on fresh weight [21]. The gluten-containing foods used for the oral challenge should be indistinguishable from the gluten-free placebo in taste, smell, texture, and appearance, and contain comparable amounts of carbohydrates, dietary fiber, fat, and protein. The challenge food should provide adequate immunoreactive protein in a reasonable portion size, be easily applicable, closely replicate the usual form of the food, and its qualitative and quantitative composition should be known [2,11]. A dose of 8 g of gluten with a defined ATI content (at least 3 g ATIs per 100 g of gluten) is recommended for diagnosis of NCGS [2]. Already in 2004, the European Academy of Allergy and Clinical Immunology demanded that challenge tests should be carried out with standardized foods guaranteeing the safety of patients, practical feasibility, and the comparability of results between different study centers [22]. Despite several meetings of expert groups, no standardized preparation has so far been developed for the diagnosis of wheat hypersensitivities, although there is a clear need, especially for NCGS where the diagnosis still relies on exclusion of all other possible causes as long as specific biomarkers for NCGS have not been identified. Therefore, the aim of this study was to thoroughly characterize wheat gluten and prepare a well-defined wheat gluten hydrolysate (called "pepgluten" in the following), which fulfills the recommendations stated above and is suited for oral food challenge in clinical and scientific studies on wheat hypersensitivities.

2. Materials and Methods

2.1. Reagents and Materials

All reagents and chemicals were purchased from Merck (Darmstadt, Germany), Sigma-Aldrich (Steinheim, Germany), AppliChem (Darmstadt, Germany), or Serva (Heidelberg, Germany) in analytical grade or higher. Water for reversed-phase high-performance liquid chromatography

(RP-HPLC) was purified with an Arium 611VF water purification system (Sartorius, Goettingen, Germany). Prolamin Working Group (PWG)-gliadin [23] used for calibration was kindly provided by Prof. Dr. Peter Koehler, chairman of the PWG. Wheat gluten "vital" (batch no. 1607220051) was obtained from Hermann Kröner GmbH (Ibbenbueren, Germany) and contained ≤8% moisture, ≤0.9% ash and ≥78% protein (nitrogen × 6.25, based on fresh weight) according to the manufacturer's product specification sheet (called "gluten" in the following). Pepsin capsules for use as a dietary supplement (153 mg pepsin, corresponding to 3×10^6 albumin digestion units per capsule) were purchased from Dr. Clark Store (Chula Vista, CA, USA). Sodium hydroxide ("baker's brine") was provided by Minerva (Calbitz, Germany). Vinegar essence (Surig®, Speyer & Grund, Meerane, Germany, 25% acetic acid), mineral water (Adelholzener, Siegsdorf, Germany, in a glass bottle) and different fruit juices and smoothies were obtained from a local supermarket. According to the label, the mineral water contained 508 mg/L salts (nitrate < 0.3 mg/L). Acetic acid (pH 3.0) was prepared by mixing 900 mL mineral water and 100 mL vinegar essence.

2.2. Standard Analyses

The moisture and ash contents were determined according to International Association for Cereal Science and Technology (ICC) Standard Methods 110/1 and 104/1, respectively. The crude protein content (nitrogen × 5.7 for wheat) was analyzed according to ICC Standard Method 167 using a TruSpec Nitrogen Analyzer (Leco, Kirchheim, Germany) calibrated with ethylenediamine- tetraacetic acid (EDTA). The content of starch was determined according to AOAC Official Method 996.11 using the Total Starch Assay Kit (Megazyme, Bray, Ireland) [24]. The analysis of total dietary fiber was carried out with the Total Dietary Fiber Assay Kit (Sigma-Aldrich, Steinheim, Germany) based on a combination of enzymatic and gravimetric methods. The fat content was determined gravimetrically after extraction in hydrochloric acid (25%, v/v) and addition of toluene [25]. All analyses were done in triplicates each for gluten and pepgluten.

2.3. Contents of Albumins/Globulins, Gliadins and Glutenins in Gluten

The extraction of modified Osborne fractions was adapted from Wieser et al. [26] as follows: Gluten (20.0 mg, $n = 3$) was first extracted with 3 × 1.5 mL of salt solution (0.4 mol/L NaCl with 0.067 mol/L Na_2HPO_4/KH_2PO_4, pH 7.6, at 20–22 °C) to obtain albumins and globulins (ALGL). In a separate experiment, gluten (20.0 mg) was stepwise extracted with 3 × 1.5 mL 60% (v/v) ethanol to obtain a mixture of ALGL and gliadins (GLIA) and then with 3 × 1.5 mL glutenin extraction solvent (50% (v/v) 1-propanol and 0.05 mol/L Tris-HCl, pH 7.5, with 2 mol/L (w/v) urea and 0.06 mol/L (w/v) dithiothreitol (DTT)) at 60 °C under nitrogen to obtain glutenin subunits (GLUT). Each extraction step was performed by vortex mixing for 2 min and magnetic stirring for 30 min followed by centrifugation (3750× g, 25 min, 22 °C). The corresponding three supernatants were combined, made up to 5.0 mL with the respective solvent and filtered (0.45 µm).

2.4. RP-HPLC for Gluten Proteins

The quantitation of protein fractions was performed by RP-HPLC on a Jasco XLC instrument (Jasco, Gross-Umstadt, Germany) with a C_{18} column (Acclaim™ 300, 2.1 × 150 mm, 3 µm, 30 nm, Thermo Fisher Scientific, Braunschweig, Germany) at 60 °C. Elution solvents were 0.1% (v/v) trifluoroacetic acid (TFA) in water (A) and 0.1% (v/v) TFA in acetonitrile (B) at a flow rate of 0.2 mL/min with the following gradient: 0 min 0% B, 0.5 min 24% B, 20 min 56% B, 20.1–24.1 min 90% B, 24.2–30 min 0% B. The injection volumes were 20 µL (ALGL, GLUT) and 10 µL (ALGL + GLIA) and protein absorbance was detected at 210 nm. PWG-gliadin [23] dissolved in 60% (v/v) ethanol was used for external calibration. The contents of ωb-gliadins, HMW-GS and LMW-GS were calculated relative to the total area of GLUT as described earlier [27]. To obtain the GLIA content, the chromatogram of the ALGL fraction was subtracted from that of the ALGL + GLIA fraction using the Chrompass software (version 1.2, Jasco, Gross-Umstadt, Germany). Then, the contents of ω5-, ω1,2-, α- and γ-gliadins were calculated from the absorbance area of each type relative to the total area.

2.5. Optimization of Gluten Hydrolysis

Different ratios of enzyme (E), gluten (G) and solvent (S) were tested. The first assay was performed according to Dorum et al. [28] (E:G:S = 1:25:1667). Gluten (3.8 g) was suspended in 260 mL HCl (0.01 mol/L, pH 2.0, 37 °C) under magnetic stirring, 153 mg pepsin (1 capsule) were added and stirred for 120 min at 37 °C. The next assays were performed with acetic acid as solvent prepared by mixing mineral water with acetic acid essence until pH 3.0 was reached. To reduce the ratio of solvent, different incubations (120 min at 37 °C each) were done using E:G:S ratios of 1:25:200, 1:25:150 and 1:25:100. Aliquots (0.5 mL) were taken from all assays for analysis before addition of the enzyme (0 min) and after 10, 20, 40, 60, 90, and 120 min and heated for 10 min at 95 °C to inactivate pepsin. The remaining portions of the hydrolysates obtained after 120 min were lyophilized. In order to reduce the amount of enzyme, different incubations at 37 °C were performed using E:G:S ratios of 1:50:200, 1:100:400 and 1:200:800. After 120 min, aliquots (0.5 mL) were taken and inactivated as described above.

2.6. Preparation of Pepgluten

Twenty-five capsules (3.8 g pepsin) were dissolved in 380 mL acetic acid (pH 3.0) at 37 °C. Gluten (95 g) was added (E:G:S = 1:25:100) and magnetically stirred for 120 min at 37 °C. The assay was cooled, frozen and lyophilized. The dried digest was mixed with boiling mineral water (200 mL) and heated for 10 min, cooled, frozen and lyophilized. The dried material was milled (A10, IKA-Werke, Staufen, Germany) and stored in a vacuum desiccator over baker's brine until a constant weight was reached.

2.7. RP-HPLC for the Gluten Hydrolysates

The 0.5 mL aliquots (see Section 2.5) were diluted 1:20 with 0.1% (*v*/*v*) TFA, filtered (0.45 μm) and 50 μL of the filtrates were analyzed on a Thermo Finnigan Spectra System (Thermo Fisher Scientific) with ChromQuest software using an Aeris Peptide XB-C_{18} column (2.1 × 150 mm, 3.6 μm, Phenomenex, Aschaffenburg, Germany). Elution solvents were 0.1% (*v*/*v*) TFA in water (A) and 0.1% (*v*/*v*) TFA in acetonitrile (B) at a flow rate of 0.2 mL/min at 22 °C and a detection wavelength of 210 nm with the following linear gradient: 0 min 0% B, 5–60 min, 0–40% B, 60.5–66.5 min 90% B, 70–76 min 0% B.

2.8. Sodium Dodecyl Sulfate-Polyacrylamide Gel Electrophoresis (SDS-PAGE)

Gluten and gluten hydrolysates were characterized by SDS-PAGE on a homogeneous NuPAGE 10% polyacrylamide-Bis-Tris gel (10 × 1 mm wells Invitrogen, Carlsbad, CA, USA) [29,30]. A mixture of proteins was used as size standard (PageRuler™ Unstained Protein Ladder, Thermo Fisher Scientific). Gluten samples (4 mg each) were mixed with 1.0 mL of extraction buffer (293.3 mmol/L sucrose, 246.4 mmol/L Tris-HCl, 69.4 mmol/L SDS, 0.51 mmol/L EDTA, 0.22 mmol/L Coomassie blue, 0.177 mmol/L phenol red, 0.105 mmol/L HCl, pH 8.5) containing DTT (50 mmol/L), incubated for 12 h, heated to 60 °C for 10 min and centrifuged (5000× *g*, 5 min, 20 °C). Ten μl of the supernatant were applied to the slots. The running buffer (MES buffer) consisted of 50 mmol/L 2-(*N*-morpholino)ethanesulfonic acid (MES), 50 mmol/L Tris-HCl, 3.5 mmol/L SDS, 1 mmol/L EDTA and 5 mmol/L DTT (pH 7.7). The running time was 30 min at 200 V and 115 mA. After the run, protein bands were fixed for 30 min in 12% (*w*/*w*) trichloroacetic acid, stained for 30 min with Coomassie blue and destained twice, first with methanol/acetic acid/water (50/10/40, *v*/*v*/*v*) and then with methanol/acetic acid/water (10/10/80, *v*/*v*/*v*). The gels were scanned, the images converted to grayscale, the lanes of interest plotted as x/y-diagrams and the peaks integrated using the Gel Doc™ EZ gel documentation system (Bio-Rad Laboratories, Munich, Germany).

2.9. Enzyme-Linked Immunosorbent Assay (ELISA)

The gluten content in the samples (gluten and pepgluten) was quantitated by a commercial competitive ELISA kit based on the R5 monoclonal antibody (RIDASCREEN® Gliadin competitive, R-Biopharm, Darmstadt, Germany). The kit is intended to measure gluten contents in the 20 mg/kg and not in the 700 g/kg range, which is why the standard extraction procedure was modified. Gluten and pepgluten (10 mg, $n = 3$) were extracted with 2.5 mL Cocktail [31] at 50 °C for 40 min followed by the addition of 7.5 mL 80% (*v*/*v*) ethanol, shaking at 22 °C for 60 min and centrifugation (3750× *g*, 10 min, 22 °C). The resulting supernatant was subsequently diluted 1:100 and 1:50 with 60% (*v*/*v*) ethanol and finally 1:50 with the diluted sample buffer of the kit, resulting in a dilution factor of 2.5×10^7. The following ELISA procedure was performed according to the kit manual in a separate, closed room where the surfaces had been cleaned with 60% ethanol (*v*/*v*) to prevent contamination with gluten. The absorbances were measured at 450 nm (Expert 96 microplate reader, Asys Hitech, Eugendorf, Austria) and the gluten concentrations calculated from the calibration curve using the cubic spline function of the RIDA®SOFT Win software (version z9996, R-Biopharm, Darmstadt, Germany).

2.10. Quantitation of ATIs

The contents of ATIs were determined based on five ATI-specific marker peptides by liquid chromatography-tandem mass spectrometry (LC-MS/MS) and stable isotope dilution assays (SIDA) with ^{13}C- and ^{15}N-labelled peptides as internal standards [32]. In brief, 10 mg of gluten and pepgluten ($n = 3$) were extracted twice with ammonium bicarbonate (0.5 mL, 50 mmol/L, pH 7.8). The combined extracts were lyophilized. After addition of the internal standards, the reconstituted ATI extract was reduced with tris(2-carboxyethyl)phosphine, alkylated with chloroacetamide, hydrolyzed with trypsin, lyophilized and re-dissolved in 1 mL of 0.1% (*v*/*v*) formic acid. Targeted LC-MS/MS was carried out with an UltiMate 3000 HPLC system (Dionex, Idstein, Germany) coupled to a triple-stage quadrupole mass spectrometer (TSQ Vantage, Thermo Fisher Scientific) exactly as described by Geisslitz et al. [32].

2.11. Descriptive Sensory Analysis

Ten healthy panelists (7 women and 3 men) with no history of known taste or smell disorders were trained in the sensory evaluation of aqueous solutions of the standard taste compounds sucralose (sweet), sodium chloride (salty), monosodium L-glutamate (umami), citric acid (sour), and caffeine (bitter) [33]. They gave written informed consent to participate in the sensory tests and had participated in sensory analyses for at least one year. The analyses were performed in a sensory panel room with separated booths at 20–22 °C. First, a descriptive analysis of the appearance, color and aroma of pepgluten was performed. Then, 2 g of pepgluten were mixed into 100 mL of different beverages with a small kitchen mixer. The beverages compared were mineral water, multivitamin juice, a mixture (70:30) of multivitamin juice and bitter lemon, grapefruit juice and different vegetable and fruit smoothies. The panel compared taste and aroma of the beverages with and without pepgluten.

2.12. Statistical Analysis

The software SigmaPlot 12.0 (Systat Software, San Jose, CA, USA) was used to assess significances of differences between the analytical parameters determined in both samples (gluten and pepgluten) with one-way analysis of variance (ANOVA) and Tukey's test at $p < 0.05$.

3. Results

3.1. Composition of Gluten

The qualitative and quantitative composition of gluten was determined to fulfill one of the most important requirements for oral food challenge materials. The nitrogen content of gluten was 126.1 mg/g, which corresponded to 718.8 mg/g crude protein using the conversion factor of

5.7 recommended for wheat proteins (ICC Standard Method 167). Further components in gluten were starch (107.7 mg/g), water (62.3 mg/g), dietary fiber (49.6 mg/g), fat (41.5 mg/g), and ash (7.9 mg/g), as seen in Table 1. The residue of 12.2 mg/g was very low (within the precision of the analytical methods used) and contained non-identified minor constituents that were not analyzed. The immunological determination of the gluten content using the R5 monoclonal antibody resulted in a gluten content of 646.6 mg/g, which corresponds to 90% of crude protein. Targeted LC-MS/MS SIDA based on five ATI-specific marker peptides revealed that 32.6 mg/g total ATIs were present in gluten, with CM3 (11.9 mg/g) and 0.19 + 0.53 (10.5 mg/g) as predominant ATI types.

Table 1. Composition of gluten and pepgluten. ATIs: α-amylase/trypsin-inhibitors.

Constituent	Gluten	Pepgluten
	(mg/g) [1]	(mg/g) [1]
Crude protein (nitrogen × 5.7)	718.8 ± 1.8^{A}	707.1 ± 2.5^{A}
Starch	107.7 ± 3.5^{A}	104.2 ± 1.0^{A}
Water	62.3 ± 0.3^{A}	59.2 ± 1.9^{B}
Fat	41.5 ± 2.7^{A}	46.6 ± 0.7^{A}
Dietary fiber	49.6 ± 4.7^{A}	40.5 ± 4.3^{A}
Ash	7.9 ± 0.1^{A}	10.9 ± 0.1^{B}
Residue	12.2	31.5
Gluten [2]	646.6 ± 34.8^{A}	372.0 ± 36.3^{B}
ATIs (sum)	32.6^{A}	22.4^{B}
ATI 0.19 + 0.53	10.5 ± 1.6^{A}	10.6 ± 1.4^{A}
ATI 0.28	2.0 ± 0.2^{A}	1.9 ± 0.1^{A}
ATI CM2	1.7 ± 0.3^{A}	1.6 ± 0.1^{A}
ATI CM3	11.9 ± 0.4^{A}	2.7 ± 0.1^{B}
ATI CM16	6.5 ± 1.1^{A}	5.6 ± 0.9^{A}

[1] Results are given as mean ± standard deviation of triplicate determinations and different superscript letters designate significant differences between the two samples (one-way analysis of variance (ANOVA), Tukey's test, $p < 0.05$, [2] Gluten content determined by R5 competitive enzyme-linked immunosorbent assay (ELISA).

3.2. Composition of the Protein Fraction in Gluten

SDS-PAGE of gluten, seen in Figure 1A, lane G, showed the typical protein bands known from wheat flours including the following gluten protein types and ranges of M_r (according to known amino acid sequences): HMW-GS (67–88 × 10^3), ω5-GLIA (49–55 × 10^3), ω1,2-GLIA (39–44 × 10^3), LMW-GS, α-GLIA and γ-GLIA (28–39 × 10^3) and ALGL (10–25 × 10^3).

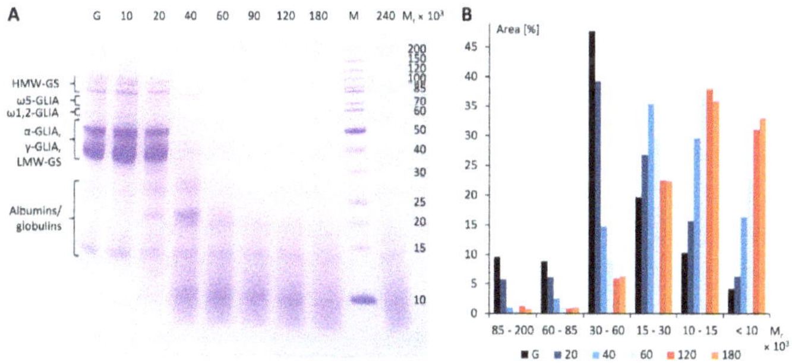

Figure 1. Sodium dodecyl sulfate-polyacrylamide gel electrophoresis (SDS-PAGE) of gluten (G) and different peptic digests incubated at 37 °C for 10 min, 20 min, 40 min, 60 min, 90 min, 120 min, 180 min and 240 min at an E:G:S ratio of 1:25:100 (**A**). Area (%) relative to the total area of selected bands according to molecular weight ranges of marker M (**B**). HMW-GS, high-molecular-weight glutenin subunits, LMW-GS, low-molecular-weight glutenin subunits, M, molecular weight marker, M_r, relative molecular weight, α-GLIA, α-gliadins, γ-GLIA, γ-gliadins, ω5-GLIA, ω5-gliadins, ω1,2-GLIA, ω1,2-gliadins.

The contents of ALGL, GLIA, and GLUT present in gluten were determined according to a combined extraction/RP-HPLC method developed for the analysis of wheat flour [26]. An advantage of RP-HPLC is that each gliadin and glutenin protein type is separated largely as a subgroup and can be quantitated without major overlap. As an example, the elution regions of ω5-, ω1,2, α-, and γ-GLIA are shown in Figure 2A for PWG-gliadin, which was used for calibration. However, the method had to be modified, because, in contrast to flour, gluten proteins strongly agglomerated after the initial extraction of ALGL with salt solution. Therefore, the following extraction of GLIA with 60% ethanol was not reproducible (coefficient of variation > 20%) and the procedure was divided into two separate experiments: First, ALGL were extracted from gluten with salt solution using three extraction steps. Second, gluten was extracted with 60% ethanol using three extraction steps to obtain a mixture of ALGL and GLIA. Then, GLUT were extracted three times with glutenin extraction solvent from the residue of ALGL + GLIA. Single corresponding extracts were combined into the three fractions ALGL, ALGL + GLIA and GLUT and analyzed by RP-HPLC, as seen in Figure 2B–D.

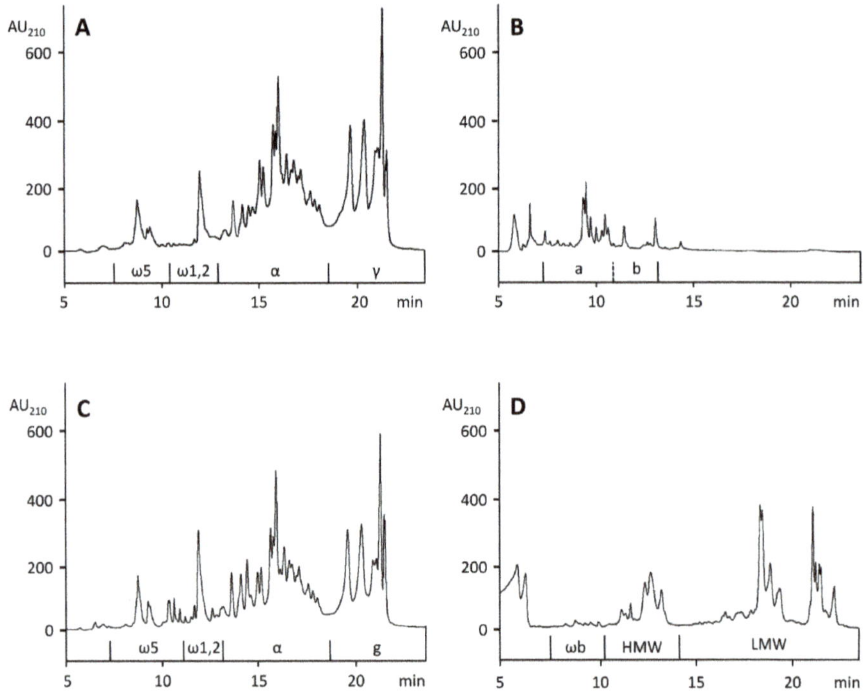

Figure 2. Reversed-phase high-performance liquid chromatography (RP-HPLC) for gluten proteins of prolamin working group (PWG)-gliadin (**A**), the ALGL fraction (**B**), the ALGL + gliadins (GLIA) fraction (**C**) and the glutenin subunits (GLUT) fraction (**D**). AU_{210}, absorbance units at 210 nm, ALGL, albumins and globulins, HMW, high-molecular-weight glutenin subunits, LMW, low-molecular-weight glutenin subunits, α, α-gliadins, γ, γ-gliadins, ω5, ω5-gliadins, ω1,2, ω1,2-gliadins, ωb, ωb-gliadins.

For the quantitation of GLIA, the value of ALGL had to be subtracted from the value of the ALGL + GLIA fraction. GLIA were predominant (402.1 mg/g), followed by GLUT (213.8 mg/g) and ALGL (27.7 mg/g), as seen in Table 2. The gluten content, as sum of GLIA and GLUT, amounted to 615.9 mg/g and the ratio of GLIA to GLUT was 1.88. The contents of gluten protein types were also calculated from the respective areas, again using the ALGL + GLIA chromatogram minus the ALGL chromatogram. The ω5-GLIA and ω1,2-GLIA were most affected by co-eluting ALGL, as 72.5% of

ALGL were eluted in the region of ω5-GLIA and 27.5% in the region of ω1,2-GLIA. Corresponding proportions of ALGL, shown in Figure 2B, areas a and b, were subtracted from ω5- and ω1,2-GLIA, respectively, as seen in Figure 2C. The elution profiles of α- and γ-GLIA from PWG-gliadin isolated from a mixture of 28 wheat cultivars [23] and of gluten (mixture of unknown cultivars), seen in Figure 2A,C, were almost identical. In total, α-GLIA (208.8 mg/g), γ-GLIA (149.2 mg/g) and LMW-GS (149.1 mg/g) belonged to the major protein types, while ω5-GLIA (16.3 mg/g), ω1,2-GLIA (27.8 mg/g), ωb-GLIA (9.7 mg/g) and HMW-GS (55.0 mg/g) were minor components, as shown in Table 2.

Table 2. Composition of the protein fraction in gluten and pepgluten.

Protein	Gluten	Gluten Digestion Assay		Pepgluten
	(mg/g) [1]	(mg/g) [2]	(%)	(mg/g)
ALGL	27.7 ± 0.8	26.3	3.6	25.4
GLIA	402.1 ± 5.4	382.0	52.1	368.6
ω5	16.3 ± 1.1	15.5	2.1	15.0
ω1,2	27.8 ± 0.6	26.4	3.6	25.5
α	208.8 ± 2.9	198.4	27.1	191.4
γ	149.2 ± 1.2	141.7	19.3	136.7
GLUT	213.8 ± 6.1	203.1	27.7	196.0
ωb	9.7 ± 0.5	9.2	1.3	8.9
HMW-GS	55.0 ± 1.5	52.3	7.1	50.5
LMW-GS	149.1 ± 3.9	141.6	19.3	136.6
Gluten [3]	615.9 ± 2.9	585.1	79.8	564.6
Residue	75.2	71.4	9.8	68.9
Capsule [4]	-	50.0	6.8	48.2
Sum	718.8 ± 1.8	732.8	100	707.1 ± 2.5

[1] Results are given as mean ± standard deviation (n = 3), [2] calculated from 95 g gluten and 5 g pepsin capsule, [3] sum of GLIA and GLUT, [4] protein content in the pepsin capsule, ALGL, albumins and globulins, HMW, high-molecular-weight glutenin subunits, LMW, low-molecular-weight glutenin subunits, α, α-gliadins, γ, γ-gliadins, ω5, ω5-gliadins, ω1,2, ω1,2-gliadins, ωb, ωb-gliadins.

3.3. Optimization of Gluten Hydrolysis

The first experiment was performed to test the activity of the commercial pepsin dietary supplement. Each capsule (203 mg weight on average) contained 153 mg pepsin (manufacturer's information). The analysis of nitrogen (177.7 mg/g) indicated that the capsules exclusively consisted of protein (101.3 ± 0.1%, n = 3), including the main component pepsin (≈75%) and also gelatin for pill preparation. Gluten was first incubated for 120 min at 37 °C at an E:G:S ratio of 1:25:1667 [28] using hydrochloric acid (0.01 mol/L, pH 2.0). The analysis of aliquots taken during the whole digestion period by RP-HPLC (for the gluten hydrolysates) indicated that gluten proteins were extensively degraded with an endpoint at 120 min. After that time, there was no further increase in absorbance areas.

Having thus confirmed the activity of the pepsin capsules, hydrochloric acid was replaced by food-grade acetic acid (acetic acid essence mixed with mineral water to obtain pH 3.0) and the solvent volume was decreased (E:G:S ratios of 1:25:200, 1:25:150 and 1:25:100) to speed up the following drying process. RP-HPLC and SDS-PAGE analyses revealed that the progress of gluten degradation was only marginally different compared to the E:G:S ratio of 1:25:1667. SDS-PAGE, shown in Figure 1A, confirmed that gluten proteins (M_r = 30–100 × 10^3 in a reduced state, according to the marker) were successively degraded during incubation and that the hydrolysis reached an endpoint at 120 min, because there was no further significant change compared to 180 min, as seen in Figure 1B. While gluten had an approximate distribution of 9% of proteins with M_r = 85–200 × 10^3 (HMW-GS), 9% (M_r = 60–85 × 10^3, ω5- and ω1,2-gliadins), 48% (M_r = 30–60 × 10^3, α- and γ-gliadins and LMW-GS), 20% (M_r = 15–30 × 10^3), 10% (M_r = 10–15 × 10^3) and 4% (M_r < 10 × 10^3), this distribution fundamentally changed to 1%, 1%, 6%, 23%, 38% and 31%, respectively, after an incubation time of 120 min. The gel thus confirmed extensive degradation of gluten proteins and revealed that about 70% of the hydrolysate was composed of gluten fragments with M_r of 15×10^3 and below.

RP-HPLC revealed that gluten did not contain any fragments, as seen in Figure 3A, whereas the gluten hydrolysate showed a complex fragment mixture after 120 min, see in Figure 3B.

To test whether the amount of pepsin could be reduced, the following E:G:S ratios were tested: 1:50:200, 1:100:400 and 1:200:800. SDS-PAGE after an incubation time of 120 min each (not shown) indicated that fragments with high M_r were generally more dominant than in the digests with E:G:S = 1:25:100. Moreover, the lyophilized material suspended in mineral water remained glutinous. Altogether, the following optimized procedure for gluten hydrolysis was used for further experiments: E:G:S ratio of 1:25:100 with food-grade acetic acid (pH 3.0) as solvent and an incubation at 37 °C for 120 min.

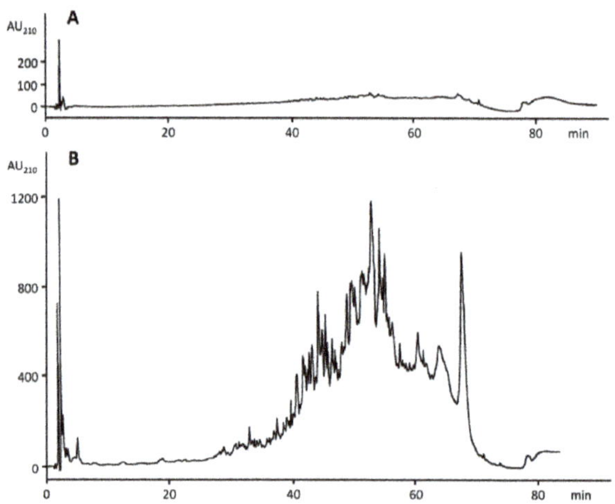

Figure 3. RP-HPLC (peptide system) of the peptic hydrolysis of gluten after incubation at 37 °C for 0 min (**A**) and 120 min (**B**). The ratio of enzyme to gluten to solvent was 1:25:100. AU_{210}, absorbance units at 210 nm.

3.4. Preparation and Characterization of Pepgluten

The final gluten hydrolysate (called "pepgluten") was prepared from 95 g gluten digested with 3.8 g pepsin (25 capsules weighing 5 g) in 380 mL acetic acid (pH 3.0) at 37 °C for 120 min (E:G:S = 1:25:100). After freezing, the preparation was lyophilized. The inactivation of the enzyme by heating was not performed in acetic acid to avoid partial deamidation of glutamine side chains, which might influence the immunoreactivity of pepgluten. Therefore, pepsin was inactivated by suspending the lyophilized digest in boiling mineral water for 10 min. An additional reason for this procedure was that heating created a more realistic material for gluten challenge tests, because most gluten-containing foods such as bread or pasta are also baked or cooked before consumption. After the second lyophilization, the dry material was milled and stored in a desiccator over sodium hydroxide (baker's brine) until constant weight. Pepgluten was not separated into soluble and insoluble parts, as had been done previously by Frazer et al. [34] (FIII and FVI) and others, who subsequently studied only the soluble part. Thus, the proportions of gluten proteins remained unchanged, which was important for the calculation of gluten equivalents in the hydrolysate.

The yield of dried pepgluten (92.6 g) was 92.2%, based on the amounts of non-volatile substances used for the digestion (95 g vital gluten, 5.1 g pepsin capsules and 0.3 g salts in the mineral water). Considering the frequent transfers of solutions and substances during the processes of digestion, freeze-drying, heating, milling and storage, the obtained yield appeared to be satisfactory. Compared to gluten as starting material, there were no significant differences between both materials for contents of protein (707.1 mg/g), starch (104.2 mg/g), fat (46.6 mg/g), dietary fiber (40.5 mg/g) and only slight differences in water (59.2 mg/g) and ash (10.9 mg/g) contents due to drying and addition of salts from the mineral water, as seen in Table 1. The gluten content of the hydrolysate (372 mg/g) determined by the R5 competitive ELISA, shown in Table 1, was reduced compared to gluten. The contents of ATIs 0.19 + 0.53, 0.28, CM2 and CM16 were not significantly different, but the content of CM3 was lower (2.7 mg/g) in pepgluten compared to the starting material (11.9 mg/g).

Finally, the contents of gluten equivalents in the hydrolysate were calculated based on its crude protein content (707 mg/g = 100%) considering the proportions of gluten proteins and pepsin capsule proteins in the digestion assay, as shown in Table 2. Accordingly, 1 g of pepgluten contained gluten equivalents derived from 369 mg GLIA and 196 mg GLUT resulting in 565 mg total gluten equivalents. Further protein components of pepgluten were derived from ALGL (25 mg/g), residual proteins (69 mg/g) and pepsin capsule proteins (48 mg/g), as seen in Table 2.

3.5. Descriptive Sensory Analysis

The pepgluten powder was slightly brownish in appearance and had a flour- and sourdough-like aroma with a residual slightly pungent note originating from acetic acid. When mixed into mineral water (2 g in 100 mL), the drink was turbid and had a dough-like aroma and bitter taste. The intensity of aroma and taste was less noticeable in a turbid multivitamin juice, which appeared to be suitable for an open challenge test. If necessary, the endogenous bitter taste can be completely covered by mixing multivitamin juice with bitter lemon (70:30 *v*/*v*) or by using grapefruit juice. Different vegetable or fruit smoothies also allowed the complete camouflage of the preparation.

4. Discussion

Due to its glutinous properties, wheat gluten is difficult to handle for oral food challenge and in cell-based assays for clinical investigations, because these only tolerate aqueous solvents. Therefore, gluten is commonly applied in form of the soluble portions of peptic [34,35], tryptic [35], chymotryptic [5], peptic-tryptic [8,36,37], peptic-chymotryptic [37] or peptic-tryptic-chymotryptic [28] hydrolysates, sometimes in combination with further enzymes such as elastase or carboxypeptidase to mimic human gastrointestinal digestion as closely as possible. Gluten contains very low amounts of arginine and lysine (preferential cleavage sites for trypsin) and cleavage after aromatic amino acid residues phenylalanine, tryptophan, and tyrosine (preferential cleavage sites for chymotrypsin) is often impeded by a following proline residue [6]. Pepsin cleaves before or after phenylalanine, tryptophan, tyrosine, and leucine and has the broadest repertoire of cleavage sites of the three enzymes, especially considering the content of repetitive sequences rich in proline and glutamine that are typical of gluten proteins [38]. Therefore, pepsin was selected to prepare pepgluten. For patient safety [11,12], the procedure was carried out in a kitchen using only food-grade ingredients: gluten (baking ingredient), pepsin (dietary supplement), acetic acid essence (for meals and salads) and mineral water in a glass bottle.

The composition of gluten proteins in the commercial gluten used as a starting material was similar to that expected from wheat flours [7]. Due to the stretched conformation of reduced gluten proteins, their SDS-PAGE mobility is known to be restricted compared to the globular proteins used in the marker, so that, e.g., HMW-GS (M_r: 67–88 × 10^3 based on known amino acid sequences) appeared between M_r: 85–120 × 10^3, as has been reported before [5,30]. The contents, elution profiles of GLIA and GLUT and their ratio (1.88) were very similar to those reported for common wheat flour [39]. In contrast, ALGL, usually present in wheat flours with contents of 150–200 mg/g, were almost absent due to the washing steps during gluten-starch separation. Judging by the overall gluten protein composition, the gluten sample appeared to be representative. The most important conclusion of the analytical characterization was, however, that commercial gluten contains a much lower amount of gluten proteins (≈62%) than is typically assumed (100%). This implies that the true amount of gluten applied would have to be reconsidered in many cases.

Pepgluten showed no significant differences to gluten in the contents of protein, starch, fat, dietary fiber, and ATIs 0.19 + 0.53, 0.28, CM2 and CM16 and only slight differences in water and ash contents due to drying and addition of mineral water. Only CM3 appeared to be susceptible to peptic hydrolysis, because the content of the marker peptide decreased to about 23%. The immunological quantitation of gluten in the hydrolysate by R5 competitive ELISA only resulted in about 58% recovery compared to the starting material. This reduced recovery after enzymatic digestion is a well-known general effect regardless of type of ELISA and antibody and has been reported for peptic-tryptic gliadin (63% recovery) [37], peptic wheat flour gluten proteins (47% recovery) [35], peptic-tryptic gliadin (56% recovery), and peptic-tryptic glutenin (23% recovery) [36]. It is uncertain whether ELISA, even in a competitive format, is the most robust assay to determine partially hydrolyzed gluten [36], which is why the calculation of gluten equivalents in the hydrolysate was performed based on results for crude protein and RP-HPLC. Further insight into the composition of pepgluten may be gained using untargeted proteomics approaches.

Pepgluten has many potential applications, e.g., as material for oral food challenge for CD patients who started a gluten-free diet prior to appropriate diagnosis [10], for wheat allergy [11] and WDEIA patients [13,40], and for NCGS and IBS patients [2,3]. It is also suitable for in vitro testing on, e.g., human monocytes [8] or for studies on small intestinal permeability with subsequent detection of gluten fragments in urine samples [41]. The commonly used lactulose/mannitol (LAMA) test [42] to assess permeability ("leaky gut") does not appear to be well suited as an indicator for the intestinal passage of larger molecules [10], so that an oral food challenge with pepgluten and detection of gluten fragments in blood, urine, or feces might be more meaningful.

5. Conclusions

Commercially available wheat gluten was extensively characterized and used as a starting material to prepare a well-defined, food-grade wheat gluten hydrolysate (pepgluten). Since no material was removed during the procedure, the peptic hydrolysate had a composition very similar to the original gluten and contained all components relevant for wheat hypersensitivities including ATIs. Based on food-grade ingredients only, it is deemed to be suitable for oral food challenge tests. Pepgluten fulfills important criteria for challenge materials, because its composition is known, it is easy to apply and, mixed with suitable beverages, it is indistinguishable from placebo samples regarding appearance, smell, taste and texture. Altogether, pepgluten is appropriate as standard preparation for oral provocation tests and clinical investigations in the field of wheat hypersensitivities.

Author Contributions: Conceptualization, Data curation, Investigation, H.W.; Methodology, Resources, Supervision, Visualization, K.A.S.; Writing—original draft, H.W.; Writing—review & editing, K.A.S.

Funding: This work was supported by the German Research Foundation (DFG) and the Technical University of Munich (TUM) in the framework of the Open Access Publishing Program.

Acknowledgments: The authors thank Alexandra Axthelm, Angelika Grassl and Stefanie Schug for excellent technical assistance, Sabine Bijewitz for help with the figures and Sabrina Geisslitz for the ATI analyses (all Leibniz-LSB@TUM) as well as Maren Wiese (Hermann Kröner GmbH) for providing the gluten sample.

Conflicts of Interest: H.W. is inventor of the utility model DE 202017005555 U1. K.A.S. declares no conflict of interest.

References

1. Sapone, A.; Bai, J.C.; Ciacci, C.; Dolinsek, J.; Green, P.H.; Hadjivassiliou, M.; Kaukinen, K.; Rostami, K.; Sanders, D.S.; Schumann, M.; et al. Spectrum of gluten-related disorders: Consensus on new nomenclature and classification. *BMC Med.* **2012**, *10*, 13. [CrossRef] [PubMed]
2. Catassi, C.; Elli, L.; Bonaz, B.; Bouma, G.; Carroccio, A.; Castillejo, G.; Cellier, C.; Cristofori, F.; De Magistris, L.; Dolinsek, J.; et al. Diagnosis of non-celiac gluten sensitivity (NCGS): The Salerno experts' criteria. *Nutrients* **2015**, *7*, 4966–4977. [CrossRef] [PubMed]

3. Catassi, C.; Alaedini, A.; Bojarski, C.; Bonaz, B.; Bouma, G.; Carroccio, A.; Castillejo, G.; De Magistris, L.; Dieterich, W.; Di Liberto, D.; et al. The overlapping area of non-celiac gluten sensitivity (NCGS) and wheat-sensitive irritable bowel syndrome (IBS): An update. *Nutrients* **2017**, *9*, 1268. [CrossRef] [PubMed]
4. Vazquez-Roque, M.I.; Camilleri, M.; Smyrk, T.; Murray, J.A.; Marietta, E.; O'Neill, J.; Carlson, P.; Lamsam, J.; Janzow, D.; Eckert, D.; et al. A controlled trial of gluten-free diet in patients with irritable bowel syndrome-diarrhea: Effects on bowel frequency and intestinal function. *Gastroenterology* **2013**, *144*, 903.e3–911.e3. [CrossRef] [PubMed]
5. Schalk, K.; Lexhaller, B.; Koehler, P.; Scherf, K.A. Isolation and characterization of gluten protein types from wheat, rye, barley and oats for use as reference materials. *PLoS ONE* **2017**, *12*, e0172819. [CrossRef] [PubMed]
6. Scherf, K.A.; Koehler, P.; Wieser, H. Gluten and wheat sensitivities—An overview. *J. Cereal Sci.* **2016**, *67*, 2–11. [CrossRef]
7. Wieser, H. Chemistry of gluten proteins. *Food Microbiol.* **2007**, *24*, 115–119. [CrossRef] [PubMed]
8. Junker, Y.; Zeissig, S.; Kim, S.J.; Barisani, D.; Wieser, H.; Leffler, D.A.; Zevallos, V.; Libermann, T.A.; Dillon, S.; Freitag, T.L.; et al. Wheat amylase trypsin inhibitors drive intestinal inflammation via activation of toll-like receptor 4. *J. Exp. Med.* **2012**, *209*, 2395–2408. [CrossRef] [PubMed]
9. Zevallos, V.; Raker, V.; Tenzer, S.; Jimenez-Calvente, C.; Ashfaq-Khan, M.; Rüssel, N.; Pickert, G.; Schild, H.; Steinbrink, K.; Schuppan, D. Nutritional wheat amylase-trypsin inhibitors promote intestinal inflammation via activation of myeloid cells. *Gastroenterology* **2017**, *152*, 1100–1113. [CrossRef] [PubMed]
10. Leffler, D.A.; Schuppan, D.; Pallav, K.; Najarian, R.; Goldsmith, J.D.; Hansen, J.; Kabbani, T.; Dennis, M.; Kelly, C.P. Kinetics of the histologic, serologic, and symptomatic responses to gluten challenge in adults with coeliac disease. *Gut* **2013**, *62*, 996–1004. [CrossRef] [PubMed]
11. Muraro, A.; Werfel, T.; Hoffmann-Sommergruber, K.; Roberts, G.; Beyer, K.; Bindslev-Jensen, C.; Cardona, V.; Dubois, A.; duToit, G.; Eigenmann, P.; et al. EAACI food allergy and anaphylaxis guidelines: Diagnosis and management of food allergy. *Allergy* **2014**, *69*, 1008–1025. [CrossRef] [PubMed]
12. Sampson, H.A.; Gerth van Wijk, R.; Bindslev-Jensen, C.; Sicherer, S.; Teuber, S.S.; Burks, A.W.; Dubois, A.E.; Beyer, K.; Eigenmann, P.A.; Spergel, J.M.; et al. Standardizing double-blind, placebo-controlled oral food challenges: American Academy of Allergy, Asthma & Immunology-European Academy of Allergy and Clinical Immunology PRACTALL consensus report. *J. Allergy Clin. Immunol.* **2012**, *130*, 1260–1274. [CrossRef] [PubMed]
13. Brockow, K.; Kneissl, D.; Valentini, L.; Zelger, O.; Grosber, M.; Kugler, C.; Werich, M.; Darsow, U.; Matsuo, H.; Morita, E.; et al. Using a gluten oral food challenge protocol to improve diagnosis of wheat-dependent exercise-induced anaphylaxis. *J. Allergy Clin. Immunol.* **2015**, *135*, 977–984. [CrossRef] [PubMed]
14. Makharia, A.; Catassi, C.; Makharia, G.K. The overlap between irritable bowel syndrome and non-celiac gluten sensitivity: A clinical dilemma. *Nutrients* **2015**, *7*, 10417–10426. [CrossRef] [PubMed]
15. Volta, U.; Pinto-Sanchez, M.I.; Boschetti, E.; Caio, G.; De Giorgio, R.; Verdu, E.F. Dietary triggers in irritable bowel syndrome: Is there a role for gluten? *J. Neurogastroenterol. Motil.* **2016**, *22*, 547–557. [CrossRef] [PubMed]
16. Di Sabatino, A.; Volta, U.; Salvatore, C.; Biancheri, P.; Caio, G.; De Giorgio, R.; Di Stefano, M.; Corazza, G.R. Small amounts of gluten in subjects with suspected nonceliac gluten sensitivity: A randomized, double-blind, placebo-controlled, cross-over trial. *Clin. Gastroenterol. Hepatol.* **2015**, *13*, 1604.e3–1612.e3. [CrossRef] [PubMed]
17. Nilsson, N.; Sjolander, S.; Baar, A.; Berthold, M.; Pahr, S.; Vrtala, S.; Valenta, R.; Morita, E.; Hedlin, G.; Borres, M.P.; et al. Wheat allergy in children evaluated with challenge and IgE antibodies to wheat components. *Pediatr. Allergy Immunol.* **2015**, *26*, 119–125. [CrossRef] [PubMed]
18. Camarca, A.; Radano, G.; Di Mase, R.; Terrone, G.; Maurano, F.; Auricchio, S.; Troncone, R.; Greco, L.; Gianfrani, C. Short wheat challenge is a reproducible in-vivo assay to detect immune response to gluten. *Clin. Exp. Immunol.* **2012**, *169*, 129–136. [CrossRef] [PubMed]
19. Ito, K.; Futamura, M.; Borres, M.P.; Takaoka, Y.; Dahlstrom, J.; Sakamoto, T.; Tanaka, A.; Kohno, K.; Matsuo, H.; Morita, E. IgE antibodies to omega-5 gliadin associate with immediate symptoms on oral wheat challenge in Japanese children. *Allergy* **2008**, *63*, 1536–1542. [CrossRef] [PubMed]

20. Catassi, C.; Fabiani, E.; Iacono, G.; D'Agate, C.; Francavilla, R.; Biagi, F.; Volta, U.; Accomando, S.; Picarelli, A.; De Vitis, I.; et al. A prospective, double-blind, placebo-controlled trial to establish a safe gluten threshold for patients with celiac disease. *Am. J. Clin. Nutr.* **2007**, *85*, 160–166. [CrossRef] [PubMed]
21. Dale, H.F.; Hatlebakk, J.G.; Hovdenak, N.; Ystad, S.O.; Lied, G.A. The effect of a controlled gluten challenge in a group of patients with suspected non-coeliac gluten sensitivity: A randomized, double-blind placebo-controlled challenge. *Neurogastroenterol. Motil.* **2018**, *30*, e13332. [CrossRef] [PubMed]
22. Bindslev-Jensen, C.; Ballmer-Weber, B.K.; Bengtsson, U.; Blanco, C.; Ebner, C.; Hourihane, J.; Knulst, A.C.; Moneret-Vautrin, D.A.; Nekam, K.; Niggemann, B.; et al. Standardization of food challenges in patients with immediate reactions to foods—Position paper from the European Academy of Allergology and Clinical Immunology. *Allergy* **2004**, *59*, 690–697. [CrossRef] [PubMed]
23. Van Eckert, R.; Berghofer, E.; Ciclitira, P.J.; Chirdo, F.; Denery-Papini, S.; Ellis, H.J.; Ferranti, P.; Goodwin, P.; Immer, U.; Mamone, G.; et al. Towards a new gliadin reference material—Isolation and characterisation. *J. Cereal Sci.* **2006**, *43*, 331–341. [CrossRef]
24. McCleary, B.V.; Solah, V.; Gibson, T.S. Quantitative measurement of total starch in cereal flours and products. *J. Cereal Sci.* **1994**, *20*, 51–58. [CrossRef]
25. Schulte, E. Simplified micro method for the gravimetric determination of fat in foods after acid treatment. *Deutsch. Lebensm. Rundsch.* **2004**, *100*, 188–189.
26. Wieser, H.; Antes, S.; Seilmeier, W. Quantitative determination of gluten protein types in wheat flour by high-performance liquid chromatography. *Cereal Chem.* **1998**, *75*, 644–650. [CrossRef]
27. Hajas, L.; Scherf, K.A.; Török, K.; Bugyi, Z.; Schall, E.; Poms, R.E.; Koehler, P.; Tömösközi, S. Variation in protein composition among wheat (*Triticum aestivum* L.) cultivars to identify cultivars suitable as reference material for wheat gluten analysis. *Food Chem.* **2018**, *267*, 387–394. [CrossRef] [PubMed]
28. Dorum, S.; Arntzen, M.O.; Qiao, S.-W.; Holm, A.; Koehler, C.J.; Thiede, B.; Sollid, L.M.; Fleckenstein, B. The preferred substrates for transglutaminase 2 in a complex wheat gluten digest are peptide fragments harboring celiac disease T-cell epitopes. *PLoS ONE* **2010**, *5*, e14056. [CrossRef] [PubMed]
29. Laemmli, U.K. Cleavage of structural proteins during assembly of head of bacteriophage T4. *Nature* **1970**, *227*, 680–685. [CrossRef] [PubMed]
30. Lagrain, B.; Rombouts, I.; Wieser, H.; Delcour, J.A.; Koehler, P. A reassessment of the electrophoretic mobility of high molecular weight subunits of wheat. *J. Cereal Sci.* **2012**, *56*, 726–732. [CrossRef]
31. Garcia, E.; Llorente, M.; Hernando, A.; Kieffer, R.; Wieser, H.; Mendez, E. Development of a general procedure for complete extraction of gliadins for heat processed and unheated foods. *Eur. J. Gastroenterol. Hepatol.* **2005**, *17*, 529–539. [PubMed]
32. Geisslitz, S.; Ludwig, C.; Scherf, K.A.; Koehler, P. Targeted LC-MS/MS reveals similar contents of α-amylase/trypsin-inhibitors as cofactors of non-celiac gluten sensitivity in all wheat species except einkorn. *J. Agric. Food Chem.* **2018**. revised.
33. Scherf, K.A.; Pflaum, T.; Koehler, P.; Hofmann, T. Salt taste perception in hydrocolloid systems is affected by sodium ion release and mechanosensory-gustatory cross-modal interactions. *Food Hydrocoll.* **2015**, *51*, 486–494. [CrossRef]
34. Frazer, A.C.; Fletcher, R.F.; Ross, C.A.; Shaw, B.; Sammons, H.G.; Schneider, R. Gluten-induced enteropathy: The effect of partially digested gluten. *Lancet* **1959**, *2*, 252–255. [CrossRef]
35. Pahlavan, A.; Sharma, G.; Pereira, M.; Williams, K.M. Effects of grain species and cultivar, thermal processing, and enzymatic hydrolysis on gluten quantitation. *Food Chem.* **2016**, *208*, 264–271. [CrossRef] [PubMed]
36. Rallabhandi, P.; Sharma, G.M.; Pereira, M.; Williams, K.M. Immunological characterization of the gluten fractions and their hydrolysates from wheat, rye and barley. *J. Agric. Food Chem.* **2015**, *63*, 1825–1832. [CrossRef] [PubMed]
37. Gessendorfer, B.; Koehler, P.; Wieser, H. Preparation and characterization of enzymatically hydrolyzed prolamins from wheat, rye, and barley as references for the immunochemical quantitation of partially hydrolyzed gluten. *Anal. Bioanal. Chem.* **2009**, *395*, 1721–1728. [CrossRef] [PubMed]
38. Scherf, K.A.; Wieser, H.; Koehler, P. Novel approaches for enzymatic gluten degradation to create high-quality gluten-free products. *Food Res. Int.* **2018**, *110*, 62–72. [CrossRef] [PubMed]
39. Lexhaller, B.; Tompos, C.; Scherf, K.A. Comparative analysis of prolamin and glutelin fractions from wheat, rye, and barley with five sandwich ELISA test kits. *Anal. Bioanal. Chem.* **2016**, *408*, 6093–6104. [CrossRef] [PubMed]

40. Matsuo, H.; Morimoto, K.; Akaki, T.; Kaneko, S.; Kusatake, K.; Kuroda, T.; Niihara, H.; Hide, M.; Morita, E. Exercise and aspirin increase levels of circulating gliadin peptides in patients with wheat-dependent exercise-induced anaphylaxis. *Clin. Exp. Allergy* **2005**, *35*, 461–466. [CrossRef] [PubMed]
41. Moreno, M.L.; Cebolla, A.; Munoz-Suano, A.; Carrillo-Carrion, C.; Comino, I.; Pizarro, A.; Leon, F.; Rodriguez-Herrera, A.; Sousa, C. Detection of immunogenic peptides in the urine of patients with coeliac disease reveals transgressions in the gluten-free diet and incomplete mucosal healing. *Gut* **2017**, *66*, 250–257. [CrossRef] [PubMed]
42. Andre, C.; Andre, F.; Colin, L.; Cavagna, S. Measurement of intestinal permeability to mannitol and lactulose as a means of diagnosing food allergy and evaluating therapeutic effectiveness of disodium cromoglycate. *Ann. Allergy* **1987**, *59*, 127–130. [PubMed]

nutrients

MDPI

Article

Social and Emotional Fears and Worries Influencing the Quality of Life of Female Celiac Disease Patients Following a Gluten-Free Diet

Wioleta Zysk [1], Dominika Głąbska [2] and Dominika Guzek [1,*]

[1] Department of Organization and Consumption Economics, Faculty of Human Nutrition and Consumer Sciences, Warsaw University of Life Sciences (SGGW-WULS), 159C Nowoursynowska Street, 02-787 Warsaw, Poland; wioleta_zysk@sggw.pl

[2] Department of Dietetics, Faculty of Human Nutrition and Consumer Sciences, Warsaw University of Life Sciences (SGGW-WULS), 159C Nowoursynowska Street, 02-787 Warsaw, Poland; dominika_glabska@sggw.pl

* Correspondence: dominika_guzek@sggw.pl; Tel.: +48-22-593-71-34

Received: 13 August 2018; Accepted: 26 September 2018; Published: 3 October 2018

Abstract: The gluten-free diet is effective in the majority of celiac disease (CD) patients, but it is burdensome and may influence quality of life (QoL). The aim of the study was to analyze the social and emotional fears and worries influencing the QoL of female CD patients following a gluten-free (GF) diet, as well as to indicate the sociodemographic interfering factors. The study was conducted on a group of 251 female CD patients, while emotional, social and worries subscales of the Celiac Disease Questionnaire (CDQ) were applied, as well as purchase-related emotions and behaviors were assessed. Respondents declaring worse economic status obtained significantly lower scores in the emotional, social and worries subscales of the CDQ than respondents declaring better economic status, while for other factors (CD duration, GFD adherence, BMI, place of residence and educational level) no significant association was stated in the multi-factor analysis. Moreover, respondents declaring worse economic status more often declared that a bad mood affected their purchase decisions than did respondents declaring better economic status. It was stated, that the economic status of CD patient could be one of the most important factors influencing their social and emotional fears and worries. It may be supposed that low economic status may lead some CD patients to choose to relieve stress by purchasing GF products instead of other products.

Keywords: celiac disease (CD); quality of life (QoL); gluten-free diet; disease duration; place of residence; educational level; economic status; body mass index (BMI)

---

1. Introduction

Celiac disease (CD) is diagnosed in almost 1% of the global population, but a high percentage of affected individuals are undiagnosed [1]. It is an autoimmune disease, defined as an inflammatory disorder of the small intestine characterized by persistent gluten protein intolerance [2,3]. In CD patients, gluten exposure leads to enteropathy with mucosal surface damage and, as a consequence, nutrient malabsorption [4]. The only therapeutic approach for CD is a gluten-free diet (GFD) [5], and strict adherence is necessary to normalize the mucous membrane of the small intestine and to improve the impaired absorption [6].

GFD is effective in the majority of CD patients, but it is burdensome and may influence the quality of life (QoL) of patients [6]. After diagnosis, some patients may feel overwhelmed and the disease itself may affect their QoL [7]. Also, following GFD is commonly associated with certain difficulties in coping with information overload and in the implementation of recommendations influencing dietary behaviors [5]. As a result, the two main aspects of the QoL of CD patients, both associated with specific eating habits, concern the quality of their social and family life.

One of the most common difficulties for CD patients is the eating-out experience. CD patients are concerned about the possibility of finding gluten-free (GF) food products or dishes in restaurants, as well as about the possibility of cross-contamination of available GF products [5]. Moreover, they may feel socially isolated when they must decline an invitation to a regular restaurant [8]. In the study by Zarkadas et al. [9], almost 80% of members of the Canadian Celiac Association stated avoiding restaurants due to this reason, while in a further study by Zarkadas et al. [10] over 70% declared being frustrated as a result of limited choices on restaurant menus, as well as almost 90% declared limited choices at fast food restaurants and almost 80%—a limited choice of restaurants. However, knowledge about GFD, as well as the GF product market has recently been increasing sharply [11]. Therefore, the situation for CD patients may be changing in the context of available restaurant GF products and dishes.

It is crucial to involve family members to prevent interference with their relationships with the CD patient, because GFD inevitably affects eating practices at home. A patient on a GFD needs assurance that gluten is absent from a product or dish, as well as that GF products are not contaminated [12]. Moreover, adherence to GFD is difficult for some patients; and therefore, the support of their relatives is also important [13].

This situation may also be gender-related, as in many countries women are responsible for their family meal preparation, and also for the family grocery shopping decisions [14]. This is observed inter alia in Poland [15] and has been indicated in Polish studies as an important determinant for consumer behaviors [16]. Given that for CD men family support in following the diet is natural, CD women may suffer from a lack of such support and thus their need for support may be higher than it is for men [17]. Furthermore, some CD patients may also experience psychological, emotional and economic stress caused by everyday implications of GFD [8]. In some studies, this percentage is higher in women than in men [17].

Many studies analyzed the gastrointestinal symptoms of CD, CD screening and management strategies, and GFD adherence in CD patients. However, only limited data describing the QoL associated with the social and emotional components of GFD are available for CD patients [18]. Therefore, the aim of the study was to analyze the social and emotional fears and worries influencing the QoL of female CD patients following a GFD, as well as to indicate the sociodemographic interfering factors.

2. Materials and Methods

2.1. Ethics Approval Statement

The study was conducted according to the guidelines laid down in the Declaration of Helsinki. The study was approved by the Ethics Committee of the Faculty of Human Nutrition and Consumer Sciences of the Warsaw University of Life Sciences (No. 20/2017; 19.06.2017). All the participants provided their informed consent to participate.

2.2. Participants

The study was conducted on a group of CD patients. Participants were recruited online by a nationwide search via local CD and GFD societies. The combined methods of purposive sampling (patients with CD diagnosed and confirmed) and network sampling (local CD and GFD societies) were applied.

Inclusion criteria were:

- women;
- aged $\geq$ 18 years old;
- CD diagnosed and biopsy-confirmed by a physician;

- declared regular meal preparation at home;
- declared regular purchase of GF products.

Exclusion criteria were:

- any data missing in the completed QoL questionnaires;
- lack of informed consent to participate.

As a result, 158 of the 409 volunteers were excluded due to not meeting the inclusion criteria (Figure 1).

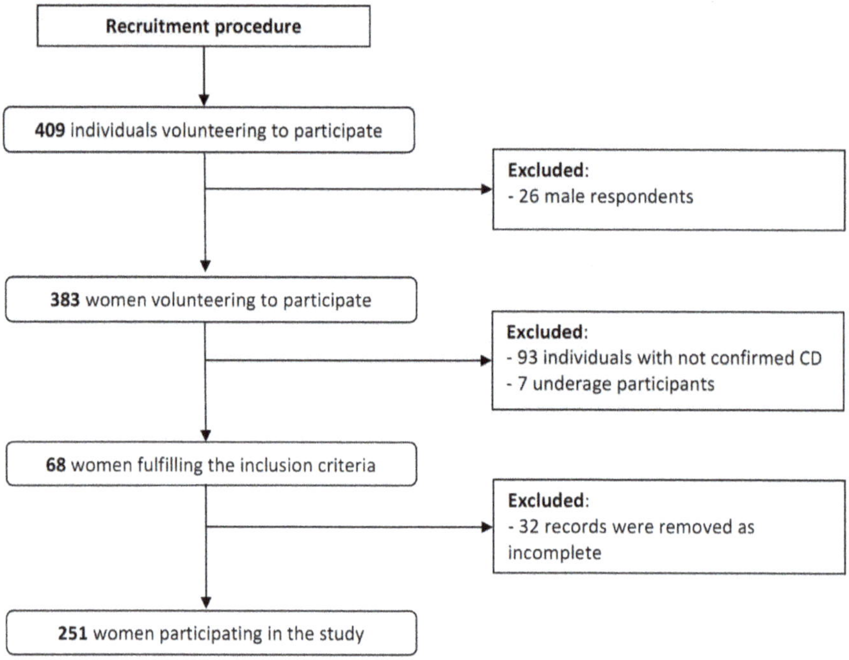

Figure 1. Participants inclusion to the study.

2.3. Study Design

Subjects were interviewed using the Computer-Assisted Web Interview (CAWI) method. The questionnaire applied was divided into two main parts. The first part included the Celiac Disease Questionnaire (CDQ), developed by Häuser et al. [19] on the basis of the Health-Related Quality of Life Questionnaire (HRQOL), as a specific form for adult CD patients. The second part included questions regarding purchase-related emotions and behaviors, as well as attitudes toward GF product attributes.

CDQ consists of four subscales–emotional subscale, social subscale, worries subscale and gastrointestinal subscale [19]. The Polish version of CDQ was applied in the present study, while it was, in some points, modified due to the aim and scope of the study. In the study, emotional, social and worries subscales were included, as the aim of the study was to assess the social and emotional fears and worries influencing the QoL, and not the gastrointestinal symptoms. Moreover, from the worries subscale, two questions directly associated with medical conditions were excluded on the basis of the pilot study so as not to cause discomfort and anxiety in the respondents and because they were not associated with the aim of the study. The excluded questions were related to cancer as a CD complication ("How many times during the last 2 weeks did you worry about or were you afraid of getting cancer as a result of your CD?") and to the possibility of CD inheritance ("How many times during the last 2 weeks were you concerned that your children could inherit or may have inherited your CD?"). A similar approach was applied in the study by Tovoli et al. [20], as a cancer-related question was also excluded. For test-retest reproducibility of the applied tool, a priori assumed criteria of Pearson correlation coefficients ($R > 0.7$, as recommended by DeVellis [21]) were obtained. The present study represents the first time the tool has been applied on a Polish population. This was based on the consent of the author of the CDQ [19] to apply the tool, obtained via e-mail.

Evaluation of the quality of data obtained on the basis of the CDQ included the floor and ceiling effects, item internal consistency and internal consistency reliability assessment (Cronbach's alpha coefficient > 0.7, as recommended by DeVellis [21]).

Among the questions regarding purchase-related emotions and behaviors, as well as attitude toward GF product attributes, there were 10 close-ended questions: Two of these were associated with purchase-related emotions and behaviors (included in the present study) and eight were associated with attitude toward GF product attributes (not related to the aim of the present study). The questions were formulated as follows: (1) "In the past 2 weeks, how many times did your mood affect your purchase decisions associated with GF products?"; (2) "In the past 2 weeks, how many times did you buy GF products to improve your mood?". For these questions, GF products were defined as products naturally free of gluten, pre-packed GF products and non-pre-packed GF products, such as those served in restaurants, according to Regulation (EU) No 828/2014 [22].

The additional part of the questionnaire included questions related to disease characteristics, including CD duration since diagnosis and GFD adherence. CD duration since diagnosis was declared by respondents in months/years. GFD adherence was assessed on a 4-point scale, as had been applied for GFD adherence in CD patients by inter alia Häuser et al. [2], van Hess et al. [23], or Kautto et al. [24]. In order to facilitate assessment, the four categories were translated into the following descriptions of adherence to GFD: (1) very poor; (2) good, but occasionally eat dishes containing gluten (at home or outside home); (3) very good, but occasionally eat dishes containing gluten (only outside home); (4) excellent. The translation of categories into descriptions was performed on the basis of commonly stated difficulties in adhering to GFD outside the home [13] and its influence on general GFD adherence [25]. An additional category was added for respondents who refused or were not able to assess their behavior.

The other questions in the additional part of the questionnaire were related to height and weight, in order to calculate Body Mass Index (BMI) [26]. Moreover, questions about the sociodemographic characteristics of respondents were included: gender, age, educational level, place of residence, occupational status and individual economic status (self-assessment).

2.4. Statistical Analysis

The statistical analysis included assessment of the normality of distribution (conducted using the Shapiro-Wilk test). Differences between groups were identified using the multi-factor analysis of variance (ANOVA) for the main effects and interaction effects. The Cronbach's alpha coefficient was applied to verify the internal reliability of data. The level of $p \leq 0.05$ was accepted as significant. The analysis was conducted using Statistica software version 8.0 (StatSoft Inc., Tulsa, OK, USA).

3. Results

3.1. Characteristics of the Analyzed Group of Patients

The characteristics of the CD patients are presented in Table 1. The median age of the patients was 33 years old (range 18–63; non-parametric distribution of data). Over half of the respondents were highly educated and they reported that they were employed (77%) or they were students (10%) while the study was being conducted. Furthermore, a high level of self-reported adherence to GFD was observed. Slightly over half of the respondents lived in big cities (cities over 100,000 inhabitants–size corresponding to the size of a Polish provincial capital).

Table 1. Characteristics of the study sample (n = 251).

Characteristics	Category	Number of Respondents (%)
CD duration	Over 3 years Below 3 years	130 (45.0) 138 (55.0)
GFD adherence [1]	1 2 3 4 0	2 (0.8) 31 (12.4) 26 (10.4) 185 (73.7) 7 (2.8)
BMI (kg/m^2) [2]	<18.5—underweight 18.5–24.9—normal weight 25–29.9—overweight	38 (15.3) 165 (66.3) 46 (18.5)
Place of residence	Village Town up to 100,000 residents Cities over 100,000 residents	49 (19.5) 72 (28.7) 130 (51.8)
Educational level	Primary and secondary Postgraduate University degree	61 (24.3) 57 (22.7) 133 (53.0)
Economic status	Very bad Bad Average Good Very good	5 (2.0) 18 (7.2) 119 (47.4) 84 (33.5) 25 (10.0)

[1] GFD (gluten-free diet) adherence: (1) very poor; (2) good, but occasionally eat dishes containing gluten (at home or outside home); (3) very good, but occasionally eat dishes containing gluten (only outside home); (4) excellent; (0) difficult to say; [2] n = 249.

3.2. Descriptive Statistics for the CDQ

The emotional, social and worries subscales data in the analyzed group of CD individuals are presented in Table 2. The floor effect was found to be negligible for all subscales, whereas the ceiling effect for the social subscale was higher, which suggests a tendency to score near the top of the subscale. The Cronbach's alpha coefficient demonstrated the good internal reliability of the data ($\geq$0.7). In the case of item-scale correlation, the results were attributed to consistency levels from acceptable to good, and this was considered satisfactory [27].

Table 2. Descriptive statistics for the CDQ.

Characteristics		Measure	Emotional (7–49)	Social (7–49)	Worries (5–35)
Score		Mean ± SD 95% CI Median Min–max 25th–75th	27.2 ± 9.6 (26.2–28.2) 26.0 [1] 7.0–49.0 22–33	36.1 ± 9.7 (34.9–37.3) 38.0 [1] 8.0–49.0 29–45	19.6 ± 6.1 (19.6–20.4) 19.0 [1] 6.0–35.0 14–24
Data quality	Floor effect	%	1	0	0
	Ceiling effect	%	1	20	2
Scaling assumptions	Item internal consistency	Item-scale correlation (corrected for overlap)	0.41–0.66	0.38–0.74	0.25–0.48
		Pearson item-scale correlation ≥ 30% [2]	100%	100%	80%
	Internal consistency reliability	Cronbach's alpha	0.88	0.88	0.74

[1] non-parametric distribution (verified using Shapiro-Wilk test—$p \leq 0.05$); [2] according to Everitt & Skrondal [28].

3.3. Social and Emotional Fears and Worries Influencing the QoL of Female CD Patients Following a GFD

The scores for emotional subscale of the CDQ categorized by CD duration, GFD adherence, BMI and sociodemographic characteristics are presented in Table 3. Respondents declaring worse economic status obtained significantly lower scores in the subscale than respondents declaring better economic status, while for other factors no significant association was stated in the multi-factor analysis.

Table 3. Emotional subscale data categorized by CD duration, GFD adherence, BMI and sociodemographic characteristics.

Categories		Mean ± SD	Median (min–max)	p-Value [1]
CD duration	Over 3 years	27.1 ± 7.8	27.0 (7.0–47.0)	0.8851
	Below 3 years	27.2 ± 8.3	26.0 (11.0–49.0)	
GFD adherence [3]	1	26.0 ± 1.4	26.0 (25.0–27.0) [2]	0.6714
	2	27.1 ± 8.5	24.5 (18.0–48.0) [2]	
	3	25.2 ± 6.9	23.0 (14.0–42.0)	
	4	27.5 ± 8.2	27.0 (7.0–49.0)	
	0	23.6 ± 7.0	22.0 (15.0–35.0)	
BMI category	Underweight	25.7 ± 9.0	25.0 (7.0–43.0)	0.5127
	Normal weight	27.3 ± 8.1	27.0 (11.0–49.0) [2]	
	Overweight	27.8 ± 7.2	27.0 (14.0–48.0)	
Place of residence	Village	28.5 ± 6.7	29.0 (13.0–49.0)	0.5299
	Town up to 100,000 residents	26.2 ± 9.1	23.5 (7.0–48.0)	
	Town over 100,000 residents	27.2 ± 7.9	26.0 (11.0–46.0)	
Educational level	Primary and Secondary	25.1 ± 7.6	23.0 (7.0–43.0) [2]	0.0594
	Postgraduate	25.9 ± 8.0	25.0 (11.0–48.0)	
	University degree	28.6 ± 8.1	28.0 (11.0–49.0)	
Economic status	Very bad and bad	21.5 ± 7.3	21.0 (11.0–42.0) [2]	0.0015
	Average	26.5 ± 7.8	25.0 (7.0–49.0)	
	Good and very good	29.1 ± 7.8	28.0 (13.0–46.0)	

[1] multifactor analysis of variance (ANOVA); [2] non-parametric distribution (verified using Shapiro-Wilk test—$p \leq 0.05$); [3] GFD (gluten-free diet) adherence: (1) very poor; (2) good, but occasionally eat dishes containing gluten (at home or outside home); (3) very good, but occasionally eat dishes containing gluten (only outside home); (4) excellent; (0) difficult to say.

The scores for social subscale of the CDQ categorized by CD duration, GFD adherence, BMI and sociodemographic characteristics are presented in Table 4. Respondents declaring worse economic status obtained significantly lower scores in the subscale than respondents declaring better economic status, while for other factors no significant association was stated in the multi-factor analysis.

The scores for worries subscale of the CDQ categorized by CD duration, GFD adherence, BMI and sociodemographic characteristics are presented in Table 5. Respondents declaring worse economic status obtained significantly lower scores in the subscale than respondents declaring better economic status, while for other factors no significant association was stated in the multi-factor analysis.

The purchase-related emotions and behaviors data regarding question about mood affecting purchase decisions categorized by CD duration, GFD adherence, BMI and sociodemographic characteristics are presented in Table 6. Respondents declaring worse economic status more often declared that their mood affected their purchase decisions (obtained significantly lower scores for the Likert scale) than did respondents declaring better economic status, while for other factors no significant association was stated in the multi-factor analysis.

Table 4. Social subscale data categorized by CD duration, GFD adherence, BMI and sociodemographic characteristics.

Categories		Mean ± SD	Median (min–max)	*p*-Value [1]
CD duration	Over 3 years	35.2 ± 9.6	36.0 (8.0–49.0) [2]	0.2012
	Below 3 years	36.9 ± 9.7	39.0 (14.0–49.0) [2]	
GFD adherence [3]	1	36.5 ± 14.9	36.0 (26.0–47.0) [2]	0.2526
	2	38.1 ± 9.6	41.0 (14.0–49.0) [2]	
	3	34.8 ± 10.8	37.0 (14.0–49.0)	
	4	36.2 ± 9.5	38.0 (8.0–49.0)	
	0	30.3 ± 10.4	27.0 (17.0–46.0)	
BMI category	Underweight	35.9 ± 10.8	38.5 (8.0–49.0) [2]	0.5055
	Normal weight	36.5 ± 9.1	38.0 (14.0–49.0) [2]	
	Overweight	35.1 ± 11.0	39.0 (11.0–49.0) [2]	
Place of residence	Village	37.4 ± 9.1	40.5 (17.0–49.0) [2]	0.2662
	Town up to 100,000 residents	34.2 ± 9.5	33.0 (15.0–49.0) [2]	
	Town over 100,000 residents	36.7 ± 9.9	39.0 (8.0–49.0) [2]	
Educational level	Primary and Secondary	33.9 ± 10.6	33.0 (8.0–49.0) [2]	0.3328
	Postgraduate	35.8 ± 9.4	39.0 (11.0–49.0) [2]	
	University degree	37.3 ± 9.3	39.0 (14.0–49.0) [2]	
Economic status	Very bad and bad	28.9 ± 11.2	27.0 (8.0–48.0)	0.0023
	Average	35.7 ± 9.6	37.0 (11.0–49.0) [2]	
	Good and very good	38.2 ± 8.7	40.0 (16.0–49.0) [2]	

[1] multifactor analysis of variance (ANOVA); [2] non-parametric distribution (verified using Shapiro-Wilk test—$p \leq 0.05$); [3] GFD (gluten-free diet) adherence: (1) very poor; (2) good, but occasionally eat dishes containing gluten (at home or outside home); (3) very good, but occasionally eat dishes containing gluten (only outside home); (4) excellent; (0) difficult to say.

Table 5. Worries subscale data categorized by CD duration, GFD adherence, BMI and sociodemographic characteristics.

Categories		Mean ± SD	Median (min–max)	*p*-Value [1]
CD duration	Over 3 years	19.1 ± 6.5	18.0 (7.0–35.0) [2]	0.3352
	Below 3 years	20.0 ± 6.7	20.0 (6.0–35.0) [2]	
GFD adherence [3]	1	18.0 ± 2.8	18.0 (16.0–20.0) [2]	0.2462
	2	21.0 ± 7.1	21.0 (8.0–34.0) [2]	
	3	19.1 ± 7.7	18.0 (8.0–34.0)	
	4	19.7 ± 6.3	19.0 (7.0–35.0)	
	0	14.3 ± 8.9	13.0 (6.0–33.0) [2]	
BMI category	Underweight	19.8 ± 7.0	19.0 (8.0–35.0)	0.7485
	Normal weight	19.6 ± 6.4	19.0 (6.0–35.0) [2]	
	Overweight	19.5 ± 7.2	20.0 (7.0–33.0)	
Place of residence	Village	20.2 ± 7.2	20.0 (8.0–35.0)	0.0816
	Town up to 100,000 residents	18.1 ± 6.0	18.0 (6.0–33.0)	
	Town over 100,000 residents	20.2 ± 6.6	20.0 (7.0–35.0)	
Educational level	Primary and Secondary	18.7 ± 6.9	17.5 (8.0–35.0) [2]	0.7919
	Postgraduate	19.7 ± 6.4	20.0 (6.0–34.0)	
	University degree	19.9 ± 6.6	19.0 (8.0–35.0) [2]	
Economic status	Very bad and bad	14.8 ± 5.1	15.0 (6.0–24.0)	0.0015
	Average	19.3 ± 6.7	19.0 (7.0–34.0) [2]	
	Good and very good	20.9 ± 6.3	21.0 (8.0–35.0)	

[1] multifactor analysis of variance (ANOVA); [2] non-parametric distribution (verified using Shapiro-Wilk test—$p \leq 0.05$); [3] GFD (gluten-free diet) adherence: (1) very poor; (2) good, but occasionally eat dishes containing gluten (at home or outside home); (3) very good, but occasionally eat dishes containing gluten (only outside home); (4) excellent; (0) difficult to say.

Table 6. Purchase-related emotions and behaviors data regarding question about mood affecting purchase decisions (*In the past 2 weeks, how many times did your mood affect your purchase decisions associated with GF products?*) categorized by CD duration, GFD adherence, BMI and sociodemographic characteristics.

Categories		Mean ± SD [4]	Median (Min–Max)	*p*-Value [1]
CD duration	Over 3 years	4.2 ± 1.8	3.0 (1.0–7.0) [2]	0.7272
	Below 3 years	4.2 ± 1.9	4.0 (1.0–7.0) [2]	
GFD adherence [3]	1	5.0 ± 0.0	5.0 (5.0–5.0) [2]	0.1981
	2	4.8 ± 1.8	5.5 (2.0–7.0) [2]	
	3	3.9 ± 1.9	3.0 (1.0–7.0) [2]	
	4	4.2 ± 1.9	4.0 (1.0–7.0) [2]	
	0	3.1 ± 1.8	3.0 (2.0–7.0) [2]	
BMI category	Underweight	4.4 ± 2.0	4.0 (1.0–7.0) [2]	0.3959
	Normal weight	4.2 ± 1.9	4.0 (1.0–7.0) [2]	
	Overweight	4.0 ± 1.9	3.0 (1.0–7.0) [2]	
Place of residence	Village	4.4 ± 1.9	4.0 (1.0–7.0) [2]	0.2567
	Town up to 100,000 residents	3.9 ± 1.8	3.0 (1.0–7.0) [2]	
	Town over 100,000 residents	4.3 ± 1.9	4.0 (1.0–7.0) [2]	
Educational level	Primary and Secondary	4.4 ± 1.8	4.0 (1.0–7.0) [2]	0.4635
	Postgraduate	3.9 ± 1.7	3.0 (1.0–7.0) [2]	
	University degree	4.2 ± 2.0	4.0 (1.0–7.0) [2]	
Economic status	Very bad and bad	3.2 ± 1.7	3.0 (1.0–6.0) [2]	0.0029
	Average	4.0 ± 1.8	3.0 (1.0–7.0) [2]	
	Good and very good	4.6 ± 1.9	5.0 (1.0–7.0) [2]	

[1] multifactor analysis of variance (ANOVA); [2] non-parametric distribution (verified using Shapiro-Wilk test—$p \leq 0.05$); [3] GFD (gluten-free diet) adherence: (1) very poor; (2) good, but occasionally eat dishes containing gluten (at home or outside home); (3) very good, but occasionally eat dishes containing gluten (only outside home); (4) excellent; (0) difficult to say; [4] seven point Likert scale, while (1) is attributed to "all of the time" and (7)—to "none of the time".

The purchase-related emotions and behaviors data regarding question about purchasing GF products because of mood categorized by CD duration, GFD adherence, BMI and sociodemographic characteristics are presented in Table 7. For the analyzed factors, no significant association was stated in the multi-factor analysis.

Table 7. Purchase-related emotions and behaviors data regarding question about purchasing GF products because of mood (*In the past 2 weeks, how many times did you buy GF products to improve your mood?*) categorized by CD duration, GFD adherence, BMI and sociodemographic characteristics.

Categories		Mean ± SD [4]	Median (min–max)	*p*-Value [1]
CD duration	Over 3 years	3.9 ± 1.5	4.0 (1.0–7.0) [2]	0.7936
	Below 3 years	3.9 ± 1.7	3.0 (1.0–7.0) [2]	
GFD adherence [3]	1	5.0 ± 0.0	5.0 (5.0–5.0) [2]	0.2695
	2	3.9 ± 1.6	3.5 (1.0–7.0) [2]	
	3	3.3 ± 1.4	3.0 (1.0–7.0) [2]	
	4	4.1 ± 1.7	4.0 (1.0–7.0) [2]	
	0	3.1 ± 1.4	3.0 (2.0–6.0) [2]	
BMI category	Underweight	4.1 ± 1.8	4.0 (1.0–7.0) [2]	0.5132
	Normal weight	4.0 ± 1.6	3.0 (1.0–7.0) [2]	
	Overweight	3.7 ± 1.6	3.0 (1.0–7.0) [2]	

Table 7. *Cont.*

Categories		Mean ± SD [4]	Median (min–max)	p-Value [1]
Place of residence	Village	4.4 ± 1.7	4.0 (1.0–7.0) [2]	0.0847
	Town up to 100,000 residents	4.0 ± 1.6	3.0 (1.0–7.0) [2]	
	Town over 100,000 residents	3.8 ± 1.6	3.0 (1.0–7.0) [2]	
Educational level	Primary and Secondary	4.1 ± 1.6	3.5 (1.0–7.0) [2]	0.3801
	Postgraduate	3.6 ± 1.7	3.0 (1.0–7.0) [2]	
	University degree	4.0 ± 1.6	4.0 (1.0–7.0) [2]	
Economic status	Very bad and bad	3.2 ± 1.2	3.0 (1.0–7.0) [2]	0.0605
	Average	3.8 ± 1.6	3.0 (1.0–7.0) [2]	
	Good and very good	4.2 ± 1.7	4.0 (1.0–7.0) [2]	

[1] multifactor analysis of variance (ANOVA); [2] non-parametric distribution (verified using Shapiro-Wilk test—$p \leq 0.05$); [3] GFD (gluten-free diet) adherence: (1) very poor; (2) good, but occasionally eat dishes containing gluten (at home or outside home); (3) very good, but occasionally eat dishes containing gluten (only outside home); (4) excellent; (0) difficult to say; [4] seven point Likert scale, while (1) is attributed to "all of the time" and (7)—to "none of the time".

4. Discussion

4.1. The Influence of CD Duration and Gender on the QoL of Patients

CD patients experience, due to their diagnosis and applied therapy, a number of problems related to their physical activity, lifestyle and eating behaviors that may affect their general QoL. However, in the review by Kurppa et al. [29], it was stated that additional factors that may affect health-related QoL of CD patients are: age at diagnosis, gender, comorbidities, dietary compliance, availability of GF products, and general knowledge about CD.

Nevertheless, the influence of some factors, e.g., age at diagnosis, on the QoL of CD patients may be contradictory, in various studies. Häuser et al. [2] and Zarkadas et al. [9] reported that diagnosis of CD at a younger age may lead to better health-related QoL, whereas Ciacci et al. [30] and Wagner et al. [31] indicated the reverse relationship.

In our own study, in order to verify the influence of CD duration, a similar assessment was conducted. Those patients with a CD duration below and over 3 years were compared, as 3 years of following a GFD is indicated as the time needed for CD adults to achieve mucosal recovery [32] and, moreover, the first 3 years of disease duration were defined in a cohort study of CD patients as a period characterized by increased mortality [33]. However, neither for emotional, social or worries subscales nor for purchase-related emotions and behaviors was the influence of disease duration reported.

Therefore, in the studied group, other factors, including sociodemographic ones, had to be considered. One of the important sociodemographic factors is gender, for which, in general, CD women experience poorer general well-being than CD men [34]. A similar situation has also been observed for other diseases or health conditions, such as hypertensive patients [35], patients undergoing coronary angiography [36], or patients with diagnosed bipolar disorder [37]. In all these studies, the QoL was measured using HRQOL questionnaires and was lower for female than for male respondents.

4.2. The Influence of GFD Adherence and BMI on the QoL of Patients

Considering the problem of the low QoL of female patients, the aim of the study was to assess the social and emotional fears and worries influencing the QoL of CD patients, in particular for the sub-group of female respondents, being those who experience especially decreased QoL, in comparison with male respondents. Moreover, as following a GFD is not only the recommended approach [38] but also influences the general QoL of CD individuals, a homogenous group of CD female patients following the GFD was studied.

In general, the majority of CD patients have a good QoL while they follow the GFD [29], but untreated patients have a significantly poorer QoL [39]. However, while general diet following influences the QoL of CD patients, dietary adherence level does not have such influence, as comparisons of non-adherent and strictly adherent patients have not demonstrated any significant differences [40]; neither were such differences confirmed in our analyzed group. This may be explained by the fact that even adherent CD patients may have some gastrointestinal symptoms, as may non-adherent ones [41]; so in general, they may be used for such symptoms.

In general, there have so far been no studies analyzing the influence of BMI on the QoL of CD patients. However, for other diseases, such an influence is sometimes stated, and in the context of CD, results observed for gastrointestinal diseases may be used for comparative purposes. For inflammatory bowel diseases, a longitudinal natural history data study showed that obesity was associated with decreasing QoL [42]. Similarly, in a study of an elderly patients group diagnosed with inflammatory bowel diseases, both being underweight and obese were associated with unfavorable health-outcomes, since being underweight was associated with a lower QoL and obesity was associated with a higher risk of depression [43]. The negative impact of both low and high body mass may be confirmed by results from a cross-sectional analysis of the Swiss Inflammatory Bowel Diseases cohort study, as QoL was globally affected in anorexic patients, while in obese ones decreases in the systemic QoL and social QoL scores were stated [44]. These observations for inflammatory bowel diseases are in agreement with the results observed for the general population, as the meta-analysis of Ul-Haq et al. [45] provided evidence that QoL is decreased in obese individuals.

However, not all studies conducted for gastrointestinal diseases indicate such associations. For women with irritable bowel syndrome, the reverse relationship was observed and normal body mass was associated with lower QoL when compared with overweight respondents [46]. Similarly, our study did not indicate any influence of BMI on the emotional, social and worries subscales, or on purchase-related emotions and behaviors in CD patients.

4.3. The Influence of Sociodemographic Characteristics on the QoL of Patients

The number of patients with diagnosed CD is constantly increasing [47] and with this the necessity for permanent changes to eating behaviors which may impacts upon lifestyles. For our group of female CD patients following the GFD, the main sociodemographic factor influencing their social and emotional fears and worries was economic status. Neither for place of residence, nor for educational level the influence was stated, while economic status influenced not only the emotional, social and worries subscales of the CDQ, but also respondents declaring worse economic status more often stated that a mood affected their purchase decisions.

In the literature, there is almost no information about the influence of socioeconomic status on the factors associated with the QoL of CD patients. This aspect is especially important, given that the prices of GF products are higher than the prices of regular ones. However, a number of people follow a strict GF diet, even if they have no specific medical conditions that require this, so the market for GF products is currently increasing [48]. Such a situation, in which the market is increasing (generating higher supply and higher accessibility) but where the prices are still high is very specific and may be burdensome for low-income CD individuals. This is confirmed by other authors, who have reported that GFD may be expensive and challenging for CD patients [49].

The results of our study suggest that not only do low economic status patients not reduce seeking stress-relief in shopping, a strategy commonly observed in the general population [50], but rather they may purchase GF products even more often to improve their mood than do other respondents. This may result from the fact that a properly followed GFD is the primary therapeutic approach [38], so CD patients consciously choose to spend extra money on GF products, instead of spending on other goods. Thus, they consciously purchase the GF products that they need, but at the same time, they sub-consciously satisfy their other needs.

At the same time, lower scores for the emotional, social and worries subscales indicate the lower QoL of CD patients of lower economic status than for those of higher economic status—a situation that is not surprising. However, lower QoL in low-income CD patients may induce the above stress-relief response, while their economic status means that they mainly go grocery shopping, especially for GF products.

The lack of influence of CD duration, GFD adherence and BMI, as well as place of residence and educational level may be associated with the prominent influence of other interfering factors in the case of CD, such as the influence of economic status. This means that economic status in CD patients must be treated as a dominant factor, creating observable associations and influencing social and emotional fears and worries.

4.4. Limitations of the Study and Future Perspectives for the Research

Although the observed associations are interesting, the potential limitations of our study should be noted. Other factors that were not analyzed in the present study may also influence the QoL of CD patients. Among such factors, age and age at diagnosis may be highlighted, as in pediatric patients it has been observed that age is associated with GFD adherence [51,52], as is age combined with educational level at diagnosis [53]. Another factor that may influence the QoL of CD patients may be dietary counseling, as GFD adherence may result from the patient's knowledge and understanding of the rules of GFD [54].

A self-report method carries with it several limitations associated with three areas—respondents, instrument of data collection and contextual factors. Moreover, our relatively small size sample does not allow generalization of our findings.

It would be interesting to conduct a similar study with a group of male CD patients, in order to compare results for men and women, as it has been claimed that there are general gender-related differences in the clinical presentation of CD [55]. Also, conducting a similar study with a group of children would be interesting, as it is especially challenging for children, in particular teenagers, to adhere to GFD [56].

5. Conclusions

1. The economic status of a CD patient could be one of the most important factors influencing their social and emotional fears and worries.
2. Although the low economic status of CD patients may lead to a lower QoL in terms of social and emotional fears and worries, it does not reduce the purchasing of GF products to improve mood.
3. It may be supposed that low economic status may lead some CD patients to choose to relieve stress by purchasing GF products instead of other products.

Author Contributions: W.Z., D.G. (Dominika Guzek) made study conception and design; W.Z. performed the research; D.G. (Dominika Głąbska), D.G. (Dominika Guzek) analyzed the data; W.Z., D.G. (Dominika Głąbska), D.G. (Dominika Guzek) interpreted the data; W.Z., D.G. (Dominika Głąbska), D.G. (Dominika Guzek) wrote the paper. All the authors read and approved the final manuscript.

Funding: This research is financed by the Polish Ministry of Science and Higher Education within funds of Faculty of Human Nutrition and Consumer Sciences, Warsaw University of Life Sciences (WULS), for scientific research.

Conflicts of Interest: The authors declare no conflict of interest.

References

1. Rubio-Tapia, A.; Murray, J.A. Celiac disease. *Curr. Opin. Gastroenterol.* **2010**, *26*, 116–122. [CrossRef] [PubMed]
2. Häuser, W.; Stallmach, A.; Caspary, W.F.; Stein, J. Predictors of reduced health-related quality of life in adults with coeliac disease. *Aliment. Pharmacol. Ther.* **2007**, *25*, 569–578. [CrossRef] [PubMed]
3. Dickson, B.C.; Streutker, C.J.; Chetty, R. Coeliac disease: An update for pathologists. *J. Clin. Pathol.* **2006**, *59*, 1008–1016. [CrossRef] [PubMed]

4. Parzanese, I.; Qehajaj, D.; Patrinicola, F.; Aralica, M.; Chiriva-Internati, M.; Stifter, S.; Elli, L.; Grizzi, F. Celiac disease: From pathophysiology to treatment. *World J. Gastrointest. Pathophysiol.* **2017**, *8*, 27–38. [CrossRef] [PubMed]
5. Ciacci, C.; Ciclitira, P.; Hadjivassiliou, M.; Kaukinen, K.; Ludvigsson, J.F.; McGough, N.; Sanders, D.S.; Woodward, J.; Leonard, J.N.; Swift, G.L. The gluten-free diet and its current application in coeliac disease and dermatitis herpetiformis. *United Eur. Gastroenterol. J.* **2015**, *3*, 121–135. [CrossRef] [PubMed]
6. Hvas, C.L.; Jensen, M.D.; Reimer, M.C.; Riis, L.B.; Rumessen, J.J.; Skovbjerg, H.; Teisner, A.; Wildt, S. Celiac disease: Diagnosis and treatment. *Dan. Med. J.* **2015**, *62*, 5051.
7. Fera, T.; Cascio, B.; Angelini, G.; Martini, S.; Guidetti, C.S. Affective disorders and quality of life in adult coeliac disease patients on a gluten-free diet. *Eur. J. Gastroenterol. Hepatol.* **2003**, *15*, 1287–1292. [CrossRef] [PubMed]
8. Makharia, G.K. Current and Emerging Therapy for Celiac Disease. *Front. Med. (Lausanne)* **2014**, *1*, 6. [CrossRef] [PubMed]
9. Zarkadas, M.; Cranney, A.; Case, S.; Molloy, M.; Switzer, C.; Graham, I.D.; Butzner, J.D.; Rashid, M.; Warren, R.E.; Burrows, V. The impact of a gluten-free diet on adults with coeliac disease: Results of a national survey. *J. Hum. Nutr. Diet.* **2006**, *19*, 41–49. [CrossRef] [PubMed]
10. Zarkadas, M.; Dubois, S.; MacIsaac, K.; Cantin, I.; Rashid, M.; Roberts, K.C.; La Vieille, S.; Godefroy, S.; Pulido, O.M. Living with coeliac disease and a gluten-free diet: A Canadian perspective. *J. Hum. Nutr. Diet.* **2013**, *26*, 10–23. [CrossRef] [PubMed]
11. Cross, C. Gluten-free industry is healthy, but is the food? *CMAJ* **2013**, *185*, 610. [CrossRef] [PubMed]
12. Ludvigsson, J.F.; Bai, J.C.; Biagi, F.; Card, T.R.; Ciacci, C.; Ciclitira, P.J.; Green, P.H.; Hadjivassiliou, M.; Holdoway, A.; van Heel, D.A.; et al. Diagnosis and management of adult coeliac disease: Guidelines from the British Society of Gastroenterology. *Gut* **2014**, *63*, 1210–1228. [CrossRef] [PubMed]
13. Samasca, G.; Sur, G.; Lupan, I.; Deleanu, D. Gluten-free diet and quality of life in celiac disease. *Gastroenterol. Hepatol. Bed Bench.* **2014**, *7*, 139–143. [PubMed]
14. Pechey, R.; Monsivais, P. Supermarket Choice, Shopping Behavior, Socioeconomic Status, and Food Purchases. *Am. J. Prev. Med.* **2015**, *49*, 868–877. [CrossRef] [PubMed]
15. Mącik, R.; Mącik, D.; Nalewajek, M. Consumer preferences for retail format choice—Case of polish consumers. In Proceedings of the Active Citizenship by Knowledge Management & Innovation Proceedings of the Management, Knowledge and Learning International Conference, Zadar, Croatia, 19–21 June 2013.
16. Olewnik-Mikołajewska, A.; Guzek, D.; Głąbska, D.; Gutkowska, K. Consumer behaviors toward novel functional and convenient meat products in Poland. *J. Sens. Stud.* **2016**, *31*, 193–205. [CrossRef]
17. Rodríguez Almagro, J.; Rodríguez Almagro, D.; Solano Ruiz, C.; Siles González, J.; Hernández Martínez, A. The experience of living with a gluten-free diet: An integrative review. *Gastroenterol. Nurs.* **2018**, *41*, 189–200. [CrossRef] [PubMed]
18. Pouchot, J.; Despujol, C.; Malamut, G.; Ecosse, E.; Coste, J.; Cellier, C. Validation of a French Version of the Quality of Life "Celiac Disease Questionnaire". *PLoS ONE* **2014**, *9*, e96346. [CrossRef] [PubMed]
19. Häuser, W.; Gold, J.; Stallmach, A.; Caspary, W.F.; Stein, J. Development and validation of the Celiac Disease Questionnaire (CDQ), a disease-specific health-related quality of life measure for adult patients with celiac disease. *J. Clin. Gastroenterol.* **2007**, *41*, 157–166. [CrossRef] [PubMed]
20. Tovoli, F.; Granito, A.; Negrini, G.; Guidetti, E.; Faggiano, C.; Bolondi, L. Long term effects of gluten-free diet in non-celiac wheat sensitivity. *Clin. Nutr.* **2017**. [CrossRef] [PubMed]
21. DeVellis, R.F. *Scale Development*; Sage Publications: Newbury Park, NJ, USA, 1991.
22. Regulation (EU) No 828/2014 of 30 July 2014 on the Requirements for the Provision of Information to Consumers on the Absence or Reduced Presence of Gluten in Food. Official Journal of the European Union L 228/5. Available online: https://eur-lex.europa.eu/eli/reg_impl/2014/828/oj (accessed on 29 September 2018).
23. Van Hees, N.J.; Van der Does, W.; Giltay, E.J. Coeliac disease, diet adherence and depressive symptoms. *J. Psychosom. Res.* **2013**, *74*, 155–160. [CrossRef] [PubMed]
24. Kautto, E.; Rydén, P.J.; Ivarsson, A.; Olsson, C.; Norström, F.; Högberg, L.; Carlsson, A.; Hagfors, L.; Hörnell, A. What happens to food choices when a gluten-free diet is required? A prospective longitudinal population-based study among Swedish adolescent with coeliac disease and their peers. *J. Nutr. Sci.* **2014**, *3*, e2. [CrossRef] [PubMed]

25. Leffler, D.A.; Dennis, M.; Edwards George, J.B.; Jamma, S.; Magge, S.; Cook, E.F.; Schuppan, D.; Kelly, C.P. A simple validated gluten-free diet adherence survey for adults with celiac disease. *Clin. Gastroenterol. Hepatol.* **2009**, *7*, 530.e2–536.e2. [CrossRef] [PubMed]
26. WHO. Body Mass Index—BMI. Available online: http://www.euro.who.int/en/health-topics/disease-prevention/nutrition/a-healthy-lifestyle/body-mass-index-bmi (accessed on 10 August 2018).
27. Kline, P.A. (Ed.) Computing test-reliability. In *Handbook of Test Construction: Introduction to Psychometric Design*; Methuen & Co.: New York, NY, USA, 1986; pp. 118–132.
28. Everitt, B.S. *The Cambridge Dictionary of Statistics*, 2nd ed.; Cambridge University Press: Cambridge, UK, 2002.
29. Kurppa, K.; Collin, P.; Mäki, M.; Kaukinen, K. Celiac disease and health-related quality of life. *Expert Rev. Gastroenterol. Hepatol.* **2011**, *5*, 83–90. [CrossRef] [PubMed]
30. Ciacci, C.; D'Agate, C.; De Rosa, A.; Franzese, C.; Errichiello, S.; Gasperi, V.; Pardi, A.; Quagliata, D.; Visentini, S.; Greco, L. Self-rated quality of life in celiac disease. *Dig. Dis. Sci.* **2003**, *48*, 2216–2220. [CrossRef] [PubMed]
31. Wagner, G.; Berger, G.; Sinnreich, U.; Grylli, V.; Schober, E.; Huber, W.D.; Karwautz, A. Quality of life in adolescents with treated coeliac disease: Influence of compliance and age at diagnosis. *J. Pediatr. Gastroenterol. Nutr.* **2008**, *47*, 555–561. [CrossRef] [PubMed]
32. Rubio-Tapia, A.; Rahim, M.W.; See, J.A.; Lahr, B.D.; Wu, T.T.; Murray, J.A. Mucosal recovery and mortality in adults with celiac disease after treatment with a gluten-free diet. *Am. J. Gastroenterol.* **2010**, *105*, 1412–1420. [CrossRef] [PubMed]
33. Corrao, G.; Corazza, G.R.; Bagnardi, V.; Brusco, G.; Ciacci, C.; Cottone, M.; Sategna Guidetti, C.; Usai, P.; Cesari, P.; Pelli, M.A.; et al. Mortality in patients with coeliac disease and their relatives: A cohort study. *Lancet* **2001**, *358*, 356–361. [CrossRef]
34. Casellas, F.; Rodrigo, L.; Vivancos, J.L.; Riestra, S.; Pantiga, C.; Baudet, J.S.; Junquera, F.; Puig Diví, V.; Abadia, C.; Papo, M.; et al. Factors that impact health-related quality of life in adults with celiac disease: A multicenter study. *World J. Gastroenterol.* **2008**, *14*, 46–52. [CrossRef] [PubMed]
35. Carvalho, M.A.; Silva, I.B.; Ramos, S.B.; Coelho, L.F.; Gonçalves, I.D.; Figueiredo Neto, J.A. Quality of life of hypertensive patients and comparison of two instruments of HRQOL measure. *Arq. Bras. Cardiol.* **2012**, *98*, 442–451. [CrossRef] [PubMed]
36. Gijsberts, C.M.; Agostoni, P.; Hoefer, I.E.; Asselbergs, F.W.; Pasterkamp, G.; Nathoe, H.; Appelman, Y.E.; de Kleijn, D.P.; den Ruijter, H.M. Gender differences in health-related quality of life in patients undergoing coronary angiography. *Open Heart* **2015**, *2*, 000231. [CrossRef] [PubMed]
37. De la Cruz, M.S.D.; Lai, Z.; Goodrich, D.E.; Kilbourne, A.M. Gender Differences in Health-Related Quality of Life in Patients with Bipolar Disorder. *Arch. Womens Ment. Health* **2013**, *16*, 317–323. [CrossRef] [PubMed]
38. Theethira, T.G.; Dennis, M. Celiac disease and the gluten-free diet: Consequences and recommendations for improvement. *Dig. Dis.* **2015**, *33*, 175–182. [CrossRef] [PubMed]
39. Viljamaa, M.; Collin, P.; Huhtala, H.; Sievänen, H.; Mäki, M.; Kaukinen, K. Is coeliac disease screening in risk groups justified? A fourteen-year follow-up with special focus on compliance and quality of life. *Aliment. Pharmacol. Ther.* **2005**, *22*, 317–324. [CrossRef] [PubMed]
40. Hopman, E.G.; Koopman, H.M.; Wit, J.M.; Mearin, M.L. Dietary compliance and health-related quality of life in patients with coeliac disease. *Eur. J. Gastroenterol. Hepatol.* **2009**, *21*, 1056–1061. [CrossRef] [PubMed]
41. Hallert, C.; Grännö, C.; Grant, C.; Hultén, S.; Midhagen, G.; Ström, M.; Svensson, H.; Valdimarsson, T.; Wickström, T. Quality of life of adult coeliac patients treated for 10 years. *Scand. J. Gastroenterol.* **1998**, *33*, 933–938. [CrossRef] [PubMed]
42. Seminerio, J.L.; Koutroubakis, I.E.; Ramos-Rivers, C.; Hashash, J.G.; Dudekula, A.; Regueiro, M.; Baidoo, L.; Barrie, A.; Swoger, J.; Schwartz, M.; et al. Impact of Obesity on the Management and Clinical Course of Patients with Inflammatory Bowel Disease. *Inflamm. Bowel Dis.* **2015**, *21*, 2857–2863. [CrossRef] [PubMed]
43. Slagboom, J.; Asscher, V.; Meijer, L.; Waars, S.; Van der Meulen-de Jong, A.; Maljaars, J. P299 Relation of body mass index and health outcomes in elderly patients with inflammatory bowel disease (IBD). *J. Crohn's Colitis* **2018**, *12*, S251–S252. [CrossRef]
44. Greuter, T.; Porchet, F.; Fournier, N.; Biedermann, L.; Schreiner, P.; Scharl, M.; Schoepfer, A.; Safroneeva, E.; Straumann, A.; Rogler, G.; et al. P192 Extreme body mass indices are frequent in inflammatory bowel disease patients and are associated with higher disease activity in Crohn's disease, but not in ulcerative colitis: A cross-sectional analysis of the Swiss IBD cohort study. *J. Crohn's Colitis* **2018**, *12*, S195. [CrossRef]

45. Ul-Haq, Z.; Mackay, D.F.; Fenwick, E.; Pell, J.P. Meta-analysis of the association between body mass index and health-related quality of life among adults, assessed by the SF-36. *Obesity* **2013**, *21*, 322–327. [CrossRef] [PubMed]
46. Sherwin, L.B.; Ozoji, O.M.; Boulineaux, C.M.; Joseph, P.V.; Fourie, N.H.; Abey, S.K.; Zhang, X.; Henderson, W.A. Gender and Weight Influence Quality of Life in Irritable Bowel Syndrome. *J. Clin. Med.* **2017**, *6*, 103. [CrossRef] [PubMed]
47. Rajpoot, P.; Makharia, G.K. Problems and challenges to adaptation of gluten free diet by Indian patients with celiac disease. *Nutrients* **2013**, *5*, 4869–4879. [CrossRef] [PubMed]
48. Singh, J.; Whelan, K. Limited availability and higher cost of gluten-free foods. *J. Hum. Nutr. Diet.* **2011**, *24*, 479–486. [CrossRef] [PubMed]
49. Pourhoseingholi, M.A.; Rostami-Nejad, M.; Barzegar, F.; Rostami, K.; Volta, U.; Sadeghi, A.; Honarkar, Z.; Salehi, N.; Asadzadeh-Aghdaei, H.; Baghestani, A.R.; et al. Economic burden made celiac disease an expensive and challenging condition for Iranian patients. *Gastroenterol. Hepatol. Bed Bench* **2017**, *10*, 258–262. [PubMed]
50. Davenport, K.; Houston, J.E.; Griffiths, M.D. Excessive eating and compulsive buying behaviours in women: An empirical pilot study examining reward sensitivity, anxiety, impulsivity, self-esteem and social desirability. *Int. J. Ment. Health Addict.* **2012**, *10*, 474–489. [CrossRef]
51. Comino, I.; Fernández-Bañares, F.; Esteve, M.; Ortigosa, L.; Castillejo, G.; Fambuena, B.; Ribes-Koninckx, C.; Sierra, C.; Rodríguez-Herrera, A.; Salazar, J.C.; et al. Fecal Gluten Peptides Reveal Limitations of Serological Tests and Food Questionnaires for Monitoring Gluten-Free Diet in Celiac Disease Patients. *Am. J. Gastroenterol.* **2016**, *111*, 1456–1465. [CrossRef] [PubMed]
52. Moreno, M.D.L.; Rodríguez-Herrera, A.; Sousa, C.; Comino, I. Biomarkers to Monitor Gluten-Free Diet Compliance in Celiac Patients. *Nutrients* **2017**, *9*, 46. [CrossRef] [PubMed]
53. Ciacci, C.; Cirillo, M.; Cavallaro, R.; Mazzacca, G. Long-term follow-up of celiac adults on gluten-free diet: Prevalence and correlates of intestinal damage. *Digestion* **2002**, *66*, 178–185. [CrossRef] [PubMed]
54. Muhammad, H.; Reeves, S.; Ishaq, S.; Mayberry, J.; Jeanes, Y.M. Adherence to a Gluten Free Diet Is Associated with Receiving Gluten Free Foods on Prescription and Understanding Food Labelling. *Nutrients* **2017**, *9*, 705. [CrossRef] [PubMed]
55. Bardella, M.T.; Fredella, C.; Saladino, V.; Trovato, C.; Cesana, B.M.; Quatrini, M.; Prampolini, L. Gluten intolerance: Gender- and age-related differences in symptoms. *Scand. J. Gastroenterol.* **2005**, *40*, 15–19. [CrossRef] [PubMed]
56. Meyer, S.; Rosenblum, S. Activities, Participation and Quality of Life Concepts in Children and Adolescents with Celiac Disease: A Scoping Review. *Nutrients* **2017**, *9*, 929. [CrossRef] [PubMed]

nutrients

MDPI

Review

The Effect of Gluten-Free Diet on Health and the Gut Microbiota Cannot Be Extrapolated from One Population to Others

Jose F. Garcia-Mazcorro [1], Giuliana Noratto [2] and Jose M. Remes-Troche [1,*]

[1] Instituto de Investigaciones Medico Biológicas, Universidad Veracruzana, Calle Agustín de Iturbide, Salvador Díaz Mirón, Veracruz 91700, Mexico; josegarcia_mex@hotmail.com

[2] Department of Nutrition and Food Science, Texas A&M University, 2253 TAMU, College Station, TX 77843, USA; gnoratto@tamu.edu

[*] Correspondence: jose.remes.troche@gmail.com; Tel.: +1-229-931-8011

Received: 27 August 2018; Accepted: 1 October 2018; Published: 4 October 2018

Abstract: Gluten-related disorders (GRD) affect millions of people worldwide and have been related to the composition and metabolism of the gut microbiota. These disorders present differently in each patient and the only treatment available is a strict life-long gluten-free diet (GFD). Several studies have investigated the effect of a GFD on the gut microbiota of patients afflicted with GRD as well as healthy people. The purpose of this review is to persuade the biomedical community to think that, while useful, the results from the effect of GFD on health and the gut microbiota cannot be extrapolated from one population to others. This argument is primarily based on the highly individualized pattern of gut microbial composition and metabolic activity in each person, the variability of the gut microbiota over time and the plethora of factors associated with this variation. In addition, there is wide variation in the composition, economic viability, and possible deleterious effects to health among different GFD, both within and among countries. Overall, this paper encourages the conception of more collaborative efforts to study local populations in an effort to reach biologically and medically useful conclusions that truly contribute to improve health in patients afflicted with GRD.

Keywords: celiac disease; gluten-free diet; gut microbiota

---

1. Introduction

Human beings are superorganisms or holobionts (i.e., hosts with associated life forms) that have evolved over millions of years collectively as a unit, yet independently [1]. From all microbial niches in the body, the digestive tract has received the mostattention in part due to its role in health and immunity [2]. Many different host-associated (e.g., age, sex, health status) and environmental factors are known to affect the composition of the gut microbiota but growing evidence suggests that diet is one of the main contributors [3–5]. Diet is particularly relevant in newborns and infants, where nutrition is not only vital for growth and development but can also have life-long consequences, a phenomenon closely linked to the gut microbiota [6,7].

The gut microbiota has been studied in a context of health and disease for over a century now. Generally, the gut microbiota is in balance with its host and shows certain resilience to change from one state to another (e.g., from healthy to diseased), although this phenomenon is still not well understood [8,9]. For example, while different diseases have been related to different states of "dysbiosis" of the gut microbiota (for example, allergies, inflammatory bowel diseases, diabetes, obesity and gluten-related disorders, see [10]), a cause–and–effect relationship can hardly be established in part because of the well-known high inter-individual variability, a phenomenon occurring even among closely related individuals [11]. Nonetheless, great progress has been achieved in understanding causal relationship between the host and its microbes [12].

The purpose of this review is to warn against extrapolation of results in the context of an effect of gluten-free diet (GFD) on health and the gut microbiota. Indeed, any metabolic response needs to be investigated specifically within population groups to increase our understanding of whether dietary treatments are effective in that group. Although the issue of extrapolation is true in all research in Nutritional Sciences, it is often overlooked and not emphasized enough among clinicians and clinical scientists.

2. Gluten-Related Disorders and Celiac Disease

Gluten-related disorders (GRD) comprise a variety of different disorders such as celiac disease (CD), non-celiac gluten sensitivity (NCGS), gluten allergy and others, where the body reacts negatively upon exposure to dietary gliadins, a class of proteins that are a component of gluten in wheat and other cereals. Clinically, GRD often range from mild presentations (such as asymptomatic CD) to very serious and life-threatening conditions in some people such as refractory CD and lymphoma [13].

From all GRD, CD has been the most studied and is currently considered to be the most common chronic enteropathy worldwide [14]. In people with CD, a significantly enhanced autoantibody response to the transglutaminase 2 (TG2) enzyme, also known as tissue transglutaminase (tTG), is a hallmark of the pathogenic process that primarily affects the architecture of the enterocyte lining of the small intestine [15] but can also affect other organs such as the liver, kidney, lymph nodes and muscles [16,17]. Interestingly, other autoantibodies may also be involved, especially in extraintestinal manifestations, such as anti-ganglioside, anti-synapsin I and anti-actin antibodies [18]. Patients with CD present either typical or atypical symptoms [19] and CD is believed to perpetuate other maladies and often presents simultaneously with other autoimmune diseases [20–23]. Despite the great progress in CD research, new key emerging findings suggest previously unknown features of CD pathogenesis, for example at the transcriptome level of immune cells [24].

The global prevalence of CD based on serologic test results is 1.4% and based on biopsy results is 0.7% [25]. The prevalence of CD varies with sex, age, and location and, in some regions and populations, it can be as high as 5.6% [26]. While different treatments are under study (e.g., using prolyl endopeptidases and vaccines [17,27]), the only effective treatment available to date for patients with CD and other GRD is a strict life-long gluten-free diet (GFD). Interestingly, GFD is being adopted worldwide by a growing number of people with and without GRD for weight control and the rather misconceived perception that this diet is healthier [28]. However, whether a GFD is healthier remains highly controversial (see Section 5.2).

3. GRD and the Gut Microbiota

The fact that genetic susceptibility is not determinant for the presentation of CD (30–40% of the population have the required genotype but the prevalence of CD is only about 1%) has prompted research to discover what other factors can predict the clinical manifestation of the disease [21]. For example, there is enough evidence to suggest that the gut microbiota (especially Bacteria) plays a role in the onset and clinical manifestations of CD [29–38] and probably other GRD. Although the exact mechanisms involved in the relationship of the gut microbiota and gut diseases are currently unknown (a relationship that is likely to be highly individualized as well), fellow colleagues have suggested an interesting proposal involving first a microbial dysbiosis (e.g., after antibiotic therapy), independent of gluten sensitivity, which then drives an activation of the innate immune system resulting in the secretion of pro-inflammatory molecules, epithelial barrier disruption, and an increased transfer of gluten peptides, a cascade that ultimately may lead to CD development [15]. Interestingly, CD may also be related with non-bacterial members of the gut microbiota such as yeasts [39,40], although the mechanisms may involve quite different mechanisms such as inter-kingdom interactions [41]. As in the case of other intestinal maladies, the main objective of these studies is to better understand the host–microbiota relationship during the disease (often compared to healthy counterparts), thus helping find new routes for treatment. For instance, the growing body of literature about host–microbiota in CD patients has prompted the use of some probiotics (e.g., *Lactobacillus* spp.) to treat GRD, particularly CD, with promising results (e.g., suppression of pro-inflammatory cytokines, reduction of mucosal damage, and enhanced production of SCFAs [31,42–45]). Other studies have shown a potential of probiotics to modulate the indigenous gut microbiota in patients with CD with inconsistent results [46,47].

4. Effect of GFD on the Gut Microbiome

The effect of GFD on the gut microbiome and related parameters has been studied in patients afflicted with GRD (particularly with CD) and in healthy subjects (Table 1). Please note that most of these studies have important limitations including small sample sizes and the use of low-throughput techniques (e.g., culturetechniques and non-sequencing based molecular techniques) that allow the analysis of a few bacterial groups that are not representative of the whole microbiota (Table 1, please note that great progress has been achieved in the field of gut microbiota culturomics [48]). The small sample sizes are particularly worrying because of the clinical variations of CD presentation. These limitations by themselves should be considered as warning signs by the biomedical community every time someone attempts to extrapolate results among different populations, especially in cases where there are patients involved because individuals are highly unique in terms of their gut microbiome (Figure 1).

Table 1. Summary of studies that have analyzed the effect of gluten-free diet (GFD) on the gut microbiota and related parameters.

Patients Characteristics	Sample Collection and Analysis	Methods	Main Finding(s)	Reference (Year of Publication)
30 subjects (21–73 years old) with CD ($n = 6$), NCGS ($n = 12$) and controls ($n = 12$) from Veracruz, México	Samples were obtained at baseline and after 4 weeks on a GFD	16S rDNA sequencing using the Illumina MiSeq platform	*Pseudomonas* was higher in duodenum of CD patients after 4 weeks on GFD	[49] (Unpublished)
21 healthy adults (16–61 years old) from Groningen, The Netherlands	Nine samples were obtained from each participant at baseline, during and after 4 weeks on GFD	16S rDNA sequencing using 454 pyrosequencing	Veillonellaceae (class Clostridia, Firmicutes) was reduced on GFD; 21 predicted pathway activity scores showed significant association to the change in diet	[50] (2016)
53 young subjects (0.5–18 years old) with CD at presentation; 74 young subjects (1–18 years old) with CD on GFD for less than 1 year; 25 subjects (3–33 years old) with CD on GFD for more than 1 year from Norrköping, Sweden	One fecal sample was obtained once from each subject	Gas liquid chromatography for SCFA measurement	Fecal SCFA levels were higher in CD patients on GFD for < 1 year compared to those on GFD > 1 year	[51] (2013)
10 untreated CD patients, 11 treated CD patients and 11 healthy adults from Leon, Spain	Samples were obtained in normal gluten diet and in GFD	DGGE and gas-liquid chromatography of SCFAs	Microbial communities of treated CD clustered together with those of healthy adults	[52] (2012)
19 CD children (6–12 years old) on GFD for at least 2 years and 15 non-celiac children from Bari, Apulia, Italy	Duodenal biopsies and fecal samples were obtained once from each subject	DGGE and culture-based methods	2 years of GFD does not fully restore the microbiota and metabolome of CD children	[53] (2010)
24 untreated CD patients (2–12 years old) on a normal-gluten containing diet; 18 treated CD patients (1–12 years old) on GFD for at least 2 years; 20 healthy children (2–11 years old) without known gluten intolerance from Valencia, Spain	One fecal sample was obtained once from each subject	FISH, flow cytometry and immunoglobulin-coated bacterial analysis	CD patients have lower levels of IgA-coated bacteria thus providing new insights into the relationship between the gut microbiota and host immune defenses	[54] (2010)
20 children with CD (1.2–16.1years old) before and after at least 9 months on GFD, and 10 controls (7.8–20.8 years old) from Rome, Italy	Biopsies from the second part of the duodenum from CD children before and after at least 9 months on GFD; duodenal biopsies from the controls undergoing upper GI endoscopy for functional dyspepsia	TGGE	Number of bands was higher in active and inactive states compared to controls, implying higher biodiversity	[55] (2010)
10 healthy adults (23–40 years old) from Valencia, Spain	One fecal sample was obtained once from each subject at baseline and after 1 month on GFD	FISH and qPCR	Reduction of "beneficial" bacteria and the ability of fecal samples to stimulate the host's immunity	[56] (2009)
34 CD patients at diagnosis and after 12 months on GFD, and 34 healthy controls from Fiorentino, Italy	Serum and urine samples were obtained once from each subject	Nuclear Magnetic Resonance (NMR) of urine and serum samples	After 12 months of GFD, all but one patient was classified as healthy	[57] (2009)

Table 1. *Cont.*

Patients Characteristics	Sample Collection and Analysis	Methods	Main Finding(s)	Reference (Year of Publication)
Group 1 (30 untreated CD patients on a normal gluten-containing diet, 56–61 months old); group 2 (18 treated CD patients with a GFD for at least 2 years, 64–58 months old); group 3 (30 control children without gluten intolerance, 45–49 months old) from Valencia, Spain	30 fecal and 25 duodenal biopsies from Group 1; 18 fecal and 8 biopsy samples from Group 2; 30 fecal and 8 biopsy samples from Group 3	qPCR for a small group of selected microbes	Duodenal and fecal microbiota is partially restored after long-term (>2 years) GFD	[58] (2009)
Seven symptom-free CD patients on GFD for at least 2 years; seven CD patients on gluten-containing diet; seven children with no known food intolerance (6–12 years old) from Bari, Apulia, Italy	Each child provided 3 fecal samples over an unknown period of time. The samples were mixed	DGGE and culture-based techniques; gas chromatography-mass spectrometry for VOCs	CD is associated with differences in fecal microbiota and biochemistry	[59] (2009)
20 CD patients (1.6–12 years old) and 10 symptom-free CD patients who had been on GFD for 1–2 years (2–8 years old) and 8 control children (2–7.8 years old) from Valencia, Spain	An unknown number of biopsy specimens was obtained once from each subject	FISH and flow cytometry for a few selected bacterial groups in duodenum	Ratio of *Lactobacillus-Bifidobacterium* to *Bacteroides-E. coli* was reduced in CD patients with either active or inactive disease compared to controls	[60] (2007)
36 children with CD at presentation, 47 patients on GFD for at least 3 months, and 42 healthy controls from Stockholm, Sweden	One fecal sample was obtained once for each subject	Gas-liquid chromatography of SCFAs in fecal samples	Difference between children on GFD and controls regarding acetic, i-butyric, i-valeric acid, and total SCFAs	[61] (2005)

CD, celiac disease; DGGE, Denaturing Gradient Gel Electrophoresis; TGGE, Temperature Gradient Gel Electrophoresis; FISH, Fluorescent in situ hybridization; SCFAs, short-chain fatty acids; VOCs, volatile organic acids; NCGS, non-celiac gluten sensitivity.

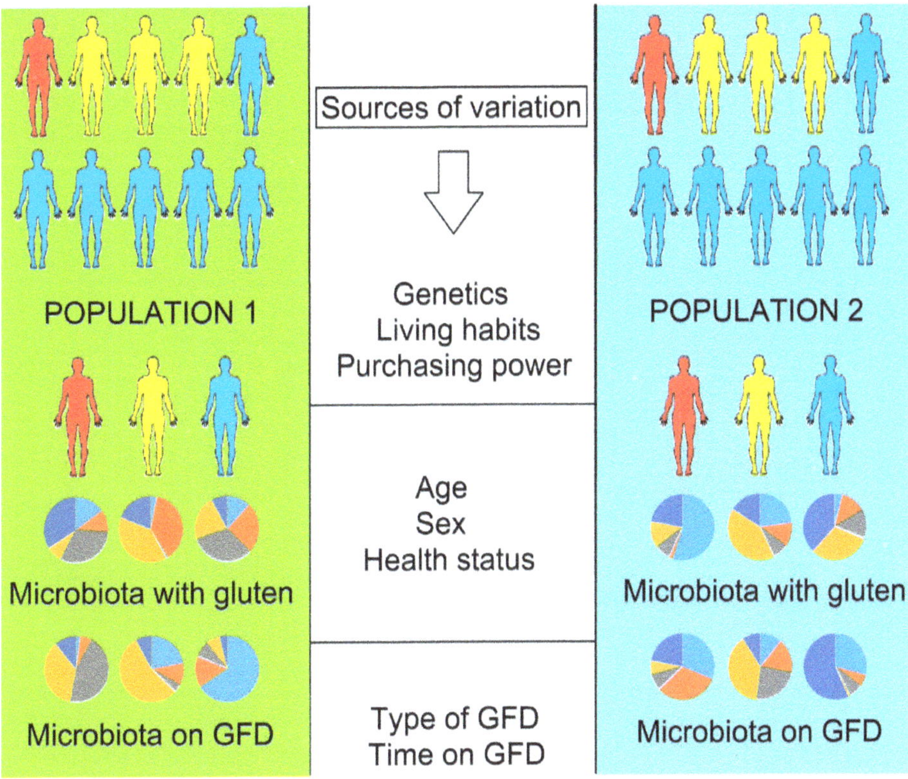

Figure 1. Results of the effect of gluten-free diet (GFD) on health and the gut microbiota cannot be extrapolated from one population to others. Genetic predisposition to CD is present in about 30–40% of the whole population (non-blue silhouettes) but affects clinically only about 1% of the population (red silhouettes). Each individual in either population harbors a highly specific microbiome in the gut (represented here by hypothetical data in pie charts where each color represents a different microbial group) that shows a unique pattern of change after consuming a GFD. The individualized microbiome and its response against dietary or therapeutic challenges is due to multiple sources of variation at the population (e.g., genetics and living habits), individual (e.g., age andsex) and experimental (e.g., type and time on GFD) level.

Before discussing the issues with extrapolation and the main arguments against extrapolation of results, it is important to briefly discuss about the nature of microbes and their identification. First, while we tend to think that members of the same "species" should share a great deal of similar characteristics, this is far from being true for most (if not all) microbial species [62]. Second, when dealing with reference gene sequences (e.g., 16S rRNA gene sequences), it has been a long tradition to group these sequences into something we call Operational Taxonomic Units (OTUs), which are simply groups of sequences based on sequence similarity, based on the belief that a given OTU would comprise similar organisms. However, OTUs show extensive mixed phylogenetic and ecological signals [63] and in fact current trends suggest that OTUs should be replaced by exact sequence variants [64]. Third, there is extensive horizontal gene transfer (i.e., movement of genetic material between different organisms, for example genes associated with antibiotic resistance) among the many members of the gut microbiota that happens at mostly unknown rates [65], a phenomenon shaped principally by ecology rather than geography or phylogeny [66] that likely generates "new" microbes de novo. Fourth, there are different techniques to identify microorganisms (e.g., culture and culture-independent), each with its own advantages and disadvantages to truly depict the real microbial ecosystem inside the gut [67]. Finally, there are technical issues that are difficult to overcome, for example the fact that bacteria are not evenly distributed in stools [68], that mucus and lumen contain widely distinct microbial ecosystems [69], and that the microbiota is different throughout the intestinal tract and different fromwhat is found in feces [70].

5. The Issue of Extrapolation

The main objective of this paper is to critically argue against extrapolation in the context of an effect of GFD on health and the gut microbiota (Figure 1). Extrapolation of results from one population to another is incorrect and risky for various reasons, both strictly statistical and scientific. As it will become clear throughout this manuscript, this concern is particularly important in the context of gut microbial ecology, health and disease. On a recent review of the relationship between the gut microbiota and dietary nutrients, Shortt et al. [71] acknowledgedthe fact that animal-derived data can hardly be extrapolated to humans, and there is a well-known bias to choose male rodents in studies from different fields of science [72], including microbial ecology [3]. However, the problem with extrapolating results among human populations is barely mentioned in the literature, even in papers from our own research group [73]. We do not generally mention this because we consider it to be common knowledge and implicit in the results of our publications. However, we strongly believe that this concern should be discussed, especially within the context of health benefits derived from a change in the gut microbial ecosystem.

5.1. Individuality and Over Time Variability of the Gut Microbiota

Each human being harbors a unique blend of trillions of microorganisms and viruses in the gut and other organs, and growing evidence suggest that colonization starts before birth [74]. The microbiota is not only highly different among individual subjects but it also shows a highly individualized response to environmental challenges such as antibiotic perturbation [75]. One study showed that variation in composition of the microbiota across different body sites was consistently larger than technical variability (e.g., PCR primers, 16S rRNA gene region, sequencing platform) across studies [76]. Overall, this means that the many different analyses showing inter-individual variation are biologically meaningful and not the result of technical artifacts.

The question of why the microbiota is so unique in each individual deserves thorough examination. The first studies on the gut microbiota soon revealed that each subject harbors a unique blend of microbes [77]. Microbial carriage varies between subjects down to the species and strain level [78,79]. Virtually all host-associated and environmental factors can have an effect on an individual's gut microbiota, either individually or collectively. Sex is also an important but often neglected topic in gut microbial ecology [80]. This is important because some GRD are known to be more prevalent in women [81]. On top of the well-known high inter-individual differences, there is considerable horizontal gene transfer happening inside the gut [64], which have the potential of increasing the uniqueness of each individual microbiome, and some microbes show bistable abundance distributions that are affected differently than the rest [82].

Another reason each individual is unique is because they live in vastly different geographic and sociocultural regions having unique foods and dietary habits. For example, Mexican people possess one of the most genome-wide variation, a fact that can affect biomedical traits as well as disease presentation, progression and response to treatment [83]. Interestingly, one seminal study about inflammatory bowel disease (IBD) and the gut microbiota showed that the patient's geographical origin was strongly associated with disease presentation and involvement of specific microbes [84].

Different studies have evaluated the gut microbiota over short periods of time but very few studies have analyzed changes in the gut microbiota over long periods of time. One study showed a pronounced variability in an individual's microbiota across months, weeks and even days, and that only a small fraction of all taxa appear to be present across all time points (in this study, 396 time points were analyzed [85]). Interestingly, baseline populations (i.e., before any major dietary or other change) can also predict the response of the gut microbiota in some situations [86].

5.2. Dietary Differences in Gluten-Containing and GFD

Gluten-containing foods provide many nutrients (e.g., prebiotics such as inulin) which may not be equally abundant in gluten-free foods. The potential issues associated with GFD have been discussed since the 1950s [87] and the concern that a GFD could produce potentially adverse effects in the microbiota solely based on a marked reduction in intake of naturally occurring prebiotics has been raised [88]. On the one hand, a recent review showed that long-term morbidities associated with CD, such as nutritional deficiencies, impaired bone health, and reproductive abnormalities, can substantially improve after strict adherence to a GFD [89]. However, a study in Italy reveals an overall low nutritional quality of gluten-free bakery products [90], and gluten-free products contribute to imbalanced diets in children from Spain [91]. In addition, a recent review showed that reduced intake of calcium, vitamins and fiber as well as enhanced consumption of fat and carbohydrates have been consistently reported in patients on GFD [92]. Moreover, there is evidence that some gluten-free foods are not enriched and may be deficient in several nutrients, including dietary fiber, folate, iron, niacin, riboflavin, and thiamine [93,94], although this would not necessarily lead to dietary deficiency of these nutrients because other gluten-free foods such as vegetables, beef, eggs and cheese are rich in these compounds. Other studies evaluating the nutritional composition of processed gluten-free products have demonstrated higher levels of lipids, trans-fat, protein, and salt compared to their gluten-containing counterparts. Furthermore, recent evidence has shown that patients under a GFD are at risk of metabolic syndrome and hepatic steatosis [95] and the concerns regarding the association between micronutrient deficiencies and increased exposure to toxins such as arsenic in GFD [96]. Moreover, some varieties of GFD do not necessarily lead to a healthier physiological state. Ercolini et al. [97], for example, showed that changing from an African-style GFD to an Italian-style GFD provoked significant changes in the salivary microbiota and metabolome of Saharawi (Western Sahara) celiac children and, more importantly, that these changes suggested metabolic dysfunction.

Another issue with GFD is its availability and costs. While some regions in the industrialized world have the luxury of having access to a wide variety of foods and dietary ingredients, most regions of the world have limited access to different foods. This translates into wide differences in GFD, even within the same geographical region. Importantly, not all gluten-free products are certified (http://www.gfco.org/) and some supposedly gluten-free products are actually contaminated with gluten [98]. Moreover, the mere availability of dietary foods in one region does not imply that all people have access to it. In México, for example, differences in income may involve as much as 27-fold difference between the average incomes of the top and the bottom deciles, a difference that stark contrasts with the average ratio of 10 to 1 in the Organization for Economic Co-operation and Development (OECD 2014, https://www.worldeconomicsassociation.org/newsletterarticles/inequality-in-mexico/). Therefore, the purchasing power is likely to be involved in the maintenance of life-long GFD.

An interesting argument emerged from one anonymous reviewer during the review process. Indeed, other grains such as corn and rice are the primary grains consumed in many different countries. In the case of maize, which is often used as an alternative to elaborate GFD for CD patients, there are some maize prolamins (called zeins) containing amino acid sequences that resemble the wheat gluten peptides that may in fact be clinically relevant [99]. The case of rice is also interesting, especially because several countries in Asia have considerably reduced their consumption of rice [100] and increased the consumption of other grains. In addition, it has been recognized that CD epidemiology has changed, in particular in areas where previously CD was unrecognized or rare such as India, China and Latin America. Several hypotheses may explain this phenomenon such as a change in the pattern of food consumption to try to beat malnutrition that has led to a wheat–rice shift in poor countries, but dysbiosis and genetic predisposition may be also related [101]. Overall, we agree with the notion that the cost and availability of GFD may be of lesser clinical importance in some regions of the world.

Aside the availability and costs, there is substantial variation in prescribing rates of gluten-free foods [102] and many GFD followers find it challenging to follow the GFD [103]. Interestingly, psychological state has been shown to predict adherence to a GFD in Australia and New Zealand [104]. Finally, a proportion of CD patients with chronic voluntary gluten ingestion do not show a relapse of clinical signs and villous atrophy despite chronic voluntary gluten ingestion [105], thus suggesting high inter-individual variability. This phenomenon is of great importance for the biomedical community, especially considering the variety of gluten-containing and GFD around the world (in other words, it is likely that not all diets have the same healing effect on regenerating enterocyte architecture and therefore health).

6. Conclusions

The microbes that inhabit the human body are unique for each individual and vary widely over time due to multiple interrelated factors. The fact that the effect of GFD on health and the gut microbiota cannot be extrapolated to other populations is often neglected in the literature but can also apply to any dietary intervention in all other gastrointestinal maladies (e.g., IBD) associated with the gut microbiota. This paper shall not be taken as a discouragement to perform more studies on this topic; on the contrary, as mentioned above, this paper ultimately seeks to encourage the conception of more collaborative efforts to study local populations in an effort to reach useful conclusions that truly contribute to improve health in patients afflicted with GRD and other maladies. This paper also strives for more awareness among the medical community regarding potential negative effects of switching patients to a GFD without adequate dietetic and medical supervision.

Author Contributions: All authors contributed equally to the conception and writing of this paper.

Funding: This research was funded by the Mexican National Council for Science and Technology (CONACYT, Mexico, FOSIS 2015-262023).

Conflicts of Interest: JF Garcia-Mazcorro is an employee of MNA de México. JM Remes-Troche has received speaker's fees, travel support, and participated in medical board meetings with Takeda Mexico, Asofarma and Menarini.

References

1. Douglas, A.E.; Werren, J.H. Holes in the hologenome: Why host-microbe symbioses are not holobionts. *mBio* **2016**, *7*. [CrossRef] [PubMed]
2. Maslowski, K.M.; Mackay, C.R. Diet, gut microbiota and immune responses. *Nat. Immunol.* **2011**, *12*, 5–9. [CrossRef] [PubMed]
3. Turnbaugh, P.J.; Ridaura, V.K.; Faith, J.J.; Rey, F.E.; Knight, R.; Gordon, J.I. The effect of diet on the human gut microbiome: A metagenomic analysis in humanized gnotobiotic mice. *Sci. Transl. Med.* **2009**, *1*. [CrossRef] [PubMed]
4. Faith, J.J.; McNulty, N.P.; Rey, F.E.; Gordon, J.I. Predicting a human gut microbiota's response to diet in gnotobiotic mice. *Science* **2011**, *333*, 101–104. [CrossRef] [PubMed]
5. Wu, G.D.; Chen, J.; Hoffmann, C.; Bittinger, K.; Chen, Y.Y.; Keilbaugh, S.A.; Bewtra, M.; Knights, D.; Walters, W.A.; Knight, R.; et al. Linking long-term dietary patterns with gut microbial enterotypes. *Science* **2011**, *334*, 105–108. [CrossRef] [PubMed]
6. Conlon, M.A.; Bird, A.R. The impact of diet and lifestyle on gut microbiota and human health. *Nutrients* **2015**, *7*, 17–44. [CrossRef] [PubMed]
7. Le Doare, K.; Holder, B.; Bassett, A.; Pannaraj, P.S. Mother's milk: A purposeful contribution to the development of the infant microbiota and immunity. *Front. Immunol.* **2018**, *9*, 361. [CrossRef] [PubMed]
8. Lozupone, C.A.; Stombaugh, J.I.; Gordon, J.I.; Jansson, J.K.; Knight, R. Diversity, stability and resilience of the human gut microbiota. *Nature* **2012**, *489*, 220–230. [CrossRef] [PubMed]

9. Sommer, F.; Anderson, J.M.; Bharti, R.; Raes, J.; Rosenstiel, P. The resilience of the intestinal microbiota influences health and disease. *Nat. Rev. Microbiol.* **2017**, *15*, 630–638. [CrossRef] [PubMed]
10. Clemente, J.C.; Ursell, L.K.; Parfrey, L.W.; Knight, R. The impact of the gut microbiota on human health: An integrative view. *Cell.* **2012**, *148*, 1258–1270. [CrossRef] [PubMed]
11. Turnbaugh, P.J.; Hamady, M.; Yatsunenko, T.; Cantarel, B.L.; Duncan, A.; Ley, R.E.; Sogin, M.L.; Jones, W.J.; Roe, B.A.; Affourtit, J.P.; et al. A core gut microbiome in obese and lean twins. *Nature* **2009**, *457*, 480–484. [CrossRef] [PubMed]
12. Turnbaugh, P.J.; Bäckhed, F.; Fulton, L.; Gordon, J.I. Diet-induced obesity is linked to marked but reversible alterations in the mouse distal gut microbiome. *Cell. Host Microbe* **2008**, *3*, 213–223. [CrossRef] [PubMed]
13. Forrest, E.A.; Wong, M.; Nama, S.; Sharma, S. Celiac crisis, a rare and profound presentation of celiac disease: A case report. *BMC Gastroenterol.* **2018**, *18*, 59. [CrossRef] [PubMed]
14. De Re, V.; Magris, R.; Cannizzaro, R. New insights into the pathogenesis of celiac disease. *Front. Med.* **2017**, *4*, 137.[CrossRef] [PubMed]
15. Cukrowska, B.; Sowińska, A.; Bierła, J.B.; Czarnowska, E.; Rybak, A.; Grzybowska-Chlebowczyk, U. Intestinal epithelium, intraepithelial lymphocytes and the gut microbiota—Key players in the pathogenesis of celiac disease. *World J. Gastroenterol.* **2017**, *23*, 7505–7518. [CrossRef] [PubMed]
16. Rampertab, S.D.; Pooran, N.; Brar, P.; Singh, P.; Green, P.H. Trends in the presentation of celiac disease. *Am. J. Med.* **2006**, *119*, 355.e9–355.e14. [CrossRef] [PubMed]
17. Gujral, N.; Freeman, H.J.; Thomson, A.B.R. Celiac disease: Prevalence, diagnosis, pathogenesis and treatment. *World J. Gastroenterol.* **2012**, *18*, 6036–6059. [CrossRef] [PubMed]
18. Yu, X.B.; Uhde, M.; Green, P.H.; Alaedini, A. Autoantibodies in the extraintestinal manifestations of celiac disease. *Nutrients* **2018**, *10*, 1123. [CrossRef] [PubMed]
19. Ramírez-Cervantes, K.L.; Remes-Troche, J.M.; Milke-García, M.P.; Romero, V.; Uscanga, L.F. Characteristics and factors related to quality of life in Mexican Mestizo patients with celiac disease. *BMC Gastroenterol.* **2015**, *15*, 4. [CrossRef] [PubMed]
20. Verdu, E.F.; Armstrong, D.; Murray, J.A. Between celiac disease and irritable bowel syndrome: The "no man's land" of gluten sensitivity. *Am. J. Gastroenterol.* **2009**, *104*, 1587–1594. [CrossRef] [PubMed]
21. Lammers, K.M.; Herrera, M.G.; Dodero, V.I. Translational chemistry meets gluten-related disorders. *Chem. Open* **2018**, *7*, 217–232. [CrossRef] [PubMed]
22. Reunala, T.; Salmi, T.T.; Hervonen, K.; Kaukinen, K.; Collin, P. Dermatitis herpetiformis: A common extraintestinal manifestation of coeliac disease. *Nutrients* **2018**, *10*, 602. [CrossRef] [PubMed]
23. Rodrigo, L.; Beteta-Gorriti, V.; Alvarez, N.; Gómez de Castro, C.; de Dios, A.; Palacios, L.; Santos-Juanes, J. Cutaneous and mucosal manifestations associated with celiac disease. *Nutrients* **2018**, *10*, 800. [CrossRef] [PubMed]
24. Ciccocioppo, R.; Panelli, S.; Conti Bellocchi, M.C.; Cangemi, G.C.; Frulloni, L.; Capelli, E.; Corazza, G.R. The transcriptomic analysis of circulating immune cells in a celiac family unveils further insights into disease pathogenesis. *Front. Med.* **2018**, *5*, 182. [CrossRef] [PubMed]
25. Singh, P.; Arora, A.; Strand, T.A.; Leffler, D.A.; Catassi, C.; Green, P.H.; Kelly, C.P.; Ahuja, V.; Makharia, G.K. Global prevalence of celiac disease: Systematic review and meta-analysis. *Clin. Gastroenterol. Hepatol.* **2018**, *16*, 823–836. [CrossRef] [PubMed]
26. Teresi, S.; Crapisi, M.; Vallejo, M.D.; Castellaneta, S.P.; Francavilla, R.; Iacono, G.; Ravelli, A.; Menegazzi, O.; Louali, M.; Catassi, C. Celiac disease seropositivity in Saharawi children: A follow-up and family study. *J. Pediatr. Gastroenterol. Nutr.* **2010**, *50*, 506–509. [CrossRef] [PubMed]
27. Haridy, J.; Lewis, D.; Newnham, E.D. Investigational drug therapies for coeliac disease—Where to from here? *Expert Opin. Investig. Drugs* **2018**, *27*, 225–233. [CrossRef] [PubMed]
28. Ontiveros, N.; Rodriguez-Bellegarrigue, C.I.; Galicia-Rodriguez, G.; Vergara-Jimenez, M.J.; Zepeda-Gomez, E.M.; Aramburo-Galvez, J.G.; Gracia-Valenzuela, M.H.; Cabrera-Chavez, F. Prevalence of self-reported gluten-related disorders and adherence to a gluten-free diet in Salvadoran adult population. *Int. J. Environ. Res. Public Health* **2018**, *15*, 786. [CrossRef] [PubMed]
29. Collado, M.C.; Calabuig, M.; Sanz, Y. Differences between the fecal microbiota of coeliac infants and healthy controls. *Curr. Issues Intest. Microbiol.* **2007**, *8*, 9–14. [PubMed]

30. Sanz, Y.; Sánchez, E.; Marzotto, M.; Calabuig, M.; Torriani, S.; Dellaglio, F. Differences in faecal bacterial communities in coeliac and healthy children as detected by PCR and denaturing gradient gel electrophoresis. *FEMS Immunol. Med. Microbiol.* **2007**, *51*, 562–568. [CrossRef] [PubMed]
31. Medina, M.; De Palma, G.; Ribes-Koninckx, C.; Calabuig, M.; Sanz, Y. *Bifidobacterium* strains suppress in vitro the pro-inflammatory milieu triggered by the large intestinal microbiota of coeliac patients. *J. Inflamm.* **2008**, *5*, 19. [CrossRef] [PubMed]
32. Sánchez, E.; Nadal, I.; Donat, E.; Ribes-Koninckx, C.; Calabuig, M.; Sanz, Y. Reduced diversity and increased virulence-gene carriage in intestinal enterobacteria of coeliac children. *BMC Gastroenterol.* **2008**, *8*, 50. [CrossRef] [PubMed]
33. Ou, G.; Hedberg, M.; Hörstedt, P.; Baranov, V.; Forsberg, G.; Drobni, M.; Sandström, O.; Wai, S.N.; Johansson, I.; Hammarström, M.L.; et al. Proximal small intestinal microbiota and identification of rod-shaped bacteria associated with childhood celiac disease. *Am. J. Gastroenterol.* **2009**, *104*, 3058–3067. [CrossRef] [PubMed]
34. Sanz, Y. Effects of a gluten-free diet on gut microbiota and immune function in healthy adult humans. *Gut Microbes* **2010**, *1*, 135–137. [CrossRef] [PubMed]
35. Cinova, J.; De Palma, G.; Stepankova, R.; Kofronova, I.; Kverka, M.; Sanz, Y.; Tuckova, L. Role of intestinal bacteria in gliadin-induced changes in intestinal mucosa: Study in germ-free rats. *PLoS ONE* **2011**, *6*, e16169. [CrossRef] [PubMed]
36. Sjöberg, V.; Sandström, O.; Hedberg, M.; Hammarström, S.; Hernell, O.; Hammarström, M.-L. Intestinal T-cell responses in celiac disease —Impact of celiac disease associated bacteria. *PLoS ONE* **2013**, *8*, e53414. [CrossRef] [PubMed]
37. Wacklin, P.; Kaukinen, K.; Tuovinen, E.; Collin, P.; Lindfors, K.; Partanen, J.; Mäki, M.; Mättö, J. The duodenal microbiota composition of adult celiac disease patients is associated with the clinical manifestation of the disease. *Inflamm. Bowel Dis.* **2013**, *19*, 934–941. [PubMed]
38. Olivares, M.; Benítez-Páez, A.; de Palma, G.; Capilla, A.; Nova, E.; Castillejo, G.; Varea, V.; Marcos, A.; Garrote, J.A.; Polanco, I.; et al. Increased prevalence of pathogenic bacteria in the gut microbiota of infants at risk of developing celiac disease: the PROFICEL study. *Gut Microbes* **2018**. [CrossRef] [PubMed]
39. Ashorn, S.; Raukola, H.; Välineva, T.; Ashorn, M.; Wei, B.; Braun, J.; Rantala, I.; Kaukinen, K.; Luukkaala, T.; Collin, P.; et al. Elevated serum anti-*Saccharomyces cerevisiae*, anti-I2 and anti-OmpW antibody levels in patients with suspicion of celiac disease. *J. Clin. Immunol.* **2008**, *28*, 486–494. [PubMed]
40. Harnett, J.; Myers, S.P.; Rolfe, M. Significantly higher faecal counts of the yeasts candida and saccharomyces identified in people with coealic disease. *Gut Pathog.* **2017**, *9*, 26. [CrossRef] [PubMed]
41. Sovran, B.; Planchais, J.; Jegou, S.; Straube, M.; Lamas, B.; Natividad, J.M.; Agus, A.; Dupraz, L.; Glodt, J.; Da Costa, G.; et al. Enterobacteriaceae are essential for the modulation of colitis severity by fungi. *Microbiome* **2018**, *6*, 152. [CrossRef] [PubMed]
42. D'Arienzo, R.; Stefanile, R.; Maurano, F.; Mazzarella, G.; Ricca, E.; Troncone, R.; Auricchio, S.; Rossi, M. Immunomodulatory effects of *Lactobacillus casei* administration in a mouse model of gliadin-sensitive enteropathy. *Scand. J. Immunol.* **2011**, *74*, 335–341. [CrossRef] [PubMed]
43. Primec, M.; Klemenak, M.; Di Gioia, D.; Aloisio, I.; BozziCionci, N.; Quagliariello, A.; Gorenjak, M.; Mičetić-Turk, D.; Langerholc, T. Clinical intervention using *Bifidobacterium* strains in celiac disease children reveals novel microbial modulators of TNF-α and short-chain fatty acids. *Clin. Nutr.* **2018**. [CrossRef] [PubMed]
44. Smecuol, E.; Hwang, H.J.; Sugai, E.; Corso, L.; Cherñavsky, A.C.; Bellavite, F.P.; González, A.; Vodánovich, F.; Moreno, M.L.; Vázquez, H.; et al. Exploratory, randomized, double-blind, placebo-controlled study on the effects of *Bifidobacteriuminfantis* natren life start strain super strain in active celiac disease. *J. Clin. Gastroenterol.* **2013**, *47*, 139–147. [CrossRef] [PubMed]
45. Pinto-Sánchez, M.I.; Smecuol, E.C.; Temprano, M.P.; Sugai, E.; González, A.; Moreno, M.L.; Huang, M.L.; Bercik, P.; Cabanne, A.; Vázquez, H.; et al. *Bifidobacteriuminfantis* NLS super strain reduces the expression of α-defensin-5, a marker of Innate Immunity, in the mucosa of active celiac disease patients. *J. Clin. Gastroenterol.* **2017**, *51*, 814–817. [PubMed]
46. Martinello, F.; Roman, C.F.; Souza, P.A. Effects of probiotic intake on intestinal bifidobacteria of celiac patients. *Arq. Gastroenterol.* **2017**, *54*, 85–90. [CrossRef] [PubMed]

47. Harnett, J.; Myers, S.P.; Rolfe, M. Probiotics and the microbiome in celiac disease: A randomised controlled trial. *Evid. Based Complement. Alternat. Med.* **2016**, *2016*, 9048574. [CrossRef] [PubMed]
48. Lagier, J.C.; Dubourg, G.; Million, M.; Cadoret, F.; Bilen, M.; Fenollar, F.; Levasseur, A.; Rolain, J.M.; Fournier, P.E.; Raoult, D. Culturing the human microbiota and culturomics. *Nat. Rev. Microbiol.* **2018**, *16*, 540–550. [CrossRef] [PubMed]
49. Garcia-Mazcorro, J.F.; Rivera-Gutierrez, X.; Cobos-Quevedo, O.J.; Grube-Pagola, P.; Meixueiro-Daza, A.; Hernandez-Flores, K.; Cabrera-Jorge, F.J.; Vivanco-Cid, H.; Dowd, S.E.; Remes-Troche, J.M. Consumption of gluten-free diet for four weeks influences the gut microbiota in patients with celiac disease and non-celiac gluten sensitivity. Unpublished work, 2018.
50. Bonder, M.J.; Tigchelaar, E.F.; Cai, X.; Trynka, G.; Cenit, M.C.; Hrdlickova, B.; Zhong, H.; Vatanen, T.; Gevers, D.; Wijmenga, C.; et al. The influence of a short-term gluten-free diet on the human gut microbiome. *Genome Med.* **2016**, *8*, 45. [CrossRef] [PubMed]
51. Tjellström, B.; Högberg, L.; Stenhammar, L.; Fälth-Magnusson, K.; Magnusson, K.-E.; Norin, E.; Sundqvist, T.; Midtvedt, T. Faecal short-chain fatty acid pattern in childhood coeliac disease is normalised after more than one year's gluten-free diet. *Microb. Ecol. Health Dis.* **2013**, *24*, 20905. [CrossRef] [PubMed]
52. Nistal, E.; Caminero, A.; Vivas, S.; Ruiz de Morales, J.M.; Sáenz de Miera, L.E.; Rodríguez-Aparicio, L.B.; Casqueiro, J. Differences in faecal bacteria populations and faecal bacteria metabolism in healthy adults and celiac disease patients. *Biochimie* **2012**, *94*, 1724–1729. [CrossRef] [PubMed]
53. Di Cagno, R.; De Angelis, M.; De Pasquale, I.; Ndagijimana, M.; Vernocchi, P.; Ricciuti, P.; Gagliaradi, F.; Laghi, L.; Crecchio, C.; Guerzoni, M.E.; et al. Duodenal and faecalmicrobiota of celiac children: Molecular, phenotype and metabolome characterization. *BMC Microbiol.* **2011**, *11*, 219. [CrossRef] [PubMed]
54. De Palma, G.; Nadal, I.; Medina, M.; Donat, E.; Ribes-Koninckx, C.; Calabuig, M.; Sanz, Y. Intestinal dysbiosis and reduced immunoglobulin-coated bacteria associated with coeliac disease in children. *BMC Microbiol.* **2010**, *10*, 63. [CrossRef] [PubMed]
55. Schippa, S.; Iebba, V.; Barbato, M.; Di Nardo, G.; Totino, V.; Checchi, M.P.; Longhi, C.; Maiella, G.; Cucchiara, S.; Conte, M.P. A distinctive 'microbial signature' in celiac pediatric patients. *BMC Microbiol.* **2010**, *10*, 175. [CrossRef] [PubMed]
56. De Palma, G.; Nadal, I.; Collado, M.C.; Sanz, Y. Effects of a gluten-free diet on gut microbiota and immune function in healthy adult human subjects. *Br. J. Nutr.* **2009**, *102*, 1154–1160. [CrossRef] [PubMed]
57. Bertini, I.; Calabrò, A.; De Carli, V.; Luchinat, C.; Nepi, S.; Porfirio, B.; Renzi, D.; Saccenti, E.; Tenori, L. The metabonomic signature of celiac disease. *J. Proteome Res.* **2009**, *8*, 170–177. [CrossRef] [PubMed]
58. Collado, M.C.; Donat, E.; Ribes-Koninckx, C.; Calabuig, M.; Sanz, Y. Specific duodenal and faecal bacterial groups associated with paediatric coeliac disease. *J. Clin. Pathol.* **2009**, *62*, 264–269. [CrossRef] [PubMed]
59. Di Cagno, R.; Rizzello, C.G.; Gagliardi, F.; Ricciuti, P.; Ndagijimana, M.; Francavilla, R.; Guerzoni, M.E.; Crecchio, C.; Gobbetti, M.; De Angelis, M. Different fecal microbiotas and volatile organic compounds in treated and untreated children with celiac disease. *Appl. Environ. Microbiol.* **2009**, *75*, 3963–3971. [CrossRef] [PubMed]
60. Nadal, I.; Donant, E.; Ribes-Koninckx, C.; Calabuig, M.; Sanz, Y. Imbalance in the composition of the duodenal microbiota of children with coeliac disease. *J. Med. Microbiol.* **2007**, *56*, 1669–1674. [CrossRef] [PubMed]
61. Tjellström, B.; Stenhammar, L.; Högberg, L.; Fälth-Magnusson, K.; Magnusson, K.E.; Midtvedt, T.; Sundqvist, T.; Norin, E. Gut microflora associated characteristics in children with celiac disease. *Am. J. Gastroenterol.* **2005**, *100*, 2784–2788. [CrossRef] [PubMed]
62. Lukjancenko, O.; Wassenaar, T.M.; Ussery, D.W. Comparison of 61 sequenced *Escherichia coli* genomes. *Microb. Ecol.* **2010**, *60*, 708–720. [CrossRef] [PubMed]
63. Koeppel, A.F.; Wu, M. Surprisingly extensive mixed phylogenetic and ecological signals among bacterial Operational Taxonomic Units. *Nucleic Acids Res.* **2013**, *41*, 5175–5188. [CrossRef] [PubMed]
64. Callahan, B.J.; McMurdie, P.J.; Holmes, S.P. Exact sequence variants should replace operational taxonomic units in marker-gene data analysis. *ISME J.* **2017**, *11*, 2639–2643. [CrossRef] [PubMed]
65. Liu, L.; Chen, X.; Skogerbø, G.; Zhang, P.; Chen, R.; He, S.; Huang, D.-W. The human microbiome: A hot spot of microbial horizontal gene transfer. *Genomics* **2012**, *100*, 265–270. [CrossRef] [PubMed]
66. Smillie, C.S.; Smith, M.B.; Friedman, J.; Cordero, O.X.; David, L.A.; Alm, E.J. Ecology drives a global network of gene exchange connecting the human microbiome. *Nature* **2011**, *480*, 241–244. [CrossRef] [PubMed]

67. Sipos, R.; Székely, A.J.; Palatinszky, M.; Révész, S.; Márialigeti, K.; Nikolausz, M. Effect of primer mismatch, annealing temperature and PCR cycle number on 16S rRNA gene-targeting bacterial community analysis. *FEMS Microbiol. Ecol.* **2007**, *60*, 341–350. [CrossRef] [PubMed]
68. Swidsinski, A.; Loening-Baucke, V.; Vaneechoutte, M.; Doerffel, Y. Active Crohn's disease and ulcerative colitis can be specifically diagnosed and monitored based on the biostructure of the fecal flora. *Inflamm. Bowel Dis.* **2008**, *14*, 147–161. [CrossRef] [PubMed]
69. Donaldson, G.P.; Lee, S.M.; Mazmanian, S.K. Gut biogeography of the bacterial microbiota. *Nat. Rev. Microbiol.* **2016**, *14*, 20–32. [CrossRef] [PubMed]
70. Hayashi, H.; Takahashi, R.; Nishi, T.; Sakamoto, M.; Benno, Y. Molecular analysis of jejunal, ileal, caecal and recto-sigmodial human colonic microbiota using 16S rRNA gene libraries and terminal restriction fragment length polymorphism. *J. Med. Microbiol.* **2005**, *54*, 1093–1101. [CrossRef] [PubMed]
71. Shortt, C.; Hasselwander, O.; Meynier, A.; Nauta, A.; Fernández, E.N.; Putz, P.; Rowland, I.; Swann, J.; Türk, J.; Vermeiren, J.; et al. Systematic review of the effects of the intestinal microbiota on selected nutrients and non-nutrients. *Eur. J. Nutr.* **2018**, *57*, 25–49. [CrossRef] [PubMed]
72. Wald, C.; Wu, C. Of mice and women: the bias in animal models. *Science* **2010**, *327*, 1571–1572. [CrossRef] [PubMed]
73. Camacho-Ortiz, A.; Gutiérrez-Delgado, E.M.; Garcia-Mazcorro, J.F.; Mendoza-Olazarán, S.; Martínez-Meléndez, A.; Palau-Davila, L.; Baines, S.D.; Maldonado-Garza, H.; Garza-González, E. Randomized clinical trial to evaluate the effect of fecal microbiota transplant for initial *Clostridium difficile* infection in intestinal microbiome. *PLoS ONE* **2017**, *12*, e0189768. [CrossRef] [PubMed]
74. Chong, C.Y.L.; Bloomfield, F.H.; O'Sullivan, J.M. Factors affecting gastrointestinal microbiome development in neonates. *Nutrients* **2018**, *10*, 74. [CrossRef] [PubMed]
75. Dethlefsen, L.; Relman, D.A. Incomplete recovery and individualized responses of the human distal gut microbiota to repeated antibiotic perturbation. *Proc. Natl. Acad. Sci. USA* **2011**, *108*, 4554–4561. [CrossRef] [PubMed]
76. Lozupone, C.A.; Stombaugh, J.; Gonzalez, A.; Ackermann, G.; Wendel, D.; Vázquez-Baeza, Y.; Jansson, J.K.; Gordon, J.I.; Knight, R. Meta-analyses of studies of the human microbiota. *Genome Res.* **2013**, *23*, 1704–1714. [CrossRef] [PubMed]
77. McCartney, A.L.; Wenzhi, W.; Tannock, G.W. Molecular analysis of the composition of the bifidobacterial and Lactobacillus microflora of humans. *Appl. Environ. Microbiol.* **1996**, *62*, 4608–4613. [PubMed]
78. The Human Microbiome Project Consortium. Structure, function and diversity of the healthy human microbiome. *Nature* **2012**, *486*, 207–214.
79. Ursell, L.K.; Clemente, J.C.; Rideout, J.R.; Gevers, D.; Caporaso, J.G.; Knight, R. The interpersonal and intrapersonal diversity of human-associated microbiota in key body sites. *J. Allergy Clin. Immunol.* **2012**, *129*, 1204–1208. [CrossRef] [PubMed]
80. Markle, J.G.M.; Frank, D.N.; Mortin-Toth, S.; Robertson, C.E.; Feazel, L.M.; Rolle-Kampczyk, U.; von Bergen, M.; McCoy, K.D.; Macpherson, A.J.; Danska, J.S. Sex differences in the gut microbiome drive hormone-dependent regulation of autoimmunity. *Science* **2013**, *339*, 1084–1088. [PubMed]
81. Ciacci, C.; Cirillo, M.; Sollazzo, R.; Savino, G.; Sabbatini, F.; Mazzacca, G. Gender and clinical presentation in adult celiac disease. *Scand. J. Gastroenterol.* **1995**, *30*, 1077–1081. [CrossRef] [PubMed]
82. Lahti, L.; Salojärvi, J.; Salonen, A.; Scheffer, M.; de Vos, W.M. Tipping elements in the human intestinal ecosystem. *Nat. Commun.* **2014**, *5*, 4344. [CrossRef] [PubMed]
83. Moreno-Estrada, A.; Gignoux, C.R.; Fernandez-Lopez, J.C.; Zakharia, F.; Sikora, M.; Contreras, A.V.; Acuña-Alonzo, V.; Sandoval, K.; Eng, C.; Romero-Hidalgo, S.; et al. The genetics of Mexico recapitulates native American substructure and affects biomedical traits. *Science* **2014**, *344*, 1280–1285. [CrossRef] [PubMed]
84. Rehman, A.; Rausch, P.; Wang, J.; Skieceviciene, J.; Kiudelis, G.; Bhagalia, K.; Amarapurkar, D.; Kupcinskas, L.; Schreiber, S.; Rosenstiel, P.; et al. Geographical patterns of the standing and active human gut microbiome in health and IBD. *Gut* **2015**, *65*, 238–248. [CrossRef] [PubMed]
85. Caporaso, J.G.; Lauber, C.L.; Costello, E.K.; Berg-Lyons, D.; Gonzalez, A.; Stombaugh, J.; Knights, D.; Gajer, P.; Ravel, J.; Fierer, N.; et al. Moving pictures of the human microbiome. *Genome Biol.* **2011**, *12*, R50. [CrossRef] [PubMed]
86. Winter, S.E.; Bäumler, A.J. Why related bacterial species bloom simultaneously in the gut: Principles underlying the 'like will to like' concept. *Cell. Microbiol.* **2014**, *16*, 179–184. [CrossRef] [PubMed]

87. Fletcher, R.F.; McCririck, M.Y. Gluten-free diets. *Br. Med. J.* **1958**, *2*, 299–301. [CrossRef] [PubMed]
88. Jackson, F.W. Effects of a gluten-free diet on gut microbiota and immune function in healthy adult human subjects—comment by Jackson. *Br. J. Nutr.* **2010**, *104*, 773. [CrossRef] [PubMed]
89. Bathrellou, E.; Kontogianni, M.D.; Panagiotakos, D.B. Celiac disease and non-celiac gluten or wheat sensitivity and health in later life: A review. *Maturitas* **2018**, *112*, 29–33. [CrossRef] [PubMed]
90. Morreale, F.; Angelino, D.; Pellegrini, N. Designing a score-based method for the evaluation of the nutritional quality of the gluten-free bakery products and their gluten-containing counterparts. *Plant Foods Hum. Nutr.* **2018**, *73*, 154–159. [CrossRef] [PubMed]
91. Larretxi, I.; Simon, E.; Benjumea, L.; Miranda, J.; Bustamante, M.A.; Lasa, A.; Eizaguirre, F.J.; Churruca, I. Gluten-free-rendered products contribute to imbalanced diets in children and adolescents with celiac disease. *Eur. J. Nutr.* **2018**. [CrossRef] [PubMed]
92. Newberry, C.; McKnight, L.; Sarav, M.; Pickett-Blakely, O. Going gluten free: The history and nutritional implications of today's most popular diet. *Curr. Gastroenterol. Rep.* **2017**, *19*, 54. [CrossRef] [PubMed]
93. Thompson, T. Thiamin, riboflavin, and niacin contents of the gluten-free diet: Is there cause for concern? *J. Am. Diet. Assoc.* **1999**, *99*, 858–862. [CrossRef]
94. Mariani, P.; Viti, M.G.; Montuori, M.; La Vecchia, A.; Cipolletta, E.; Calvani, L.; Bonamico, M. The gluten-free diet: A nutritional risk factor for adolescents with celiac disease? *J. Pediatr. Gastroenterol. Nutr.* **1998**, *27*, 519–523. [CrossRef] [PubMed]
95. Tortora, R.; Capone, P.; De Stefano, G.; Imperatore, N.; Gerbino, N.; Donetto, S.; Monaco, V.; Caporaso, N.; Rispo, A. Metabolic syndrome in patients with coeliac disease on a gluten-free diet. *Aliment. Pharmacol. Ther.* **2015**, *41*, 352–359. [CrossRef] [PubMed]
96. Potter, M.D.E.; Brienesse, S.C.; Walker, M.M.; Boyle, A.; Talley, N.J. Effect of the gluten-free diet on cardiovascular risk factors in patients with coeliac disease: A systematic review. *J. Gastroenterol. Hepatol.* **2018**, *33*, 781–791. [CrossRef] [PubMed]
97. Ercolini, D.; Francavilla, R.; Vannini, L.; De Filippis, F.; Capriati, T.; Di Cagno, R.; Iacono, G.; De Angelis, M.; Gobbetti, M. From an imbalance to a new imbalance: Italian-style gluten-free diet alters the salivary microbiota and metabolome of African celiac children. *Sci. Rep.* **2015**, *5*, 18571. [CrossRef] [PubMed]
98. Verma, A.K.; Gatti, S.; Galeazzi, T.; Monachesi, C.; Padella, L.; Del Baldo, G.; Annibali, R.; Lionetti, E.; Catassi, C. Gluten contamination in naturally or labeled gluten-free products marketed in Italy. *Nutrients* **2017**, *9*, 115. [CrossRef] [PubMed]
99. Cabrera-Chaves, F.; Iametti, S.; Miriani, M.; de la Barca, A.M.; Mamone, G.; Bonomi, F. Maize prolamins resistant to peptic-tryptic digestion maintain immune-recognition by IgA from some celiac disease patients. *Plant Foods Hum. Nutr.* **2012**, *67*, 24. [CrossRef] [PubMed]
100. Hossain, M. *Long-Term Prospects for the Global Rice Economy, in Rice in Global Markets and Sustainable Production Systems*; Food and Agriculture Organization of the United Nations: Rome, Italy, 2004.
101. Catassi, C.; Gatti, S.; Fasano, A. The new epidemiology of celiac disease. *J. Pediatr. Gastroenterol. Nutr.* **2014**, *59*, S7–S9. [CrossRef] [PubMed]
102. Walker, A.J.; Curtis, H.J.; Bacon, S.; Croker, R.; Goldacre, B. Trends, geographical variation and factors associated with prescribing of gluten-free foods in English primary care: A cross-sectional study. *BMJ Open* **2018**, *8*, e021312. [CrossRef] [PubMed]
103. Lu, Z.; Zhang, H.; Luoto, S.; Ren, X. Gluten-free living in China: The characteristics, food choices and difficulties in following a gluten-free diet—An online survey. *Appetite* **2018**, *127*, 242–248. [CrossRef] [PubMed]
104. Halmos, E.P.; Deng, M.; Knowles, S.R.; Sainsbury, K.; Mullan, B.; Tye-Din, J.A. Food knowledge and psychological state predict adherence to a gluten-free diet in a survey of 5310 Australians and New Zealanders with coeliac disease. *Aliment. Pharmacol. Ther.* **2018**. [CrossRef] [PubMed]
105. Norsa, L.; Branchi, F.; Bravo, M.; Ferretti, F.; Roncoroni, L.; Somalvico, F.; Conte, D.; Bardella, M.T.; Fabiano, S.; Barigelletti, G.; et al. Celiac disease 30 years after diagnosis: Struggling with gluten-free adherence or gaining gluten tolerance? *J. Pediatr. Gastroenterol. Nutr.* **2018**. [CrossRef] [PubMed]

nutrients

MDPI

Article

Adherence to Gluten-Free Diet in Children with Celiac Disease

Grażyna Czaja-Bulsa [1,*] and Michał Bulsa [2]

[1] Department of Pediatric Diseases and Pediatric Nursing, Clinic of Pediatrics, Gastrology and Childrens Rheumatology, Pomeranian Medical University, 71-454 Szczecin, Poland

[2] Department of Gynecological Surgery and Gynecological Oncology of Adults and Adolescents, Pomeranian Medical University, 71-454 Szczecin, Poland; michal.bulsa@gmail.com

* Correspondence: grazyna.bulsa@pum.edu.pl

Received: 27 August 2018; Accepted: 28 September 2018; Published: 4 October 2018

Abstract: Celiac disease (CD) can only be treated by rigorous life-long gluten-free diet (GFD). The study included 102 mothers and their CD children treated with GFD for at least two years. Frequency and cause of diet failure in children treated at present (54 children) and 10 years ago (48 children) were compared. Dietary adherence was evaluated serologically (tTG), while diet management difficulties were examined by means of a questionnaire. The study shows that one-third of patients fail to follow GFD, more often 10 years ago than now (40% vs. 26%; $p < 0.05$), mainly children aged 13–18 (54% vs. 40% now; $p < 0.05$). Younger children (up to 12) are less likely to abandon the diet (27% vs. 8%; $p < 0.05$). In this age group non-intentional diet failure prevails, while teenagers interrupt their diet intentionally (45% vs. 33%; p = ns (small population of children in this groups)). Currently, the most common causes of teenage diet failure are the absence of symptoms after consuming a small amount of gluten and, even more often, troublesome diet administration. Previously, the absence of peer acceptance prevailed. With this study we found that: 1. In West Pomerania, every fourth CD child does not follow GFD. 2. For years, teenagers have failed to follow GFD due to the absence of symptoms after consuming small amounts of gluten. 3. The incidence of non-intentional failure to follow GFD has significantly decreased over years, which indicates better dietary care.

Keywords: gluten-free diet; celiac disease; children; teenagers

---

1. Background

Celiac disease (CD) is a genetically conditioned, immunologically mediated chronic intestinal disease, in which in genetically predisposed people the consumption of gluten leads to the disappearance of intestinal flora [1]. This results in reduced nutrient absorption. The disease frequency is steadily increasing—in Europe and America it affects 1% of people. The only effective way of its treatment is life-long strict adherence to a gluten-free diet (GFD) [1]. The gluten-free diet consists in the complete elimination of products derived from wheat, rye, and barley and products processed from these cereals. They are replaced by naturally gluten-free products (maize, rice, oats, buckwheat, lamb, meat, fish, vegetables, fruit) or by products from which gluten has been removed. Adherence to GFD leads to the regeneration of intestinal villi after a period of 6 to 24 months. The life-long GFD secures a child's proper development and protects them from ailments such as abdominal pain, flatulence, loose stools, constipation, iron deficiency anemia, low stature, and osteoporosis. In adults with CD, it also reduces the risk of cardiovascular diseases and intestinal tumors [1,2].

The most reliable method to control GFD adherence are serological tests and small intestine biopsy [1]. It is recommended to determine serum tissue transglutaminase concentration in IgA class (IgA-tTG), while in patients with selective IgA deficiency—in IgG class (IgG-tTG) [1]. The determination of tTG concentration in patients treated with GFD is commonly referred to as the 'lie test' because it allows to identify people who do not follow the diet. Being an invasive test, endoscopic small intestine biopsy is not recommended to confirm non-adherence to GFD.

Some researchers suggest using nutritional history to assess the GFD adherence. However, it does not allow to identify patients who non-intentionally fail to adhere to GFD, therefore its importance for monitoring procedures is low. Leffler et al. proposed a seven-point questionnaire to identify patients who did not adhere to GFD (Celiac Dietary Adherence Test, CDAT). The test assesses their knowledge of the disease, which, according to Leffler, is highly correlated with serological test results [3]. In 2017, a new method was proposed to confirm the consumption or nibbling of gluten by people with CD. The method consists in determination of gluten immunogenic proteins in urine [4]. This is a very attractive proposal as the test is non-invasive.

Adherence to GFD is troublesome [5]. The patients or their guardians are required to have extensive knowledge about CD and the GFD requirements. The changes in eating habits affect not only the patient, but often their whole family. According to Meyer et al., in order to better manage CD the daily routines of young patients should be carefully examined to help them strictly comply with GFD [6]. The GFD preparation time is much longer than that of a diet containing gluten [7]. Also, it is much more expensive than traditional nutrition, which limits its availability to many patients. Fortunately, in some countries the costs of GFD are partially refunded [8,9]. It was noted that in such countries the patients who receive products free of charge follow the GFD requirements more often [7,10]. For the low-income adult patients the high cost of GFD products is a barrier to diet adherence [11]. On the other hand, the studies of Humayun et al. and Leffler et al. did not confirm the significant influence of the GFD price on the frequency of the GFD adherence, except for those CD adult patients who openly declared that the high price of products made it difficult for them to follow the diet [3,7].

In the opinion of some authors, the following factors contribute to the better adherence to GFD: good knowledge of the disease and its treatment, higher education level, better social situation of the family, female sex, young age, high self-esteem, good grades at school, good availability and labelling of products, good contact with a doctor and a dietitian, and finally, membership in the Coeliac Society [5,7,11–13]. The Coeliac Society members understand the disease better and know how to prepare gluten-free meals. They also receive stronger day-to-day support (meetings, help in obtaining GFD products, partially reimbursed youth camps) [7,10,14].

The factors responsible for not adhering to GFD are: poor taste of gluten-free products, their high price and low availability (especially during travel and social meetings), the patient's adolescence, the absence of immediate symptoms after consuming small amounts of gluten, and low awareness of the disease [5,11,13].

Better awareness of the factors that have significant impact on the GFD adherence can improve the supervision of CD patients.

The aim of this study was to determine the incidence and causes of non-adherence to GFD by children with CD treated now and 10 years ago.

The first analysis of the causes of failure to adhere to GFD was carried out in 2006–2007 with a view to improving the effectiveness of CD treatment, as it had been observed that many patients discontinued GDF after years of adherence. In recent years, GFD has become popular in Poland and therefore the conclusions concerning the patients' failure to adhere to GFD 10 years ago are no longer relevant. Unfortunately, it has been observed that teenagers still tend to discontinue their GFD. Therefore, in the 2016–2017 study, the questions about the reason for failure to follow GFD were again included in the CD patients' medical history.

2. Materials and Methods

The study covered 102 children (64 girls) with coeliac disease (CD) treated with GFD. All patients were diagnosed in accordance with the applicable criteria: elevated antibodies anti–endomysium (EMA) and anti-tissue transglutaminase (tTG) as well as duodenal atrophy of intestinal mucosa [1].

There were no patients with selective IgA deficiency in the study group, therefore antibodies were determined only in the IgA class. At the time of their CD diagnosis the mean IgA-EMA concentration was 1:120 (range: 1:170–1:10) and IgA-tTG was 171 RU/mL (range: 297 RU/mL–38 RU/mL). During the first two years after the diagnosis, serological indicators (EMA and tTG) normalized in all patients, in most of them already in the first year of treatment. It is believed that in patients treated with GFD, a two-year period is sufficient to fully normalize the antibodies concentration and the intestinal mucosa [15].

The patients were recruited during their GFD treatment, two years or more after the diagnosis, during control tests performed routinely twice a year. The mean time of the GFD treatment before their inclusion in the study was 104 months (28 months–208 months).

During the medical interview, patients made a declaration concerning their dietary adherence. If they reported that they did not follow the diet, they were asked to give reasons. Five probable causes were specified: poor taste of the diet, its high price, troublesome dietary regime (understood as problems with the purchase of gluten-free diet, its labelling, the inability to eat outside the home), difficulties in relationships with peers (due to being rejected by the peer group) and the absence of symptoms after consuming gluten products. Each patient was asked to choose which of the reasons was the most relevant to them, i.e., which led to deliberately abandoning of GFD. In the case of the youngest children (under seven years of age), dietary declarations were made by their guardians (in this study all of them were mothers). Older children with CD and their guardians jointly chose the most important reason for their failure to follow GFD.

The tests performed during each control visit included serum assays of tissue transglutaminase (tTG) in the IgA class. The presence of tTG antibodies in serum confirmed that the CD patient had consumed gluten. Patients who claimed to adhere to GFD and in whose blood tTG antibodies were found were considered as those who non-intentionally failed to adhere to GFD. In 33 children who did not follow GFD, the average IgA-tTG concentration was 126 RU/mL (264 RU/mL–22 RU/mL). In children adhering to GFD the IgA-tTG concentration was below 20 RU/mL.

Patients were divided into two groups: children (0–12 years old) and teenagers (13–18 years old) (Table 1). The frequency and reason for non-adherence to GFD was compared between children treated now (54 children) and 10 years before (48 children).

Table 1. Number of children covered by the study in 2006–2007 and in 2016–2017.

Child's Age (years)	Number of Children		Σ
2006–2007	2006–2007	2016–2017	
0–12	26	24	50
13–18	22	30	52
0–18	48	54	102

EMA was determined by indirect immunofluorescence test (standard < 1:10), while IgA-tTG was assayed by ELISA (standard < 20 RU/mL). The obtained results were subjected to statistical analysis. The Student's *t*-test was used for independent trials.

The survey did not require the permission of the PUM (Pomeranian Medical University) Bioethical Committee. The relevant opinion was obtained from the Chairman of the Committee in 2006. All subjects had given their informed consent for inclusion before they were included in the study.

3. Results

It has been shown that children with CD are now more likely to adhere to GFD than before. In 2016–2017, 26% of children did not adhere to GFD, whereas 10 years earlier, in 2006–2007, as many as 40% failed to do so ($p < 0.05$) (Figure 1). Those were mainly children aged 13–18 (40%) by age (cumulative assessment of 2006–2007 and 2016–2017 studies) now and 54% a decade ago; $p < 0.05$). Younger children (up to 12 years) were less likely to miss the diet (8% at present and 27% a decade ago; $p < 0.05$). At that age, the incidence of non-intentional GFD failure was larger: 4% at present (1 of 24 children) and 19% previously (5 of 26 children) (Figure 2). Teenagers often intentionally interrupt their diet: 33% now (10 of 30 children) and 45% a decade ago (10 of 22 children) (Figure 2). Currently, the most common reason for the teenage diet failure is the lack of symptoms after consuming a small amount of gluten products, while the inconvenience of GFD regime is less common (Figures 3 and 4). In 2006–2007, the main reason for GFD non-adherence was the difficulty in peer relations (rejection by peer groups), while the absence of symptoms after occasional gluten intake or troublesome dietary regime were less common (Figures 3 and 4).

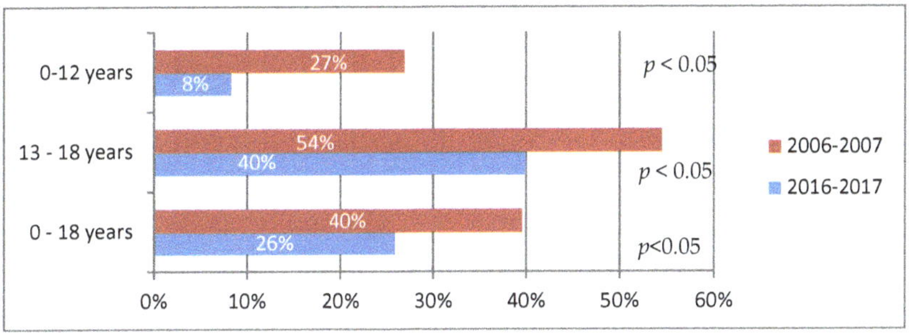

Figure 1. Proportion of children failing to adhere to gluten-free diet (GFD) by age and time of study.

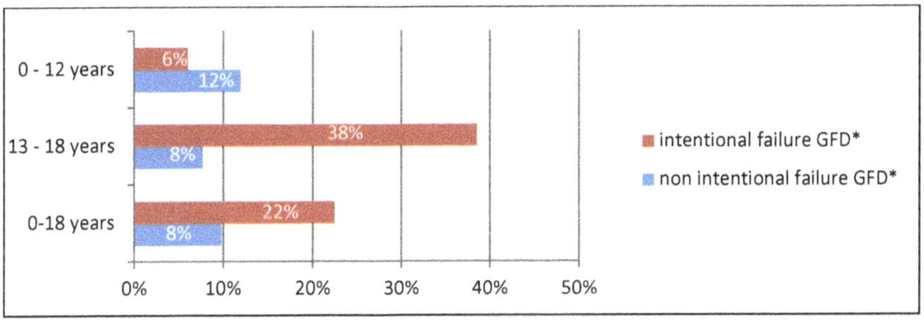

Figure 2. Incidence to intentional and non-intentional failure to adhere to gluten-free diet (GFD). * GFD—gluten-free diet.

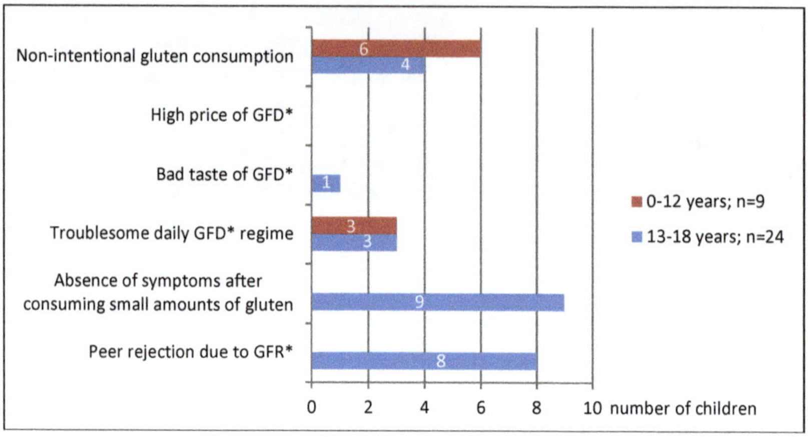

Figure 3. Reasons for non-adherence to gluten-free diet (GFD) by age. * GFD—gluten free diet.

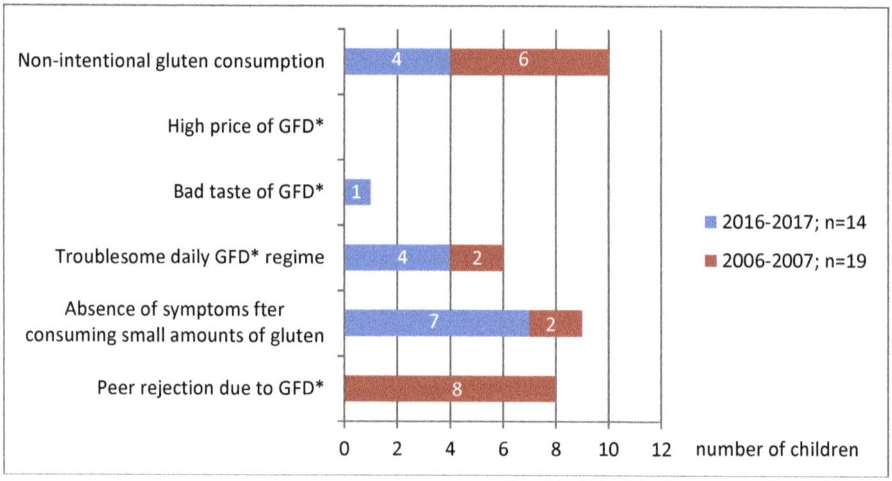

Figure 4. Reasons for GFD non-adherence by time of study. * GFD—gluten-free diet.

4. Discussion

The analysis shows that currently every fourth child with CD does not adhere to GFD (Figure 1). Ten years ago, in 2006–2007, the failure to adhere to GFD was more common, and was reported by as many as 40% of the respondents. Studies in other countries have shown that between 30% and 75% of patients fail to follow GFD [7,11,14,16]. In Polish multi-center studies conducted in 2010—2013 and covering 277 children with CD, it was found that GFD was not observed by 25% of patients, of whom 19% had abandoned the diet intentionally [17].

Currently, teenagers are five times more likely not to adhere to GFD than younger children (40% vs. 8%). In 2006–2007, teenagers consumed gluten only twice as often as younger children (54% vs. 27%). Similar observations were made by other researchers [5,12,18]. What has clearly decreased in recent years is the incidence of dietary failure among younger children, who most often fail to follow GFD unintentionally (Figure 2). In this group, the intentional failure to adhere to the diet was primarily a consequence of their parents' inability to provide them with a sufficient amount of gluten-free products. In those years, the access to such products was much more difficult than today. Currently, CD families are better prepared to adopt GFD. The improved ability of parents and children to identify gluten-free products is a consequence of better dietary support, greater involvement of the Coeliac Society (regular meetings, publications), improved labelling of gluten-free products and a more convenient way to obtain them (online shopping).

Both 10 years ago and now, the majority of CD teenagers intentionally fail to adhere to GFD (Figure 2), which has also been found out by other authors [5]. Currently, the main reason for their failure to adhere to GFD is that they believe that the systematic low intake of gluten does not affect their health, as it does not cause any intestinal symptoms which they experienced before (Figures 3 and 4). Unfortunately, non-adherence to GFD at this age does not correlate well with the presence of the CD symptoms.

In younger children (<3 years), the consumption of even the smallest amounts of gluten usually result in intestinal symptoms, most commonly abdominal pain or abnormal stools. Teenagers, seeing that such a co-incidence no longer occurs, start to believe that they can consume gluten in small amounts. There are patients who are able to precisely define the amount of gluten that cause the symptoms. Therefore, they try to consume smaller amounts, which in their opinion does not harm their health. In this group of patients, dietary errors are caused by insufficient knowledge of CD and its treatment. They need to be informed about the CD again. It seems that such information should be provided to every juvenile patient once they enter adolescence. It should be particularly pointed out that, at this age, eating small amounts of gluten may not cause such intestinal discomfort as previously, but it still remains detrimental to their health. We try to persuade these patients to adhere strictly to GFD by showing them that their growth rate has been slowed down, anemia induced by iron deficiency has occurred, bone density has decreased (in densitometric evaluation), and antibodies indicating CD activity have appeared in serum. In some cases, we repeat endoscopic tests of fragments from the duodenum in order to show that intestinal villi atrophy has reoccurred in their duodenum. We explain that these are the complications due to the young patient's failure to adhere to GFD and that they have appeared independently from the absence of intestinal discomfort. Systematic monitoring of teenagers' dietary adherence is absolutely essential, even if they have had a history of strict GFD adherence. Other authors also believe that the lack of immediate symptoms after consumption of small amounts of gluten is an important factor in teenagers' failure to adhere to GFD [5].

Ten years earlier, in 2006–2007, the main cause of non-adherence to GFD by teenagers was peer rejection due to their different dietary regime. These children were stigmatized by other children and isolated from the group. In order not to be socially excluded, teenagers with CD intentionally consumed gluten products while in social situations. None of these children changed their behavior throughout the treatment period (up to 18 years), despite having been informed about the adverse effects of such behavior. Similar teenagers' attitudes have also been described by other authors [5,6,16,19]. Swedish studies have found that girls are more likely than boys to follow GFD [20].

In our 2016–2017 study, none of the children reported the above as a reason for non-adherence to GFD. This is a consequence of a change in social customs. Today, GFD has become popular in Poland and it is used by many people who do not suffer from CD. Similar trends have also been observed in other countries where the frequency of GFD consumption far exceeds the number of CD patients [19,21,22].

Younger children have never reported this problem. In kindergartens and schools, they consumed gluten-free products and that fact did not have any negative impact on their peer relations.

At present, just like 10 years ago, the second most frequent reason for non-adherence to GFD is its troublesome administration, as reported by both younger children and adolescents (Figures 3 and 4). By the troublesome use of GFD we mean a number of difficulties encountered by a patient in everyday life. These are: problems with buying GFD and with label reading, as well as the inability to eat out, which makes travelling and social gatherings more difficult. In the years 2006–2007 in Poland the purchase of gluten-free products was possible only in specialist shops located in large cities. That significantly hindered access to gluten-free food for the residents of small towns and villages. It forced people to prepare gluten-free products (bread, cakes, pasta) on their own at home. There were no possibilities to order gluten-free meals outside one's place of residence. The children went on trips with their own bread, which significantly limited their ability to travel. The only form of organized tourism were camps organized by the Coeliac Society, but they were not widely available. The situation is now much better. Most families buy gluten-free products online, and in many towns and cities there are gluten-free food stands in supermarkets. There is a wide offer of children and youth camps serving gluten-free menu that are organized not only by the Coeliac Society. However, the possibility of eating out is still very limited, even though the situation has improved considerably in recent years. Currently, GFD has become 'trendy' in Poland, it is chosen by many people, not only by the CD patients. In many restaurants you can order gluten-free menu. Unfortunately, most of such places are usually located in large towns, which still hampers the CD patients' mobility. Similar difficulties are also highlighted by other authors from other countries [5,7,13,23]. In Wolf et al. studies, difficulties with eating outside the home were more frequently reported by teenagers than by adults (87% vs. 74%) [24]. In our study on teenagers, that was the main factor indicating the troublesome character of the diet. Parents of younger children (<12 years old) reported difficulty in reading labels on gluten-free products, their high price, and difficult access.

When buying gluten-free products, patients can benefit from a mobile application containing an inventory of gluten-free products available in a given country [25]. Such an application has been available in Poland since spring 2017. It is free of charge for patients with CD belonging to the Coeliac Society. In Canada, as many as a quarter of patients reported that it would be very helpful to include a list of 100 most frequently purchased gluten-free products in their mobile applications. Silvester et al. have shown that in the USA only 25% of adults with CD are able to recognize the majority of gluten products from the list (14 out of 17 products) [14].

In our studies none of the CD patients gave a high GFD price as the main reason for not following it. That was another, but not the most important, reason. During the 2006–2007 study, all Polish children with CD received a cash allowance to buy GFD. Unfortunately, today the allowance is not available to the majority of children. Many authors point out that the high price of GFD is an important reason for not adhering to GFD by many patients [11,13,26]. It is also an essential factor affecting the quality of life of adult patients with CD [27].

None of the examined groups of children indicated the illegible labelling of the gluten-free products as the most important reason for not adhering to GFD, which has also been reported by other researchers [7,8,13].

Strict adherence to GFD is most common among patients with greater knowledge of their disease [24]. They are 'extremely vigilant' in selecting the right products. They eat meals only at home, as they are afraid to eat out. They are constantly using the Internet and mobile applications to help them buy GFD products. They are more likely to experience anxiety and fatigue. Their quality of life (QoL) is significantly lower than that of patients who are 'less vigilant' in the choice of GFD [24]. This applies to teenagers as much as to adults, more often to women [27]. This is a negative consequence of strict adherence to the diet and points to the need to provide psychological and emotional support for the patients with CD. The opposite results were obtained by other researchers in their studies on adults which revealed better quality of life reported by patients strictly adhering to GFD [5,28]. The discrepancies between the two findings have been explained by Nachman et al. who showed that in the first year of strict adherence to GFD the quality of life of adult CD patients was higher (symptoms disappeared), but then it significantly decreased (probably due to the difficulty in strict maintenance of GFD) [29]. Mazzone et al. demonstrated that children and teenagers with CD were more likely to experience emotional and behavioral problems, particularly loneliness and depression, than their healthy peers [30]. Parents rated the quality of life of their CD children lower than the children themselves [31].

5. Conclusions

Over the last 10 years, an increase in the number of children with celiac disease adhering to the gluten-free diet has been observed in the West Pomeranian region. Similarly, to other countries, today every fourth child with celiac disease does not follow a gluten-free diet.

For years, it was teenagers who most often failed to adhere to the gluten-free diet. The lack of awareness of the course of the disease, the increasing independence from parents, the need to buy food and prepare meals for themselves, the need to better organize everyday life as well as the environmental pressure are the factors resulting in more frequent failure to follow GFD. Teenagers require psychological support and repeated instruction explaining to them that they cannot eat even the smallest amounts of gluten, even though it does not cause any intestinal symptoms at this age, but unfortunately is harmful to their health.

Over the years, the frequency of non-intentional non-adherence to the gluten-free diet has significantly decreased as a result of better dietary care.

Systematic medical and dietary supervision contributes to more effective treatment of children with celiac disease, which in turn ensures their proper development and prevents complications.

Author Contributions: G.C.-B.—work concept, data interpretation and analysis, writing the manuscript. M.B.—summary of results, writing the article.

Conflicts of Interest: The authors declare no conflict of interest.

References

1. Husby, S.; Koletzko, S.; Korponay-Szabó, I.R.; Mearin, M.L.; Phillips, A.; Shamir, R.; Troncone, R.; Giersiepen, K.; Branski, D.; Catassi, C.; et al. European Society for Pediatric Gastroenterology, Hepatology, and Nutrition guidelines for the diagnosis of coeliac disease. *J. Pediatr. Gastroenterol. Nutr.* **2012**, *54*, 136–160. [CrossRef] [PubMed]
2. Bathrellou, E.; Kontogianni, M.D.; Panagiotakos, D.B. Celiac disease and nonb-celic gluten or wheat sensitivity and health in later life: A review. *Maturotas* **2018**, *112*, 29–33. [CrossRef] [PubMed]
3. Leffler, D.A.; Dennis, M.; Edwards George, J.B.; Jamma, S.; Magge, S.; Cook, E.F.; Schuppan, D.; Kelly, C.P. A Simple Validated Gluten-Free Diet Adherence Survey for Adult with Celiac disease. *Clin. Gastroenterol. Hepatol.* **2009**, *7*, 530–536. [CrossRef] [PubMed]
4. Moreno, M.; Cebolla, A.; Muñoz-Suano, A.; Carrillo-Carrion, C.; Comino, I.; Pizarro, Á.; León, F.; Rodríguez-Herrera, A.; Sousa, C. Detection of gluten immunogenic peptides in the urine of patients with coeliac disease reveals transgression in the gluten gluten-free diet and incomplete mucosal healing. *Gut* **2017**, *66*, 250–257. [CrossRef] [PubMed]
5. Freeman, H.J. Dietary compliance in celiac disease. *World J. Gastroenterol.* **2017**, *23*, 2635–2639. [CrossRef] [PubMed]
6. Muhammad, H.; Reeves, S.; Ishag, S.; Mayberry, J.; Jeanes, Y.M. Adherence to a Gluten Free Diet is Associated with Receiving Gluten Free Foods on Prescripion and Understanding Food Labelling. *Nutrients* **2017**, *9*. [CrossRef] [PubMed]
7. Silvester, J.A.; Weiten, D.; Graff, L.A.; Walker, J.R.; Duerksen, D.R. Is it gluten-free? Relationship between self-reported gluten-free diet adherence and knowledge of gluten content of foods. *Nutrition* **2016**, *32*, 777–783. [CrossRef] [PubMed]
8. Silvester, J.A.; Weiten, D.; Graff, L.A.; Walker, J.R.; Duerksen, D.R. Living gluten-free: adherence, knowledge, lifestyle adaptations and feelings towards a gluten-free diet. *J. Hum. Nutr. Diet.* **2016**, *29*, 374–382. [CrossRef] [PubMed]
9. Villafuerte-Galvez, J.; Vanga, R.R.; Dennis, M.; Hansen, J.; Leffler, D.A.; Kelly, C.P.; Mukherjee, R. Factors governing long-term adherence to a gluten-free diet in adult patients with coeliac disease. *Aliment. Pharmacol. Ther.* **2015**, *42*, 753–760. [CrossRef] [PubMed]
10. Stolarczyk, A.; Matuszczyk, M.; Rybak, A.; Socha, P.; Oralewska, B.; Szaflarska-Popławska, A.; Jarocka-Cyrta, E.; Iwańczak, B.; Grzybowska-Chlebowczyk, U.; Cichy, W.; et al. Dietary assessment of

children with coeliac disease—Is diet a risk factor of atherosclerosis? *Med. Stand. Pediatr.* **2014**, *11*, 428–439. (In Polish)
11. Greco, L.; Mayer, M.; Ciccarelli, G.; Troncone, R.; Auricchio, S. Compliance to a gluten-free diet in adolescents, or, "what do 300 coeliac adolescents eat every day?". *Ital. J. Gastroenterol. Hepatol.* **1997**, *29*, 305–310. [PubMed]
12. White, L.E.; Bannerman, E.; Gillet, P.M. Coeliac disease and the gluten-free diet: A review of the burdens; factors associated with adherence and impact on health-related quality of live, with specific focus on adolescence. *J. Hum. Nutr. Diet.* **2016**, *29*, 593–606. [CrossRef] [PubMed]
13. Kurppa, K.; Lauronen, O.; Collin, P.; Ukkola, A.; Laurila, K.; Huhtala, H.; Mäki, M.; Kaukinen, K. Factors associated with dietary adherence in celiac disease: A nationwide study. *Digestion* **2012**, *86*, 309–314. [CrossRef] [PubMed]
14. Meyer, S.; Rosenblum, S. Activities, Participation and Quality of Life Concepts in Children and Adolescents with Celiac Disease: A Scoping Review. *Nutrients* **2017**, *24*. [CrossRef]
15. Bulka, C.M.; Davis, M.A.; Karagas, M.R.; Ahsan, H.; Argos, M. The Unintended Consequences of a Gluten-Free Diet. *Epidemiology* **2017**, *28*, e24–e25. [CrossRef] [PubMed]
16. Ljungman, G.; Myrdal, U. Compliance in teenagers with coeliac disease—A Swedish follow-up study. *Acta Paediatr.* **1993**, *82*, 235–238. [CrossRef] [PubMed]
17. Choung, R.S.; Ditah, I.C.; Nadeau, A.M.; Rubio-Tapia, A.; Marietta, E.V.; Brantner, T.L.; Camilleri, M.J.; Rajkumar, S.V.; Landgren, O.; Everhart, J.E.; et al. Trends and racial/ethnic disparities in gluten-sensitive problems in the United States: Findings from National Health and Nutrition Examination Surveys from 1988 to 2012. *Am. J. Gastroenterol.* **2015**, *110*, 455–461. [CrossRef] [PubMed]
18. Choung, R.S.; Unalp-Arida, A.; Ruhl, C.E.; Brantner, T.L.; Everhart, J.E.; Murray, J.A. Less Hidden Celiac Disease but Increased Gluten Avoidance without a Diagnosis in the United States: Findings from the National Health and Nutrition Examination Surveys from 2009 to 2014. *Mayo Clin. Proc.* **2016**. [CrossRef]
19. Roma, E.; Roubani, A.; Kolia, E.; Panayiotou, J.; Zellos, A.; Syriopoulou, V.P. Dietary compliance and life style of children with coeliac disease. *J. Hum. Nutr. Diet.* **2010**, *23*, 176–182. [CrossRef] [PubMed]
20. Olson, H.C.; Lyon, P.; Hörnell, A.; Ivarsson, A.; Sydner, Y.M. Food that makes you different: The stigma experienced by adolescents with celiac disease. *Qual. Health Res.* **2009**, *19*, 976–984. [CrossRef] [PubMed]
21. Wolf, R.L.; Lebwohl, B.; Lee, A.R.; Zybert, P.; Reilly, N.R.; Cadenhead, J.; Amengual, C.; Green, P.H.R. Hypervigilance to a Gluten-Free Diet and Decreased Quality of Life in Teenagers and Adults with Celiac Disease. *Dig. Dis. Sci.* **2018**, *63*, 1438–1448. [CrossRef] [PubMed]
22. Dowd, A.J.; Jackson, C.; Tang, K.T.Y.; Nielsen, D.; Clarkin, D.H.; Culos-Reed, S.N. MyHealthyGut: Development of a theory-based self-regulatory app to effectievely manage celiac disease. *Mhealth* **2018**, *4*, 19. [CrossRef] [PubMed]
23. Singh, J.; Whelan, K. Limited availability and higher cost of gluten-free foods. *J. Hum. Nutr. Diet.* **2011**, *24*, 479–486. [CrossRef] [PubMed]
24. Martinez-Martinez, M.I.; Alegre-Martinez, A.; Garcia-Ibanez, J.; Cauli, O. Quality of life in people with coeliac disease: Psychological and social-economic aspects. *Endocr. Metab. Immune. Disord. Drug Targets* **2018**. [CrossRef] [PubMed]
25. Verrill, L.; Zhang, Y.; Kane, R. Food label usage and reported difficulty with following a gluten-free diet among individuals in the USA with coeliac disease and those with noncoeliac gluten sensitivity. *J. Hum. Nutr. Diet.* **2013**, *26*, 479–487. [CrossRef] [PubMed]
26. Burden, M.; Mooney, P.D.; Blanshard, R.J.; White, W.L.; Cambray-Deakin, D.R.; Sanders, D.S. Cost and availability of gluten-free foods in the UK: In store and online. *Postgrad. Med. J.* **2015**, *91*, 622–626. [CrossRef] [PubMed]
27. Hall, N.J.; Rubin, G.P.; Charnock, A. Intentional and inadvertent non-adherence in adult coeliac disease. A cross-sectional survey. *Appetite* **2013**, *68*, 56–62. [PubMed]
28. Burger, J.P.W.; de Brouver, B.; IntHout, J.; Wahab, P.J.; Tummers, M.; Drenth, J.P.H. Systematic review with meta-analysis: Dietary adherence influences normalization of health-related quality of life in coeliac disease. *Clin. Nutr.* **2017**, *36*, 399–406. [CrossRef] [PubMed]
29. Nachman, F.; del Campo, M.; González, A.; Corzo, L.; Vázquez, H.; Sfoggia, C.; Smecuol, E.; Sánchez, M.I.; Niveloni, S.; Sugai, E.; et al. Long-term deterioration of quality of live in adult patients with celiac disease is associated with treatment noncompliance. *Dig. Liver Dis.* **2010**, *42*, 685–691. [CrossRef] [PubMed]

30. Mazzone, L.; Reale, L.; Spina, M.; Guarnera, M.; Lionetti, E.; Martorana, S.; Mazzone, D. Compliant gluten-free children with celiac disease: an evaluation of psychological distress. *BMC Pediatr.* **2011**, *11*, 46. [CrossRef] [PubMed]
31. Byström, I.M.; Hollen, E.; Fälth-Magnusson, K.; Johansson, A.K. Health-Related Quality of Life in Children and Adolescents with Celiac disease: From the Perspectives of Children and Parents. *Gastroenterol. Res. Pract.* **2012**. [CrossRef] [PubMed]

nutrients

MDPI

Article

First Insights into the Gut Microbiota of Mexican Patients with Celiac Disease and Non-Celiac Gluten Sensitivity

Jose F. Garcia-Mazcorro [1], Xaira Rivera-Gutierrez [1], Orestes De Jesus Cobos-Quevedo [1], Peter Grube-Pagola [1], Arturo Meixueiro-Daza [1], Karina Hernandez-Flores [1], Francisco J. Cabrera-Jorge [1], Hector Vivanco-Cid [1], Scot E. Dowd [2] and Jose M. Remes-Troche [3,*]

1 Instituto de Investigaciones Medico Biológicas, Universidad Veracruzana, Calle Agustín de Iturbide, Salvador Díaz Mirón, 91700 Veracruz, México; josegarcia_mex@hotmail.com (J.F.G.-M.); xaai.rg@gmail.com (X.R.-G.); orestes.cq7@gmail.com (O.D.J.C.-Q.); grubejr78@gmail.com (P.G.-P.); arturomeixueiro@hotmail.com (A.M.-D.); karinahernandezflores@gmail.com (K.H.-F.); fco-javier-cj@hotmail.com (F.J.C.-J.); hvivanco@uv.mx (H.V.-C.)

2 Molecular Research LP, 503 Clovis Rd, Shallowater, TX 79363, USA; sdowd@mrdnalab.com

3 Laboratorio de Fisiología Digestiva y Motilidad Gastrointestinal, Instituto de Investigaciones Medico Biológicas, Universidad Veracruzana, Calle Agustín de Iturbide, Salvador Díaz Mirón, 91700 Veracruz, México

* Correspondence: josegarcia_mex@hotmail.com or jose.remes.troche@gmail.com; Tel.: +1-229-931-8011

Received: 5 October 2018; Accepted: 31 October 2018; Published: 2 November 2018

Abstract: Gluten-related disorders (GRDs) are common chronic enteropathies and increasing evidence suggests an involvement of the gut microbiota. We examined the gut microbiota in Mexican people afflicted with GRDs. Ultra-high-throughput 16S marker sequencing was used to deeply describe the duodenal and fecal microbiota of patients with celiac disease (CD, $n = 6$), non-celiac gluten sensitivity (NCGS, $n = 12$), and healthy subjects ($n = 12$) from our local area. Additionally, we also investigated the changes in gut microbiota after four weeks on a gluten-free diet (GFD) in a subset of patients from whom paired samples were available. Despite a high inter-individual variability, significant differences in various microbial populations were identified. The linear discriminant analysis (LDA) effect size (LEfSe) method revealed that the genus *Actinobacillus* and the family Ruminococcaceae were higher in the duodenal and fecal microbiota of NCGS patients, respectively, while *Novispirillum* was higher in the duodenum of CD patients ($p < 0.05$, LDA score > 3.5). Interestingly, paired samples from NCGS patients showed a significant difference in duodenal *Pseudomonas* between the baseline period (median: 1.3%; min/max: 0.47–6.8%) and the period after four weeks on GFD (14.8%; 2.3–38.5%, $p < 0.01$, Wilcoxon signed-rank test). These results encourage more research on GRDs in México.

Keywords: gluten-related disorders; celiac disease; gut microbiota; gluten-free diet; *Pseudomonas*

1. Introduction

The gut microbiota is comprised of thousands of microbial species that vary widely among individuals [1] and also over time within the same individual due to environmental factors such as dietary patterns [2]. The gut microbiota helps modulate the immune system [3] and has been associated with diseases related to the alimentary tract such as obesity and inflammatory bowel diseases [4]. Given the close relationship between the immune system and microorganisms inside the gut, it is believed that most disorders of the digestive tract bear some relationship with the gut microbiota although a cause-effect relationship can hardly be established [5].

Gluten-related disorder (GRD) is a general term to describe all maladies triggered by gluten, with celiac disease (CD) being the most studied. CD is an autoimmune disorder where the consumption of gluten leads to an abnormal T cell-mediated immune response and damage to epithelial cells in genetically susceptible individuals [6,7]. Other factors related to CD include perinatal environmental factors such as the duration of breastfeeding as well as gut-microbiota interactions [8] and the only available treatment for GRDs is a life-long consumption of a gluten-free diet (GFD). On the other hand, non-celiac gluten sensitivity (NCGS) is a different GRD yet it also responds to a gluten-free diet (GFD) [9,10]. The diagnosis of NCGS is based on the clinical response to GFD and the exclusion of other syndromes as there is no NCGS-specific biomarker yet identified like in wheat's allergy (e.g., the presence of IgE) or CD (e.g., the presence of TG2 antibodies) [11].

Growing evidence suggests that the gut microbiota is closely related to GRDs, particularly CD [8,12]; however, a disease-specific microbial signature of GRDs has not yet been defined and there is a lack of consensus with respect to the specific changes involved in these disorders with or without dietary gluten [12–15], partly due to the well-known high interindividual variation of the gut microbiota [16,17]. One study used culture techniques to investigate the effect of GFD on fecal *Bifidobacterium* and showed that CD patients have a lower load of this microorganism [18]. However, it is more informative to analyze all (or most) members of the gut microbiota to reach biologically feasible and clinically useful conclusions. In this regard, several studies have used massive high-throughput sequencing technologies to do so but have mostly focused on child populations [19,20]. Another study analyzed the fecal microbiota in 21 adults from the Netherlands before, during and after four weeks on GFD but did so in healthy control volunteers only [21]. Interestingly, the authors showed that a decreased abundance of Veillonellaceae was a distinctive feature during the consumption of GFD [21].

In México, CD has a prevalence of ~1% (~1.2 million people) [22], yet we know very little about CD in terms of its genetic predisposition, clinical presentation, treatment and involvement of the gut microbiota in Mexican patients [17,23–27]. The purpose of this research is to investigate the gut microbiota composition and predicted functional profile in Mexican patients with GRDs. To our knowledge, this work represents the first effort to investigate the gut microbiota in these important clinical conditions in México. Additionally, we also investigated the changes in the gut microbiota after four weeks on a gluten-free diet (GFD) in a subset of patients from whom paired samples were available.

2. Materials and Methods

2.1. Ethical Considerations

This study was conceived with the combined knowledge and expertise of clinical and biomedical scientists from the Instituto de Investigaciones Medico Biologicas at the Universidad Veracruzana. Informed consent was obtained from all subjects and the study was approved by the local ethics committee (IIMB-UV 2016/011).

2.2. Recruitment of Participants

Consecutive newly diagnosed CD and NCGS subjects were recruited and evaluated over six months from patients attending the Department of Gastroenterology of the Universidad Veracruzana in Veracruz, México. CD diagnosis was based on the presence of CD-specific antibodies, genetic markers and histological examination; NCGS diagnosis was made during the patient's consultation if subjects had symptoms related to the ingestion of gluten (e.g., bloating, flatulence, altered bowel habits, and muscle pains) but no CD-specific antibodies and negative biopsies at the baseline (see "2.1 Subject enrollment" in Supplementary Information for more detailed explanations). Healthy volunteers with no history of digestive pathologies, lack of CD-specific antibodies and normal biopsies at baseline, were also included in the study. Blood samples, small bowel (i.e., proximal duodenum) mucosal biopsies, and fecal samples were obtained from the majority of the subjects although many patients refused to provide stool samples. As mentioned before, we additionally sought to investigate the potential microbial signatures associated with the consumption of certified gluten-free foods, where adherence to the GFD was defined if the subjects kept the diet >90% of the recorded time using diary records (see "2.2 GFD intervention" in Supplementary Information).

2.3. DNA Extraction, PCR, and 16S rDNA Sequencing

Biopsy and fecal samples were used to obtain the total genomic DNA samples for further PCR and sequencing of the 16S rRNA gene (16S rDNA) as shown elsewhere [28,29]. Briefly, we used a bead-beating coupled with a commercial DNA extraction kit (Wizard® Genomic DNA Purification, PROMEGA, Madison, WI, USA) and samples were normalized to 100 ng/uL for further analysis. We used primers 515F (GTGYCAGCMGCCGCGGTAA) and 806R (GGACTACNVGGGTWTCTAAT) to amplify the V4 region of the 16S rDNA as suggested by the Earth Microbiome Project. Purified PCR products were used to prepare the DNA libraries using the Illumina TruSeq DNA library preparation protocol. Sequencing was performed in a MiSeq instrument (Illumina) at Molecular Research LP (MR DNA, Shallowater, TX, USA) following the manufacturer's instructions.

2.4. Bioinformatics

The open-source bioinformatics pipeline Quantitative Insights into Microbial Ecology [30] v.1.8 was used for most of the core analyses. Operational Taxonomic Units (OTUs) were chosen using two approaches. First, using the pick_open_reference_otus.py accordingly to the suggestions by Rideout et al. [31]. This approach is capable of detecting OTUs that are not necessarily represented in the reference databases. Further taxonomic and diversity analyses were performed using all OTUs (i.e., the full OTU table) and a filtered OTU table (OTUs with <0.005% of all sequences were removed as suggested by Navas et al. [32]. Second, using the pick_closed_reference_otus.py to then be able to use the OTU table for the prediction of functional metagenome using Phylogenetic Investigation of Communities by Reconstruction of Unobserved States (PICRUSt) [33]. The GreenGenes database [34] at 97% similarity was used as the reference 16S database. All sequence and metadata information are publicly available (NCBI, PRJNA401920).

2.5. Statistical Analysis

A chi-squared test was used to compare the frequencies (e.g., the proportion of women, number of patients showing a clinical improvement) and the non-parametric Kruskal–Wallis test was used for comparison of health parameters (e.g., blood parameters) and microbial groups. The linear discriminant analysis (LDA) effect size (LEfSe, [35]) was used to determine the organisms that explain the differences in microbiota. Please note that in LEfSe, the idea is that the significant biomarkers (in this case microbial phylogroups) are ranked based on the effect size (the magnitude of the variation) rather than on the statistical significance. When comparing two sets of data (e.g., before and after GFD), the Wilcoxon signed-rank test or the Mann–Whitney test were used. The unique fraction metric (UniFrac) was used to measure the phylogenetic distance among taxa [36]. Both weighted and unweighted UniFrac were calculated and analyzed using Principal Coordinate Analyses (PCoA) because they can lead to different insights into the factors that shape the composition of bacterial communities [37,38]. The ANOSIM and Adonis tests were used to determine whether the grouping of samples by a given category (e.g., health status) is statistically significant based on the UniFrac distances. Two age groups (young < 35 years; old > 35 years) and two body mass index (BMI) groups (low < 24.5; high > 24.5) were created to evaluate the potential contribution of these factors to the similarity of bacterial communities. STAMP [39] was used to analyze PICRUSt data using non-parametric tests.

3. Results

3.1. Subjects

A total of six patients with CD, twelve patients with NCGS and twelve control subjects were successfully enrolled over the six months enrollment period (Table 1). Please note that not all samples were obtained from all subjects mainly because of the lack of compliance, especially with the submission of stool samples. Among the CD patients, one had a Marsh I classification, two had Marsh II and three had Marsh IIIa. The impact of these varying baseline scores on clinical development and gut microbiota is uncertain but something to look for in future studies. The history of CD among relatives was more common in CD patients, CD patients had lower BMIs and hemoglobin levels and higher intraepithelial lymphocyte counts (Table 2). There was no difference between the CD and NCGS patients at baseline with regards to abdominal pain and bloating (Table 2).

Table 1. The health status, age (in years), BMI, sex, and sampling information for all our group of 30 subjects [1].

ID	Health Status	Age	BMI	Sex	Paired Duodenal Samples?	Paired Fecal Samples?
9	CD	35	27	Woman	Yes	Yes
16	CD	36	20	Woman	Yes	Yes
18	CD	62	18	Woman	Yes	Yes
19	CD	25	23	Woman	Yes	NA
20	CD	47	25	Woman	Yes	NA
23	CD	73	21	Woman	Yes	Only on GFD
1	NCGS	23	28	Woman	Yes	Yes
3	NCGS	21	24	Woman	Only baseline	NA
5	NCGS	24	25	Woman	Yes	Only on GFD
6	NCGS	23	29	Woman	Yes	Yes
7	NCGS	22	25	Woman	Yes	NA
8	NCGS	24	27	Woman	Yes	NA
10	NCGS	27	23	Man	Yes	Yes
11	NCGS	23	29	Man	Yes	Only baseline
13	NCGS	37	31	Woman	Yes	Yes
17	NCGS	59	19	Woman	Yes	Yes
22	NCGS	34	26	Woman	Only baseline	NA
24	NCGS	38	24	Woman	Yes	Only baseline
2	Control	23	33	Man	Only baseline	NA
4	Control	24	33	Man	Only baseline	NA
12	Control	23	24	Woman	Only baseline	NA
14	Control	25	23	Woman	Only baseline	NA
15	Control	26	21	Woman	Yes	Yes
21	Control	24	29	Man	Yes	NA
25	Control	45	28	Woman	Yes	Only baseline
26	Control	64	24	Man	Yes	Yes
27	Control	23	25	Man	Yes	Only baseline
28	Control	39	25	Man	Yes	NA
29	Control	58	26	Woman	Yes	NA
30	Control	42	27	Woman	Yes	NA

[1] ID: patients' internal identification number useful for retrieval of sequence information from the SRA (NCBI). CD: Celiac Disease; NCGS: non-celiac gluten sensitivity; GFD: gluten-free diet; BMI: body mass index. NA: not available for analysis.

Table 2. The baseline clinical, physiological, and other parameters among the groups of subjects [1].

	CD (n = 6)	NCGS (n = 12)	Controls (n = 12)	p Value
Proportion of women	100%	92%	50%	0.017
CD in family, %	67%	17%	8%	0.017
DQ2 or DQ8 positive, %	83%	50%	42%	0.217
Severe abdominal bloating (Likert), %	66%	81%	NA	0.121
Severe abdominal pain (Likert), %	50%	42%	NA	0.862
Age in years (median, range)	41.5 (25–73)	24 (21–59)	25.5 (23–64)	0.077
BMI, kg/m^2, median (range)	21.8 (18–27)	25.3 (21–30)	25.2 (19–31)	0.050
Hemoglobin, g/dL, median (range)	12.3 (10.7–12.6)	13.8 (12.1–14.6)	13.8 (12.7–16)	0.050
Total cholesterol, mg/dL, median (range)	151 (110–222)	207 (116–323)	198 (136–299)	0.100
HDL, mg/dL, median (range)	38 (35–47)	43 (29–51)	36 (34–70)	0.013
LDL, mg/dL, median (range)	91.8 (63–161)	109 (75–143)	106 (79–186)	0.409
Triglycerides, mg/dL, median (range)	69.5 (40–230)	108 (62–270)	154 (83–277)	0.182
AST, median (range) UI/mL	29 (19–37)	23 (8–44)	26 (8–53)	0.523
ALT, median (range) UI/mL	22 (10–39)	19 (11–85)	24 (11–51)	0.895
Eosinophils DLP, median (range)	5 (0–22)	1.5 (0–13)	3.8 (0–11)	0.392
IEL in duodenum, median (range)	24 (15–39)	8 (0–22)	6 (0–12)	0.001

[1] p values come from the chi-squared test when comparing proportions (e.g., proportion of women) or the non-parametric Kruskal–Wallis test when comparing all other values. CD: Celiac disease; NCGS: non-celiac gluten sensitivity; DQ2 and DQ8 are haplotypes within the HLA-DQ serotyping system; BMI: body mass index; HDL: high density lipoprotein; LDL: low density lipoprotein; AST: aspartate aminotransferase; ALT: alanine aminotransferase; IEL: intraepithelial lymphocytes; DLP: duodenal lamina propria. NA: not applicable.

3.2. 16S Sequencing and Taxonomic Classification of Sequence Reads

A total of 2.3 million (biopsies, n = 30) and 1.5 million (fecal, n = 14, many patients refused to provide a stool sample) good-quality 16S rDNA sequences (median length: 300 base pairs) were obtained from the baseline samples and used for OTU picking and further analyses. A total of 32,800 OTUs were originally detected using the open OTU picking approach (unfiltered OTU table); the removal of low-abundant OTUs (i.e., OTUs with <0.005% of total reads) yielded 975 and 916 OTUs (only ~3% of all original OTUs) in biopsy and fecal samples, respectively. It is outside the scope of this current work to discuss the consequences of removing low abundant OTUs but please be aware that the so-called rare microbes may in fact be keystone species regulating the function of different microbial environments, including host-associated microbiomes [40].

3.3. Microbiota at Baseline

3.3.1. Microbiota in Duodenal Biopsy Samples at Baseline

Overall 16S reads were assigned to a total of 27 phyla in all samples but only five phyla (Proteobacteria, Firmicutes, Actinobacteria, Bacteroidetes, and Fusobacteria) comprised the vast majority (>90%) of reads in most samples (Figure 1), as shown elsewhere. At the phylum level, there was a significantly lower abundance of Bacteroidetes ($p = 0.022$, Kruskal–Wallis test) and Fusobacteria ($p = 0.052$) in duodenal biopsies from CD patients ($n = 30$, Figure 2). This lower abundance of Bacteroidetes and Fusobacteria in CD patients was also true when analyzing the duodenal microbiota of women only ($n = 22$, $p = 0.028$ and $p = 0.067$, respectively).

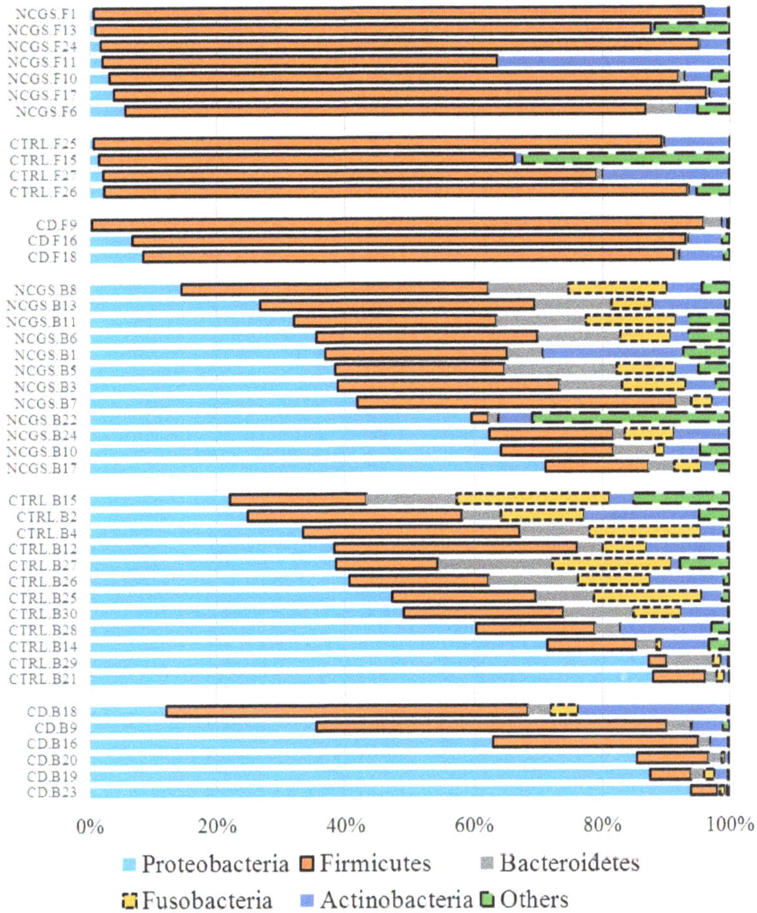

Figure 1. The taxonomic composition of duodenal ($n = 30$) and fecal ($n = 14$) microbiota at baseline at the phylum level. Please note that the samples were organized based on the highest abundant phylum for each subset of subjects. This figure was created using data from the full (i.e., unfiltered) OTU table, thus, allowing for a more complete taxonomic view of the samples. In the samples IDs: CD (celiac disease), NCGS (non-celiac gluten sensitivity), CTRL (control subjects), B: duodenal biopsy, F: fecal.

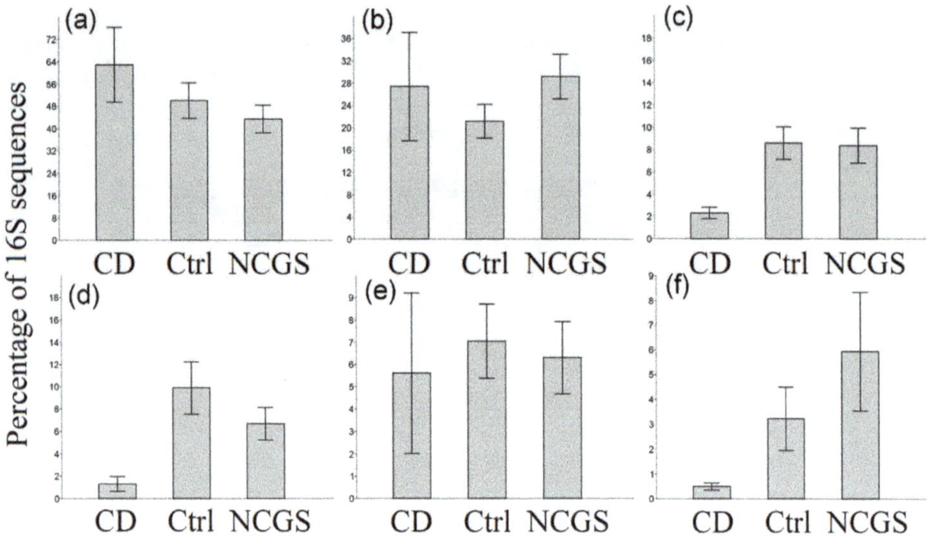

Figure 2. Bar charts showing the relative proportions of the 16S rDNA reads from the duodenal microbiota for all the main phyla. (**a**) Proteobacteria, (**b**) Firmicutes, (**c**) Bacteroidetes, (**d**) Fusobacteria, (**e**) Actinobacteria, (**f**) Others. Significant differences were only found in Bacteroidetes (**c**) and Fusobacteria (**d**), see main text. Bars represent the mean ± SE.

LEfSe analysis confirmed the finding of statistically significant differences in various bacterial groups among the three groups of subjects at the baseline (Figure 3). For instance, there was a higher abundance of *Actinobacillus* (Gammaproteobacteria), *Finegoldia* (Clostridia), and the phylum TM7 in NCGS patients, while *Sphingobacterium* (Bacteroidetes) was higher in the healthy subjects (Figure 3). The separate LEfSe analysis of samples from women confirmed the higher abundance of TM7 in NCGS patients and *Sphingobacterium* in healthy subjects and also revealed significant differences in various other bacterial groups (e.g., women with CD were deprived of Campylobacterales, Paraprevotellaceae, and Fusobacteriaceae; see Supplementary Figure S1). The health status of the patients was not related to significant differences in any index of richness or diversity with the exception of Shannon diversity index (lower in CD patients; Table 3 and Supplementary Table S1). This overall lack of difference in alpha diversity was also true when only analyzing samples from women (n = 22).

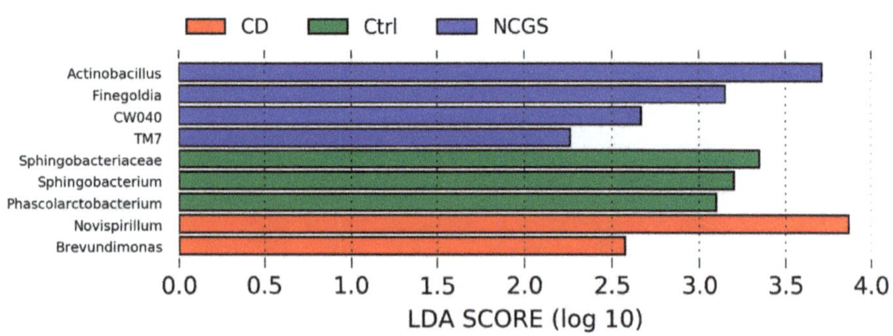

Figure 3. The LEfSe results from the comparison of the baseline duodenal microbiota. Please note that the bigger the LDA score, the bigger the contribution to the magnitude of the variation.

Table 3. The summary of the alpha-diversity indices from the analysis of all OTUs (full OTU table) from the duodenal microbiota accordingly to the diet and health status [1].

Biopsy Samples	Baseline (n = 30)	On GFD (n = 24)	p Value	Control (n = 20)	CD (n = 12)	NCGS (n = 22)	p Value
Richness	1127	1177	0.9562	1695	1687	1917	0.8450
PD whole tree	87	91	0.8961	1113	1057	1231	0.8426
Chao1	1746	1831	0.9924	88	86	91	0.9327
Shannon	5.5	5.5	0.8954	5.6 ^{a}	4.8 ^{a,b}	5.9 ^{a,c}	0.0193
Fecal samples	Baseline (n = 14)	On GFD (n = 12)	p value	Control (n = 6)	CD (n = 7)	NCGS (n = 13)	p value
Richness	1692	1341	0.2519	1696	1347	1552	0.7946
PD whole tree	101	89	0.3217	99	86	98	0.6694
Chao1	2205	1826	0.2519	2192	1783	2088	0.8086
Shannon	5.5	5.2	0.7425	4.6	5.8	5.4	0.7551

[1] p values come from the Kruskal–Wallis test (same superscripts indicate lack of statistically significant difference). GFD: gluten-free diet; CD: celiac disease; NCGS: non-celiac gluten sensitivity. For clarity and lack of statistical significant difference for most values, only median values are presented.

The differences in duodenal microbiota at the phylum (e.g., Bacteroidetes) and lower taxonomic levels (e.g., *Actinobacillus*) were not enough to differentiate the bacterial communities as a whole, as evaluated by the PCoA plots of weighted and unweighted UniFrac distances (Supplementary Figure S2) and this was also true when only analyzing the samples from women. The PICRUSt predicted metabolic features with the lowest uncorrected p values were flavonoid biosynthesis, dioxin degradation, and riboflavin metabolism (Figure 4) but after the Bonferroni correction, there was no significant difference in any metabolic feature.

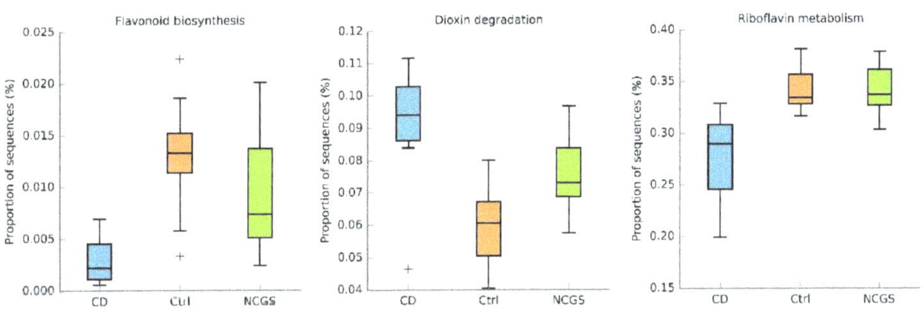

Figure 4. The box plots showing proportions of sequences for three metabolic features from the duodenal microbiota at the baseline. Plus (+) symbols represent outliers. Please note that there was no difference in any metabolic feature. CD: celiac disease, Ctrl: control, NCGS: non-celiac gluten sensitivity.

To summarize the results for the baseline duodenal microbiota, we found significant differences in the relative abundance of several bacterial groups but these differences were not enough to modify the diversity parameters (with the exception of Shannon diversity indexes) or predicted metabolic features.

3.3.2. Microbiota in Fecal Samples at the Baseline

Only 14 samples were available for the analysis of fecal microbiota at the baseline. Fecal samples showed an unexpected high abundance of Firmicutes (~85%) and a low abundance of Bacteroidetes (~1%) regardless of the disease status (Figure 1). Despite the low number of samples, there was a clear higher abundance of fecal Ruminococcaceae in NCGS patients, and this difference was significant according to the LEfSe analysis (Supplementary Figure S3).

3.4. *Effect of GFD on the Gut Microbiota*

3.4.1. Effect of GFD on Duodenal Microbiota

All subjects had a GFD adherence above 90%. Sixty-seven percent of CD patients (4/6) and ninety percent of NCGS patients (9/10) reported a global improvement of symptoms after four weeks on GFD but this difference was not significant ($p = 0.247$, chi-squared test). There was also no difference in any other clinical or physiological parameter with the exception of abdominal pain (lower during GFD in CD patients, Table 4).

Table 4. The clinical, physiological, and other parameters before and after four weeks of consumption of a gluten-free diet[1].

	CD ($n = 6$)		NCGS ($n = 12$)		Controls ($n = 12$)	
	Baseline	**On GFD**	**Baseline**	**On GFD**	**Baseline**	**On GFD**
Hemoglobin, g/dL, median (range)	12.3 (10.7–12.6)	12.4 (12.2–13.3)	13.8 (12.1–14.6)	13.5 (11.6–12.10)	13.8 (12.7–16)	13.7 (12.7–14.5)
Total cholesterol, mg/dL, median (range)	151 (110–222)	160.5 (103–210)	207 (116–323)	185 (140–245)	198 (136–299)	175 (189–207)
HDL, mg/dL, median (range)	38 (35–47)	37.4 (35–37)	43 (29–51)	41 (14–53.5)	36 (34–70)	46 (15–65)
LDL, mg/dL, median (range)	91.8 (63–161)	104 (65–130)	109 (75–143)	121 (76–135)	106 (79–186)	120 (82–157)
Triglycerides, mg/dL, median (range)	69.5 (40–230)	118 (38–157)	108 (62–270)	93 (70–217)	154 (83–277)	194 (73–247)
AST, UI/mL, median (range)	29 (19–37)	21 (13–40)	23 (8–44)	20 (12–52)	26 (8–53)	19 (13–28)
ALT, UI/mL, median (range)	22 (10–39)	25 (16–38)	19 (11–85)	22 (9–V61)	24 (11–51)	26 (19–33)
Severe abdominal bloating (Likert), %	66%	0%	81%	25%	NA	NA
Severe abdominal pain (Likert), %	50%	0%	42%	14%	NA	NA
Eosinophils DLP, median (range)	5 (0–22)	10 (0–14)	1.5 (0–13)	1.5 (0–15)	3.8 (0–11)	4 (0–22)
Intraepithelial lymphocytes in duodenum, median (range)	12 (0–29)	11 (0–43)	0 (0–22)	7.5 (0–22)	5 (0–20)	7.5 (5–33)

[1] The only parameter that showed statistically significant difference was severe abdominal pain ($p < 0.05$, chi-squared test). CD: Celiac disease; NCGS: non-celiac gluten sensitivity; GFD: gluten-free diet; HDL: high density lipoprotein; LDL: low density lipoprotein; AST: aspartate aminotransferase; ALT: alanine aminotransferase; DLP: duodenal lamina propria. NA: not applicable.

An additional 2.9 million sequences (1.8 million from a total of 24 biopsy samples, and 1.1 million from a total of 12 fecal samples) were obtained from subjects on GFD. Paired samples were not obtained for all subjects mainly because of the lack of compliance, especially with the submission of stool samples (Table 1). Despite an apparently clear distinctive abundance and distribution of phyla in duodenum between the periods with and without dietary gluten (Figure 5), there was no significant difference in the abundance of any taxa between the two periods of time ($p > 0.1$), likely due to the high inter-individual variability. Additional analyses of relative abundances in paired samples revealed that each group of patients (controls, CD, and NCGS) displayed a distinctive variation over-time after consuming the GFD for four weeks (for example, most NCGS patients displayed little change after the GFD period, Figure 6). Interestingly, and despite a relatively more stable division-wide composition, 9 out of 10 paired samples of patients with NCGS showed an increase in the duodenal *Pseudomonas* on the GFD (Figure 7, baseline median: 1.3%, min/max: 0.47–6.8%; median after four weeks on GFD: 14.8%, 2.3–38.5%, $p < 0.01$, Wilcoxon signed-rank test, only subject 7 showed a decrease in this group, from 4.3% to 2.5%). This difference in most individuals was specific for *Pseudomonas* and not for other members of the duodenal microbiota (Figure 7). In contrast, only half of the paired samples (3 out of 6) from CD patients showed increases in *Pseudomonas* but these increases were so pronounced that they also affected median values (Figure 7). Additional analyses revealed that the 16S sequences from *Pseudomonas* were not different among the groups of subjects (see Figure S4 in "3.1 *Pseudomonas* in duodenum" in the Supplementary Information), thus suggesting that taxonomically similar *Pseudomonas* populations react differently in the presence of similar environmental conditions, in this case, in the absence of dietary gluten. This is particularly relevant in a context of the ecological significance of microdiversity [41].

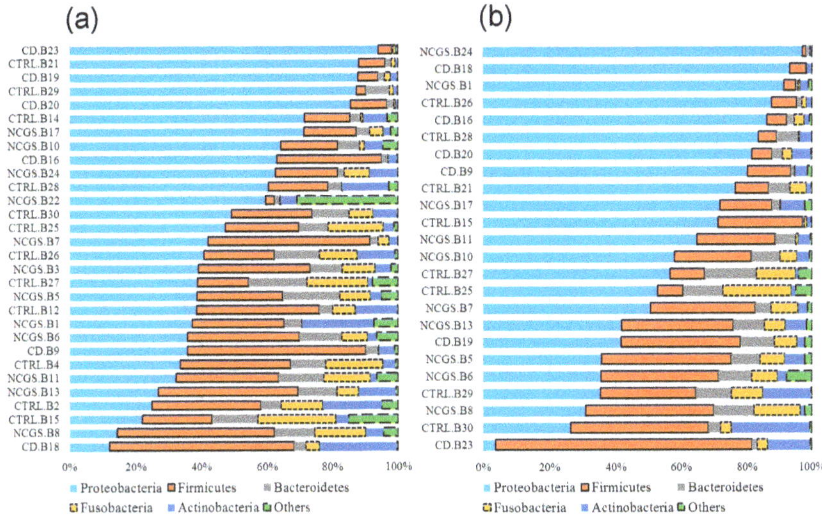

Figure 5. The taxonomic composition of duodenal microbiota between the baseline period ((**a**), $n = 30$) and the period after four weeks on GFD ((**b**), $n = 24$). Please note that the samples were organized based on the abundance of the most abundant phylum (i.e., Proteobacteria). In the samples IDs: CD (celiac disease), NCGS (non-celiac gluten sensitivity), CTRL (control subjects).

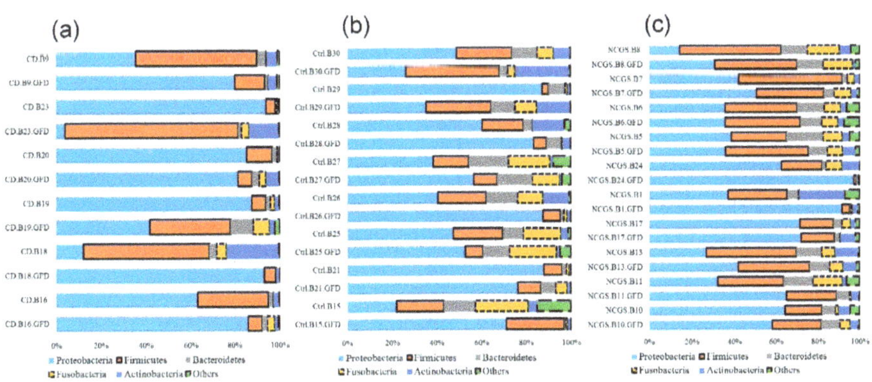

Figure 6. The taxonomic composition of duodenal microbiota for all paired samples from the CD patients (**a**), controls (**b**) and patients with NCGS (**c**). The purpose of this plot is to illustrate the over time variation within individuals. In samples IDs: CD (celiac disease), NCGS (non-celiac gluten sensitivity), Ctrl (control subjects).

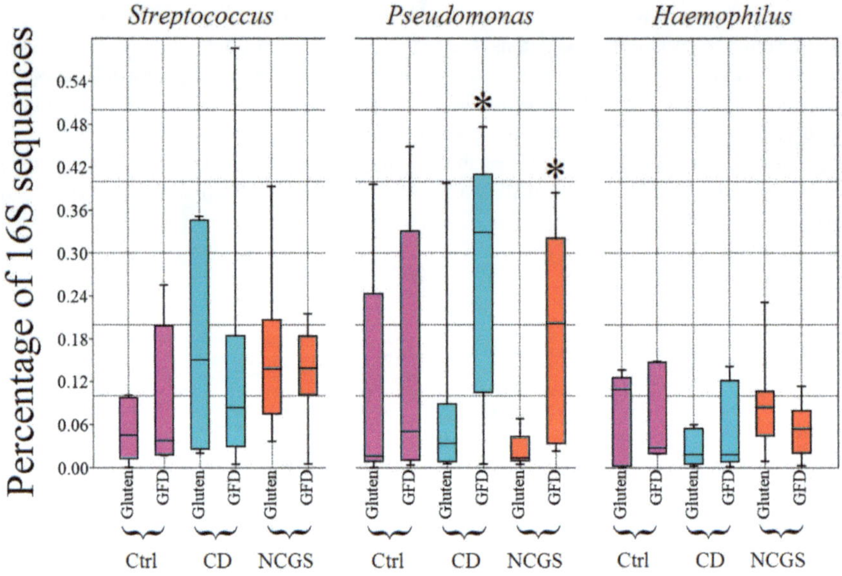

Figure 7. The box plots showing the relative abundance of 16S rDNA reads corresponding to the three most abundant bacterial groups in the duodenum at the genus level. * Significantly higher compared to the period of gluten consumption ($p < 0.05$, Wilcoxon signed-rank test). Please note that 90% (9 out of 10) and 50% (3 out of 6) of paired samples of patients with NCGS and CD (respectively) showed an increase in *Pseudomonas* (see main text for more details on this). CD: celiac disease, Ctrl: controls, NCGS: non-celiac gluten sensitivity, GFD: gluten-free diet.

LEfSe analysis of the taxa at the genus level confirmed the results on *Pseudomonas* and showed that other Proteobacteria (e.g., *Stenophomonas* and *Novosphingobium*) were significantly more abundant on the GFD, while Actinomycetaceae was lower before the GFD (Figure 8). On the other hand, LEfSe did not reveal any taxa significantly associated with either a specific health status or with diet as class and health status as a subclass. Interestingly, LEfSe analysis revealed that *Brevundimonas* (a very low abundant group, <0.5% of all reads) was significantly enriched in CD patients when analyzing health status as class and diet as a subclass. This result was mainly due to a higher abundance of *Brevundimonas* in CD patients on the GFD. Other factors such as age, sex, or BMI were not significantly associated with the abundance of any bacterial taxa accordingly to the LEfSe analysis; however, this lack of significance must be taken cautiously because of the low sample size in each subgroup of patients.

There was no significant difference in the bacterial richness or diversity in the duodenum when comparing the period at baseline and after four weeks on GFD or health status using either the full OTU table (Table 3) or the filtered OTU table (Table S1). The ANOSIM and Adonis tests revealed interesting results to the factors associated with the differences in microbial composition among the samples based on UniFrac distances (Table 5 and Supplementary Table S2). For example, the diet factor almost reached a level of significance when analyzing the weighted UniFrac distances (Table 5 and Table S2). Additionally, the grouping of duodenal samples based on health status was found to be statistically significant when using unweighted UniFrac distances and almost reached a level of significance when using weighted UniFrac distances (Adonis test, Table 5 and Table S2). The age of the patients also seemed to contribute to the separation of duodenal communities, especially when using the filtered OTU table (Table S2). These results were supported by significance in the ANOSIM test but the associated R values were very low ($R < 0.10$), indicating that the clustering of samples was relatively weak (Table 5 and Table S2). Please note that the analysis of both the full and the filtered OTU table revealed similar results, thus suggesting that low-abundant OTUs did not play an important role in the separation or lack thereof of communities.

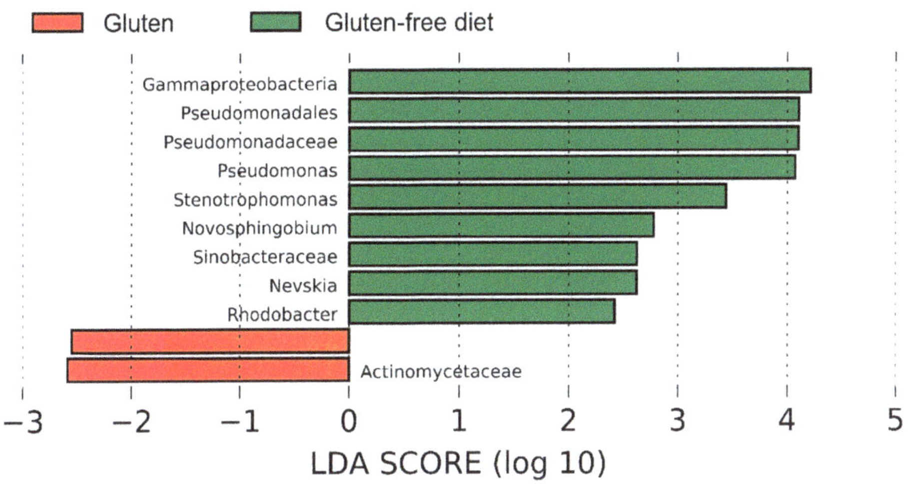

Figure 8. The LEfSe results of the duodenal microbiota from the comparison of the baseline and the period after four weeks on a GFD. These results are interesting because they also point out a potential difference in the *Pseudomonas* populations.

Table 5. The *R* and *p* values resulting from the Adonis and ANOSIM tests from the analysis of all OTUs (full OTU table) for each variable.

	Biopsy Samples		Fecal Samples	
Adonis Test Results	**Weighted**	**Unweighted**	**Weighted**	**Unweighted**
Diet	$p = 0.053$	$p = 0.293$	$p = 0.406$	$p = 0.877$
Disease	$p = 0.072$	$p = 0.006$	$p = 0.323$	$p = 0.195$
Group	$p = 0.067$	$p = 0.080$	$p = 0.417$	$p = 0.494$
Age	$p = 0.119$	$p = 0.060$	$p = 0.299$	$p = 0.201$
BMI	$p = 0.401$	$p = 0.082$	$p = 0.007$	$p = 0.010$
	Biopsy Samples		**Fecal Samples**	
ANOSIM Test Results	**Weighted**	**Unweighted**	**Weighted**	**Unweighted**
Diet	$R = 0.038$ $p = 0.106$	$R = 0.014$ $p = 0.262$	$R = 0.009$ $p = 0.333$	$R = -0.071$ $p = 0.952$
Disease	$R = 0.078$ $p = 0.026$	$R = 0.058$ $p = 0.058$	$R = 0.082$ $p = 0.136$	$R = 0.055$ $p = 0.221$
Group	$R = 0.082$ $p = 0.039$	$R = 0.035$ $p = 0.174$	$R = 0.039$ $p = 0.307$	$R = -0.001$ $p = 0.482$
Age	$R = 0.083$ $p = 0.034$	$R = 0.081$ $p = 0.032$	$R = 0.009$ $p = 0.349$	$R = 0.009$ $p = 0.392$
BMI	$R = 0.034$ $p = 0.230$	$R = -0.050$ $p = 0.800$	$R = 0.132$ $p = 0.024$	$R = 0.155$ $p = 0.018$

The variables included Diet (gluten/GFD), Disease (Control/CD/NCGS), Group (six groups of samples comprise this category: Control, CD and NCGS before and after four weeks of GFD), Age (Young/Old), BMI (high/low). *p* values that reached statistical significance ($p < 0.05$) or were close to reaching significance ($p < 0.1$) are highlighted in bold for better visualization.

Considering the differences in relative abundance among the different bacterial groups of the duodenal microbiota (e.g., the higher *Pseudomonas* on GFD in CD and NCGS patients), we hypothesized that the beta diversity analyses for different bacterial populations may offer clues regarding the effect on different factors such as the diet and health status. Therefore, we used the Adonis and ANOSIM tests to compare UniFrac distances for either all non-Proteobacteria OTUs and *Pseudomonas* OTUs only (Supplementary Table S3). Despite obtaining low R values, thus suggesting the weak clustering of communities, this additional analysis revealed that the effect of these factors is different in distinct populations of microbes. For example, the effect of the BMI was stronger for *Pseudomonas* populations (Table S3).

3.4.2. Effect of GFD on Fecal Microbiota

Gluten proteins are not completely digested in the small intestine and several members of the fecal microbiota have the capacity to metabolize gluten [42]; therefore, the removal of gluten from the diet may also affect the distal gut microbiota. In this study, however, both diet and health status were not associated with differences in fecal bacterial richness or diversity (Table 3 and Supplementary Table S1). LEfSe analysis did not find any indication to suggest a difference in fecal microbial communities according to diet as the class or diet as a class and health status as a subclass. Interestingly, the LEfSe approach revealed a diverse group of microorganisms that were significantly enriched in each of the disease states when using health status as the main class (Figure 9). The family Veillonellaceae, which was found to be lower in the feces of healthy subjects on GFD [21] and contains sulfite reducer members [43], was included in this group (higher in CD patients, Figure 9). The analysis of health status as class and diet as subclass revealed that Proteobacteria (in general, without an indication of a particular taxon within) was more abundant in CD patients. Beta-diversity analyses of UniFrac distances showed a significant grouping of fecal samples accordingly to BMIs and this relationship was also independent of low-abundant OTUs (Adonis test, Table 5 and Table S2).

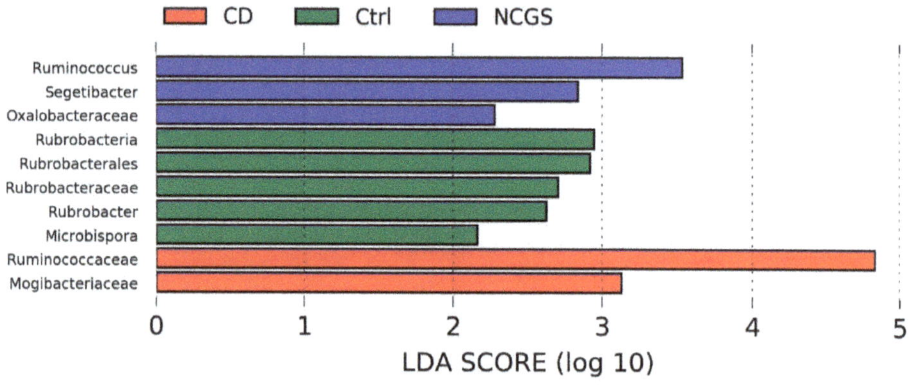

Figure 9. The LEfSe results of fecal microbiota from the comparison of all three groups of patients regardless of diet.

3.4.3. Effect of GFD on the Predicted Functional Profile

The closed OTU picking approach yielded a total of 4958 OTUs in biopsies and fecal samples. PICRUSt revealed no significant difference in the predicted functional profile of duodenal or fecal microbiota accordingly to diet or health status. Interesting results were found (for fecal samples only) when analyzing the group factor (six groups, control, CD and NCGS patients before and on GFD). For example, the proportions of genes related to the propanoate metabolism were higher in CD patients on a GFD (see "3.2 Predicted functional profile" in Supplementary Information) but caution must be exerted because of the low sample size in each subgroup of patients.

4. Discussion

Increasing evidence suggests a role of the gut microbiota in the onset and clinical development of GRDs but this phenomenon has been mostly studied in Europe. This study sheds light for the first time into the complex host-microbiota interactions in control subjects and patients with CD and NCGS from México. Additionally, this study offers relevant clues regarding the potential effect of GFD on health and gut microbiota.

The gluten metabolism is an interesting physiological phenomenon and growing evidence suggests a strong involvement of the gut microbiota [44]. However, each individual carries a highly specific group of microorganisms even at the strain level [1], and therefore such an involvement must be highly individualized. More importantly, the response of these unique communities to environmental factors (e.g., dietary changes, antibiotic administration) is also unique and may never return to the exact same baseline state before the challenge [45]. Finally, the region where the individuals live is an important factor, in fact, one study showed important interactions between the patients' geographical location and the clinical and microbiological manifestations of inflammatory bowel disease [16]. In this study, for example, our results are unlikely to apply to patients with GRDs from other cities, even within the same state of Veracruz.

From a clinical perspective, four weeks on GFD often improves symptoms and the quality of life in patients with CD or NCGS and this paper shows that this period of time was also enough to change the gut microbiota in our group of subjects, for example, duodenal *Pseudomonas* in NCGS patients. In contrast, Tjellström et al. [46] showed that fecal short-chain fatty acids output (a direct result of microbial activity) in CD patients with more than one year on GFD was significantly different compared to the output in CD patients with less than one year on GFD and CD patients at the presentation, thus suggesting that a long period of time on GFD may be necessary to fully re-establish the functioning of the gut microbial ecosystem in some patients. It has also been shown that a subgroup of patients does not respond positively even while adhering to a strict GFD and that these patients seem to harbor distinctive microbiota [47]. Here we showed that each individual carries a highly specific gut microbial composition, that the microbiota is different between healthy subjects and people with GRDs, and that this microbiota can experience variation due to the removal of gluten. It is important to note that this change also varies widely among individuals (the most significant and consistent change was associated with duodenal *Pseudomonas* in NCGS patients but every individual showed a unique increase or decrease in the abundance of these and other microorganisms).

The (unexpected) finding of higher abundance of *Pseudomonas* in some patients during GFD deserves special attention. For instance, whether the increase in *Pseudomonas* is beneficial or not to the integrity of the duodenal mucosa is uncertain. Clinicians often associate *Pseudomonas* with diseases because of the pathogenic nature of some strains of *P. aeruginosa* and other species. However, *Pseudomonas* is a highly heterogenic bacterial genus that includes thousands of non-pathogenic, highly divergent strains inhabiting a wide variety of environments [48]. Unfortunately, very few studies have paid attention to native gut-associated *Pseudomonas* [49–52]. The finding that a GFD is associated with a higher abundance of *Pseudomonas* in the duodenum could be explained using at least two hypotheses. First, gluten may lead to a given immunological status in the mucosa that interferes negatively with the presence of autochthonous *Pseudomonas*, thus explaining the lower abundance at baseline. Second, some members of *Pseudomonas* may act as a protective microbe and its low abundance may prompt a more sensitive state to dietary allergens. This is supported by the relatively lower abundance of *Pseudomonas* in CD and NCGS patients before the GFD (Figure 7).

The possibility that some members of *Pseudomonas* can act as protective agents suggest that some strains of *Pseudomonas* may even be considered as probiotics for patients with some GRDs. Interestingly, Gao et al. [53] showed that *Pseudomonas* and other bacteria were reduced in cancerous tissues compared to adjacent non-cancerous tissues, thus suggesting a protective role in the gut mucosa. Wei et al. [54] identified an interesting aciduric gluten-degrading enzyme from *P. aeruginosa* with a therapeutic potential for CD; yet this does not explain whether GFD would lead to a higher or lower abundance of gluten-degrading *Pseudomonas* (we reasoned that gluten-degrading *Pseudomonas* populations would grow preferentially only if gluten consumption offers a selective advantage). One study showed higher abundances of *Pseudomonas* in the duodenum of adult CD patients on a GFD compared to controls but this finding was not discussed at all [55]. This current study also suggests that other non-*Pseudomonas* Proteobacteria (e.g., *Stenophomonas*) deserve attention in terms of gluten degradation and gut health.

This study also shows that the health status in terms of gluten sensitivity may be related to differences in the distal digestive microbiota. For example, this study showed a higher abundance of Ruminococcaceae in the fecal microbiota of NCGS patients. Additionally, Veillonellaceae, a pro-inflammatory taxon that has been shown to be increased in patients with inflammatory bowel disease and inflammatory bowel syndrome [56–58], was shown to be increased in fecal samples from CD patients. This adds valuable information to a growing literature showing that the distal microbiota is also worth looking at in gluten-related disorders [59].

This study has limitations that are relevant to future studies. First, this and other studies lack a large enough sample size to generalize phenomena and even with bigger samples sizes the results cannot be extrapolated from one population to others [17]. Second, gluten-free diets vary widely around the world and these may or may not lead to a microbial state more similar to healthy controls [13]. Third, 16S sequencing does not inform about the microbe-immune system interaction at the cell level. In this regard, De Palma et al. [60] showed interesting differences in IgA-coated fecal bacteria in treated and untreated CD patients, thus suggesting that a simple molecular characterization of microbes is not enough to fully capture the complex relationship. Fourth, one study showed that serum concentrations of short-chain fatty acids were similar in the control and CD patients; however, the authors found an interesting difference between genders [61]. This is particularly important because the reasons explaining the differences between genders with regards to the clinical presentation and severity of GRDs and other autoimmune disorders have not been fully clarified. One hypothesis suggests that infections can induce autoimmune diseases [62]. Finally, we only looked at the bacterial microbiota here, yet non-bacterial organisms (e.g., yeasts) may play a role in these disorders [63].

5. Conclusions

In summary, this study generates valuable preliminary data about the relationship between the gut microbiota and gluten-related disorders in Mexican people. Interestingly, the four-week consumption of GFD was associated with an increased abundance of *Pseudomonas* in duodenal biopsies of patients with these disorders, particularly in NCGS patients. This change was noticed despite a general lack of differences in richness or diversity. *Pseudomonas* comprises strains with gluten-degrading capabilities that deserves more attention. It is our hope that these results can contribute to starting to visualize alternatives for the more effective treatment of afflicted patients in our area.

Supplementary Materials: The following are available online at http://www.mdpi.com/2072-6643/10/11/1641/s1, Detailed information about recruitment of participants, the diagnosis of CD and NCGS, as well as GFD intervention, Figure S1: LEfSe results from the separate analysis of baseline samples from women only, Figure S2: PCoA plots of unweighted and weighted UniFrac using the original OTU table and the filtered OTU table, Figure S3: relative abundance of fecal Ruminococcaceae at baseline, Figure S4: jackknifed tree based on weighted UniFrac distances, Table S1: summary of alpha-diversity indices from the analysis of the filtered OTU table accordingly to diet and health status, Table S2: R and p values resulting from Adonis and ANOSIM tests from the analysis of the filtered OTU table, Table S3: R and p values resulting from Adonis and ANOSIM tests from the analysis of the OTU table containing all non-Proteobacteria OTUs and *Pseudomonas* OTUs only in duodenal biopsies.

Author Contributions: Conceptualization, X.R.-G., O.D.J.C.-Q., P.G.-P., A.M.-D., and J.M.R.-T.; Data Curation, J.F.G.-M., S.E.D. and J.M.R.-T.; Formal Analysis, J.F.G.-M., K.H.-F., H.V.-C., S.E.D., and J.M.R.-T.; Funding Acquisition, J.M.R.-T.; Investigation, J.F.G.-M., X.R.-G., O.D.J.C.-Q., P.G.-P., A.M.-D., F.J.C.-J., H.V.-C. and J.M.R.-T.; Methodology, J.F.G.-M., X.R.G., O.D.J.C.-Q., P.G.-P., A.M.-D., K.H.-F., F.J.C.-J., H.V.-C., and J.M.R.-T.; Project Administration, A.M.-D., H.V.-C., and J.M.R.-T.; Resources, H.V.-C., S.E.D., and J.M.R.-T.; Software, J.F.G.-M., and S.E.D.; Supervision, X.R.-G., O.D.J.C.-Q., P.G.-P., A.M.-D., K.H.-F., F.J.C.-J., H.V.-C. and J.M.R.-T.; Validation, J.F.G.-M., X.R.-G., O.D.J.C.-Q., P.G.-P., K.H.-F., F.J.C.-J., and J.M.R.-T.; Visualization, J.F.G.-M., X.R.-G., K.H.-F., S.E.D., and J.M.R.-T.; Writing-Original Draft Preparation, J.F.G.-M., and J.M.R.-T.; Writing-Review & Editing,

J.F.G.-M., X.R.-G., P.G.-P., A.M.-D., K.H.-F., H.V.-C., and J.M.R.-T. All authors reviewed and approved the final manuscript.

Funding: This research was funded by the Mexican National Council for Science and Technology (CONACYT, Mexico, FOSIS 2015-262023).

Acknowledgments: We thank all participants from the city of Veracruz (México) and the staff from the Universidad Veracruzana for their help throughout the study.

Conflicts of Interest: J.M.R.-T. has received speaker's fees, travel support, and participated in medical board meetings with Takeda Mexico, Asofarma and Menarini. The remaining authors declare no conflict of interest. The funders had no role in the design of the study; in the collection, analyses, or interpretation of data; in the writing of the manuscript, and in the decision to publish the results.

References

1. The Human Microbiome Project Consortium. Structure, function and diversity of the healthy human microbiome. *Nature* **2012**, *486*, 207–214. [CrossRef] [PubMed]
2. Wu, G.D.; Chen, J.; Hoffmann, C.; Bittinger, K.; Chen, Y.-Y.; Keilbaugh, S.A.; Bewtra, M.; Knights, D.; Walters, W.A.; Knight, R.; et al. Linking long-term dietary patterns with gut microbial enterotypes. *Science* **2011**, *334*, 105–108. [CrossRef] [PubMed]
3. Hasegawa, M.; Inohara, N. Regulation of the gut microbiota by the mucosal immune system in mice. *Int. Immunol.* **2014**, *26*, 481–487. [CrossRef] [PubMed]
4. Walters, W.A.; Xu, Z.; Knight, R. Meta-analyses of human gut microbes associated with obesity and IBD. *FEBS Lett.* **2014**, *588*, 4223–4233. [CrossRef] [PubMed]
5. Sun, J.; Chang, E.B. Exploring gut microbes in human health and disease: Pushing the envelope. *Genes Dis.* **2014**, *1*, 132–139. [CrossRef] [PubMed]
6. Ludvigsson, J.F.; Leffler, D.A.; Bai, J.; Biagi, F.; Fasano, A.; Green, P.H.; Hadjivassiliou, M.; Kaukinen, K.; Kelly, C.P.; Leonard, J.N.; et al. The Oslo definitions for coeliac disease and related terms. *Gut* **2013**, *62*, 43–52. [CrossRef] [PubMed]
7. Galipeau, H.J.; Verdu, E.F. Gut microbes and adverse food reactions: Focus on gluten related disorders. *Gut Microbes* **2014**, *5*, 594–605. [CrossRef] [PubMed]
8. Gutierrez-Achury, J.; Zhernakova, A.; Pulit, S.L.; Trynka, G.; Hunt, K.A.; Romanos, J.; Raychaudhuri, S.; van Heel, D.A.; Wijmenga, C.; de Bakker, P.I. Fine mapping in the MHC region accounts for 18% additional genetic risk for celiac disease. *Nat. Genet.* **2015**, *47*, 577–578. [CrossRef] [PubMed]
9. Escudero-Hernandez, C.; Peña, A.S.; Bernardo, D. Immunogenetic pathogenesis of celiac disease and non-celiac gluten sensitivity. *Curr. Gastroenterol. Rep.* **2016**, *18*, 36. [CrossRef] [PubMed]
10. Rotondi Aufiero, V.; Fasano, A.; Mazzarella, G. Non-celiac gluten sensitivity: How its gut immune activation and potential dietary management differ from celiac disease. *Mol. Nutr. Food. Res.* **2018**, *62*, e1700854. [CrossRef] [PubMed]
11. Catassi, C.; Elli, L.; Bonaz, B.; Bouma, G.; Carroccio, A.; Castillejo, G.; Cellier, C.; Cristofori, F.; de Magistris, L.; Dolinsek, J.; et al. Diagnosis of non-celiac gluten sensitivity (NCGS): The Salerno experts' criteria. *Nutrients* **2015**, *7*, 4966–4977. [CrossRef] [PubMed]
12. Verdu, E.F.; Galipeau, H.J.; Jabri, B. Novel players in coeliac disease pathogenesis: Role of the gut microbiota. *Nat. Rev. Gastroenterol. Hepatol.* **2015**, *12*, 497–506. [CrossRef] [PubMed]
13. Ercolini, D.; Francavilla, R.; Vannini, L.; De Filippis, F.; Capriati, T.; Di Cagno, R.; Iacono, G.; De Angelis, M.; Gobbetti, M. From an imbalance to a new imbalance: Italian-style gluten-free diet alters the salivary microbiota and metabolome of African celiac children. *Sci. Rep.* **2015**, *5*, 18571. [CrossRef] [PubMed]
14. Verdu, E.F.; Armstrong, D.; Murray, J.A. Between celiac disease and irritable bowel syndrome: The "no man's land" of gluten sensitivity. *Am. J. Gastroenterol.* **2009**, *104*, 1587–1594. [CrossRef] [PubMed]
15. Volta, U.; Caio, G.; Tovoli, F.; De Giorgio, R. Non-celiac gluten sensitivity: Questions still to be answered despite increasing awareness. *Cell. Mol. Immunol.* **2013**, *10*, 383–392. [CrossRef] [PubMed]
16. Rehman, A.; Rausch, P.; Wang, J.; Skieceviciene, J.; Kiudelis, G.; Bhagalia, K.; Amarapurkar, D.; Kupcinskas, L.; Schreiber, S.; Rosenstiel, P.; et al. Geographical patterns of the standing and active human gut microbiome in health and IBD. *Gut* **2015**, *65*, 238–248. [CrossRef] [PubMed]
17. Garcia-Mazcorro, J.F.; Noratto, G.; Remes-Troche, J.M. The effect of gluten-free diet on health and the gut microbiota cannot be extrapolated from one population to others. *Nutrients* **2018**, *10*, 1421. [CrossRef]

18. Golfetto, L.; de Senna, F.D.; Hermes, J.; Soares Beserra, B.T.; da Silva França, F.; Martinello, F. Lower bidifobacteria counts in adult patients with celiac disease on a gluten-free diet. *Arq. Gastroenterol.* **2014**, *51*, 139–143. [CrossRef]
19. Cheng, J.; Kalliomäki, M.; Heilig, H.G.H.J.; Palva, A.; Lähteenoja, H.; de Vos, W.M.; Salojärvi, J.; Satokari, R. Duodenal microbiota composition and mucosal homeostasis in pediatric celiac disease. *BMC Gastroenterol.* **2013**, *13*, 113. [CrossRef] [PubMed]
20. Sánchez, E.; Donat, E.; Ribes-Koninckx, C.; Fernandez-Murga, M.L.; Sanz, Y. Duodenal-mucosal bacteria associated with celiac disease in children. *Appl. Environ. Microbiol.* **2013**, *79*, 5472–5479. [CrossRef] [PubMed]
21. Bonder, M.J.; Tigchelaar, E.F.; Cai, X.; Trynka, G.; Cenit, M.C.; Hrdlickova, B.; Zhong, H.; Vatanen, T.; Gevers, D.; Wijmenga, C.; et al. The influence of a short-term gluten free diet on the human gut microbiota. *Genome Med.* **2016**, *8*, 45. [CrossRef] [PubMed]
22. Remes-Troche, J.M. Doctor, why am I celiac if I'm Mexican? Breaking another paradigm of celiac disease in Mexico. *Rev. Gastroenterol. Mex.* **2018**, *83*, 77–78. [CrossRef] [PubMed]
23. Ramírez-Cervantes, K.L.; Remes-Troche, J.M.; Milke-García, M.P.; Romero, V.; Uscanga, L.F. Characteristics and factors related to quality of life in Mexican mestizo patients with celiac disease. *BMC Gastroenterol.* **2015**, *15*, 4. [CrossRef] [PubMed]
24. Remes-Troche, J.M.; Nuñez-Alvares, C.; Uscanga-Dominguez, L.F. Celiac disease in Mexican population: An update. *Am. J. Gastroenterol.* **2013**, *108*, 283–284. [CrossRef] [PubMed]
25. Sotelo Cruz, N.; Calderon de la Barca, A.M.; Hurtado Valenzuela, J.G. Celiac disease in children from the northwest of Mexico: Clinical characteristics of 24 cases. *Rev. Gastroenterol. Mex.* **2013**, *78*, 211–218. [CrossRef] [PubMed]
26. Cerda-Contreras, E.; Duarte-Rojo, A.; Granados, J.; Vargas, F.; Uscanga-Dominguez, L.F. Frecuencia de antígenos de histocompatibilidad DQ2 DQ8 en sujetos con diarrea crónica y enfermedad celiaca (EC). *Rev. Gastroentol. Mex.* **2008**, *73* (Suppl. 2), 131–132.
27. Remes-Troche, J.M.; Uscanga-Domínguez, L.F.; Aceves-Tavares, R.G.; Calderón de la Barca, A.M.; Carmona-Sánchez, R.I.; Cerda-Contreras, E.; Coss-Adame, E.; Icaza-Chávez, M.E.; Lopez-Colombo, A.; Milke-García, M.P.; et al. Clinical guidelines on the diagnosis and treatment of celiac disease in Mexico. *Rev. Gastroenterol. Mex.* **2018**. [CrossRef]
28. Caporaso, J.G.; Lauber, C.L.; Walters, W.A.; Berg-Lyons, D.; Lozupone, C.A.; Turnbaugh, P.J. Global patterns of 16S rRNA diversity at a depth of millions of sequences per sample. *Proc. Natl. Acad. Sci. USA* **2011**, *108*, 4516–4522. [CrossRef] [PubMed]
29. Garcia-Mazcorro, J.F.; Lage, N.N.; Mertens-Talcott, S.; Talcott, S.; Chew, B.; Dowd, S.E.; Kawas, J.R.; Noratto, G.D. Effect of dark sweet cherry powder consumption on the gut microbiota, short-chain fatty acids, and biomarkers of gut health in obese db/db mice. *PeerJ* **2018**, *6*, e4195. [CrossRef] [PubMed]
30. Caporaso, J.G.; Kuczynski, J.; Stombaugh, J.; Bittinger, K.; Bushman, F.D.; Costello, E.K.; Fierer, N.; Peña, A.G.; Goodrich, J.K.; Gordon, J.I.; et al. QIIME allows analysis of high-throughput community sequencing data. *Nat. Meth.* **2010**, *7*, 335–336. [CrossRef] [PubMed]
31. Rideout, J.R.; He, Y.; Navas-Molina, J.A.; Walters, W.A.; Ursell, L.K.; Gibbons, S.M.; Chase, J.; McDonald, D.; Gonzalez, A.; Robbins-Pianka, A.; et al. Subsampled open-reference clustering creates consistent, comprehensive OTU definitions and scales to billions of sequences. *PeerJ* **2014**, *2*, e545. [CrossRef] [PubMed]
32. Navas-Molina, J.A.; Peralta-Sanchez, J.M.; Gonzalez, A.; McMurdie, P.J.; Vazquez-Baeza, Y.; Xu, Z.; Ursell, L.K.; Lauber, C.; Zhou, H.; Song, S.J.; et al. Advancing our understanding of the human microbiome using QIIME. *Methods Enzymol.* **2013**, *531*, 371–444. [CrossRef] [PubMed]
33. Langille, M.G.I.; Zaneveld, J.; Caporaso, J.G.; McDonald, D.; Knights, D.; Reyes, J.A.; Clemente, J.C.; Burkepile, D.E.; Vega Thurber, R.L.; Knight, R.; et al. Predictive functional profiling of microbial communities using 16S rRNA marker gene sequences. *Nat. Biotechnol.* **2013**, *31*, 814–823. [CrossRef] [PubMed]
34. DeSantis, T.Z.; Hugenholtz, P.; Larsen, N.; Rojas, M.; Brodie, E.L.; Keller, K.; Huber, T.; Dalevi, D.; Hu, P.; Andersen, G.L. Greengenes, a chimera-checked 16S rRNA gene database and workbench compatible with ARB. *Appl. Environ. Microbiol.* **2006**, *72*, 5069–5072. [CrossRef] [PubMed]
35. Segata, N.; Izard, J.; Wladron, L.; Gevers, D.; Miropolsky, L.; Garrett, W.S.; Huttenhower, C. Metagenomic biomarker discovery and explanation. *Genome Biol.* **2011**, *12*, R60. [CrossRef] [PubMed]
36. Lozupone, C.; Knight, R. UniFrac: A new phylogenetic method for comparing microbial communities. *Appl. Environ. Microbiol.* **2005**, *71*, 8228–8235. [CrossRef] [PubMed]

37. Lozupone, C.A.; Hamady, M.; Kelley, S.T.; Knight, R. Quantitative and qualitative β diversity measures lead to different insights into factors that structure microbial communities. *Appl. Environ. Microbiol.* **2007**, *73*, 1576–1585. [CrossRef] [PubMed]
38. Garcia-Mazcorro, J.F.; Mills, D.A.; Murphy, K.; Noratto, G. Effect of barley supplementation on the fecal microbiota, caecal biochemistry, and key biomarkers of obesity and inflammation in obese db/db mice. *Eur. J. Nutr.* **2017**. [CrossRef] [PubMed]
39. Parks, D.H.; Beiko, R.G. Identifying biologically relevant differences between metagenomic communities. *Bioinformatics* **2010**, *26*, 715–721. [CrossRef] [PubMed]
40. Jousset, A.; Bienhold, C.; Chatzinotas, A.; Gallien, L.; Gobet, A.; Kurm, V.; Küsel, K.; Rillig, M.C.; Rivett, D.W.; Salles, J.F.; et al. Where less may be more: How the rare biosphere pulls ecosystems strings. *ISME J.* **2017**, *11*, 853–862. [CrossRef] [PubMed]
41. Jaspers, A.; Overmann, J. Ecological significance of microdiversity: Identical 16S rRNA gene sequences can be found in bacteria with highly divergent genomes and ecophysiologies. *Appl. Environ. Microbiol.* **2004**, *70*, 4831–4839. [CrossRef] [PubMed]
42. Caminero, A.; Herrán, A.R.; Nistal, E.; Pérez-Andrés, J.; Vaquero, L.; Vivas, S.; Ruiz de Morales, J.M.; Albillos, S.M.; Casqueiro, J. Diversity of the cultivable human gut microbiome involved in gluten metabolism: Isolation of microorganisms with potential interest for coeliac disease. *FEMS Microbiol. Ecol.* **2014**, *88*, 309–319. [CrossRef] [PubMed]
43. Feng, Y.; Stams, A.J.M.; de Vos, W.M.; Sánchez-Andrea, I. Enrichment of sulfidogenic bacteria from the human intestinal tract. *FEMS Microbiol. Lett.* **2017**, *364*. [CrossRef] [PubMed]
44. Caminero, A.; Nistal, E.; Herrán, A.R.; Pérez-Andrés, J.; Vaquero, L.; Vivas, S.; Ruíz de Morales, J.; Casqueiro, J. Gluten Metabolism in Humans. Involvement of the Gut Microbiota. In *Wheat and Rice in Disease Prevention and Health*, 1st ed.; Watson, R.R., Preedy, V.R., Zibadi, S., Eds.; Elsevier Inc.: Atlanta, GA, USA, 2014; pp. 157–170.
45. Modi, S.R.; Collins, J.J.; Relman, D.A. Antibiotics and the gut microbiota. *J. Clin. Investig.* **2014**, *124*, 4212–4218. [CrossRef] [PubMed]
46. Tjellström, B.; Högberg, L.; Stenhammar, L.; Fälth-Magnusson, K.; Magnusson, K.-E.; Norin, E.; Sundqvist, T.; Midtvedt, T. Faecal short-chain fatty acid pattern in childhood coeliac disease is normalized after more than one year's gluten-free diet. *Microb. Ecol. Health Dis.* **2013**, *24*, 20905. [CrossRef]
47. Wacklin, P.; Laurikka, P.; Lindfors, K.; Collin, P.; Salmi, T.; Lähdeaho, M.L.; Saavalainen, P.; Mäki, M.; Mättö, J.; Kurppa, K.; et al. Altered duodenal microbiota composition in celiac disease patients suffering from persistent symptoms on a long-term gluten-free diet. *Am. J. Gastroenterol.* **2014**, *109*, 1933–1941. [CrossRef] [PubMed]
48. Silby, M.W.; Winstanley, C.; Godfrey, S.A.C.; Levy, S.B.; Jackson, R.W. Pseudomonas genomes: Diverse and adaptable. *FEMS Microbiol. Rev.* **2011**, *35*, 652–680. [CrossRef] [PubMed]
49. Aujoulat, F.; Roudière, L.; Picaud, J.C.; Jacquot, A.; Filleron, A.; Neveu, D.; Baum, T.P.; Marchandin, H.; Jumas-Bilak, E. Temporal dynamics of the very premature infant gut dominant microbiota. *BMC Microbiol.* **2014**, *14*, 325. [CrossRef] [PubMed]
50. Mao, B.; Li, D.; Zhao, J.; Liu, X.; Gu, Z.; Chen, Y.Q.; Zhang, H.; Chen, W. In vitro fermentation of lactulose by human gut bacteria. *J. Agric. Food Chem.* **2014**, *62*, 10970–10977. [CrossRef] [PubMed]
51. Petriz, B.A.; Castro, A.P.; Almeida, J.A.; Gomes, C.P.; Fernandes, G.R.; Kruger, R.H.; Pereira, R.W.; Franco, O.L. Exercise induction of gut microbiota modifications in obese, non-obese and hypertensive rats. *BMC Genom.* **2014**, *15*, 511. [CrossRef] [PubMed]
52. Scales, B.S.; Dickson, R.P.; LiPuma, J.J.; Huffnagle, G.B. Microbiology, genomics, and clinical significance of the Pseudomonas fluorescens species complex, an unappreciated colonizer of humans. *Clin. Microbiol.* **2014**, *27*, 927–948. [CrossRef] [PubMed]
53. Gao, Z.; Guo, B.; Gao, R.; Zhu, Q.; Qin, H. Microbiota disbiosis is associated with colorectal cancer. *Front. Microbiol.* **2015**, *6*, 20. [CrossRef] [PubMed]
54. Wei, G.; Tian, N.; Valery, A.C.; Zhong, Y.; Schuppan, D.; Helmerhorst, E.J. Identification of pseudolysin (lasB) as an aciduric gluten-degrading enzyme with high therapeutic potential for celiac disease. *Am. J. Gastroenterol.* **2015**, *110*, 899–908. [CrossRef] [PubMed]
55. D'Argenio, V.; Casaburi, G.; Precone, V.; Pagliuca, C.; Colicchio, R.; Sarnataro, D.; Discepolo, V.; Kim, S.M.; Russo, I.; Del Vecchio Blanco, G.; et al. Metagenomics reveals dysbiosis and a potentially pathogenic N.

flavescens strain in duodenum of adult celiac patients. *Am. J. Gastroenterol.* **2016**, *111*, 879–890. [CrossRef] [PubMed]

56. Gevers, D.; Kugathasan, S.; Denson, L.A.; Vázquez-Baeza, Y.; Van Treuren, W.; Ren, B.; Schwager, E.; Knights, D.; Song, S.J.; Yassour, M.; et al. The treatment-naive microbiome in new-onset Crohn's disease. *Cell. Host Microbe* **2014**, *15*, 382–392. [CrossRef] [PubMed]
57. Haberman, Y.; Tickle, T.L.; Dexheimer, P.J.; Kim, M.O.; Tang, D.; Karns, R. Pediatric Crohn disease patients exhibit specific ileal transcriptome and microbiome signature. *J. Clin. Investig.* **2014**, *124*, 3617–3633. [CrossRef] [PubMed]
58. Shukla, R.; Ghoshal, U.; Dhole, T.N.; Ghoshal, U.C. Fecal microbiota in patients with irritable bowel syndrome compared to healthy controls using real-time polymerase chain reaction: An evidence of dysbiosis. *Dig. Dis. Sci.* **2015**, *60*, 2953–2962. [CrossRef] [PubMed]
59. Nistal, E.; Caminero, A.; Vivas, S.; Ruiz de Morales, J.M.; Saenz de Miera, L.E.; Rodríguez-Aparicio, L.B.; Casqueiro, J. Differences in faecal bacteria populations and faecal bacteria metabolism in healthy adults and celiac disease patients. *Biochimie* **2012**, *94*, 1724–1729. [CrossRef] [PubMed]
60. De Palma, G.; Nadal, I.; Medina, M.; Donat, E.; Ribes-Koninckx, C.; Calabuig, M.; Sanz, Y. Intestinal dysbiosis and reduced immunoglobulin-coated bacteria associated with coeliac disease in children. *BMC Microbiol.* **2010**, *10*, 63. [CrossRef] [PubMed]
61. Jakobsdottir, G.; Bjerregaard, J.H.; Skovbjerg, H.; Nyman, M. Fasting serum concentration of short-chain fatty acids in subjects with microscopic colitis and celiac disease: No difference compared with controls, but between genders. *Scand. J. Gastroenterol.* **2013**, *48*, 696–701. [CrossRef] [PubMed]
62. Fairweather, D.; Rose, N.R. Women and autoimmune diseases. *Emerg. Infect. Dis.* **2004**, *10*, 2005–2011. [CrossRef] [PubMed]
63. Harnett, J.; Myers, S.P.; Rolfe, M. Significantly higher faecal counts of the yeasts candida and saccharomyces identified in people with coealic disease. *Gut Pathog.* **2017**, *9*, 26. [CrossRef] [PubMed]

nutrients

MDPI

Review

The Handbook of Minerals on a Gluten-Free Diet

Iga Rybicka

Faculty of Commodity Science, Poznań University of Economics and Business, 61-875 Poznań, Poland; iga.rybicka@ue.poznan.pl

Received: 13 October 2018; Accepted: 29 October 2018; Published: 5 November 2018

Abstract: The importance of a gluten-free diet (GFD) in the treatment of celiac disease and other gluten-related disorders is undisputable. However, strict GFD often lead to nutritional imbalances and, therefore, to deficiencies. One of the most common deficiencies from a GFD are an insufficient amount of Ca, Fe, Mg, and Zn. This is mainly because the most of popular gluten-free (GF) raw materials are poor in minerals. Although the popularity of GFD is constantly growing, the data on minerals in GF products are still limited. More importantly, an access to the data is even more restricted. Therefore, the paper reviews the Ca, Fe, Mg, and Zn contents in hundreds of grain GF products available worldwide. The data for 444 products from categories of flours, mixes for cooking, bakery products, cereals, groats, rice, and pasta are obtained from research papers and nutritional databases. The calculation of the realization of mineral requirements from a portion of each product with its graphical classification as rich/average/poor source of each mineral is given. The review is a handbook of minerals for people on a GFD, dietitians, and food producers.

Keywords: gluten-free diet; mineral; deficiency; calcium; iron; magnesium; zinc

1. Introduction

A gluten-free diet (GFD) has been the most popular elimination diet for more than a decade. The number of people on a GFD is constantly increasing [1]. It results primarily from a "free from" trend [2] and not from the higher prevalence of gluten-related disorders [3]. In the United States, more than 100 million people consume gluten-free (GF) products with most of these people lacking any gluten-related disorders [4].

Although GFD is associated with being more healthy [5], epidemiological studies indicate nutritional imbalances for people following GFD. They refer both to macronutrients and micronutrients including minerals. Vici [6] and Gobbetti [7] with coauthors reviewed data from clinical studies on a nutritional status on a GFD indicating too high intake of energy, sugars, lipids, and saturated lipids and too low intake of fiber, vitamin D, B-group vitamins, and minerals—Ca, Fe, Mg, and Zn.

Despite the huge popularity of GFD, the data on mineral content in GF products are still limited. More importantly, an access to such data is even more restricted. The improvement of the nutritional quality of GFD, which is mentioned by many researchers [7–10], should start in the quality assessment of available products. The constant expansion of the GF nutritional data together with alimentary education are key elements for successful therapy in gluten-related disorders. Therefore, the aim of the study was to develop a database of Ca, Fe, Mg, and Zn in grain gluten-free products available worldwide. The results are presented in separate tables for each mineral in a way that allows quick recognition for the products of high content of the nutrient from different categories. The review is a handbook of minerals not only for people on a gluten-free diet but also for food producers and dietitians who play a crucial role in the education of patients with gluten-related disorders.

2. Materials and Methods

2.1. Methods

The data were electronically searched for keywords in different national databases and literature data. The keywords included in the study were: "gluten-free" ("gluten free") plus "mineral" (including "calcium" or "iron" or "magnesium" "or "zinc" or "element" or "microelement" or "macroelement"). The study was restricted to the publications after 1 January 2005.

Data from nutritional databases are presented as they were found. When producer or ingredients were given, they are presented. The data obtained from research articles included only products with detailed material's description or ingredients or the recipe.

2.2. Data Extraction

Data selection under the study is presented in Scheme 1.

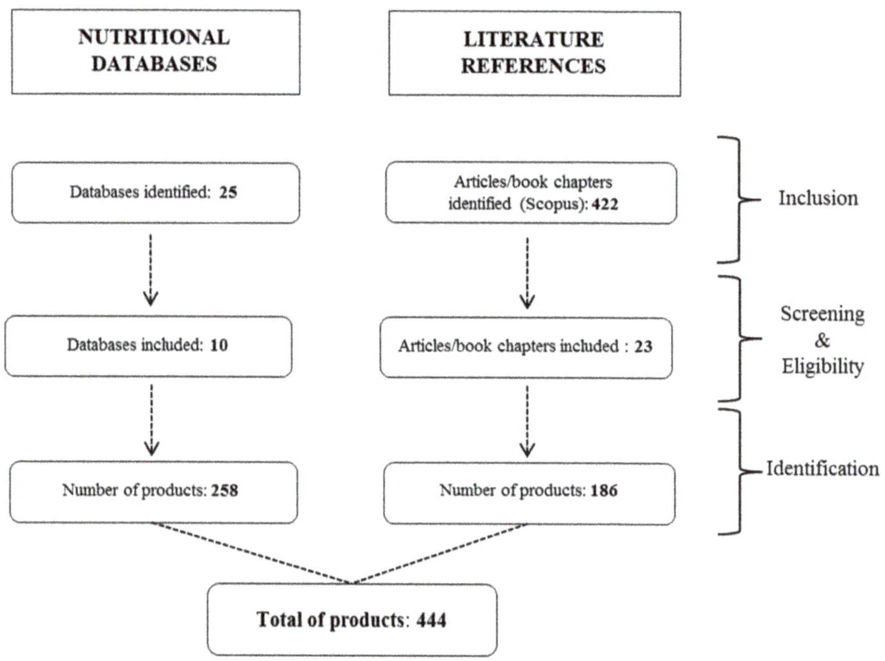

Scheme 1. Data selection scheme.

Literature references were searched in the Scopus while the nutritional databases under the study were those found on the FAO website [11]. The study includes databases from the United States [12,13], Australia [14], Canada [15], and several European countries [16–21]. Records with at least one mineral of interest were analyzed. All commercial products selected from the nutritional databases were described as "gluten-free" or were signed with the Cross Grain symbol. Products from research studies had to be described as GF. Raw materials and naturally gluten-free products not described as a GF, e.g., rice, buckwheat, and groats were omitted.

3. Results & Discussion

A total of 444 GF products were incorporated into the study including 186 products from literature data (23 articles and book chapters) and 258 GF products from 10 databases. Databases included in the study were from the United States (212 products) [12,13], Germany (14 products) [16], Norway (10 products) [17], Holland (7 products) [18], Australia (6 products) [14], Finland (6 products) [19], Belgium (2 products) [20], Canada (2 products) [15], and Estonia (1 product) [21].

No GF hits for minerals of interest were found in databases form: Armenia [22], the Czech Republic [23], Denmark [24], France [25], Greece [26], Iceland [27], Italy [28], Latvia [29], Serbia [30], Slovakia [31], Spain [32], Sweden [33], Switzerland [34], Turkey [35], and the United Kingdom [36].

The handbook replies only to grain GF products since they should partially consist of the everyday diet. Even though grain products are not the best source of all analyzed minerals (e.g., Ca), due to their substantial daily consumption, they significantly realize daily requirements for nutrients.

Moreover, different studies indicate that the proportion of the main nutrients on GFD is improper and that people on a GFD often omit some assortment of grain products like commercial bakery products [37]. Only grain products that should consist of the everyday diet were included in the study. Cookies and snacks, e.g., crackers, were not taken into account. The total number of grain GF products was significant. Therefore, they were divided into categories shown below.

I—flours
II—mixes for cooking
III—bakery products (e.g., breads, rolls, dinner rolls, crack bread)
IV—cereals (plain and musli flakes)
V—grains and rice
VI—pasta

All included products were described as GF. When the manufacturer or a brand was known, the ingredients were not presented since consumers can easily recognize these products. When the producer was unknown, the main ingredients were presented (if applicable).

The daily portion for each category was established. For the I, II, and IV category, it was 30 g, for V and VI, it was 50 g, and, for III, it was 100 g. The percent of Reference Nutrient Intakes (RNIs) were calculated for 800 mg, 14 mg, 375 mg, and 10 mg for Ca, Fe, Mg, and Zn, respectively [38].

Moreover, different colors were given to show the contribution of the portion of each product to realization of daily requirements for minerals (Figure 1). Dark green indicated that these products are a good source of nutrients (>25% of RNI), bright green indicates a moderate source (10% to 25% of RNI), and white indicates a poor source (<10% of RNI).

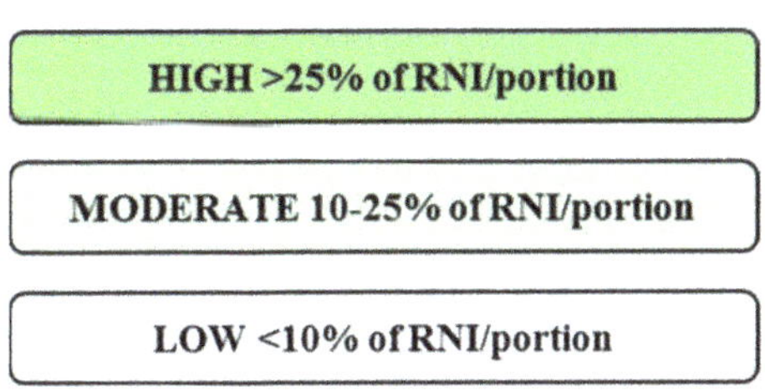

Figure 1. The criteria of product classification to high, moderate, and low contribution to realization of daily requirements for Ca, Fe, Mg, and Zn.

Tables S1–S4 present the data for Ca, Fe, Mg, and Zn, respectively, in a range of GF products separately for each category. The data were expressed in mg for 100 g of the edible product (fresh matter). The data were sorted from the highest to the lowest content of each mineral. If original data are presented in dry matter and the moisture is given, data were calculated into fresh matter. The authors of dry matter data were asked for water content data. When they did not answer or the data were unavailable, the data were calculated for the average moisture of 10% for VI category, 15% for I, II, IV, and V category, and 40% for III category [39,40]. The data for equal products from different references were averaged, e.g., the content of Ca in amaranth flour presented in Table S1 was calculated from values from four references. For these products, the minimum and maximum contents were presented.

As presented in Table S1, only three products were characterized by high content of Ca. These were crisp bread [17] and white and brown breads included in the Dutch database [18]. Additionally, 34 were of moderate contribution to the daily intake of Ca and most of them were bakery products. No data for calcium were found for a quarter of GF products (113 products). As mentioned above, because of significant daily consumption of grain products, they contribute to the daily intake of Ca even though they are not considered a good source of that mineral.

Databases and literature references were well-supplied with Fe data. Only 36 out of 444 products did not deliver data on iron content (Table S2). A total of 23 products were classified as an important source of Fe including most from categories of bakery products and pasta. Additionally, 112 products from all categories were of moderate contribution to daily intake of Fe.

In addition, 63% of selected products (278 items) were not characterized by the content of Mg (Table S3). From the remaining 166 products, only six bakery products (e.g., crisp breads) were classified as an important source of magnesium [12,14,16,18,19]. A total of 53 products for the I, III, IV, and VI category were of moderate content of Mg. None of the products from the II and V category were regarded as of high or moderate impact on the realization of Mg requirements.

Most of the products (372 items) did not deliver data on Zn content (Table S4). Only eight products (mostly crisp breads) were classified as of high impact on daily intake of zinc [12,17,19,41–43]. Twenty-nine products from 5 out 6 categories were described as a moderate source of Zn. All products from category II were assigned as a poor source of zinc.

The content of minerals in food product primarily results from its ingredients especially raw materials. Thus, in Table 1, contents of Ca, Fe, Mg, and Zn in the most popular GF raw materials—amaranth, buckwheat, chickpea, corn, millet, quinoa, rice, sorghum, tapioca, and teff were given. Original data expressed in dry matter were calculated into fresh matter at the level of 15% water [44]. As shown in Tables S1–S4, most of the GF products available in the worldwide market were produced from rice and corn, which are not a good source of macro-elements and microelements. Pseudo cereals like amaranth, quinoa, or teff are e.g., excellent sources of Fe and Mg, but their characteristic aroma and flavor limit their application in significant quantities in food products. For example, the most preferable amount of teff in breads should not exceed 10% [45]. Many researchers underline the necessity of the improvement of nutritional quality of GFD by replacing the low-nutritional GF raw materials with pseudo cereals with high nutritive value or by fortification with minerals [7–10]. The presented data on the mineral composition in commercial GF products (Tables S1–S4) along with information on the abundance of cereals and pseudo cereals in minerals (Table 1) prompt how to mix them in order to obtain nutritionally balanced food or meal. For example, 5% of an addition of acorn flour to the Gluten Free Cornbread Mix produced by The King Arthur Flour Company Inc. (Norwich, VT, USA) [12] will enrich it in iron by approximately 10%.

Nevertheless, review on recent literature revealed several important drawbacks. One of the most worrisome is the lack of data on Mg and Zn contents in the majority of GF products. Most of the total 444 foods included in the study did not have data on zinc (84% products). The data on magnesium was also very limited. In fact, 63% of products had no data on that mineral. Another problem was the quality of some of the presented results. Data presented from the largest database, USDA, is open for everybody and it allows manufacturers to describe their products. It can lead to the overestimation of their products. Thus, the ideal situation is building the databases based on the analytical determinations like those presented by e.g., Mazzeo and co-authors [56].

In addition, the problem is that the average consumer does not have access to literature references. Therefore, the actualization of online nutritional databases is the most preferable way to achieve this goal. The data should be developed at national levels and should be easily accessed. Nutritional databases should be free, on-line, and regularly updated. Providing the free-of-charge nutritional databases should be one of the key responsibilities for national food and nutrition institutes. The availability and quality of nutritional databases is even more crucial for the assortment of GF products since GFD is the only efficient treatment for celiac disease and other gluten-related disorders.

Table 1. The content of Ca, Fe, Mg, and Zn in GF cereals and pseudo cereals.

	Ca [mg/100 g]	Fe [mg/100 g]	Mg [mg/100 g]	Zn [mg/100 g]	Literature Source
Amaranth	61 [4] 153 [5] 159 [3] 165 [1] 170 [6] 497 [2]	6.2 [6] 7.6 [3] 7.8 [5] 8.9 [4] 9.6 [1] 16 [2]	129 [2] 231 [1] 237 [5] 248 [3] 279 [6] 313 [4]	1.4 [5] 2.2 [2] 2.9 [3] 3.9 [6] 5.6 [1] n.a. * [4]	1 [46] 2 [47] 3 [48] 4 [49] 5 [50] 6 [51]
Buckwheat	15 [2] 52 [1]	2.4 [2] 4.0 [1]	173 [1] 204 [2]	0.9 [1] 1.6 [2]	1 [50] 2 [51]
Chickpea	93–197 [1]	4.6–6.7 [1]	125–159 [1]	3.7–7.4 [1]	1 [52]
Corn	Purple < LOQ [1] Yellow 7 [2]	Purple 2.78 [1] Yellow 2.7 [2]	Purple 118 [1] Yellow 127 [2]	Purple 2.5 [1] Yellow 2.2 [2]	1 [46] 2 [12]
Millet	8 [2] 9 [1]	3 [2] 4.8 [1]	103 [1] 114 [2]	1.7 [2] 3.4 [1]	1 [21] 2 [12]
Quinoa	24–127 [2] 26 [4] 28 [6] 44 [1] 61 [5] 66 [7] 80 [3]	1.2–14 [2] 3.6 [7] 3.7 [4] 4.7 [6] 5.5 [1] 8 [3] 8.9 [5]	22–427 [2] 131 [4] 167 [7] 176 [6] 197 [1] 275 [3] 313 [5]	1.5 [6] 2.4–4.1 [2] 2.5 [3] 2.5 [7] 2.9 [1] 3.3 [4] n.a. [5]	1 [46] 2 [53] 3 [21] 4 [36] 5 [49] 6 [50] 7 [51]
Rice	Brown 32 [1] White < LOQ [1] 10 [3]	White 0.22 [1] 0.8 [3] 1.2 [2]	White n.d. * [2] 13 [3] 27 [1]	White n.d. * [3] 0.5 [2] 1.0 [1]	1 [46] 2 [53] 3 [49]
	19 [2]	Wholegrain 1.3 [1]	Wholegrain 115 [1]	Wholegrain 2.1 [1]	1 [21]
	Wholegrain 11 [1]	Red 2.2 [1]	Red 106 [1]	Red 1.5 [1]	1 [21]
	Red 15 [1] Wild 8 [1]	Wild 1.27 [1] Brown 1.3 [1]	Wild 108 [1] Brown 110 [1]	Wild 4.3 [1] n.a. [1]	1 [21] 1 [49]
	Indica/Japonica 3.6/4.3 [4]	Indica/Japonica 0.1/0.1 [4]	Indica/Japonica 24/17 [4]	Indica/Japonica 0.9/0.7 [4]	4 [51]
Sorghum	13 [2] 28 [1]	3.4 [2] 4.4 [1]	162 [1] 165 [2]	n.a. * [1] 1.7 [2]	1 [49] 2 [12]
Tapioca	16 [1] 20 [2]	1.3 [1] 1.6 [2]	1 [2] 2 [1]	n.a. * [1] 0.1 [2]	1 [49] 2 [12]
Teff	White/Red 32/44 [1] 180 [2]	White/Red 1.1/1.4 [1] 7.6 [2]	White/Red 54/44 [1] 184 [2]	White/Red 1.0/1.0 [1] 3.6 [2]	1 [54] 2 [55]

* 1–7 the superscript numbers refer to references from the last column, n.a.—not available, n.d.—not detected.

4. Conclusions

The handbook of minerals on GFD allows for the quick recognition of the best sources of Ca, Fe, Mg, and Zn. These are elements that are often deficient when excluding gluten. When analyzing the mineral composition of GF grain products, it is common to identify that they are rarely rich or moderate source of minerals. It applies in particular to the most popular GF products made with starches and refined flours. What is even more disturbing is the limited data on Mg and Zn contents in GF products. Additionally, access to this information is very restricted. The easily accessed nutritional databases for GF products should by developed at a national level and at international levels. Only then nutritional education, which is a crucial element of treating gluten-related disorders, would be credible and effective.

Supplementary Materials: The following are available online at http://www.mdpi.com/2072-6643/10/11/1683/s1, Table S1: Calcium in gluten-free I—flours, II—mixes for cooking, III—bakery products, IV—cereals and flakes, V—groats and rice, VI—pasta. Table S2: Iron in gluten-free I—flours, II—mixes for cooking, III—bakery products, IV—cereals and flakes, V—groats and rice, VI—pasta. Table S3: Magnesium in gluten-free I—flours, II—mixes for cooking, III—bakery products, IV—cereals and flakes, V—groats and rice, VI—pasta. Table S4: Zinc in gluten-free I—flours, II—mixes for cooking, III—bakery products, IV—cereals and flakes, V—groats and rice, VI—pasta.

Funding: This research was funded by the National Science Center Poland grant number 2017/01/X/NZ9/00669.

Conflicts of Interest: The author declares no conflict of interest.

References

1. Topper, A. Non-Celiacs Drive Gluten-Free Market Growth. Mintel Group Ltd. 2014. Available online: http://www.mintel.com/blog/food-market-news/gluten-free-consumption-trends (accessed on 7 November 2018).
2. Priven, M.; Baum, J.; Vieira, E.; Fung, T.; Herbold, N. The influence of a factitious free-from food product label on consumer perceptions of healthfulness. *J. Acad. Nutr. Diet.* **2015**, *115*, 1808–1814. [CrossRef] [PubMed]
3. Kim, H.; Patel, K.G.; Orosz, E.; Kothari, N.; Demyen, M.F.; Pyrsopoulos, N.; Ahlawat, S.K. Time trends in the prevalence of celiac disease and gluten-free diet in the us population: Results from the national health and nutrition examination surveys 2009–2014. *JAMA Intern. Med.* **2016**, *176*, 1716–1717. [CrossRef] [PubMed]
4. Richardson, B. Food Trends and Gluten. Know the Facts. Nutrition Foodservice Edge. 2018. Available online: https://www.anfponline.org/docs/default-source/legacy-docs/docs/ce-articles/nc012018.pdf (accessed on 7 November 2018).
5. Christoph, M.J.; Larson, N.; Hootman, K.C.; Miller, J.M.; Neumark-Sztainer, D. Who values gluten-free? Dietary intake, behaviors, and sociodemographic characteristics of young adults who value gluten-free food. *J. Acad. Nutr. Diet.* **2018**, *118*, 1389–1398. [CrossRef] [PubMed]
6. Vici, G.; Belli, L.; Biondi, M.; Polzonetti, V. Gluten free diet and nutrient deficiencies: A review. *Clin. Nutr.* **2016**, *35*, 1236–1241. [CrossRef] [PubMed]
7. Gobbetti, M.; Pontonio, E.; Filannino, P.; Rizzello, C.G.; De Angelis, M.; Di Cagnoa, R. How to improve the gluten-free diet: The state of the art from a food science perspective. *Food Res. Int.* **2018**, *11*, 22–32. [CrossRef] [PubMed]
8. Pellegrini, N.; Agostoni, C. Nutritional aspects of gluten-free products. *J. Sci. Food Agric.* **2015**, *95*, 2380–2385. [CrossRef] [PubMed]
9. Bascuñán, K.A.; Vespa, M.C.; Araya, M. Celiac disease: Understanding the gluten-free diet. *Eur. J. Nutr.* **2017**, *56*, 449–459. [CrossRef] [PubMed]
10. Foschia, M.; Horstmann, S.; Arendt, E.K.; Zannini, E. Nutritional therapy–Facing the gap between coeliac disease and gluten-free food. *Int. J. Food Microbiol.* **2016**, *239*, 113–124. [CrossRef] [PubMed]
11. FAO. 2018. Available online: http://www.fao.org/infoods/infoods/tables-and-databases/europe/en/ (accessed on 10 October 2018).
12. USDA Food Composition Database. Release April 2018. Available online: https://ndb.nal.usda.gov/ndb/search/list (accessed on 10 October 2018).
13. Nutritionix. 2018. Available online: https://www.nutritionix.com/ (accessed on 10 October 2018).
14. Nutrient Reference Values for Australia and New Zealand. 2018. Available online: https://www.nrv.gov.au/nutrients-energy-calculation/nutrients-energy-calc-result-1531402860 (accessed on 10 October 2018).
15. Canadian Nutrient File. 2018. Available online: https://food-nutrition.canada.ca/cnf-fce/search-rechercher.do;jsessionid=C82C3179ABE8F09D19D8F621E5D3CC9C (accessed on 10 October 2018).
16. Bundeslebensmittelschlüssel BLS, Version 3.02. 2018. Available online: https://www.blsdb.de/ (accessed on 10 October 2018).
17. Norwegian Food Composition Table Matvaretabellen. 2018. Available online: http://www.matvaretabellen.no/ (accessed on 10 October 2018).
18. The Dutch Food Composition Database (NEVO) Online Version 2016/5.0. 2016. Available online: https://nevo-online.rivm.nl/ (accessed on 10 October 2018).

19. Fineli, Version 29.06.2018. 2018. Available online: https://fineli.fi/fineli/en/index? (accessed on 10 October 2018).
20. Internubel 2018. Available online: http://www.internubel.be (accessed on 10 October 2018).
21. NutriData Estonian Food Composition Database, Version 8. 2018. Available online: http://tka.nutridata.ee/index.action?request_locale=en (accessed on 10 October 2018).
22. Armenian Food Composition Table. 2010. Available online: http://www.fao.org/fileadmin/templates/food_composition/documents/ArmenianFoodCompositionTable2010.pdf (accessed on 10 October 2018).
23. Czech Food Composition Database, Version 7.16. 2016. Available online: https://www.nutridatabaze.cz/en/ (accessed on 10 October 2018).
24. Danish Food Composition Databank, Revision 7.0. 2018. Available online: https://frida.fooddata.dk/?lang=en (accessed on 10 October 2018).
25. ANSES-CIQUAL Food Composition Table. 2017. Available online: https://ciqual.anses.fr/ (accessed on 10 October 2018).
26. Medical School of Crete: Food Composition Tables of Greek Foods 2018. Available online: http://www.hhf-greece.gr/tables/Dishes.aspx?l=en (accessed on 10 October 2018).
27. Icelandic Food Composition Database Matís. 2018. Available online: http://www1.matis.is/ISGEM/default_en.aspx (accessed on 10 October 2018).
28. Food Composition Database for Epidemiological Studies in Italy BDA 2015. Available online: http://www.bda-ieo.it/wordpress/en/?page_id=27 (accessed on 10 October 2018).
29. Latvian Food Composition Database. 2018. Available online: http://www.partikasdb.lv/ (accessed on 10 October 2018).
30. Serbian Food and Nutrition Database. 2018. Available online: http://104.155.19.23/serbianfood/index.php (accessed on 10 October 2018).
31. Slovak Food Composition Data Bank. 2018. Available online: http://www.pbd-online.sk/en (accessed on 10 October 2018).
32. Spanish Food Composition Database. 2018. Available online: http://www.bedca.net/bdpub/index_en.php (accessed on 10 October 2018).
33. Swedish Food Composition Database. 2015. Available online: https://www.livsmedelsverket.se/en/food-and-content/naringsamnen/livsmedelsdatabasen (accessed on 10 October 2018).
34. Swiss Food Composition Database 2018. Available online: http://www.naehrwertdaten.ch/request?xml=MessageData&xml=MetaData&xsl=Start&lan=en&pageKey=Start (accessed on 10 October 2018).
35. National Food Composition Database Türkomp. 2018. Available online: http://www.turkomp.gov.tr/main (accessed on 10 October 2018).
36. McCance and Widdowson's the Composition of Foods Integrated Dataset. 2015. Available online: https://www.gov.uk/government/publications/composition-of-foods-integrated-dataset-cofid?utm_source=MW7+List+March+2015&utm_campaign=947c9d4b28-Newsletter_2_December_2013_FINAL12_13_2013&utm_medium=email&utm_term=0_3b8ecbdaea-947c9d4b28-95444717 (accessed on 10 October 2018).
37. Lu, Z.; Zhang, H.; Luoto, S.; Ren, X. Gluten-free living in China: The characteristics, food choices and difficulties in following a gluten-free diet—An online survey. *Appetite* **2018**, *127*, 242–248. [CrossRef] [PubMed]
38. Regulation (EU) No 1169/2011 of the European Parliament and of the Council of 25 October 2011 on the Provision of Food Information to Consumers, Amending Regulations (EC) No 1924/2006 and (EC) No 1925/2006 of the European Parliament and of the Council, and Repealing Commission Directive 87/250/EEC, Council Directive 90/496/EEC, Commission Directive 1999/10/EC, Directive 2000/13/EC of the European Parliament and of the Council, Commission Directives 2002/67/EC and 2008/5/EC and Commission Regulation (EC) No 608/2004 Text with EEA Relevance. Available online: https://www.tul.cz/en/document/2471 (accessed on 10 October 2018).
39. Bradley, R.L. Moisture and total solids analysis. In *Food Analysis*, 4th ed.; Nielsen, S.S., Ed.; Food Science Texts Series; Springer: Berlin, Germany, 2010; pp. 85–104.
40. Skendi, A.; Mouselemidou, P.; Papageorgiou, M.; Papastergiadis, E. Effect of acorn meal-water combinations on technological properties and fine structure of gluten-free bread. *Food Chem.* **2018**, *253*, 119–126. [CrossRef] [PubMed]
41. Gull, A.; Prasad, K.; Kumar, P. Nutritional, antioxidant, microstructural and pasting properties of functional pasta. *J. Saudi Soc. Agric. Sci.* **2018**, *17*, 147–153. [CrossRef]

42. Cabrera-Chávez, F.; Calderón de la Barca, A.M.; Islas-Rubio, A.R.; Marti, A.; Marengo, M.; Pagani, M.; Bonomi, F.; Iametti, S. Molecular rearrangements in extrusion processes for the production of amaranth-enriched, gluten-free rice pasta. *LWT Food Sci. Technol.* **2012**, *47*, 421–426. [CrossRef]
43. Orecchio, S.; Amorello, S.; Raso, M.; Barreca, S.; Lino, C.; Di Gaudio, F. Determination of trace elements in gluten-free food for celiac people by ICP-MS. *Microchem. J.* **2014**, *116*, 163–172. [CrossRef]
44. Risius, H.; Prochnow, A.; Ammon, C.; Mellmann, J.; Hoffmann, T. Appropriateness of on-combine moisture measurement for the management of harvesting and postharvest operations and capacity planning in grain harvest. *Biosyst. Eng.* **2017**, *156*, 120–135. [CrossRef]
45. Campo, E.; del Arco, L.; Urtasun, L.; Oria, R.; Ferrer-Mairal, A. Impact of sourdough on sensory properties and consumers' preference of gluten-free breads enriched with teff flour. *J. Cereal Sci.* **2016**, *67*, 75–82. [CrossRef]
46. Nascimento, A.C.; Mota, C.; Coelho, I.; Gueifão, S.; Santos, M.; Matos, A.S.; Gimenez, A.; Lobo, M.; Samman, N.; Castanheira, I. Characterisation of nutrient profile of quinoa (*Chenopodium quinoa*), amaranth (*Amaranthus caudatus*), and purple corn (*Zea mays* L.) consumed in the North of Argentina: Proximates, minerals and trace elements. *Food Chem.* **2014**, *148*, 420–426. [CrossRef] [PubMed]
47. Kumar, K.V.P.; Dharmaraj, U.; Sakhare, S.D.; Inamdar, A.A. Preparation of protein and mineral rich fraction from grain amaranth and evaluation of its functional characteristics. *J. Cereal Sci.* **2016**, *69*, 358–362. [CrossRef]
48. Jimoh, M.O.; Afolayan, A.J.; Lewu, F.B. Suitability of Amaranthus species for alleviating human dietary deficiencies. *S. Afr. J. Bot.* **2018**, *115*, 65–73. [CrossRef]
49. Kunachowicz, H. (Ed.) *Gluten-Free Diet—What to Choose?* 2nd ed.; Wydawnictwo Lekarskie PZWL: Warsaw, Poland, 2015; pp. 99–170. ISBN 978-83-200-4965-7.
50. Alvarez-Jubete, L.; Arendt, E.K.; Gallagher, E. Nutritive value and chemical composition of pseudocereals as gluten-free ingredients. *Int. J. Food Sci. Nutr.* **2009**, *60*, 240–257. [CrossRef] [PubMed]
51. Mota, C.; Nascimento, A.C.; Santos, M.; Delgado, I.; Coelho, I.; Rego, A.; Matos, A.S.; Torres, D.; Castanheira, I. The effect of cooking methods on the mineral content of quinoa (*Chenopodium quinoa*), amaranth (*Amaranthus* sp.) and buckwheat (*Fagopyrum esculentum*). *J. Food Compos. Anal.* **2016**, *49*, 57–64. [CrossRef]
52. Thavarajah, D.; Thavarajah, P. Evaluation of chickpea (*Cicer arietinum* L.) micronutrient composition: Biofortification opportunities to combat global micronutrient malnutrition. *Food Res. Int.* **2012**, *49*, 99–104. [CrossRef]
53. Vilcacundo, R.; Hernandez-Ledesma, B. Nutritional and biological value of quinoa (*Chenopodium quinoa* Willd.). *Curr. Opin. Food Sci.* **2017**, *14*, 1–6. [CrossRef]
54. Dame, Z.T. Analysis of major and trace elements in teff (*Eragrostis tef*). *J. King Saud Univ. Sci.* **2018**. [CrossRef]
55. Zhu, F. Chemical composition and food uses of teff (*Eragrostis tef*). *Food Chem.* **2018**, *239*, 402–415. [CrossRef] [PubMed]
56. Mazzeo, T.; Cauzzi, S.; Brighenti, F.; Pellegrini, N. The development of a composition database of gluten-free products. *Public Health Nutr.* **2014**, *18*, 1353–1357. [CrossRef] [PubMed]

nutrients

MDPI

Review

Motility Disorders in Celiac Disease and Non-Celiac Gluten Sensitivity: The Impact of a Gluten-Free Diet

Paolo Usai-Satta [1,*], Francesco Oppia [1], Mariantonia Lai [2] and Francesco Cabras [1]

1 Gastroenteorlogy Unit, Brotzu Hospital, 09121 Cagliari, Italy; f.oppia@tiscali.it (F.O.); francescocabras@aob.it (F.C.)
2 Gastroenterology Unit, University of Cagliari, 09042 Monserrato, Italy; toninalai@medicina.unica.it
* Correspondence: paolousai@aob.it; Tel.: +39-070-539-395

Received: 25 September 2018; Accepted: 5 November 2018; Published: 7 November 2018

Abstract: Background: There is evidence that digestive motor disorders are frequently present in untreated celiac disease (CD) patients. Similarly, non-celiac gluten sensitivity (NCGS) can be associated with gut motor disorders. In both cases, gut dysmotility can improve or be completely reversed with a gluten-free diet (GFD). **Methods:** A literature search for motility disorders in CD and NCGS patients was carried out using the online databases PubMed, Medline and Cochrane. **Results:** Esophageal, gastric, small bowel and gallbladder motor disorders are common in both children and adults with CD. Although the clinical consequences of these disorders are not clearly defined, gastric dysfunction could affect drug absorption and metabolism in the thyroid and neurological conditions associated with CD. The impact of a GFD on motility disorders is, however, controversial. No systematic studies are available on NCGS. NCGS frequently overlaps with irritable bowel syndrome (IBS) and similar pathophysiological mechanisms may be hypothesized. **Conclusions:** Mucosal damage may affect gut motility in untreated CD through perturbation of hormonal and neuro-immunomodulatory regulation. A persistent low-grade mucosal inflammation could explain the cases of persistent motor disorders despite a GFD. Further studies are needed to definitely assess the role of gut motor disorders in NCGS.

Keywords: celiac disease; non-celiac gluten sensitivity; gut motility; gluten-free diet

1. Introduction

Celiac disease (CD) is a permanent, chronic, gluten-sensitive disorder characterized by small intestinal mucosal injury and malabsorption in genetically predisposed individuals [1]. Self-reported wheat sensitivity without the diagnostic features of CD or wheat allergy has recently been named non-celiac gluten sensitivity (NCGS) [2]. Unlike CD, NCGS has no specific diagnostic test available. There is evidence suggesting that abnormal gut motility may frequently be present in CD and that all of the gastro-intestinal tract, including the gallbladder, can be involved. Several studies have shown that a gluten-free diet (GFD) can improve or normalize these disorders [3–10]. Not surprisingly, the data on motility disorders in NCGS are just emerging. In addition, a possible overlap between intestinal bowel syndrome (IBS) and gluten related disorders have been clearly demonstrated [11]. The aim of this review was to provide an overview of gut motility abnormalities in these gluten related disorders and to establish the real clinical impact of a GFD on these functional diseases.

2. Materials and Methods

A review of the literature on motility disorders in CD and NCGS patients was conducted using the online databases PubMed, Medline and Cochrane. Original research, reviews, and relevant books were included in the search. All the validated motility methods, manometry, pH-metry, gastric emptying studies (scintigraphy, octanoic acid breath testing and ecography), gallbladder ecography and lactulose breath testing for oro-cecal transit time, were included in this review.

3. Celiac Disease

3.1. Esophageal Motor Disorders

In two successive studies, using standard esophageal manometry, we found motor abnormalities in 67% of the adult patients examined [5,12]. These alterations consisted of nutcracker esophagus, a hypotonic lower esophageal sphincter (LES) and frequent repetitive (>3 peaks) contractions. Interestingly, 50% of celiac patients complained of dysphagia compared with only 9% of controls ($p < 0.001$) [12]. In addition, we performed esophageal pH-metry and the acid score was abnormal in 30% of celiac patients [5]. In 1998, Iovino et al. [13] confirmed that adult celiac patients with steatorrhea presented a higher prevalence of esophageal symptoms and a lower LES pressure when compared with celiac patients without steatorrhea and control subjects. Preliminary results from a more recent South American study demonstrated motility alterations in 83% of CD patients using esophageal manometry and pH-impedance [14].

3.2. Gastric Emptying Dysfunction

There is evidence suggesting that gastric emptying (GE) may frequently be delayed in CD patients, although a direct correlation to specific dyspeptic symptoms is not clear. To assess gastric emptying, different methods are available and they generally agree to demonstrate an altered gastric function in both children and adults with CD. In 1997, we documented delayed gastric emptying in 50% of the adult celiac patients examined in a scintigraphic study [5]. Similar results were observed by Perri et al. in a pediatric population of CD patients by using octanoic acid breath testing (OBT) [7]. Further studies using ecography and OBT confirmed that gastric emptying was constantly delayed in CD patients compared with that in healthy controls [8–10]. Recently, we performed OBT on a group of untreated adult celiac patients and 75% of them showed delayed gastric emptying with no significant correlation to specific dyspeptic symptoms [15].

3.3. Small Bowel Motility Disorders

Bassotti et al. [3] were the first to manometrically display fasting motor abnormalities, represented by discrete clustered contractions, giant jejunal contractions and bursts of non-propagated contractions in both adults and children with CD. Cucchiara et al. [4] evaluated 14 untreated pediatric CD patients by manometric study, and found that 90% had a reduced postprandial antral motility index, shorter activity fronts, prolonged small bowel phasic activity and uncoordinated peristalsis. In the study of 1997 we also performed a gastro-intestinal manometry to assess gastric and small bowel motility in CD patients [5]. During the fasting period 75% of celiac patients showed abnormal propagation of activity fronts and clustered contractions. The duration of antral contractile response to the standard meal was reduced compared with that of control subjects. A more recent study by Bassotti et al. confirmed that more than 80% of untreated celiac patients had discrete motor abnormalities of the upper gut in both fasting and fed periods [16].

3.4. Oro-Cecal Transit and Colonic Motor Disorders

Delayed oro-cecal transit in CD patients has been frequently demonstrated by the breath test method. Spiller et al. [17] first showed increased transit time in CD patients with steatorrhea compared with that in healthy controls. More recently, Chiarioni et al. [6] found delayed oro-cecal time in 16 adult CD patients by way of lactulose breath testing. Bai et al. [18] confirmed the results of oro-cecal transit while colonic transit measured by radiopaque markers (Metcalf method) showed faster transit times in untreated CD patients. In 2012, Benini et al. [19] showed that mouth-to-cecum transit time was more prolonged in CD patients than in controls. The same study performed colonic transit with radiopaque markers but no differences were found between celiac patients and controls. No studies are available on ano-rectal motility disorders in CD patients.

3.5. Gallbladder Motility

Gallbladder (GB) motility in CD patients has been studied since the 1970s. The scintigraphy performed in earlier studies and more recent ultrasonography agree upon delayed GB emptying in untreated celiac patients [20,21]. These abnormalities were associated with decreased peak plasma CCK levels and increased basal plasma somatostatin values. Benini et al. [19] performed a study to assess GB motility by means of ultrasonography and found that GB fasting volume and postprandial residual volume were significantly higher in CD patients than in controls.

3.6. Pathophysiological Mechanisms of Motility Disorders in CD Patients

It has been hypothesized that mucosal damage and inflammation may affect contractile gut motility through perturbations of the complex hormonal and neuro-immunomodulatory regulation of the intestinal mucosa. Low-grade mucosal inflammation and mast-cell infiltration could play an important role in untreated CD [22], as well as having been observed in patients with irritable bowel syndrome (IBS) [23]. Earlier studies showed that the secretion of several hormones regulating gastrointestinal motility could be altered as a consequence of intestinal mucosal damage [24,25]. A decrease in cholecystokinin and an increase in somatostatin have been implicated in gallbladder dysmotility, while an increase in neurotensin and plasma peptide Y levels has been suggested as a cause of delayed gastric emptying and esophageal abnormalities [9].

Another underlying mechanism for motor disorders in CD patients may relate to autonomic nervous system dysfunction [26]. In particular, we observed that extrinsic autonomic neuropathy could play a role in provoking upper-gut motor disorders in untreated CD patients [5].

3.7. Clinical Consequences of Motility Disorders in CD Patients

As already described dysphagia is a frequent complaint of celiac patients [12,13], although severe motor disorders and serious nutritional consequences have not been described in these cases. In addition, gastro-esophageal reflux may be more frequent in CD patients than in the general population [5], which could suggest a specific therapeutic approach.

Surprisingly, a direct correlation to specific dyspeptic symptoms has not been demonstrated in the presence of delayed gastric emptying either in children or in adults with CD [5,7,10]. Similarly, small bowel dysmotility and altered oro-cecal transit have not been associated with specific clinical or nutritional problems.

On the other hand, special attention should be paid to the therapeutic implications of neurological conditions and thyroid dysfunction frequently associated with CD [27,28]. In these cases, gut dysmotility and, in particular, delayed gastric emptying could affect drug absorption and metabolism.

3.8. The Impact of GFD on Digestive Motor Disorders

Several articles have assessed the effects of a GFD on gut motor disorders, with conflicting results (Table 1). The majority of these studies showed that motor disorders can be completely reversible with a GFD.

Iovino et al. [13] showed that the prevalence of esophageal symptoms was significantly reduced in celiac patients after a year of a GFD. According to manometric evaluation, LES pressure was also significantly greater while on a GFD rather than on free diet.

Using OBT, Perri et al. [7] demonstrated that delayed gastric emptying could be normalized in the pediatric population afflicted by CD by means of a GFD. Similarly, a more recent OBT study showed that gluten withdrawal was effective in normalizing the gastric emptying time in all adult CD patients [10]. Benini et al. [8], using ultrasonography, showed that, after jejunal recovery, gastric emptying of the meal containing gluten remained unchanged, whereas emptying of the gluten-free meal was significantly shortened.

In a manometric small bowel study, four pediatric patients repeated the manometry after six months of a GFD and the traces had normalized [4]. Furthermore, a GFD normalized mouth-to-cecum transit in adult patients with CD in the study by Chiarioni et al. [6]. Finally, ecographic studies proved a GFD normalizes gallbladder motility [19,21].

On the other hand, we recently showed that delayed gastric emptying did not normalize on a GFD, despite the improved symptom score [15]. In addition, patients on a GFD showed motor abnormalities, albeit to a lesser extent than untreated CD subjects, in a small bowel manometric study [16]. In these patients, histological evaluation displayed the persistence of mild mucosal inflammation. Mouth-to-cecum transit time remained unchanged or more prolonged in CD patients than in controls after the introduction of a GFD in a lactulose breath testing study [19]. The same authors observed that duodenal infiltration with lymphocytes and mast cells remained higher than that in controls after gluten withdrawal.

Table 1 summarizes gut motility results in untreated and treated CD patients.

Table 1. Summary of more significant studies on gut motility in celiac disease (CD).

Authors [Ref]	Organs	Subjects	Methods	Findings	on GFD
Bassotti [3]	Small bowel	Adult and children CD	Manometry	Major frequence of migrating motor complex	No detected
Cucchiara [4]	Small bowel	Children CD	Manometry	Shorter activity front	Motor disorders normalized
Usai [5]	Esophagus, stomach, small bowel	Adult CD	Manometry pH-metry Scintigraphy	Nutcracker esophagus, esophageal reflux, delayed GE, abnormal small bowel activity front	No detected
Chiarioni [6]	OCT	Adult CD	Lactulose BT	Increased OCT	OCT normalized
Perri [7]	Stomach	Children CD	Octanoic BT	Delayed GE	GE normalized
Benini L [8]	Stomach	Adult CD	Ecography	Delayed GE	GE partially normalized
Rocco [10]	Stomach	Adult CD	Octanoic BT	Delayed GE	GE normalized
Usai [12]	Esophagus	Adult CD	Manometry pH-metry	Hypotonic LES, repetitive waves	No detected
Iovino [13]	Esophagus	Adult CD	Manometry	Hypotonic LES	Increased LES pressure
Usai Satta [15]	Stomach	Adult CD	Octanoic BT	Delayed GE	Unchanged GE
Bassotti [16]	Small bowel	Adult CD	Manometry	Shorter activity front	Unchanged data
Spiller [17]	OCT	Adult CD	Lactulose BT	Delayed OCT	No detected
Benini F [19]	Gallbladder, OCT	Adult CD	Ecography Lactulose BT	Delayed GB emptying and OCT	GB emptying normalized; OCT unchanged
Fraquelli [21]	Gallbladder	Adult CD	Ecography	Delayed GB emptying	GB emptying normalized

Notes: CD: celiac disease; GFD: gluten free diet; OCT: oro-cecal transit; LES: lower esophageal sphincter; BT: breath test; GE: gastric emptying; GB: gallbladder.

4. Non-Celiac Gluten Sensitivity (NCGS)

Digestive Motor Disorders and NCGS

Although no systematic studies have assessed overall gastro-intestinal and gallbladder motor disorders in NCGS, some indirect evidences support the hypothesis of a possible derangement of digestive motor function in these patients [29].

Preliminary results by a pilot study suggest that patients with NCGS can present with colonic motility alterations that improve after implementation of a GFD [30].

The complex of symptoms associated with gluten-related disorders and in particular NCGS, such as diarrhea, constipation or abdominal pain, may overlap and be similar to those caused by irritable bowel syndrome with diarrhea (IBS-D) [11]. IBS complaints are often part of the NCGS clinical picture. For subjects diagnosed with NCGS, the ingestion of gluten exerts a direct effect on the onset of digestive symptoms and the exclusion of gluten is the treatment of choice. Only a portion of the patients with IBS relate their symptoms to a gluten-containing diet. In a randomized controlled trial, a gluten-containing diet provoked an increase in the number of bowel movements per day and higher small bowel permeability compared with a GFD in IBS-D patients [31]. No differences in overall gastro-intestinal motility were observed after one month of a GFD. Experimental data showed that transgenic mice, sensitized by gluten, had an altered barrier function and enhanced muscle contractility [32]. Furthermore, gluten-induced symptoms in IBS-D patients were associated with increased myosin light chain kinase activity and claudin-15 expression, as described in a recent trial [33].

On the other hand, it was recently demonstrated that gluten ingestion can exert objective effects on gastric and gallbladder motility in healthy subjects [34]. The potential role of proteins other than gluten on gastric and gallbladder motility has been hypothesized. In fact, other wheat components, such as amylase-tripsin inhibitors or fructans, have been linked to the development of gastrointestinal symptoms in both patients with NCGS and IBS [35,36].

5. Conclusions

Gut motility is frequently abnormal in untreated CD in both children and adults. Most pediatric studies address gastro-intestinal motor disorders and show similar findings to those of adult CD patients. These abnormalities may be independent of the presence and grading of symptoms. Special attention should be paid to possible nutritional and pharmacological consequences. In the majority of studies, a GFD improved or normalized these abnormalities. In the case of these disorders persisting while the patient is on a GFD, the presence of a chronic low-grade mucosal inflammation with permanent perturbation of the neuro-immunomodulatory regulation may be hypothesized.

Due to the absence of structured studies, data on motility disorders in NCGS are just emerging. The clinical picture of IBS can overlap with NCGS. Further studies are needed to definitely assess the role of gut motor disorders in NCGS.

Author Contributions: All authors provided input on the content of the manuscript. All authors read and approved the final manuscript.

Funding: This review received no external funding.

Conflicts of Interest: The authors declare no conflicts of interest.

References

1. Kelly, C.P.; Bai, J.C.; Liu, E.; Leffler, D.A. Advances in diagnosis and management of celiac disease. *Gastroenterology* **2015**, *148*, 1175–1186. [CrossRef] [PubMed]
2. Catassi, C.; Elli, L.; Bonaz, B.; Bouma, G.; Carroccio, A.; Castillejo, G.; Cellier, C.; Cristofori, F.; De Magistris, L.; Dolinsek, J.; et al. Diagnosis of non-celiac gluten sensitivity (NCGS): The Salerno experts' criteria. *Nutrients* **2015**, *7*, 4966–4977. [CrossRef] [PubMed]
3. Bassotti, G.; Castellucci, G.; Betti, C.; Fusaro, C.; Cavalletti, M.L.; Bertotto, A.; Spinozzi, F.; Morelli, A.; Pello, M.A. Abnormal gastrointestinal motility in patients with celiac sprue. *Dig. Dis. Sci.* **1994**, *39*, 1947–1954. [CrossRef] [PubMed]
4. Cucchiara, S.; Bassotti, G.; Castellucci, G.; Minella, R.; Betti, C.; Fusaro, C.; Morelli, A.; Bertotto, A.; Auricchio, S. Upper gastrointestinal motor abnormalities in children with active celiac disease. *J. Pediatr. Gastroenterol. Nutr.* **1995**, *21*, 435–442. [CrossRef] [PubMed]
5. Usai, P.; Usai Satta, P.; Lai, M.; Corda, M.G.; Piras, E.; Calcara, C.; Boy, M.F.; Morelli, A.; Balestrieri, A.; Bassotti, G. Autonomic dysfunction and upper digestive functional disorders in untreated adult celiac disease. *Eur. J. Clin. Investig.* **1997**, *27*, 1009–1015. [CrossRef]

6. Chiarioni, G.; Bassotti, G.; Germani, U.; Battaglia, E.; Brentegani, M.T.; Morelli, A.; Vantini, I. Gluten-free diet normalizes mouth-to-cecum transit of a caloric meal in adult patients with celiac disease. *Dig. Dis. Sci.* **1997**, *42*, 2100–2105. [PubMed]
7. Perri, F.; Pastore, M.; Zicolella, A.; Annese, V.; Quitadamo, M.; Andriulli, A. Gastric emptying of solids is delayed in celiac disease and normalizes after gluten withdrawal. *Acta Paediatr.* **2000**, *89*, 921–925. [CrossRef] [PubMed]
8. Benini, L.; Sembenini, C.; Salandini, L.; Dall'O, E.; Bonfante, F.; Vantini, I. Gastric emptying of realistic meals with and without gluten in patients with coeliac disease. Effect of jejunal mucosal recovery. *Scand. J. Gastroenterol.* **2001**, *36*, 1044–1048. [PubMed]
9. Elli, L.; Bardella, M.T. Motility disorders in patients with celiac disease. *Scand. J. Gastroenterol.* **2005**, *40*, 743–749. [CrossRef] [PubMed]
10. Rocco, A.; Sarnelli, G.; Compare, D.; De Colibus, P.; Micheli, P.; Somma, P.; Marotti, B.; Cuomo, R.; Nardone, G. Tissue ghrelin level and gastric emptying rate in adult patients with celiac disease. *Neurogastroenterol. Motil.* **2008**, *20*, 884–890. [CrossRef] [PubMed]
11. Catassi, C.; Alaedini, A.; Bojarski, C.; Bonaz, B.; Bouma, G.; Carroccio, A.; Castillejo, G.; De Magistris, L.; Dieterich, W.; Di Liberto, D.; et al. The Overlapping Area of Non-Celiac Gluten Sensitivity (NCGS) and Wheat-Sensitive Irritable Bowel Syndrome (IBS): An Update. *Nutrients* **2017**, *9*, E1268. [CrossRef] [PubMed]
12. Usai, P.; Bassotti, G.; Usai Satta, P.; Cherchi, M.; Plesa, A.; Boy, F.; Morelli, A.; Balestrieri, A. Oesophageal motility in adult coeliac disease. *Neurogastroenterol. Motil.* **1995**, *7*, 239–244. [CrossRef] [PubMed]
13. Iovino, P.; Ciacci, C.; Sabbatini, F.; Acioli, D.M.; D'Argenio, G.; Mazzacca, G. Esophageal impairment in adult celiac disease with steatorrhea. *Am. J. Gastroenterol.* **1998**, *93*, 1243–1249. [CrossRef] [PubMed]
14. Nachman, F.; Pinto-Sanchez, M.I.; Salím, S.; Hwang, H.J.; Costa, F.; Longarini, G.; Ditaranto, A.; Fuxman, C.; Vazquez, H.; Moreno, M.L.; et al. Disfuncion esofágica en pacientes con enfermedad celiaca (abstract). *Acta Gastroenterol. Latinoam.* **2014**, *44*, S10.
15. Usai-Satta, P.; Oppia, F.; Scarpa, M.; Giannetti, C.; Cabras, F. Delayed gastric emptying does not normalize after gluten withdrawal in adult celiac disease. *Scand. J. Gastroenterol.* **2016**, *51*, 923–926. [CrossRef] [PubMed]
16. Bassotti, G.; Villanacci, V.; Mazzocchi, A.; Mariano, M.; Incardona, P.; Clerici, C.; Morelli, A. Antroduodenojejunal motor activity in untreated and treated celiac disease patients. *J. Gastroenterol. Hepatol.* **2008**, *23*, e23–e28. [CrossRef] [PubMed]
17. Spiller, R.C.; Lee, Y.C.; Edge, C.; Ralphs, D.N.L.; Stewart, J.S.; Bloom, S.R.; Silk, D.B. Delayed mouth-caecum transit of a lactulose labelled liquid test meal in patients with steatorrhea caused by partially treated coeliac disease. *Gut* **1987**, *28*, 1275–1282. [CrossRef] [PubMed]
18. Bai, J.C.; Mauriño, E.; Martínez, C.; Vasquez, H.; Niveloni, S.; Solfer, G.; Flores, D.; Boerr, L.A. Abnormal colonic transit time in untreated celiac sprue. *Acta Gastroenterol. Latinoam.* **1995**, *25*, 277–284. [PubMed]
19. Benini, F.; Mora, A.; Turini, D.; Bertolazzi, S.; Lanzarotto, F.; Ricci, C.; Villanacci, V.; Barbara, G.; Stanghellini, V.; Lanzini, A. Slow gallbladder emptying reverts to normal but small intestinal transit of a physiological meal remains slow in celiac patients during gluten-free diet. *Neurogastroenterol. Motil.* **2012**, *24*, e79–e80. [CrossRef] [PubMed]
20. Low-Beer, T.S.; Harvey, R.F.; Davies, E.R.; Read, A.F. Abnormalities of serum cholecystokinin and gallbladder emptying in celiac disease. *N. Engl. J. Med.* **1975**, *292*, 961–963. [CrossRef] [PubMed]
21. Fraquelli, M.; Bardella, M.T.; Peracchi, M.; Cesana, B.M.; Bianchi, P.A.; Conte, D. Gallbladder emptying and somatostatin and cholecystokinin plasma levels in celiac disease. *Am. J. Gastroenterol.* **1999**, *94*, 1867–1870. [CrossRef] [PubMed]
22. Strobel, S.; Busuttil, A.; Ferguson, A. Human intestinal mucosal mast cells: Expanded population in untreated coeliac disease. *Gut* **1983**, *24*, 222–227. [CrossRef] [PubMed]
23. Barbara, G.; Stanghellini, V.; De Giorgio, R.; Corinaldesi, R. Functional gastrointestinal disorders and mast cells: Implications for therapy. *Neurogastroenterol. Motil.* **2006**, *18*, 6–17. [CrossRef] [PubMed]
24. Besterman, H.S.; Bloom, S.R.; Sarson, D.L.; Blackburn, A.M.; Johnston, D.I.; Patel, H.R.; Stewart, J.S.; Modigliani, R.; Guerin, S.; Mallinson, C.N. Gut-hormone profile in coeliac disease. *Lancet* **1978**, *1*, 785–788. [CrossRef]

25. Sjolund, K.; Alumets, J.; Berg, N.O.; Hakanson, R.; Sundler, F. Duodenal endocrine cells in adult coeliac disease. *Gut* **1979**, *20*, 547–552. [CrossRef] [PubMed]
26. Gibbons, C.H.; Freeman, R. Autonomic neuropathy and coeliac disease. *J. Neurol. Neurosurg. Psychiatr.* **2005**, *76*, 579–581. [CrossRef] [PubMed]
27. Casella, G.; Bordo, B.M.; Schalling, R.; Villanacci, V.; Salemme, M.; Di Bella, C.; Baldini, V.; Bassotti, G. Neurological disorders and celiac disease. *Minerva Gastroenterol. Dietol.* **2016**, *62*, 197–206. [PubMed]
28. Centanni, M.; Benvenga, S.; Sachmechi, I. Diagnosis and management of treatment-refractory hypothyroidism: An expert consensus report. *J. Endocrinol. Investig.* **2017**, *40*, 1289–1301. [CrossRef] [PubMed]
29. Pinto-Sanchez, M.I.; Bercik, P.; Verdu, E.F. Motility alterations in celiac disease and non-celiac gluten sensitivity. *Dig. Dis.* **2015**, *33*, 200–207. [CrossRef] [PubMed]
30. Pinto-Sanchez, M.I.; Basra, D.; McCarville, J.; Deng, Y.; Hansen, S.; Nardelli, A.; Niveloni, S.; Smecuol, E.; Armstrong, D.; Moayyedi, P.; et al. Improvement of gastrointestinal symptoms and motility in non-celiac gluten sensitive patients after the gluten free diet (abstract FS193_0136). Presented at Celiac Disease and Other Small Bowel Disorders, Falk Symposium 193. Amsterdam, The Netherlands, 5–6 September 2014; 156. Symposia and Workshops 2014. Available online: http://www.falk-foundation-symposia.org/symposia-and-workshops/2014/?L=1 (accessed on 10 September 2018).
31. Vazquez-Roque, M.I.; Camilleri, M.; Smyrk, T.; Murray, J.A.; Marietta, E.; O'Neill, J.; Carlson, P.; Lamsam, J.; Janzow, D.; Eckert, D.; et al. A controlled trial of gluten-free diet in patients with irritable bowel syndrome-diarrhea: Effects on bowel frequency and intestinal function. *Gastroenterology* **2013**, *144*, 903–911. [CrossRef] [PubMed]
32. Natividad, J.M.; Huang, X.; Slack, E.; Jury, J.; Sanz, Y.; David, C.; Denou, E.; Yang, P.; Murray, J.; McCoy, K.D.; et al. Host responses to intestinal microbial antigens in gluten-sensitive mice. *PLoS ONE* **2009**, *4*, e6472. [CrossRef] [PubMed]
33. Wu, R.L.; Vazquez-Roque, M.I.; Carlson, P.; Burton, D.; Grover, M.; Camilleri, M.; Turner, J.R. Gluten-induced symptoms in diarrhea-predominant irritable bowel syndrome are associated with increased myosin light chain kinase activity and claudin-15 expression. *Lab. Investig.* **2017**, *97*, 14–23. [CrossRef] [PubMed]
34. Massironi, S.; Branchi, F.; Fraquelli, M.; Baccarin, A.; Somalvico, F.; Ferretti, F.; Conte, D.; Elli, L. Effects of a Gluten-Containing Meal on Gastric Emptying and Gallbladder Contraction. *Nutrients* **2018**, *10*, 910. [CrossRef] [PubMed]
35. Biesiekierski, J.R.; Peters, S.L.; Newnham, E.D.; Rosella, O.; Muir, J.G.; Gibson, P.R. No effects of gluten in patients with self-reported non-celiac gluten sensitivity after dietary reduction of fermentable, poorly absorbed, short-chain carbohydrates. *Gastroenterology* **2013**, *145*, 320–328. [CrossRef] [PubMed]
36. Mansueto, P.; Seidita, A.; D'Alcamo, A.; Carroccio, A. Role of FODMAPs in patients with irritable bowel syndrome. *Nutr. Clin. Pract.* **2015**, *30*, 665–682. [CrossRef] [PubMed]

nutrients

MDPI

Review

Mood Disorders and Gluten: It's Not All in Your Mind! A Systematic Review with Meta-Analysis

Eleanor Busby [1], Justine Bold [1,*], Lindsey Fellows [1] and Kamran Rostami [2]

[1] The School of Allied Health and Community, University of Worcester, Worcester WR2 6AJ, UK; busel_17@uni.worc.ac.uk (E.B.); l.fellows@worc.ac.uk (L.F.)

[2] Department of Gastroenterology, Mid-Central District Health Board, Palmerston North Hospital, Palmerston North 4442, New Zealand; kamran.rostami@midcentraldhb.govt.nz

* Correspondence: j.bold@worc.ac.uk; Tel.: +44-1905-855-391

Received: 14 October 2018; Accepted: 6 November 2018; Published: 8 November 2018

Abstract: Gluten elimination may represent an effective treatment strategy for mood disorders in individuals with gluten-related disorders. However, the directionality of the relationship remains unclear. We performed a systematic review of prospective studies for effects of gluten on mood symptoms in patients with or without gluten-related disorders. Six electronic databases (CINAHL, PsycINFO, Medline, Web of Science, Scopus and Cochrane Library) were searched, from inception to 8 August 2018, for prospective studies published in English. Meta-analyses with random-effects were performed. Three randomised-controlled trials and 10 longitudinal studies comprising 1139 participants fit the inclusion criteria. A gluten-free diet (GFD) significantly improved pooled depressive symptom scores in GFD-treated patients (Standardised Mean Difference (SMD) −0.37, 95% confidence interval (CI) −0.55 to −0.20; $p < 0.0001$), with no difference in mean scores between patients and healthy controls after one year (SMD 0.01, 95% CI −0.18 to 0.20, $p = 0.94$). There was a tendency towards worsening symptoms for non-coeliac gluten sensitive patients during a blinded gluten challenge vs. placebo (SMD 0.21, 95% CI −0.58 to 0.15; $p = 0.25$). Our review supports the association between mood disorders and gluten intake in susceptible individuals. The effects of a GFD on mood in subjects without gluten-related disorders should be considered in future research.

Keywords: gluten-related disorders; gluten-free diet; coeliac disease; non-coeliac gluten sensitivity; irritable bowel syndrome; mood disorders; affective disorders; depression; major depressive disorder; mental health; nutrition

1. Introduction

Mood disorders are a global healthcare burden, with 300 million people now suffering from depression worldwide [1]. In 2015, the World Health Organisation (WHO) estimated that 4.4% of the global population were suffering from clinical depression—a 18.4% increase in prevalence since 2005. On top of this, around 61 million antidepressants are prescribed in a single year in the UK alone [2], while depressive disorders were ranked as the largest contributor to global non-fatal health loss, as well as increased suicide risk [3].

Wheat products are now the main source of carbohydrate in the Western diet and contain high amounts of the protein, gluten. In recent years, reports of gastrointestinal and extra-intestinal symptoms, due to gluten-containing foods have been on the increase [4]. Coeliac disease (CD) is characterised by intestinal mucosal damage due to an immune response to gluten peptides, with clinical improvement after following a gluten-free diet (GFD) [5]. This involves the elimination of gluten-containing foods from the diet, such as wheat, rye and barley products. CD affects about 1% of the UK population [6] and its global prevalence is on the rise [7]. Moreover, around 10% of CD patients are affected by psychiatric disorders [8], with a higher proportion of CD patients exhibiting depression compared to the general population [9]. However, CD can manifest in a variety of ways, with symptomatically atypical and silent patient subgroups [10], and hence is thought to be underdiagnosed [5]. Therefore, it is a possibility that CD may be misdiagnosed, as depression for example, due to a lack of classical symptoms.

A growing body of evidence suggests that mood symptoms are associated with a spectrum of gluten-related disorders [9,11,12]. Reports of health improvements after following a GFD in the absence of CD has led to non-coeliac gluten sensitivity (NCGS) becoming increasingly recognised as its own clinical entity [13], with evidence indicating a higher prevalence than CD [14]. In contrast to CD, specific serological markers for NCGS are lacking; only some patients exhibit increased antibodies to gluten peptides and no mucosal damage is generally observed [15]. Nonetheless, in 1956 it was suggested that gluten may be associated with mood and psychiatric symptoms in a case series of subjects without CD [16]. More recently, mood symptoms are frequently reported as a result of wheat ingestion [17] with 'low mood' being a common motivation for gluten avoidance [18] in the absence of both CD and wheat allergy. Furthermore, recent clinical studies have found raised gluten-related antibodies in patients with bipolar, major depressive disorder, and schizophrenia [19–21], while episodes of acute mania may be associated with increased serum levels of antibodies against gliadin [22]. Hence, there is mounting evidence for a, potentially bidirectional, relationship between gluten sensitivity and psychiatric disorders.

Numerous theories regarding the aetiology of mood symptoms in those with gluten-related disorders exist. One theory suggests that an immune response to gluten may lead to depressive symptoms [23]. Further evidence suggests social exclusion could lead to depression in CD [6] while another study relates mood symptoms to adjusting to the chronic nature of a physical disease in general [24]. Contrary to this, Roos et al. found no relationship between gastrointestinal symptoms and psychological well-being in CD [25], although antidepressants have interestingly been found to reduce abdominal pain in irritable bowel syndrome (IBS) [26]. Conversely, nutritional deficiencies may be a causative factor for reduced mood; for instance, B-vitamin supplementation was found to significantly improve depression in adults with longstanding CD on a GFD [27]. Finally, the ingestion of FODMAPs (Fermentable Oligo-, Di-, Mono-saccharides And Polyols—short chain carbohydrates also present in wheat, rye and barley, as well as beans, pulses and certain vegetables), have also been suggested to increase both physical and psychological symptoms in those thought to be gluten sensitive [28,29]. Hence, there appears to be a complex and multifactorial relationship between mood and gluten-related disorders.

Regardless, a GFD has been shown to improve mental health in susceptible individuals. Significant improvements in mood disorders and psychological well-being have been recognised in patients with CD [30–32], IBS [33] and NCGS [34] following a GFD, although the magnitude of improvement is found to be dependent on good dietary adherence [11,35]. Moreover, anti-gliadin IgG antibodies disappeared in NCGS patients [34] and markers of systemic inflammation were reduced in IBS patients [36], as well as healthy mice [37] following initiation of a GFD. Hence, a GFD may reduce inflammation and improve mood, although a relationship between these outcomes remains theoretical.

Whilst the GFD for autism spectrum disorders has been well reviewed [38,39], other reviews of psychiatric and mood disorders in relation to gluten have focussed on CD and epidemiological, rather than interventional, evidence [12,40]. Meanwhile, a review on extra-intestinal symptoms in NCGS [41] included only one study considering psychiatric outcomes [42]. However, a search of registered protocols did not reveal that any systematic reviews on gluten and mood are planned or currently in progress. Therefore, we conducted a systematic review of prospective studies with a gluten challenge or GFD intervention on the prevalence and/or severity of mood symptoms in patients with or without gluten-related disorders. Our study was underpinned by the following objectives: To establish whether a relationship exists between mood and gluten; to explore the outcomes of severity mood symptoms and the prevalence of mood disorders; to assess the impact of the level of adherence to a GFD on the severity of mood symptoms; to highlight gaps in the research literature; and to determine implications for practice in terms of implementing a GFD in those with gluten-related and mood disorders.

2. Materials and Methods

2.1. Eligibility Criteria

The eligibility criteria for inclusion of studies into our systematic review consisted of the following:

1. All studies evaluating the effect of gluten ingestion or elimination on the presence or severity of depressive symptoms and other mood disorders, with any gluten-related intervention for any length of time.
2. As evidence suggests a correlation between mood and level of adherence to a GFD [35,43,44], dietary adherence must be defined using a validated measure and either specify good adherence or report data for adherent and non-adherent participants separately.
3. All prospective intervention studies—randomised, non-randomised, longitudinal—which investigated the change in the severity of mood symptoms as a primary or secondary outcome using a validated questionnaire. We excluded retrospective and cross-sectional studies, as we aimed to investigate the relationship between mood and gluten over a specified amount of time while measuring adherence.
4. Published studies in English.

Further to this, we defined the following eligibility criteria for inclusion of study data into meta-analysis:

1. Data must be reported as means and standard deviations (SDs), or these values must be calculatable or estimable using the available data by methods outlined in the Cochrane Handbook [45].
2. Each study should report a different sample; for different studies utilising the same sample, as part of a follow-up study or ad-hoc analysis for example, only data from the most relevant study or the study reporting the largest sample were included.
3. For comparisons between patients and healthy controls, control and patient groups must be demographically matched by age and gender.

2.2. Search Strategy and Selection Criteria

The scientific databases CINAHL, PsycINFO, Medline, Web of Science, Scopus and the Cochrane Library were searched using the strategies outlined in Tables S1–S6 in Supplementary File 1. These were designed using keywords, Medical Subject Heading (MeSH) terms and free text words, such as gluten-free diet and depression, combined using Boolean operators. The strategies were piloted for each database and three authors (E.B., J.B. and L.F.) reviewed and amended the search strategy before E.B. commenced the final search. To ensure all relevant studies were captured, two authors (E.B. and J.B.) independently screened and selected the studies. In cases of disagreement, a third author (L.F.) was consulted for the final decision. Reference lists of relevant studies were also searched.

2.3. Data Extraction and Quality Assessment

One reviewer (E.B.) extracted the data according to a data extraction form developed to collect information regarding study design, population, intervention, controls and outcomes. The data extraction form included information on authors, country, recruitment methods, number of participants, methods of measuring adherence, level of dietary adherence, commercial funding and/or conflicts of interest, study/intervention duration and analysis strategy (ITT—intention-to-treat; PP—per-protocol). Further data was extracted in order to assess risk of bias (ROB) according to tools developed by the Cochrane Collaboration; Cochrane's ROB 2.0 (University of Bristol, Bristol, UK) [46] was used for randomised controlled trials (RCTs) and the Risk Of Bias In Non-randomized Studies of Interventions (ROBINS-I) tool (University of Bristol, Bristol, UK) [47] for all types of non-randomised studies. The bias domains included in ROBINS-I overlap with the Cochrane ROB 2.0 tool, but instead of assessing the randomisation process, include the additional domains: Confounding, selection of participants into the study and classification at intervention. Specific criteria for assessing the risk of bias in each of the domains in the context of our review are described in Table S7 in Supplementary File 2.

2.4. Statistical Analysis

We performed all meta-analyses with Review Manager (RevMan) 5.3 (The Nordic Cochrane Centre, Copenhagen, Denmark, 2014). Outcomes are based on random-effects models using mean differences. Results from the analysis are presented as mean differences along with the 95% confidence intervals. Statistical significance was set at 0.05 for two-sided p-values. Data was synthesised by meta-analysis when there was a consistent comparison in two or more studies measuring depressive outcomes. Where possible, only depressive outcome data from questionnaires not biased towards physical illness, with no questions related to gastrointestinal health and eating habits, were synthesised in meta-analysis; data from studies using biased questionnaires containing these types of questions were reported separately. For continuous data, scores from depression scales were reported as means and the standardised mean difference (SMD) was used as a summary statistic. The means of psychometric scales that increased with severity of depression were multiplied by -1 to ensure that all the scales point in the same direction. Dichotomous data were presented as the percentage of patients who were depressed with a score above a specified cut-point, which we reported only when the cut-point score used in the study was based on a validated rather than arbitrary figure. Risk difference (RD) was used to report the results as this is a measure of absolute effect and more intuitive to interpret [45], especially for change of scores from baseline. Funnel plots were used to evaluate publication bias. All forest plots were stratified according to risk of detection bias. We have highlighted this domain as the key risk of bias domain for our study due to our outcome of interest being a subjective measurement. We used the Grades of Recommendation, Assessment, Development and Evaluation Working Group (GRADE Working Group) system [48,49] for grading the quality of evidence for each outcome according to study design, consistency, directness, imprecision and reporting bias. We used GRADEpro GTD to build the Summary of Findings (SoF) and GRADE profile tables [50].

2.5. Heterogeneity and Sensitivity Analyses

Heterogeneity between studies was interpreted according to general guidance [51], which suggest that I^2 values of 25%, 50%, and 75% may indicate low, medium and high heterogeneity, respectively, while a value of 0% indicates no observed heterogeneity. To address the most important sources of heterogeneity, we performed planned subgroup analyses considering the effect of CD (CD vs. non-CD participants), gastrointestinal symptoms (symptomatic vs. asymptomatic), and the presence of the CD-associated HLA-DQ2/8 genotype (positive vs. negative) on depressive outcome measures. We also retrospectively performed a subgroup analysis into population sample country of origin after extracting and analysing the data in order to further investigate heterogeneity. The effect of dietary adherence (compliant vs. noncompliant participants) was analysed as a separate comparison so as to include data from Nachman et al. (2010). Sensitivity analyses were performed for: Study searching, by including abstracts whose results could not be confirmed in subsequent publications; data selection, by excluding results from studies utilising an ITT approach; study methods, by analysing only studies with an average intervention time of one year; study quality, by excluding studies at a high risk of bias in key domain(s); and analysis methods by changing random-effects (RE) for fixed-effects (FE) and risk differences (RD) for risk ratios (RR) and odds ratios (OR).

2.6. Missing Data

All studies reporting the necessary outcome data as mean values with SDs were included in meta-analysis. If the necessary data was not reported in the correct format for meta-analysis, the corresponding author of the relevant study was contacted via email to request the required data. If no reply was received, a reminder email was sent three weeks after the initial request and other study authors were contacted if emails could be retrieved. As a final resort, and if possible, means and SDs were calculated from the available information (as long as the data were determined to be normally distributed) according to the methods outlined in Chapter 7 of the Cochrane Handbook version 5.1.0 [45]. Some scores were derived from graphs by optical plot reading using WebPlotDigitizer (Version 4.1, Ankit Rohatgi, Austin, TX, USA) [52].

3. Results

3.1. Literature Search

The final literature search for all databases was conducted on 8 August 2018 by E.B. These searches identified 236 papers, three additional citations were identified by a recursive bibliography search [34,53,54], one study was referred by an expert in the field [55] and one study was already known by the authors [29]. After excluding records based on duplicate data, title or abstract, fifty-one were fully reviewed. Finally, 13 studies met the inclusion criteria (Figure 1). The characteristics of these included studies are summarised in Table 1. A summary of reasons for the studies excluded by full-text screening are provided in Table S8 in Supplementary File 3.

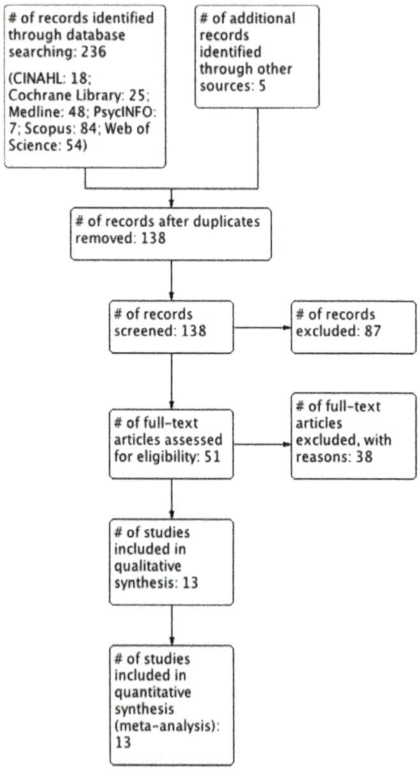

Figure 1. Flow diagram of study selection. #, number.

3.2. Characteristics of the Included Studies

Of the 13 studies, three were RCTs [42,53,56]. Study participants were subjects with self-reported NCGS with [42] and without [56] diagnosed IBS, and asymptomatic EmA-positive subjects [53]. Each of these studies excluded CD either by previous diagnosis [53] or study screening [42,56]. The remaining 10 studies were single arm before-after studies; one of these was a time-interrupted study and one was a follow-up study. Of these, two reported on the same group of participants; Nachman et al. (2009) reported the initial study period from baseline to one year at intervals of three months for all participants, while Nachman et al. (2010) reported baseline, one-year and four-year follow-up results for a subset of the same participants (n = 53) who continued to follow a GFD for the full four years. Although using the same sample, both studies were included as they elucidate the short and long-term effects of a GFD on depressive symptoms. Nevertheless, results from these studies were not pooled in meta-analysis as they report on the same participants, and hence were analysed separately.

There were differences in the questionnaires utilised to measure the severity of depression between the included studies. Three studies used questionnaires containing questions related to gastrointestinal health and eating habits; two used the Beck Depression Inventory (BDI) [57,58], and one the Hamilton Depression Rating Scale (HDRS) [59]. However, one of these studies reported some data from a sub-analysis removing these questions [58]. Conversely, nine studies used questionnaires containing no such questions; four used the Psychological General Well-Being Index (PGWB) [53,60–62], one the Hospital Anxiety and Depression Scale (HADS) [63], one the Crown-Crisp Experiential Index (CCEI) [64], one the Children's Depression Inventory (CDI) [11] and one the State-Trait Personality Inventory (STPI) [42], while one further study [65] used a modified version of the Zung Self-Rating Depression Scale (SDS) with such questions removed. Finally, one study simply asked participants to grade depression as present or absent on each day [56].

3.3. Quality Assessment

Of the RCTs, one study was found to have a low risk of bias and two were found to have a high risk of bias. Of the non-randomised studies, three were found to have a moderate risk of bias while the remaining seven were found to have a serious risk of bias. Graphical representations of the summary of risk of bias for individual studies and across all studies are given in Figure 2, and the analysis of each domain is detailed in Supplementary File 4.

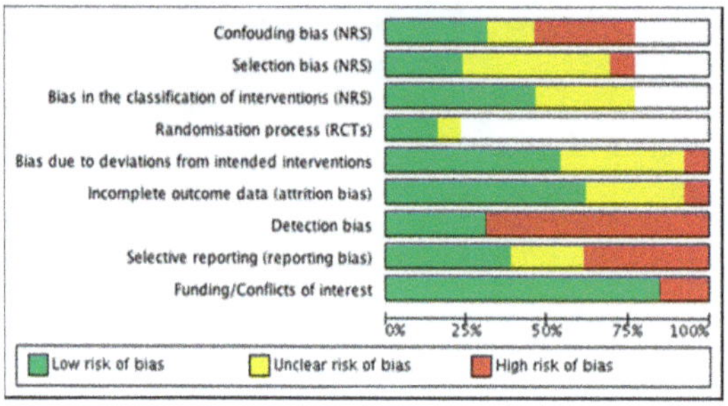

A

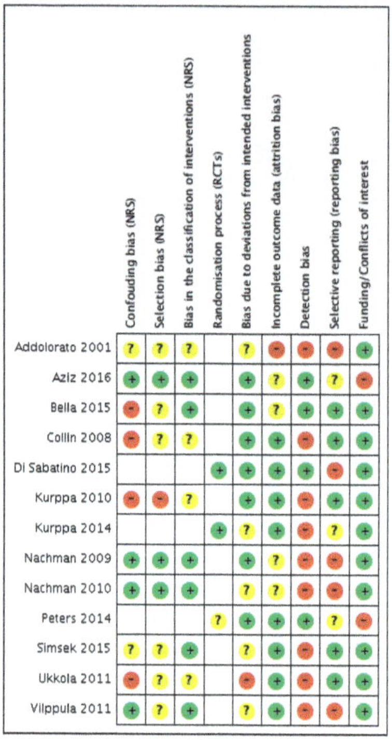

B

Figure 2. (**A**) Risk of bias graph: Review authors' judgements about each risk of bias item presented as percentages across all included studies. (**B**) Risk of bias summary: Review authors' judgements about each risk of bias item for each included study.

Table 1. Characteristics of included studies.

Author (Year)	Country of Origin/Study Design	Participants	Healthy Controls	Interventions	Outcomes	Method of Measuring Adherence *	Notes
Addolorato et al. (2001) [65]	Italy Single centre BA comparison	35 newly diagnosed classical CD patients	59 HC recruited from hospital staff members	GFD for 1 y	Changes in depression score BA a GFD (M-SDS) Changes in no. patients positive for depression BA a GFD (M-SDS score > 49)	1—validated 2—family member interview 3—AGA, EmA 4—biopsy at 6–8 mo	
Aziz et al. (2016) [63]	UK Single centre BA comparison	41 IBS-D patients; 20 HLA-DQ2/8+ and 21 HLA-DQ2/8−	NC	GFD for 6 wk; FU at 18 mo for those who continued on GFD	Changes in HADS before and after a GFD Difference between HLA-DQ2/8+/− groups	1—validated ("Patients scoring 0 or 1 do not follow a strict GFD. Patients scoring 2 follow a GFD but with errors necessitating correction. Finally, patients scoring three or four follow a strict GFD.")	Educational grant from Dr. Schär (a gluten-free food manufacturer) to undertake investigator-conceived and -led research on gluten sensitivity
Bella et al. (2015) [59]	Italy Single centre BA comparison (FU study from Pennisi et al. (2014))	13 CD patients	NC	GFD for 16 mo	Changes in depression score BA a GFD (HDRS) Changes in no. patients positive for depression (dysthymia) BA a GFD (SCID-I)	1—validated 3—EmA, tTG	
Collin et al. (2008) [64]	Finland Single centre BA comparison	20 biopsy-proven CD patients	HCs not recruited from same community (female students/male workers)	GFD for 1 y	Changes in depression score BA a GFD (sub-score of CCEI/Middlesex Hospital Questionnaire)	3—EmA 4—Vh/CrD	
Di Sabatino et al. (2015) [56]	Italy Multicentre DB, PC, CO RCT	59 patients suspected of having NCGS (CD and WA excluded)	NA	2 arms; GFD (1 wk baseline period) followed by 1 wk: (a) 4.375 g/day gluten (b) rice starch placebo with 1 wk wash-out periods inbetween	Difference in mean daily depression scores (unvalidated questionnaire) between gluten and placebo groups	1—validated 6—unused capsules counted	
Kurppa et al. (2010) [60]	Finland Single centre Cohort	73 EmA-positive adults; 27 mild enteropathy (Marsh I-II), 46 CD (Marsh III)	110 HCs (age and gender matched)	GFD for 1 y	Changes in depression score BA a GFD (sub-score of PGWB)	3—EmA, tTG 4—Vh/CrD	
Kurppa et al. (2014) [53]	Finland Multicentre DB, CO RCT	40 asymptomatic EmA-positive adults (CD excluded)	NA	2 arms; participants randomised to a GFD or gluten-containing diet for 1 y then cross-over	Difference in mean depression score between gluten and GFD groups at 1 y (sub-score of PGWB)	2—NI on who conducted 3—EmA, tTG 4—Vh/CrD	Deviations from protocol: No-one in GFD group willing to restart gluten-containing diet so only data from 1 y FU used

Table 1. *Cont.*

Author (Year)	Country of Origin/Study Design	Participants	Healthy Controls	Interventions	Outcomes	Method of Measuring Adherence *	Notes
Nachman et al. (2009) [58]	Argentina Single centre BA comparison/time-interrupted study	84 newly diagnosed biopsy-proven CD patients; 62 classical, 14 atypical and 8 asymptomatic	70 HCs recruited from hospital staff members (age and gender matched)	GFD for 1 y	At baseline, 3, 6, 9 and 12 mo: Changes in depression score BA a GFD (BDI) Changes in no. patients positive for depression BA a GFD (BDI score $\geq$ 18) Subgroup analysis: Compliant vs. noncompliant	Opinion of physician in charge, based on: 1—self-rated questionnaire 2—"meticulous enquiry by an experienced dietician" 3—tTG, DGP, EmA, AGA 4—Vh/CrD 5—4 day (self-reported)	
Nachman et al. (2010) [57]	Argentina Single centre BA comparison/FU from Nachman et al. (2009)	53 CD patients; 37 classical and 16 atypical/asymptomatic	70 HCs recruited from hospital staff members (age and gender matched) (same as Nachman et al. (2009))	GFD for 4 y	At baseline, 1 y and 4 y: Changes in depression score BA a GFD (BDI) Changes in no. patients positive for depression BA a GFD (BDI score $\geq$ 18) Subgroup analysis: Compliant vs. noncompliant	Opinion of physician in charge, based on: 1—self-rated questionnaire 2—"meticulous enquiry by an experienced dietician" 3—tTG, DGP, EmA, AGA 4—Vh/CrD 5—4 day (self-reported)	
Peters et al. (2014) [42]	Australia Single centre DB, PC, CO RCT	20 IBS patients (CD excluded by biospy); recruited from a preceding study in which subjects with self-reported NCGS were challenged with diets containing varying amounts of gluten (Biesiekierski et al., 2013)	NA	3 arms; low-FODMAPs + GFD (3 day baseline period) followed by 3 day: (a) gluten (16 g/day) (b) whey (16 g/day) (protein control) (c) placebo with 3–14 day washout period in between	Difference in depression scores following each dietary challenge (sub-score of STPI)	1—validated 5—3 day (self-reported) 6—unused/additional food counted	Peter R. Gibson has published two books on a diet for IBS. This study was supported by George Weston Foods as part of a partnership in an Australian Research Council Linkage Project and the National Health and Medical Research Council (NHMRC) of Australia.
Simsek et al. (2015) [11]	Turkey Single centre BA comparison	24 newly diagnosed biopsy-proven paediatric CD patients; age limit 9–16 y	25 HCs recruited from same centre; EmA-negative	GFD for 6–20 mo	Changes in depression score BA a GFD (CDI) Subgroup analysis: Compliant vs. noncompliant	3—EmA, tTG	
Ukkola et al. (2011) [61]	Finland Nationwide BA comparison	698 newly diagnosed (within 1 y) biopsy-proven CD patients; 490 classical, 62 atypical and 146 screen-detected	110 HCs (age and gender matched)	GFD for 1 y	Changes in depression score BA a GFD (subscore of PGWB)	1—unvalidated FU question ("strict diet" or "dietary lapses")	

Table 1. *Cont.*

Author (Year)	Country of Origin/Study Design	Participants	Healthy Controls	Interventions	Outcomes	Method of Measuring Adherence *	Notes
Vilppula et al. (2011) [62]	Finland Nationwide BA comparison	32 screen-detected biopsy-proven CD patients; age > 50 y	110 HCs recruited from neighbourhoods of CD patients (age and gender matched)	GFD for 1–2 y	Changes in depression score BA a GFD (subscore of PGWB)	2—with dietician 3—tTG, EmA 4—Vh/CrD ("Diet considered strict when there were no signs of dietary transgressions upon the interview. Occasional GFD defined as a gluten intake occurring less often than once in the month.")	

NOTE: Studies in alphabetical order. Abbreviations: RCT, randomised controlled trial; BA, before-after; DB, double-blind; PC, placebo controlled; CO, cross-over; CD, coeliac disease; WA, wheat allergy; GFD, gluten-free diet; HC, healthy control; NC, no control group; IBS(-D), irritable bowel syndrome (diarrhoea-predominant); NCGS, non-coeliac gluten sensitivity; y, year; mo, month; wk, week; FU, follow-up; M-SDS, modified Zung Self-reported Depression Scale; HADS, Hospital Anxiety and Depression Scale; HDRS, Hamilton Depression Rating Scale; SCID-I, Structured Clinical Interview for DSM-IV Axis I Disorders; CCEI, Crown-Crisp Experiential Index; PGWB, Psychological General Well-Being Index; BDI, Beck Depression Inventory; STPI, State-Trait Personality Inventory; CDI, Children's Depression Inventory; AGA, Anti-gliadin antibodies; EmA, anti-endomysial antibodies; tTG, Anti-tissue transglutaminase antibodies; Vh/CrD, villous height:crypt depth ratio; DGP, Deamidated Gliadin Peptide; NI, no information; NA, not applicable. * 1, Self-rated questionnaire; 2, Interview; 3, Serology; 4, Histology; 5, Food diary/record; 6, Other.

3.4. *Data and Analyses*

A summary of our findings are presented in Tables S9–S12 in Supplementary File 5.

3.4.1. A GFD vs. A Gluten-Containing Diet

3.4.1.1. Difference in Mean Depression Scores

One RCT compared a GFD to a normal gluten-containing diet in a two-arm study [53] and ten reports of nine single-arm before-after studies compared depression scores for participants at baseline (on a gluten-containing diet) and after following a GFD. However, two studies were not eligible for meta-analysis [59,65] and one study [57] was a follow-up of the same sample from another study [58]. Hence, eight studies with a total of 953 participants were included in meta-analysis. We found that a GFD significantly reduced depressive symptoms in 953 participants overall (SMD −0.37, 95% CI −0.55 to −0.20; $p < 0.0001$) (Figure 3A). There was low-medium heterogeneity between the studies overall ($I^2 = 38\%$), but zero heterogeneity between the non-randomised studies and RCTs. Subgroup analyses (Figure S1, Supplementary File 6) revealed no difference in effect between those with and without diagnosed CD ($p = 0.73$) or between those HLA-DQ2/8-positive and HLA-DQ2/8-negative ($p = 0.49$). Conversely, there was a significant difference in effect between those with classical, atypical and silent CD ($p = 0.003$) with high heterogeneity between subgroups ($I^2 = 82.5\%$) (Figure 3B); while classical CD patients exhibited a significant effect (SMD −0.65, 95% CI −0.96 to −0.34; $p < 0.0001$), the effect for silent CD patients was nonsignificant (SMD −0.06, 95% CI −0.38 to 0.26; $p = 0.71$) and one study reported a significant effect for atypical CD patients.

Of the studies not eligible for meta-analysis, one reported non-normally distributed data as medians and IQRs as opposed to means and SDs [59] and one only reported mean scores for patients positive for depression rather than all participants [65]. One study included in meta-analysis did not report SDs for the PGWB subcategories [61], so SDs for the mean depression values were estimated using methods described in the Cochrane Handbook [45] and 95% CI values imputed from an ad-hoc analysis of the same population sample [66]. Only data for the classical CD patients from Nachman et al. [58] were used because this was the only data reported for the modified BDI removing questions to avoid bias due to illness. Moreover, only scores for adherent participants ($n = 7$) were used from Simsek et al. [11] as noncompliance was high with 17/24 participants (71%) found not to follow a strict GFD. Finally, one study providing data for a second follow-up at four years [57] suggests an insignificant trend towards worsening depressive symptoms relative to one year ($p = 0.39$), which remained significant relative to baseline ($p < 0.0001$) (Figure S2, Supplementary File 6).

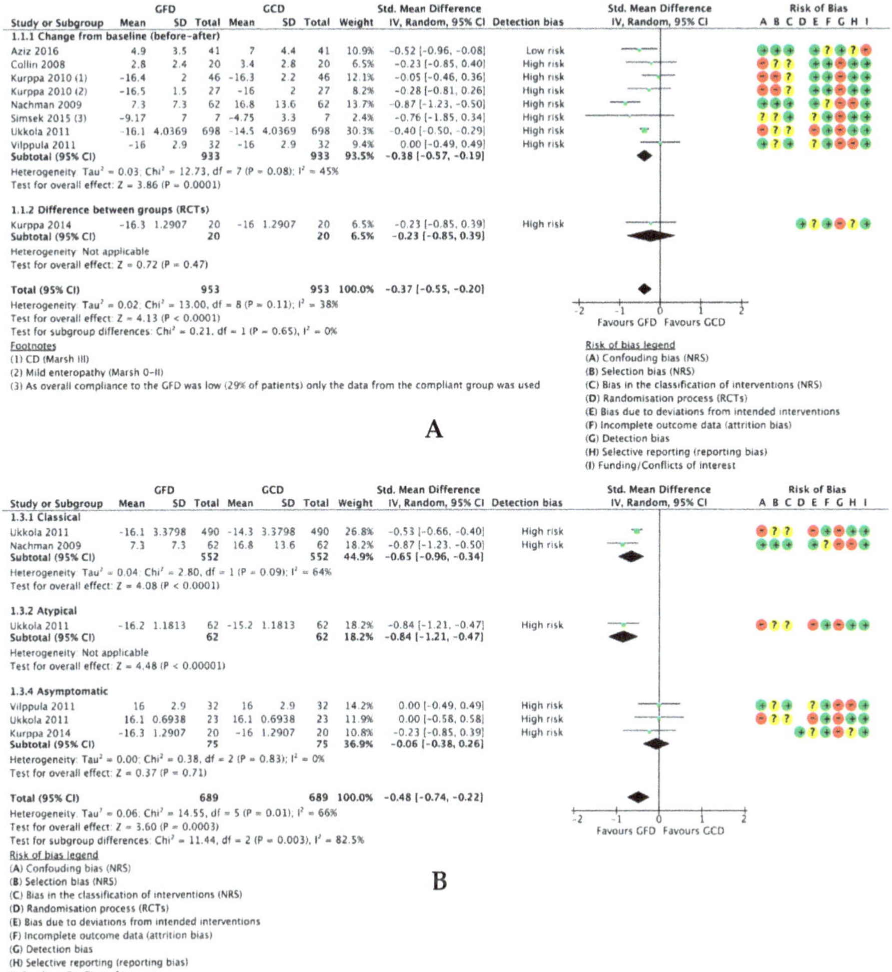

Figure 3. Forest plot demonstrating the difference in mean depression scores between following a GFD and a gluten-containing diet for (**A**) all studies (1 RCT comparing two intervention groups and seven BA studies comparing participant scores at baseline) and (**B**) subgroup analysis based on symptoms (classical, atypical and asymptomatic). CI, confidence interval; df, degrees of freedom; GFD, gluten-free diet; GCD, gluten-containing diet; I^2, heterogeneity; IV, inversed variance; Random, random effects model; SD, standard deviation; Std., standardised; total, number of patients.

3.4.1.2. Change in Number of Participants Positive for Depression

Four reports of three studies compared the number of participants positive for depression at baseline and after following a GFD. Three were included in meta-analysis (Figure 4). For 110 classical CD patients, there was a reduction of 31% of patients positive for depression after following a GFD (RD −0.31, 95% CI −0.52 to −0.10; $p = 0.003$). All the included data is for classical CD patients following a GFD for one year; no studies reported this outcome for non-CD patients. We found a significant difference in effect between the studies reporting results from modified and unmodified questionnaires, with a significant effect seen for the unmodified questionnaires and a nonsignificant effect in studies using an unmodified questionnaire.

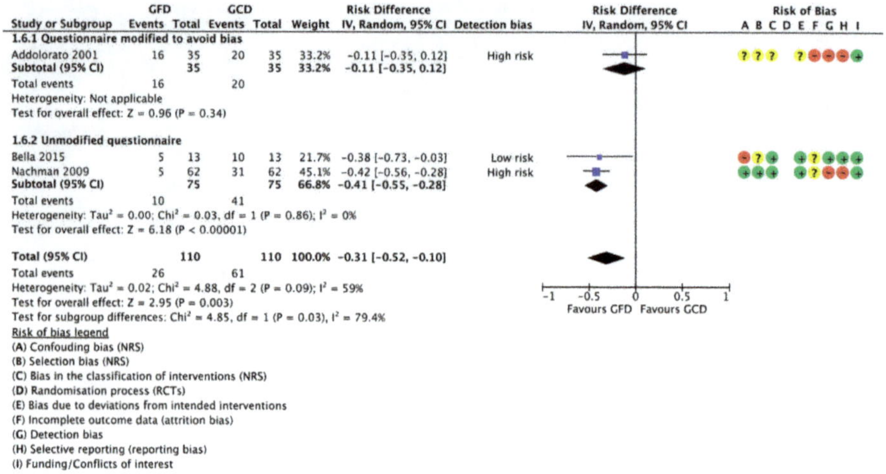

Figure 4. Forest plot demonstrating the change the number of CD participants with depression after following a GFD for one year.

3.4.2. Gluten Challenge vs. Placebo (GFD)

Two RCTs compared the mean depression scores of subjects during the gluten and placebo challenge periods and were included in meta-analysis [42,56] (Figure 5). We found a trend towards worsened depressive symptoms during the gluten challenge period compared to placebo, although this did not reach significance (SMD 0.21, 95% CI −0.58 to 0.15; $p = 0.25$). Heterogeneity was low ($I^2 = 19\%$). Both used a cross-over trial design with participants acting as their own controls and both adequately described blinding of participants and researchers. Moreover, both used a per-protocol (PP) approach in their analyses. Depression scores were derived from a graph by optical plot reading using WebPlotDigitizer [52].

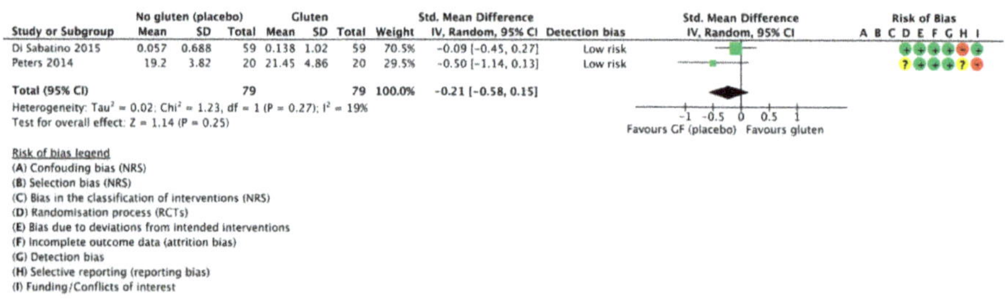

Figure 5. Forest plot demonstrating the difference in participant depression scores between gluten and placebo challenges in subjects with self-reported NCGS.

3.4.3. Compliant vs. Noncompliant Participants

Three publications of two studies reported depression scores separately for CD patients compliant and noncompliant to the GFD; no studies reported separate data for these subgroups in non-CD patients. However, two of the three studies used the same sample at different follow-up timepoints [57,58]. Moreover, as there is considerable variation in results and inconsistency in the direction of effect, no meta-analysis was conducted (Figure 6). Firstly, Nachman et al. [58] found a nonsignificant difference in mean depression scores between 59 compliant (M −7.9, 95% CI 4.8 to 11.0) and 25 noncompliant patients (M −6.3, 95% CI 3.6 to 9.5) at year one, although there was a slightly lower severity of depressive symptoms in the noncompliant subgroup. Nevertheless, they reported a significantly higher severity of depression in the noncompliant subjects after four years on a GFD ($p = 0.04$), with 27 compliant and 26 noncompliant CD patients having mean scores of 5.8 (95% CI 2.1 to 9.5) and 11.3 (95% CI 7.6 to 15.0), respectively [57]. Conversely, when comparing the number of patients positive for depression (Figure S3, Supplementary File 6), they consistently reported a nonsignificant trend towards a lower number of depressed patients in the compliant group, with no difference between the proportion of depressed patients at one year and four year follow-ups ($p = 0.86$; $I^2 = 0\%$). On the contrary, Simsek et al. [11] found the severity of depressive symptoms to be significantly higher in noncompliant, compared to compliant, CD children after only one year on a GFD ($p = 0.005$), with seven compliant patients and 17 noncompliant patients achieving mean CDI scores of 4.75 (SD 3.3) and 12.33 (SD 5.8), respectively.

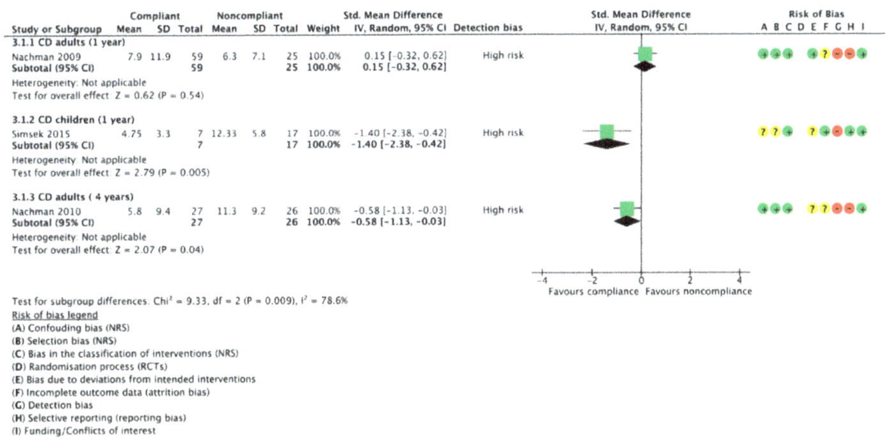

Figure 6. Mean depression scores in compliant vs. noncompliant CD adults at one year, CD children at one year, and CD adults at four years after following a GFD.

3.4.4. GFD-Treated Patients vs. Healthy Controls

3.4.4.1. Difference in Mean Depression Scores

Five publications reporting on four studies included an eligible healthy control group, of which four were included in meta-analysis (Figure 7A). As Nachman et al. [57,58] used the same sample and healthy controls, the results for the four year follow-up [57] were reported separately. Overall, we found no difference between the depressive outcome scores between 868 GFD-treated patients and 400 healthy controls at one year follow-up (SMD 0.01, 95% CI −0.18 to 0.20, $p = 0.94$) and zero heterogeneity between the studies ($I^2 = 0\%$). Similarly, there was no significant difference at the four year follow-up between 27 strictly adherent patients and 70 healthy controls (SMD −0.08, 95% CI −0.52 to 0.36, $p = 0.72$). Two studies with a healthy control group were not eligible for meta-analysis; Simsek et al. [11] reported depressive outcome data for their healthy controls as medians and IQRs, but similarly reported an insignificant difference between patients and controls, while Collin et al. [64] did not demographically match patients and healthy controls, hence we have not reported their data.

3.4.4.2. Difference in Number Participants Positive for Depression

Three studies [57,58,65] reported the number of GFD-treated participants and healthy controls positive for depression, of which two were meta-analysed and data from Nachman et al. [57] were reported as separately (Figure 7B). Only data from patients strictly adherent to the GFD were included. We found a trend towards an increased prevalence of depression in GFD-treated patients compared to healthy controls at one year (RD 0.21, 95% CI −0.16 to 0.58; $p = 0.26$) and four years (RD 0.10, 95% CI −0.02 to 0.22; $p = 0.12$), although these were nonsignificant. There was no significant difference between the results at one year and four years ($p = 0.56$), and heterogeneity was zero between all studies and subgroups.

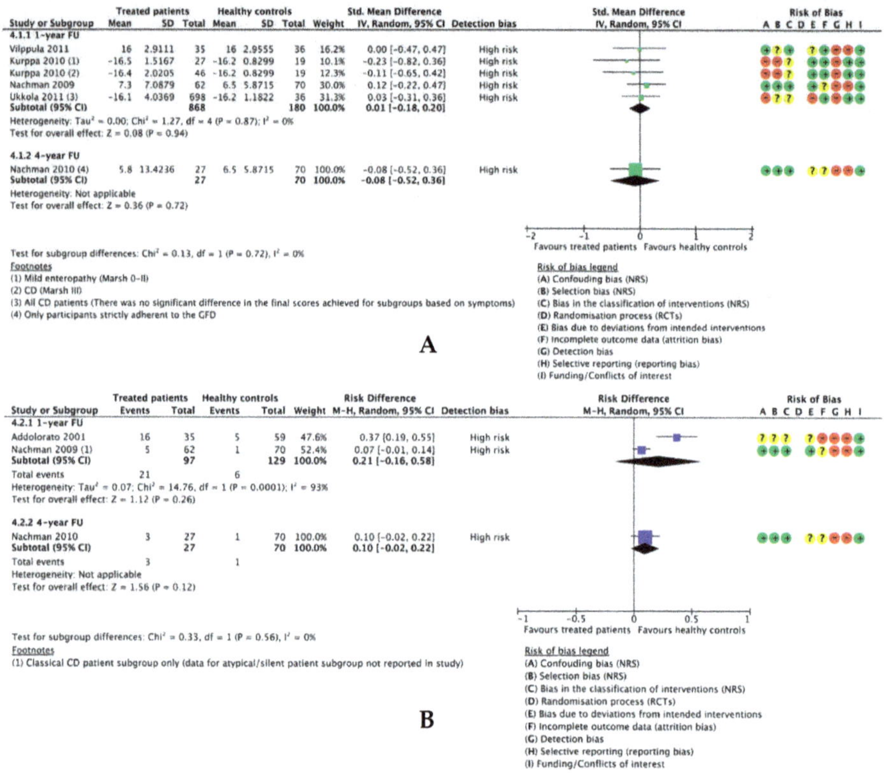

Figure 7. Forest plots comparing: (**A**) Mean depression scores in treated patients and healthy controls and (**B**) the difference in the no. treated patients and healthy controls positive for depression at one year and four years after following a GFD.

3.5. Sensitivity Analyses

Various sensitivity analyses were untaken to ensure significant differences were not as a result of arbitrary decisions throughout the study process (Figures S4–S6 and Tables S13–S14, Supplementary File 7). Firstly, no significant differences in meta-analysis results were found when interchanging random-effects for fixed-effects, or risk difference for odds ratio and risk ratio, for the majority of analyses (Tables S13 and S14). However, there was a difference in the final results for analysis Section 3.4.4.2. at one year, which became significant when using fixed-effects, as opposed to random-effects, and odds ratio or risk ratio, as opposed to risk difference. Secondly, removing studies at an unclear/high risk of detection bias, leaving only those at low risk, did not produce substantially different results for any applicable comparison (Figure S4). Thirdly, while removing data from Nachman et al. [58] from our meta-analyses did not significantly alter the results, overall heterogeneity was reduced from $I^2 = 38\%$ to $I^2 = 0\%$ for the main analysis (Figure S5) and from $I^2 = 52\%$ to $I^2 = 13\%$ for the CD subgroup. On the other hand, there was no difference in results or heterogeneity between using outcome data from Nachman et al. for classical CD patients from the modified BDI and the unmodified BDI [58], or all CD patient subgroups from the unmodified BDI [57] (Figure S6). Finally, the results from a potential conference abstract for a cross-over RCT [67], excluded from our study due to the lack of a published final article, could not be included in a sensitivity analysis as only the mean change in the STPI state depression sub-score was reported between gluten and placebo groups (mean change 0.69, 95% CI −2.15 to 3.53, $p = 0.61$). Nevertheless, these results for NCGS patients are in agreement with our meta-analysis in Section 3.4.2.

3.6. Publication Bias

Inspection from the funnel plot that arose from our main analysis (Figure 8) suggests the presence of publication bias due to location biases [68], with published studies from Finland less likely to find to find a large effect from a GFD on reducing depressive symptom scores relative to published studies from other countries.

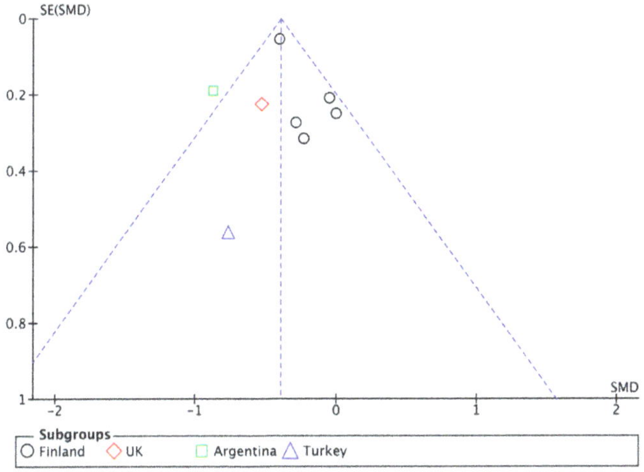

Figure 8. Funnel plot.

4. Discussion

Our systematic review involved a total of 13 studies and 1139 patients, with meta-analysis on an eligible sample of 933 patients from non randomised studies and 99 patients from RCTs, as well as 180 healthy controls. Although we generally found a low level of heterogeneity, a limitation of our review was the small number of studies available for subgroup analyses that limited our ability to investigate any heterogeneity. Moreover, despite the fact that we contacted authors for missing data, no additional data was retrieved. This was either because: The data was no longer available; authors had retired or moved to another area of research; or a lack of response. Nevertheless, we adhered to the Preferred Reporting Items for Systematic Reviews and Meta-Analyses (PRISMA) statement [69] guidelines wherever possible (see PRISMA checklist, Table S15 in Supplementary File 8) and assessed the quality of the individual studies using tools developed and recommended by the Cochrane Collaboration for both the RCTs and non-randomised studies. Moreover, we applied the GRADE process [48] to assess the certainty of our conclusions and recommendations based on the evidence across the studies for each outcome.

A further strength of our systematic review was our comprehensive search strategy, which we piloted and tailored to numerous databases, and strict application of inclusion and exclusion criteria. Therefore, we are relatively certain that all relevant studies have been included in our review. Although diagnosed conditions or disorders were not an exclusion criteria for our study, only studies on populations with CD, IBS or NCGS were identified through our searches; no other gluten-related disorder, such as dermatitis herpetiformis or gluten ataxia, nor any other condition, such as major depressive disorder, were identified. Moreover, our searches only identified studies assessing depression, or depression as a subcategory of quality of life; no studies were found that assessed other determinants of mood or mood disorders. We conducted further, broader searches for other mood disorders as a sensitivity analysis in attempts to find studies we may have missed in our search strategy, but identified no further relevant studies. As we found no studies that attempted a GFD intervention on a sample of patients with depression, despite evidence for significantly higher levels of gluten-related antibodies in patients with major depressive disorder [19], this would be an interesting topic for future studies to address in order to help assess the directionality of the relationship between depression and gluten.

Our first objective was to establish whether a relationship exists between mood and gluten in those with and without gluten-related disorders. We found that a long-term GFD may significantly reduce and normalise the severity of depressive symptoms for subjects with CD, IBS and NCGS, with a medium-large effect for both symptomatic and atypical CD patients, but no effect for asymptomatic/silent cases [70]. However, the criteria for what constitutes silent CD remains uncertain; although neuropsychiatric disorders are likely to be included in the definition of atypical CD [71], there are a variety of pathophysiological differences underlying the clinical spectrum of depressive disorders [72]. Hence, it is uncertain whether those with depression, but no other symptoms, at baseline would be classified as having atypical or silent CD. Moreover, one of our included studies found that the significant improvement in depressive symptoms for the atypical/silent combined subgroup was no longer significant when the questionnaire was modified to remove questions based on gastrointestinal symptoms [58]. Conversely, another one of our included studies reported that all asymptomatic CD participants randomised to the GFD group for the first year of the study refused to crossover to a follow a gluten-containing diet again, due to a fear of worsening symptoms [53], suggesting that even subjects who did not report any symptoms at baseline experienced improvements after following a GFD. Hence, although we established an overall effect, is it difficult to draw many conclusions based on symptom classification at this time.

Further to this, we assessed the impact of the level of adherence to a GFD on mood symptom severity. Interestingly, we found a significant difference in mean depression scores in favour of strict compliance for CD children after one year, whereas the difference for CD adults was nonsignificant at the same timepoint. This, nevertheless, became significant in favour of compliance at the four year follow-up. Previous systematic reviews and meta-analyses have consistently found a moderate association between poorer GFD adherence and worsened depressive symptoms [35,73], though with high heterogeneity between the studies. However, our nonsignificant finding for adults after the first year does not support this relationship described by others. On one hand, a standardised method for measuring adherence to the GFD does not yet exist, and hence there were differences in the methods utilised by each studies. Alternatively, recent cross-sectional studies suggest that hypervigilance to a GFD, associated with greater knowledge, was significantly associated with reduced quality of life [44], and that those with worse economic status were at an increased risk of lower quality of life while following a GFD [74]. Conversely, the presence of depression has been suggested to weaken the correlation between GFD adherence and symptoms [43], implying that symptoms may be driven by factors other than gluten exposure. To summarise, further studies with standardised measurements of adherence are required before definitive conclusions may be drawn on the effects of gluten-free dietary adherence on the severity of depressive symptoms.

On the other hand, we found the proportion of participants testing positive for depression tended to be higher in GFD-treated patients compared to healthy controls at both one and four years, which was unaffected by the level of compliance. In line with this, previous studies suggest that up to 30% of CD patients show persistent enteropathy after one year on a GFD [75], potentially due to consuming trace amounts of gluten via cross-contamination [76,77]. Despite this, recent RCTs suggest that a low-FODMAPs diet can further reduce the severity of depressive symptoms in those with NCGS [29] and CD [78] already on a GFD, although further research is needed in this area. In addition, while it has been suggested that altered gut microbiota may contribute to the psychiatric effects of a GFD [29,79,80], results should not be extrapolated from one population to another, due to the highly individualised pattern of gut microbial composition [81]. In any case, future studies should be mindful of the shortcomings of only considering mean scores of the sample as a whole, and closer attention should be paid to patients who may be unresponsive to a GFD in research and practice.

In terms of the short-term effects for gluten on mood, the trend towards increased severity of depressive symptoms in NCGS patients after only a few days of a blinded gluten challenge further reinforces our findings that the ingestion of gluten plays a role in the presence of depressive symptoms—even in those without mucosal gut damage. Although one of our included studies reported no concurrent differences in gastrointestinal symptom severity between gluten, whey and placebo challenges [42], other clinical trials on non-CD participants report a significant increase in physical symptoms when challenging with foods containing wheat [82] and fructans [83]. Additionally, despite the fact that another RCT found no gluten-specific gastrointestinal symptoms when challenging NCGS patients already on a low-FODMAPs diet, all patients returned to a GFD at the end of the trial as they subjectively reported "feeling better" [28]. However, the weaknesses of this study have been discussed in a previous paper [84]; while the sample is unlikely to be representative of the NCGS population, the crossover design could have also produced an anticipatory nocebo response [85]. Nonetheless, a proposed mechanism requiring further investigation is that FODMAPs predominantly trigger GI symptoms whereas gluten is a trigger for neurological and psychiatric symptoms by having direct effects on the brain [86].

Unfortunately, the overall quality of the evidence base was poor and confounding factors were problematic. Firstly, while a few studies stated subject antidepressant use as an exclusion criteria, other studies did not consider this. Secondly, seasonal affective disorder (SAD), a type of depression with a seasonal pattern, may overlap with other depressive disorders [87], but was not considered or controlled for in any of the studies. Although the majority of the non-randomised studies planned the follow-up to be one year after the start of the GFD, this timespan varied between clients, as well as between studies and none specified the time of year. Moreover, some of the questionnaires utilised, namely the SDS, HDRS and BDI, contained questions related to gastro-intestinal symptoms and eating habits, which are likely to introduce bias due to physical illness. Finally, our sample is dominated by Finnish participants (75.8%), with only 9.4% participants from Italy and 3.6% from the UK, significantly reducing the applicability of our findings; a GFD may be easier to follow in Finland as there is good knowledge of CD and easy availability of gluten-free products [88], which may lead to a lower risk of depression, due to isolation and other issues associated with following a GFD.

Nonetheless, we set out to determine implications for future research, as well as implementation of GFDs in practice. Firstly, our included studies varied in their criteria for CD diagnosis; whereas one study relied on EmA-positivity [53], another used biopsy [61] as their criteria for inclusion of silent CD patients. Moreover, broad subcategories, such as 'atypical', were problematic when attempting to assess specific atypical symptoms, such as depression. Hence, specific standardised criteria for the classification of the different subtypes of CD, as well as other gluten-sensitive disorders, should be developed to aid further research in terms of comparability, as well as identification and suitable treatment of those with CD. Secondly, our finding that the proportion of adults strictly adherent to the GFD decreased significantly over time is supported by a large recent meta-analysis [35], and is likely related to the amount of support received by patients. For instance, a RCT found that six months of psychological counselling improved GFD adherence and reduced depression in CD patients with depression at baseline [89]. While no studies exist that support or repute our findings that a lower proportion of children achieved strict adherence than adults, practical tools have been shown to promote self-management, dietary adherence and well-being in children and adolescents with CD [90]. Hence, the development of both standardised measurement methods and tools to promote dietary adherence would be useful for future research, as well as patient management. Moreover, a balance between dietary adherence and well-being appears important for those following a GFD, with careful consideration of the level of support available for specific populations in maintaining a GFD diet over time.

5. Conclusions

Our study confirms that gluten elimination may represent an effective treatment strategy for mood disorders in individuals with gluten-related disorders, while highlighting specific considerations for future research and implications for practice. Firstly, standardisation of methods to measure dietary adherence and mood symptoms with no bias, due to physical illness would greatly increase the validity and comparability of future research. Secondly, future studies focusing on gluten and mood in participants without a gut-related disorder, for example, in a population sample with depression, would contribute to the evidence necessary to determine the directionality of the relationship. Nevertheless, authors should be mindful of the shortcomings of only considering mean scores of a sample, with potentially GFD-resistant participants requiring closer attention. In practice, implementation of a gluten-contamination elimination diet, such as that detailed by Hollon et al. [76], in which processed foods are eliminated, could prove beneficial for some individuals. Thirdly, standardisation of the classification for the subtypes of CD, as well as other gluten-sensitive disorders, should be developed to aid further research in terms of comparability, as well as identification and suitable treatment of those with CD. Finally, the level of support available to help a patient in maintaining a GFD diet over time should be carefully considered when recommending a GFD in practice.

Supplementary Materials: The following are available online at http://www.mdpi.com/2072-6643/10/11/1708/s1, Figure S1: Forest plots demonstrating the difference in mean depression scores between following a GFD and a gluten-containing diet for the following subgroup analyses: (A) population country of origin. (B) CD diagnosis—CD and non-CD patients; and (C) HLA-DQ2/8 genotype – positive and negative, Figure S2: Forest plot demonstrating the relative difference in change of mean depression scores between baseline + year one and baseline + year four for participants following a GFD for four years, Figure S3: Forest plots comparing the no. CD adult patients positive for depression at one year and four years, Figure S4: Sensitivity analysis removing studies at unclear or high risk of detection bias, Figure S5. Sensitivity analysis removing data from Nachman et al., Figure S6. Sensitivity analysis swapping Nachman et al. (2009) outcome data for classical CD patients from the modified BDI to that for (A) 62 classical CD patients from the unmodified BDI (Nachman et al., 2009), and (B) 53 CD patients from the unmodified BDI (Nachman et al., 2010), Tables S1–S6: Search strategies, Table S7: Specific criteria for assessing the risk of bias for each of the domains from Cochrane's ROB 2.0 and ROBINS-I tools in the context of our review, Table S8: Studies excluded by full-text screening, Tables S9–S12: Summary of findings, Table S13: Sensitivity analysis comparing random-effects (RE) and fixed-effects (FE) models, Table S14: Sensitivity analysis comparing risk difference (RD), risk ratio (RR) and odds ratio (OR) for dichotomous outcomes, Table S15: PRISMA checklist.

Author Contributions: All authors provided input on the content of the manuscript. Conceptualisation: E.B., J.B. and K.R.; Search and Data Collection: E.B.; Software: E.B.; Validation: J.B., L.F. and K.R.; Formal Analysis: E.B.; Investigation: E.B.; Writing—Original Draft Preparation: EB; Writing—Review and Editing: J.B., L.F. and K.R.; Supervision: J.B.; Project Administration: E.B. All authors read and approved the final manuscript.

Funding: This research received no external funding.

Acknowledgments: Research undertaken as part of a postgraduate degree in Nutritional Therapy at the University of Worcester.

Conflicts of Interest: The authors declare no conflict of interest.

References

1. Depression. Available online: http://www.who.int/news-room/fact-sheets/detail/depression (accessed on 22 October 2018).
2. NHS. *Statistics for England, 2002–2012;* Prescriptions Dispensed in the Community; NHS: London, UK, 2013.
3. World Health Organization. *Depression and Other Common Mental Disorders;* Global Health Estimates; World Health Organization: Geneva, Switzerland, 2017.

4. Sapone, A.; Bai, J.C.; Ciacci, C.; Dolinsek, J.; Green, P.H.; Hadjivassiliou, M.; Kaukinen, K.; Rostami, K.; Sanders, D.S.; Schumann, M.; et al. Spectrum of gluten-related disorders: Consensus on new nomenclature and classification. *BMC Med.* **2012**, *10*, 13. [CrossRef] [PubMed]
5. NIH. In Proceedings of the NIH Consensus Development Conference on Celiac Disease, Bethesda, MD, USA, 28–30 June 2004; Volume 21, pp. 1–23.
6. Black, J.L.; Orfila, C. Impact of coeliac disease on dietary habits and quality of life. *J. Hum. Nutr. Diet.* **2011**, *24*, 582–587. [CrossRef] [PubMed]
7. Tack, G.J.; Verbeek, W.H.M.; Schreurs, M.W.J.; Mulder, C.J.J. The spectrum of celiac disease: Epidemiology, clinical aspects and treatment. *Nat. Rev. Gastroenterol. Hepatol.* **2010**, *7*, 204–213. [CrossRef] [PubMed]
8. Addolorato, G.; Di Giuda, D.; De Rossi, G.; Valenza, V.; Domenicali, M.; Caputo, F.; Gasbarrini, A.; Capristo, E.; Gasbarrini, G. Regional cerebral hypoperfusion in patients with celiac disease. *Am. J. Med.* **2004**, *116*, 312–317. [CrossRef] [PubMed]
9. Smith, D.F.; Gerdes, L.U. Meta-analysis on anxiety and depression in adult celiac disease: Anxiety and depression in celiac disease. *Acta Psychiatr. Scand.* **2012**, *125*, 189–193. [CrossRef] [PubMed]
10. Ludvigsson, J.F.; Leffler, D.A.; Bai, J.; Biagi, F.; Fasano, A.; Green, P.H.; Hadjivassiliou, M.; Kaukinen, K.; Kelly, C.; Leonard, J.N.; et al. The Oslo definitions for coeliac disease and related terms. *Gut* **2013**, *62*, 43. [CrossRef] [PubMed]
11. Simsek, S.; Baysoy, G.; Gencoglan, S.; Uluca, U. Effects of Gluten-Free Diet on Quality of Life and Depression in Children with Celiac Disease. *J. Pediatr. Gastroenterol. Nutr.* **2015**, *61*, 303. [CrossRef] [PubMed]
12. Liester, M.B.; Liester, M.G. A Review of Psychiatric Disorders Associated with Celiac Disease. *Dual Diagn. Open Access* **2017**, *3*. [CrossRef]
13. Catassi, C.; Elli, L.; Bonaz, B.; Bouma, G.; Carroccio, A.; Castillejo, G.; Cellier, C.; Cristofori, F.; de Magistris, L.; Dolinsek, J.; et al. Diagnosis of Non-Celiac Gluten Sensitivity (NCGS): The Salerno Experts' Criteria. *Nutrients* **2015**, *7*, 4966–4977. [CrossRef] [PubMed]
14. Catassi, C. Gluten Sensitivity. *Ann. Nutr. Metab.* **2015**, *67* (Suppl. S2), 16–26. [CrossRef] [PubMed]
15. Volta, U.; Tovoli, F.; Cicola, R.; Parisi, C.; Fabbri, A.; Piscaglia, M.; Fiorini, E.; Caio, G. Serological tests in gluten sensitivity (nonceliac gluten intolerance). *J. Clin. Gastroenterol.* **2012**, *46*, 680–685. [CrossRef] [PubMed]
16. Daynes, G. Bread and Tears—Naughtiness, Depression and Fits Due to Wheat Sensitivity. *Proc. R. Soc. Med.* **1956**, *49*, 391–394. [PubMed]
17. Carroccio, A.; Giambalvo, O.; Blasca, F.L.; Iacobucci, R.; D'Alcamo, A.; Mansueto, P. Self-Reported Non-Celiac Wheat Sensitivity in High School Students: Demographic and Clinical Characteristics. *Nutrients* **2017**, *9*, 771. [CrossRef] [PubMed]
18. Harper, L.; Bold, J.S. An exploration into the motivation for gluten avoidance in the absence of coeliac disease. *Gastroenterol. Hepatol. Bed Bench* **2018**. [CrossRef]
19. Porcelli, B.; Verdino, V.; Ferretti, F.; Bizzaro, N.; Terzuoli, L.; Cinci, F.; Bossini, L.; Fagiolini, A. A study on the association of mood disorders and gluten-related diseases. *Psychiatry Res.* **2018**, *260*, 366–370. [CrossRef] [PubMed]
20. Karakula-Juchnowicz, H.; Gałęcka, M.; Rog, J.; Bartnicka, A.; Łukaszewicz, Z.; Krukow, P.; Morylowska-Topolska, J.; Skonieczna-Zydecka, K.; Krajka, T.; Jonak, K.; et al. The Food-Specific Serum IgG Reactivity in Major Depressive Disorder Patients, Irritable Bowel Syndrome Patients and Healthy Controls. *Nutrients* **2018**, *10*, 548. [CrossRef] [PubMed]
21. Jackson, J.; Eaton, W.; Cascella, N.; Fasano, A.; Santora, D.; Sullivan, K.; Feldman, S.; Raley, H.; McMahon, R.P.; Carpenter, W.T.J.; et al. Gluten sensitivity and relationship to psychiatric symptoms in people with schizophrenia. *Schizophr. Res.* **2014**, *159*, 539–542. [CrossRef] [PubMed]
22. Dickerson, F.; Stallings, C.; Origoni, A.; Vaughan, C.; Khushalani, S.; Yolken, R. Markers of gluten sensitivity in acute mania: A longitudinal study. *Psychiatry Res.* **2012**, *196*, 68–71. [CrossRef] [PubMed]
23. Karakuła-Juchnowicz, H.; Szachta, P.; Opolska, A.; Morylowska-Topolska, J.; Gałęcka, M.; Juchnowicz, D.; Krukow, P.; Lasik, Z. The role of IgG hypersensitivity in the pathogenesis and therapy of depressive disorders. *Nutr. Neurosci.* **2017**, *20*, 110–118. [CrossRef] [PubMed]
24. Fera, T.; Cascio, B.; Angelini, G.; Martini, S.; Guidetti, C. Affective disorders and quality of life in adult coeliac disease patients on a gluten-free diet. *Eur. J. Gastroenterol. Hepatol.* **2003**, *15*, 1287–1292. [CrossRef] [PubMed]

25. Roos, S.; Kärner, A.; Hallert, C. Gastrointestinal symptoms and well-being of adults living on a gluten-free diet: A case for nursing in celiac disease. *Gastroenterol. Nurs.* **2009**, *32*, 196–201. [CrossRef] [PubMed]
26. Ruepert, L.; Quartero, A.O.; de Wit, N.J.; van der Heijden, G.J.; Rubin, G.; Muris, J.W. Bulking agents, antispasmodics and antidepressants for the treatment of irritable bowel syndrome. *Cochrane Database Syst. Rev.* **2011**, CD003460. [CrossRef] [PubMed]
27. Hallert, C.; Svensson, M.; Tholstrup, J.; Hultberg, B. Clinical trial: B vitamins improve health in patients with coeliac disease living on a gluten-free diet. *Aliment. Pharmacol. Therapeut.* **2009**, *29*, 811–816. [CrossRef] [PubMed]
28. Biesiekierski, J.R.; Peters, S.L.; Newnham, E.D.; Rosella, O.; Muir, J.G.; Gibson, P.R. No effects of gluten in patients with self-reported non-celiac gluten sensitivity after dietary reduction of fermentable, poorly absorbed, short-chain carbohydrates. *Gastroenterology* **2013**, *145*, 320–328. [CrossRef] [PubMed]
29. Dieterich, W.; Schuppan, D.; Schink, M.; Schwappacher, R.; Wirtz, S.; Agaimy, A.; Neurath, M.F.; Zopf, Y. Influence of low FODMAP and gluten-free diets on disease activity and intestinal microbiota in patients with non-celiac gluten sensitivity. *Clin. Nutr.* **2018**. [CrossRef] [PubMed]
30. Horvath-Stolarczyk, A.; Sidor, K.; Dziechciarz, P.; Siemińska, J. Assessment of emotional status, selected personality traits and depression in young adults with celiac disease. *Pediatr. Wspolczesna* **2002**, *4*, 241–246.
31. Cicarelli, G.; Della Rocca, G.; Amboni, M.; Ciacci, C.; Mazzacca, G.; Filla, A.; Barone, P. Clinical and neurological abnormalities in adult celiac disease. *Neurol. Sci.* **2003**, *24*, 311–317. [CrossRef] [PubMed]
32. Burger, J.P.W.; de Brouwer, B.; IntHout, J.; Wahab, P.J.; Tummers, M.; Drenth, J.P.H. Systematic review with meta-analysis: Dietary adherence influences normalization of health-related quality of life in coeliac disease. *Clin. Nutr.* **2017**, *36*, 399–406. [CrossRef] [PubMed]
33. Shahbazkhani, B.; Sadeghi, A.; Malekzadeh, R.; Khatavi, F.; Etemadi, M.; Kalantri, E.; Rostami-Nejad, M.; Rostami, K. Non-Celiac Gluten Sensitivity Has Narrowed the Spectrum of Irritable Bowel Syndrome: A Double-Blind Randomized Placebo-Controlled Trial. *Nutrients* **2015**, *7*, 4542–4554. [CrossRef] [PubMed]
34. Caio, G.; Volta, U.; Tovoli, F.; De Giorgio, R. Effect of gluten free diet on immune response to gliadin in patients with non-celiac gluten sensitivity. *BMC Gastroenterol.* **2014**, *14*, 26. [CrossRef] [PubMed]
35. Sainsbury, K.; Marques, M.M. The relationship between gluten free diet adherence and depressive symptoms in adults with coeliac disease: A systematic review with meta-analysis. *Appetite* **2018**, *120*, 578–588. [CrossRef] [PubMed]
36. Vazquez-Roque, M.I.; Camilleri, M.; Smyrk, T.; Murray, J.A.; Marietta, E.; O'Neill, J.; Carlson, P.; Lamsam, J.; Janzow, D.; Eckert, D.; et al. A controlled trial of gluten-free diet in patients with irritable bowel syndrome-diarrhea: Effects on bowel frequency and intestinal function. *Gastroenterology* **2013**, *144*, 903–911. [CrossRef] [PubMed]
37. Soares, F.L.P.; de Oliveira Matoso, R.; Teixeira, L.G.; Menezes, Z.; Pereira, S.S.; Alves, A.C.; Batista, N.V.; de Faria, A.M.C.; Cara, D.C.; Ferreira, A.V.M.; et al. Gluten-free diet reduces adiposity, inflammation and insulin resistance associated with the induction of PPAR-alpha and PPAR-gamma expression. *J. Nutr. Biochem.* **2013**, *24*, 1105–1111. [CrossRef] [PubMed]
38. Mulloy, A.; Lang, R.; O'Reilly, M.; Sigafoos, J.; Lancioni, G.; Rispoli, M. Gluten-free and casein-free diets in the treatment of autism spectrum disorders: A systematic review. *Res. Autism Spectr. Disord.* **2010**, *4*, 328–339. [CrossRef]
39. Piwowarczyk, A.; Horvath, A.; Łukasik, J.; Pisula, E.; Szajewska, H. Gluten- and casein-free diet and autism spectrum disorders in children: A systematic review. *Eur. J. Nutr.* **2018**, *57*, 433–440. [CrossRef] [PubMed]
40. Brietzke, E.; Cerqueira, R.O.; Mansur, R.B.; McIntyre, R.S. Gluten related illnesses and severe mental disorders: A comprehensive review. *Neurosci. Biobehav. Rev.* **2018**, *84*, 368–375. [CrossRef] [PubMed]
41. Losurdo, G.; Principi, M.; Iannone, A.; Amoruso, A.; Ierardi, E.; Leo, A.D.; Barone, M. Extra-intestinal manifestations of non-celiac gluten sensitivity: An expanding paradigm. *World J. Gastroenterol.* **2018**, *24*, 1521–1530. [CrossRef] [PubMed]
42. Peters, S.L.; Biesiekierski, J.R.; Yelland, G.W.; Muir, J.G.; Gibson, P.R. Randomised clinical trial: Gluten may cause depression in subjects with non-coeliac gluten sensitivity—An exploratory clinical study. *Aliment. Pharmacol. Therapeut.* **2014**, *39*, 1104–1112. [CrossRef] [PubMed]
43. Joelson, A.M.; Geller, M.G.; Zylberberg, H.M.; Green, P.H.R.; Lebwohl, B. The Effect of Depressive Symptoms on the Association between Gluten-Free Diet Adherence and Symptoms in Celiac Disease: Analysis of a Patient Powered Research Network. *Nutrients* **2018**, *10*, 538. [CrossRef] [PubMed]

44. Wolf, R.L.; Lebwohl, B.; Lee, A.R.; Zybert, P.; Reilly, N.R.; Cadenhead, J.; Amengual, C.; Green, P.H.R. Hypervigilance to a Gluten-Free Diet and Decreased Quality of Life in Teenagers and Adults with Celiac Disease. *Digest. Dis. Sci.* **2018**, *63*, 1438–1448. [CrossRef] [PubMed]
45. The Cochrane Collaboration. *Cochrane Handbook for Systematic Reviews of Interventions*; Higgins, J., Green, S., Eds.; The Cochrane Collaboration: London, UK, 2011.
46. Higgins, J.; Sterne, J.A.; Savović, J.; Page, M.; Hróbjartsson, A.; Boutron, I.; Reeves, B.C.; Eldridge, S. A revised tool for assessing risk of bias in randomized trials. *Cochrane Database Syst. Rev.* **2016**, *10* (Suppl. S1). [CrossRef]
47. Sterne, J.A.; Hernán, M.A.; Reeves, B.C.; Savović, J.; Berkman, N.D.; Viswanathan, M.; Henry, D.; Altman, D.G.; Ansari, M.T.; Boutron, I.; et al. ROBINS-I: A tool for assessing risk of bias in non-randomised studies of interventions. *BMJ* **2016**, *355*, i4919. [CrossRef] [PubMed]
48. Guyatt, G.H.; Oxman, A.D.; Vist, G.E.; Kunz, R.; Falck-Ytter, Y.; Alonso-Coello, P.; Schünemann, H.J. GRADE: An emerging consensus on rating quality of evidence and strength of recommendations. *BMJ* **2008**, *336*, 924–926. [CrossRef] [PubMed]
49. The GRADE Working Group. *GRADE Handbook for Grading Quality of Evidence and Strength of Recommendations*; Updated October 2013; Schünemann, H., Brożek, J., Guyatt, G., Oxman, A., Eds.; The GRADE Working Group: Hamilton, ON, Canada, 2013.
50. Evidence Prime, Inc. *GRADEpro GDT: GRADEpro Guideline Development Tool [Software]*; McMaster University: Hamilton, ON, Canada, 2015.
51. Higgins, J.P.T.; Thompson, S.G.; Deeks, J.J.; Altman, D.G. Measuring inconsistency in meta-analyses. *BMJ* **2003**, *327*, 557–560. [CrossRef] [PubMed]
52. Rohatgi, A. WebPlotDigitizer. Available online: https://automeris.io/WebPlotDigitizer/ (accessed on 22 October 2018).
53. Kurppa, K.; Paavola, A.; Collin, P.; Sievänen, H.; Laurila, K.; Huhtala, H.; Saavalainen, P.; Mäki, M.; Kaukinen, K. Benefits of a gluten-free diet for asymptomatic patients with serologic markers of celiac disease. *Gastroenterology* **2014**, *147*, 610–617. [CrossRef] [PubMed]
54. Elli, L.; Tomba, C.; Branchi, F.; Roncoroni, L.; Lombardo, V.; Bardella, M.T.; Ferretti, F.; Conte, D.; Valiante, F.; Fini, L.; et al. Evidence for the Presence of Non-Celiac Gluten Sensitivity in Patients with Functional Gastrointestinal Symptoms: Results from a Multicenter Randomized Double-Blind Placebo-Controlled Gluten Challenge. *Nutrients* **2016**, *8*. [CrossRef] [PubMed]
55. Paavola, A.; Kurppa, K.; Ukkola, A.; Collin, P.; Lähdeaho, M.-L.; Huhtala, H.; Mäki, M.; Kaukinen, K. Gastrointestinal symptoms and quality of life in screen-detected celiac disease. *Dig. Liver Dis.* **2012**, *44*, 814–818. [CrossRef] [PubMed]
56. Di Sabatino, A.; Volta, U.; Salvatore, C.; Biancheri, P.; Caio, G.; De Giorgio, R.; Di Stefano, M.; Corazza, G.R. Small Amounts of Gluten in Subjects With Suspected Nonceliac Gluten Sensitivity: A Randomized, Double-Blind, Placebo-Controlled, Cross-Over Trial. *Clin. Gastroenterol. Hepatol.* **2015**, *13*, 1604–1612. [CrossRef] [PubMed]
57. Nachman, F.; del Campo, M.P.; González, A.; Corzo, L.; Vázquez, H.; Sfoggia, C.; Smecuol, E.; Sánchez, M.I.P.; Niveloni, S.; Sugai, E.; et al. Long-term deterioration of quality of life in adult patients with celiac disease is associated with treatment noncompliance. *Dig. Liver Dis.* **2010**, *42*, 685–691. [CrossRef] [PubMed]
58. Nachman, F.; Mauriño, E.; Vázquez, H.; Sfoggia, C.; Gonzalez, A.; Gonzalez, V.; del Campo, M.P.; Smecuol, E.; Niveloni, S.; Sugai, E.; et al. Quality of life in celiac disease patients. Prospective analysis on the importance of clinical severity at diagnosis and the impact of treatment. *Dig. Liver Dis.* **2009**, *41*, 15–25. [CrossRef] [PubMed]
59. Bella, R.; Lanza, G.; Cantone, M.; Giuffrida, S.; Puglisi, V.; Vinciguerra, L.; Pennisi, M.; Ricceri, R.; D'Agate, C.C.; Malaguarnera, G.; et al. Effect of a Gluten-Free Diet on Cortical Excitability in Adults with Celiac Disease. *PLoS ONE* **2015**, *10*, 1–11. [CrossRef] [PubMed]
60. Kurppa, K.; Collin, P.; Sievänen, H.; Huhtala, H.; Mäki, M.; Kaukinen, K. Gastrointestinal symptoms, quality of life and bone mineral density in mild enteropathic coeliac disease: A prospective clinical trial. *Scand. J. Gastroenterol.* **2010**, *45*, 305–314. [CrossRef] [PubMed]
61. Ukkola, A.; Mäki, M.; Kurppa, K.; Collin, P.; Huhtala, H.; Kekkonen, L.; Kaukinen, K. Diet Improves Perception of Health and Well-being in Symptomatic, but Not Asymptomatic, Patients With Celiac Disease. *Clin. Gastroenterol. Hepatol.* **2011**, *9*, 118–123. [CrossRef] [PubMed]

62. Vilppula, A.; Kaukinen, K.; Luostarinen, L.; Krekelä, I.; Patrikainen, H.; Valve, R.; Luostarinen, M.; Laurila, K.; Mäki, M.; Collin, P. Clinical benefit of gluten-free diet in screen-detected older celiac disease patients. *BMC Gastroenterol.* **2011**, *11*. [CrossRef] [PubMed]
63. Aziz, I.; Trott, N.; Briggs, R.; North, J.R.; Hadjivassiliou, M.; Sanders, D.S. Efficacy of a Gluten-Free Diet in Subjects With Irritable Bowel Syndrome-Diarrhea Unaware of Their HLA-DQ2/8 Genotype. *Clin. Gastroenterol. Hepatol.* **2016**, *14*, 696–703. [CrossRef] [PubMed]
64. Collin, P.; Kaukinen, K.; Mattila, A.K.; Joukamaa, M. Psychoneurotic symptoms and alexithymia in coeliac disease. *Scand. J. Gastroenterol.* **2008**, *43*, 1329–1333. [CrossRef] [PubMed]
65. Addolorato, G.; Capristo, E.; Ghittoni, G.; Valeri, C.; Mascianà, R.; Ancona, C.; Gasbarrini, G. Anxiety but not depression decreases in coeliac patients after one-year gluten-free diet: A longitudinal study. *Scand. J. Gastroenterol.* **2001**, *36*, 502–506. [CrossRef] [PubMed]
66. Fuchs, V.; Kurppa, K.; Huhtala, H.; Mäki, M.; Kekkonen, L.; Kaukinen, K. Delayed celiac disease diagnosis predisposes to reduced quality of life and incremental use of health care services and medicines: A prospective nationwide study. *United Eur. Gastroenterol. J.* **2018**, *6*, 567–575. [CrossRef] [PubMed]
67. Peters, S.; Yelland, G.; Moore, J.; Ward, M. No effect of gluten on anxiety or depression in patients with NCGS, but could it be brain fog? *J. Gastroenterol. Hepatol.* **2016**, *31*, 175–176. [CrossRef]
68. Sterne, J.A.C.; Sutton, A.J.; Ioannidis, J.P.A.; Terrin, N.; Jones, D.R.; Lau, J.; Carpenter, J.; Rücker, G.; Harbord, R.M.; Schmid, C.H.; et al. Recommendations for examining and interpreting funnel plot asymmetry in meta-analyses of randomised controlled trials. *BMJ* **2011**, *343*, d4002. [CrossRef] [PubMed]
69. Moher, D.; Liberati, A.; Tetzlaff, J.; Altman, D.G. Preferred reporting items for systematic reviews and meta-analyses: The PRISMA statement. *BMJ* **2009**, *339*, b2535. [CrossRef] [PubMed]
70. Cohen, J. *Statistical Power Analysis in the Behavioral Sciences*, 2nd ed.; Routledge: Hillsdale, MJ, USA, 1988; ISBN 978-0-8058-0283-2.
71. Admou, B.; Essaadouni, L.; Krati, K.; Zaher, K.; Sbihi, M.; Chabaa, L.; Belaabidia, B.; Alaoui-Yazidi, A. Atypical Celiac Disease: From Recognizing to Managing. *Gastroenterol. Res. Pract.* **2012**, *2012*. [CrossRef] [PubMed]
72. Concerto, C.; Lanza, G.; Cantone, M.; Pennisi, M.; Giordano, D.; Spampinato, C.; Ricceri, R.; Pennisi, G.; Aguglia, E.; Bella, R. Different patterns of cortical excitability in major depression and vascular depression: A transcranial magnetic stimulation study. *BMC Psychiatry* **2013**, *13*, 300. [CrossRef] [PubMed]
73. Hall, N.J.; Rubin, G.; Charnock, A. Systematic review: Adherence to a gluten-free diet in adult patients with coeliac disease. *Aliment. Pharmacol. Therapeut.* **2009**, *30*, 315–330. [CrossRef] [PubMed]
74. Zysk, W.; Głąbska, D.; Guzek, D.; Zysk, W.; Głąbska, D.; Guzek, D. Social and Emotional Fears and Worries Influencing the Quality of Life of Female Celiac Disease Patients Following a Gluten-Free Diet. *Nutrients* **2018**, *10*, 1414. [CrossRef] [PubMed]
75. Leonard, M.; Cureton, P.; Fasano, A.; Leonard, M.M.; Cureton, P.; Fasano, A. Indications and Use of the Gluten Contamination Elimination Diet for Patients with Non-Responsive Celiac Disease. *Nutrients* **2017**, *9*, 1129. [CrossRef] [PubMed]
76. Hollon, J.R.; Cureton, P.A.; Martin, M.L.; Puppa, E.L.L.; Fasano, A. Trace gluten contamination may play a role in mucosal and clinical recovery in a subgroup of diet-adherent non-responsive celiac disease patients. *BMC Gastroenterol.* **2013**, *13*, 40. [CrossRef] [PubMed]
77. Rostami, K.; Bold, J.; Parr, A.; Johnson, M.; Rostami, K.; Bold, J.; Parr, A.; Johnson, M.W. Gluten-Free Diet Indications, Safety, Quality, Labels, and Challenges. *Nutrients* **2017**, *9*, 846. [CrossRef] [PubMed]
78. Roncoroni, L.; Bascuñán, K.; Doneda, L.; Scricciolo, A.; Lombardo, V.; Branchi, F.; Ferretti, F.; Dell'Osso, B.; Montanari, V.; Bardella, M.; et al. A Low FODMAP Gluten-Free Diet Improves Functional Gastrointestinal Disorders and Overall Mental Health of Celiac Disease Patients: A Randomized Controlled Trial. *Nutrients* **2018**, *10*, 1023. [CrossRef] [PubMed]
79. Jiang, H.; Ling, Z.; Zhang, Y.; Mao, H.; Ma, Z.; Yin, Y.; Wang, W.; Tang, W.; Tan, Z.; Shi, J.; et al. Altered fecal microbiota composition in patients with major depressive disorder. *Brain Behav. Immun.* **2015**, *48*, 186–194. [CrossRef] [PubMed]
80. Majeed, M.; Nagabhushanam, K.; Arumugam, S.; Majeed, S.; Ali, F. Bacillus coagulans MTCC 5856 for the management of major depression with irritable bowel syndrome: A randomised, double-blind, placebo controlled, multi-centre, pilot clinical study. *Food Nutr. Res.* **2018**, *62*. [CrossRef] [PubMed]

81. Garcia-Mazcorro, J.; Noratto, G.; Remes-Troche, J.; Garcia-Mazcorro, J.F.; Noratto, G.; Remes-Troche, J.M. The Effect of Gluten-Free Diet on Health and the Gut Microbiota Cannot Be Extrapolated from One Population to Others. *Nutrients* **2018**, *10*, 1421. [CrossRef] [PubMed]
82. Biesiekierski, J.R.; Newnham, E.D.; Irving, P.M.; Barrett, J.S.; Haines, M.; Doecke, J.D.; Shepherd, S.J.; Muir, J.G.; Gibson, P.R. Gluten Causes Gastrointestinal Symptoms in Subjects Without Celiac Disease: A Double-Blind Randomized Placebo-Controlled Trial. *Am. J. Gastroenterol.* **2011**, *106*, 508–514. [CrossRef] [PubMed]
83. Skodje, G.I.; Sarna, V.K.; Minelle, I.H.; Rolfsen, K.L.; Muir, J.G.; Gibson, P.R.; Veierød, M.B.; Henriksen, C.; Lundin, K.E.A. Fructan, Rather Than Gluten, Induces Symptoms in Patients With Self-Reported Non-Celiac Gluten Sensitivity. *Gastroenterology* **2018**, *154*, 529–539. [CrossRef] [PubMed]
84. Catassi, C.; Alaedini, A.; Bojarski, C.; Bonaz, B.; Bouma, G.; Carroccio, A.; Castillejo, G.; De Magistris, L.; Dieterich, W.; Di Liberto, D.; et al. The Overlapping Area of Non-Celiac Gluten Sensitivity (NCGS) and Wheat-Sensitive Irritable Bowel Syndrome (IBS): An Update. *Nutrients* **2017**, *9*, 1268. [CrossRef] [PubMed]
85. Aziz, I.; Hadjivassiliou, M.; Sanders, D.S. The spectrum of noncoeliac gluten sensitivity. *Nat. Rev. Gastroenterol. Hepatol.* **2015**, *12*, 516–526. [CrossRef] [PubMed]
86. Ford, R.P.K. The gluten syndrome: A neurological disease. *Med. Hypotheses* **2009**, *73*, 438–440. [CrossRef] [PubMed]
87. Morales-Muñoz, I.; Koskinen, S.; Partonen, T. Differences in clinical and cognitive variables in seasonal affective disorder compared to depressive-related disorders: Evidence from a population-based study in Finland. *Eur. Psychiatry* **2017**, *44*, 9–16. [CrossRef] [PubMed]
88. Kurppa, K.; Lauronen, O.; Collin, P.; Ukkola, A.; Laurila, K.; Huhtala, H.; Mäki, M.; Kaukinen, K. Factors Associated with Dietary Adherence in Celiac Disease: A Nationwide Study. *DIG* **2012**, *86*, 309–314. [CrossRef] [PubMed]
89. Addolorato, C.; De Lorenzi, C.; Abenavoli, L.; Leccio, L.; Capristo, E.; Casbarrini, C. Psychological support counselling improves gluten-free diet compliance in coeliac patients with affective disorders. *Aliment. Pharmacol. Therapeut.* **2004**, *20*, 777–782. [CrossRef] [PubMed]
90. Fueyo-Díaz, R.; Magallón-Botaya, R.; Gascón-Santos, S.; Asensio-Martínez, Á.; Palacios-Navarro, G.; Sebastián-Domingo, J.J. Development and Validation of a Specific Self-Efficacy Scale in Adherence to a Gluten-Free Diet. *Front. Psychol.* **2018**, *9*. [CrossRef] [PubMed]

nutrients

MDPI

Article

Celiac Male's Gluten-Free Diet Profile: Comparison to that of the Control Population and Celiac Women

Teba González [1,†], Idoia Larretxi [2,†], Juan Carlos Vitoria [1,3], Luis Castaño [1], Edurne Simón [2], Itziar Churruca [2,*], Virginia Navarro [2,*] and Arrate Lasa [2]

1 Instituto de Investigación Sanitaria Biocruces Bizkaia, Hospital Universitario Cruces, UPV/EHU, CIBERDEM, CIBERER, 48903 Barakaldo, Spain; teba.gonzalez@gmail.com (T.G.); jcvitoria45@gmail.com (J.C.V.); lcastano@osakidetza.eus (L.C.)

2 Gluten Analysis Laboratory of the University of the Basque Country, Department of Nutrition and Food Science, Faculty of Pharmacy, University of the Basque Country (UPV/EHU), Paseo de la Universidad, 7, 01006 Vitoria-Gasteiz, Spain; ilarretxi@hotmail.com (I.L.); edurne.simon@ehu.eus (E.S.); arrate.lasa@ehu.eus (A.L.)

3 Servicio de Gastroenterología Pediátrica, Hospital Universitario Cruces, UPV/EHU, 48903 Barakaldo, Spain

* Correspondence: itziar.txurruka@ehu.eus (I.C.); virginia.navarros@ehu.eus (V.N.); Tel.: +34-945-013071 (I.C.); +34-945-013923 (V.N.); Fax: +34-945-013014 (I.C. & V.N.)

† González and Larretxi contributed equally and should be considered as first authors.

Received: 16 October 2018; Accepted: 5 November 2018; Published: 8 November 2018

Abstract: The aim of the present work was to analyze the body composition and dietary profile of Spanish celiac men and to compare them to control men and celiac women from our previous studies. Forty-two celiac men (31.5 ± 11.9 years) were recruited and anthropometric measurements were taken. Analysis of energy consumption, macro- and micronutrient intake and food frequency consumption was carried out. Celiac men were more overweight and obese than celiac women, but less than the control population, reporting the same energy intake and macronutrient distribution. Most micronutrient deficiencies in celiac men were not directly related to a gluten free diet; these were also observed for the entire population. The least adherence to Dietary Reference Intakes in women was reported for iron, iodine, potassium and selenium, whereas magnesium intake was higher than in men. Among celiac participants (both genders), cereal, vegetable and legume consumption was poor and meat intake was contrastingly excessive. In conclusion, the dietary profile of celiac men is as unbalanced as that of control men but slightly more than that of celiac women. General nutritional education should be given to both general and celiac populations, and specific advices to celiac men, in order to decrease the risk of celiac disease-related pathologies.

Keywords: celiac disease; gluten-free diet; diary recommended intake; food habit; body composition

1. Introduction

Celiac disease (CD) is described as a permanent intolerance to gluten and is the most common chronic intestinal disease in Europe. Its estimated prevalence in Europe is around 1%, and this only refers to those that are diagnosed, since a significant number of patients have not been diagnosed yet [1,2].

This intestinal disease is more frequent in women than in men in a 2:1 ratio [3] and thus, in the vast majority of studies carried out in celiac people, it is common to find a larger number of female participants than males. Moreover, it must be pointed out that, in general, the male population is less likely to take part in health promotion programs than women are. Different reasons for this have been put forward, such as their low recruitment, delayed help-seeking behavior, and less interest and knowledge about health-related topics and habits [4,5]. As a result, this population cohort is often undervalued and does not always receive gender-specific healthcare.

The only effective treatment for celiac disease is a strict lifelong gluten-free diet (GFD). In fact, small amounts of gluten ingestion can cause important damage-causing disorders in the intestinal mucosa. Apart from gluten absence, a GFD must guarantee nutritional balance and so prevent deficiencies. However, when the nutritional composition of GFD of celiac people has been assessed, imbalanced proportions of macronutrients and several deficiencies in vitamin and mineral content have been observed [6–11]. Specifically, a GFD is usually accompanied by a low intake of carbohydrates, iron, calcium, folate, niacin, zinc and fiber and excess of saturated fats.

Some aspects of the GFD profile could be linked to a higher risk of several diseases. For instance, the relationship between low fiber, high saturated fat intake and cardiovascular diseases and obesity has been widely described [12,13]. Micronutrient deficiencies are related to comorbidities such as ferropenic anemia and osteopenia. This fact enhances the importance of complying with not only the intake recommendations of some key nutrients such as iron, calcium, vitamin D, but also those of other important molecules that regulate the immune system and help metabolic status to be balanced (zinc, magnesium, selenium, folate and so on), either in women or in men. In fact, it has been described that these deficiencies persist in some of these patients, even if they follow a strict GFD [8,10,14,15].

Bearing in mind all the above mentioned, the aim of the present work was to evaluate the body composition of adult celiac men from a region in Spain and the nutritional composition of the GFD they followed, as well as compare it with international recommendations, and with dietary habits of the general population (Spanish adult men). As a second objective, energy and nutrient intake and dietary habits of celiac men were compared to those reported in our previous studies for celiac women from the same region.

2. Materials and Methods

2.1. Participants and Procedure

The present study used data from a celiac men cohort recruited between 2007 and 2013 from three regions of the Basque Country (Araba, Gipuzkoa, and Bizkaia), in the north of Spain, as part of a prospective SUSFOOD study conducted in collaboration with the Gastroenterology and Endocrinology Units of Cruces University Hospital and Coeliac Association from the Basque Country. Forty-two celiac men took part in the study (mean age $\pm$ SD: 31.5 $\pm$ 11.9); all participants were diagnosed with celiac disease according to ESPGHAN guidelines and followed a GFD for at least one year. Exclusion criteria included a history of chronic diseases such as cardiovascular disease, diabetes, hyperthyroidism/hypothyroidism, hypercholesterolemia, hypertriglyceridemia or high blood pressure levels, other digestive pathologies that need specific dietary advice, and lack of motivation to participate in the study. Written informed consent was obtained from all participants, after receiving information about the survey. This study was approved by the Ethical Committee of Cruces Hospital (CEIC E-08/66) and the Ethical Committee of the University of The Basque Country (CEISH/76/2011).

Celiac women were recruited simultaneously and their data were collected in the same way as results from men; in fact, the woman cohort is part of the SUSFOOD study mentioned, which has already been published [6]. Control men data were obtained from the ENIDE nutritional survey carried out in Spain, based on 1589 adult men and conducted over the same period of time as the present work (ENIDE).

2.2. Anthropometric Measurements

Anthropometric measurements were collected by trained personnel. Body weight ($\pm$10 g) was measured after voiding using a digital integrating scale (SECA 760). Height was determined to the nearest 5 mm using a stadiometer (SECA 220). Body Mass Index (BMI) was calculated from weight and height (kg/m^2). The BMI values were categorized according to the World Health Organization (WHO) criteria as follows: Below 18.5 kg/m^2 considered as underweight, 18.5–24.9 kg/m^2 as normal weight, 25–29.9 kg/m^2 as overweight and >30 kg/m^2 as obese (WHO).

2.3. Body Composition and Energy Expenditure

Fat mass was estimated by a direct segmental multiple-frequency bioelectrical impedance analysis method (Inbody 230; Biospace, Seoul, Korea). Two skin electrodes were placed on the feet and two on the hands. Following the standard procedure, whole-body resistance and reactance were measured. Fat mass was evaluated from total-body impedance (Z). The guidelines of Gallagher et al. were used as reference for body fat mass [16].

Weight, height and age were used to calculate individual energy expenditure according to the Harris-Benedict formula. Standard activity level value was applied.

2.4. Dietary Assessment

Dietary intake was assessed using 3-day 24-h food recalls (24 HR), two on weekdays and one at the weekend. Sixteen participants filled out a food frequency questionnaire (FFQ). Trained nutritionist-dieticians recorded the answers of participants. Food portions and amounts were determined by using photographs of rations and sizes described in the Photo Album, as per the author of [17]. Energy and nutrient intakes were calculated by the nutritional software program "Alimentación y Salud" (AyS, Software, Tandem Innova, Inc., Huesca, Spain). The composition of specific gluten-free products for celiac people consumed by the participants was collected from the manufacturers and added into the food composition database of the program before calculations. As gluten-free product labels did not indicate micronutrient content (vitamins and minerals), an estimation with homologous gluten-containing products was carried out.

Dietary reference intakes (DRI) for Spanish population issued by the Spanish Societies of Nutrition, Feeding and Dietetics (FESNAD) in 2010 were taken as references for the interpretation of the 24 HR [18]. In the case of FFQ, Spanish Society of Community Nutrition (SENC) recommendations were used for the correct interpretation of the results [19].

Moreover, the results were compared to energy, nutrient and food intake of celiac women [6] and those of the mentioned Spanish reference population (ENIDE) [20].

2.5. Statistical Analysis

Statistical analyses of results were performed by using the IBM SPSS statistical program, version 23 (IBM Inc., Armonk, NY, USA). Normality in the distribution was assessed by the Kolmogorov-Smirnov test, and homogeneity by Levene's test. Statistical analyses were performed in order to calculate differences between celiac men and control population were performed with summary *t* Student's test, and those between celiac men and celiac women with Chi-square test. p values < 0.05 were accepted as significant.

3. Results

3.1. Anthropometric Measurements

Anthropometric data of celiac men from the present study are shown in Table 1.

57.1% of the participants showed normal BMI values and only 4.8% were underweight. In contrast, 38.1% of them were above normal BMI values, 26.2% were overweight, and 11.9% obese. Fat mass measurements indicated that 52% of the participants had excessive adiposity and 41% were between normal values. Only three participants (7%) had very low fat mass values.

Table 1. Characteristic of celiac participants included in the survey.

Characteristic	Men
N	42
Age (year)	31.5 ± 11.9
Mean duration of GFD (year)	20.9 ± 11.9
Height (cm)	176.2 ± 6.2
Weight (kg)	75.8 ± 13.9
Fat mass (%)	24.1 ± 8.1
Body-Mass Index	
Mean (kg/m^2)	24.7 ± 4.1
Underweight < 18.5—no. (%)	4.8
Normal 18.5–24.9—no. (%)	57.1
Overweight 25–29.9—no. (%)	26.2
Obese > 30—no. (%)	11.9

Notes: Values are mean ± SD or percentages; SD, standard deviation; *N*: sample size; no, number of subjects; GFD, gluten-free diet.

3.2. Dietary Intakes

3.2.1. Energy, Macronutrients, Fiber and Cholesterol Intake in Celiac Men

Daily energy intake was comparable to that observed in control men in ENIDE study. Energy distribution among macronutrients was not balanced in celiac men. To be specific, proteins and fats were consumed in excess (17% and 41% respectively) accompanied by a small amount of carbohydrates (42%) (Figure 1). When these data were compared to those of the ENIDE study, no significant differences were observed in energy and macronutrient consumption.

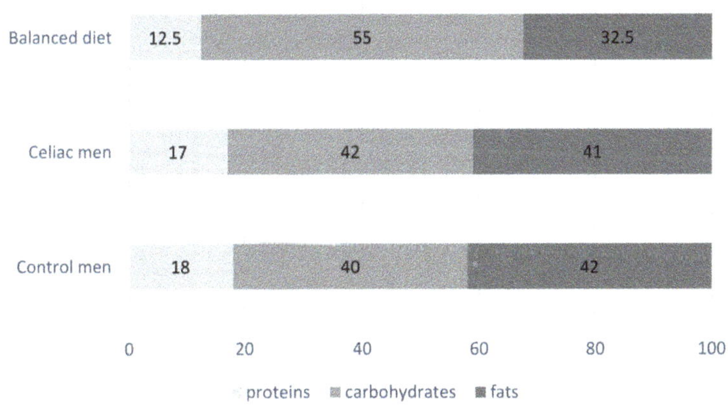

Figure 1. Mean contribution of macronutrients to energy in Spanish celiac (n = 42) and control men (n = 1589) (ENIDE study, representative at national level of the adult population) compared to the recommended contribution in a balanced diet proposed by the Federation of Spanish Societies of Nutrition and Dietetics (FESNAD).

In order to evaluate fat sources, dietary lipid profile was calculated. While saturated fatty acid (SFA) and monounsaturated fatty acid (MUFA) consumption was similar in celiac men and control men, polyunsaturated fatty acid (PUFA) consumption of celiac men was lower. In general terms, saturated and unsaturated fatty acids ratios were reached, as in the ENIDE survey (Table 2) [21]. Cholesterol ingestion was also similar in both groups, higher than that recommended [18].

Table 2. Energy and nutrient distribution in celiac and Spanish control men and results from recent studies.

Characteristic	Celiac Men (n = 42)	Spanish Men (ENIDE Study) (n = 1589)	p Value	Sheperd 2013 (11 Men)	Martin 2013 (18 Men)	Wild 2010 (31 Men)
Energy (kcal)	2355.4 ± 659.0	2546.8 ± 860.9	NS	2697 ± 445	2401 ± 592	2500 ± 717
Protein (g)	100.2 ± 30.1	109.4 ± 47.7	NS	98.8 ± 22.83	92.4 ± 17.5	92.7 ± 24.9
Carbohydrate (g)	220.7 ± 84.7	242.7 ± 101.8	NS	294 ± 72.3	267 ± 95	315.6 ± 98.5
Fat (g)	114.0 ± 32.2	114.9 ± 46.0	NS	67.9 ± 50.58	97.4 ± 29.7	93.2 ± 36.6
MUFA (g)	52.4 ± 16.1	48.29 ± 22.2	NS	-	-	-
PUFA (g)	13.2 ± 5.8	15.5 ± 8.5	<0.05	-	-	-
SFA (g)	34.5 ± 11.2	32.71 ± 15.55	NS	34.7 ± 7.7	-	-
(PUFA + MUFA)/SFA	1.93	1.95	-	-	-	-
PUFA/SFA	0.38	0.47	-	-	-	-
Cholesterol (mg)	421.2 ± 132.8	423.82 ± 181.25	NS	-	-	-
Fiber (g)	20.3 ± 7.1	20.94 ± 11.38	NS	30.2 ± 7.7	22.3 ± 6.0	13.7 ± 5.3

Notes: Values are means ± SD; Spanish adult men data were taken from the Spanish dietary nutritional assessment (ENIDE study, representative of the adult population at national level); SD, standard deviation; NS: non-significant; PUFA, polyunsaturated fatty acids; MUFA, monounsaturated fatty acids; SFA, saturated fatty acids.

Regarding dietary fiber consumption, celiac men were below recommendations (25–35 g/day). In fact, fiber consumption of 28% of participants was below 15 g per day and that of 43% between 15.1 and 25 g per day. A similar intake of fiber was also reported in control men, taken from the ENIDE survey (Table 2).

A comparison of energy intake between celiac men from the present study and celiac women from our previous studies [6] revealed that while the majority of women (65%) consumed the correct amounts of calories in their diet, less than half the men (46%) did so (Table 3). Moreover, only 6% of women consumed calories in excess, which, by contrast, 14% of men did. However, macronutrient distribution, similar in both genders, was higher than recommendations for proteins and fat intakes, and lower in the case of carbohydrates.

Table 3. Percentage of celiac men (n = 42) and women (n = 54) that fulfilled energy and macronutrient recommendation and their comparison.

	Recommended Intake *	Celiac Men			Celiac Women [6]			p Value
		Low	Adequate	Excessive	Low	Adequate	Excessive	
Energy intake	±20% of EE	40	46	14	30	65	6	<0.001
Protein	10–15%	0	19	81	0	20	81	NS
Carbohydrate	50–60%	98	2	0	91	9	0	NS
Total Fat	30–35%	0	5	95	4	11	85	NS
SFA	<10%	0	17	83	0	33	67	<0.05
MUFA	15–20%	14	31	55	31	37	28	NS

Notes: * Recommended energy and nutrient intake in a balanced diet proposed by the Federation of Spanish Societies (FESNAD). EE: energy expenditure; SFA, saturated fatty acids; MUFA, monounsaturated fatty acids; NS: non-significant. p value corresponds to differences between celiac males' and females' suitable intakes.

Dietary lipid profiles were similar between celiac men and women. In both groups, the highest percentage of participants consumed excessive SFA and cholesterol, though even more so in men.

Although both groups contained a high proportion of subjects with low fiber intakes (71% in men vs. 96% in women), there were more men that achieved adequate fiber consumption (26% in men vs. 4% in women).

3.2.2. Micronutrients Intake in Celiac Men

When vitamin and mineral mean intake of celiac participants was compared to that of control men, differences in eight micronutrient mean consumption were observed (Table 4). Celiac men consumed lower amounts of vitamin E, niacin and magnesium than the control group. By contrast, their riboflavin, B6, zinc, potassium and selenium mean intake was higher.

Table 4. Micronutrients mean intake in celiac and Spanish men.

	Celiac Men (n = 42)	Control Men (ENIDE Study) (n = 1589)	DRI: FESNAD (2010)	p Celiac Men vs. Spanish Men (ENIDE Study)
Vitamin A (ug)	802 ± 340	748 ± 338	700 [a]	NS
Thiamin (mg)	2.0 ± 1.4	2.1 ± 6.7	1.2 [b]	NS
Riboflavin (mg)	2.2 ± 1.1	1.5 ± 0.8	1.6	<0.001
Vitamin B6 (mg)	2.7 ± 0.9	2.0 ± 0.9	1.5 [c]	<0.001
Vitamin B12 (ug)	8.1 ± 5.6	7.9 ± 6.1	2	NS
Vitamin C (mg)	143 ± 82	131 ± 81	60 [d]	NS
Vitamin D (ug)	4.4 ± 4.5	4.3 ± 4.5	5 [e]	NS
Vitamin E (mg)	10.8 ± 5.1	14.9 ± 8.4	15	<0.001
Niacin (mg)	38.5 ± 13.6	45.7 ± 39.5	18 [f]	<0.01
Folate (ug)	302 ± 115	296 ± 121	300	NS
Calcium (mg)	939 ± 295	886 ± 345	900 [g]	NS
Iron (mg)	16.5 ± 5.1	16.1 ± 6.5	9 [h]	NS
Magnesium (mg)	323 ± 107	396 ± 139	350	<0.001
Iodine (ug)	117 ± 88	100 ± 50.5	150	NS
Phosphorus (mg)	1580 ± 442	1535 ± 471	700 [i]	NS
Zinc (mg)	12 ± 4.0	10.5 ± 3.7	9.5 [j]	<0.01
Potassium (mg)	3481 ± 980	3045 ± 917	3100	<0.01
Selenium (ug)	93.8 ± 53.5	63.5 ± 35.1	55	<0.001

Notes: Values are means ± SD. Spanish adult men data were taken from the Spanish dietary nutritional assessment (ENIDE study, representative at national level of the adult population). SD, standard deviation; DRI, dietary reference intake; FESNAD, Federation of Spanish Societies of Nutrition and Dietetics; NS: non-significant. [a] Vitamin A, 800 mg for 16–19 year range men; [b] Thiamin, 1.1 mg for >60 years old men; [c] Vitamin B6, 1.4 mg for 16–18 years old and 1.6 mg for >60 years old men; [d] Vitamin C, 70 mg for >60 years old men; [e] Vitamin D, 7.5 mg for >60 years old men; [f] Niacin, 17 mg for 50–69 years old men; [g] Calcium, 1000 mg 16–19 years old and for >60 years old men; [h] Iron, 10 mg for >60 years old men; [i] Phosphorus, 800 mg for 16–19 years old men; [j] Zinc: 10 mg for >60 years old men.

A 67% (2/3) DRI cutoff value for deficient micronutrient intake was set as reported by the literature [22,23]. According to this cutoff, vitamin A, D and E, iodine, folate and magnesium were deficient, as a small amount (41–81%) of participants accomplished it (Table 5). In the case of calcium, zinc, selenium and vitamin C, most participants (around 90% of them) fulfilled 2/3 of the DRIs. None of the celiac men showed low intakes of vitamin B6, B12, niacin, riboflavin, thiamine, phosphorus and iron.

Table 5. Percentage of celiac men (n = 42) and women (n = 54) that fulfilled at least 2/3 of DRI (FESNAD, 2010) and their comparison.

	Celiac Men	Celiac Women [6]	p Value
	% of Participants that Fulfilled at Least 67% of Recommendations	% of Participants that Fulfilled at Least 67% of Recommendations	
Vitamin A (ug)	81	89	NS
Thiamin (mg)	98	100	NS
Riboflavin (mg)	98	98	NS
Vitamin B6 (mg)	100	100	NS
Vitamin B12 (ug)	100	100	NS
Vitamin C (mg)	93	96	NS
Vitamin D (ug)	45	52	NS
Vitamin E (mg)	48	61	NS

Table 5. *Cont.*

	Celiac Men	Celiac Women [6]	*p* Value
	% of Participants that Fulfilled at Least 67% of Recommendations	% of Participants that Fulfilled at Least 67% of Recommendations	
Niacin (mg)	100	100	NS
Folate (ug)	76	82	NS
Calcium (mg)	86	87	NS
Iron (mg)	100	69	<0.001
Magnesium (mg)	71	91	<0.05
Iodine (ug)	50	20	<0.01
Phosphorus (mg)	100	100	NS
Zinc (mg)	91	98	0.093
Potassium (mg)	98	85	<0.05
Selenium (ug)	93	69	<0.01

Notes: Recommended intake of vitamins and minerals proposed by the Federation of Spanish Societies (FESNAD). NS: non-significant. *p* value correspond to differences between celiac men and celiac women's appropriate intakes.

Several differences were found in mineral intake accomplishment, but not in vitamins, when comparing celiac men and women habits (Table 5). Celiac women fulfilled magnesium requirements better than celiac men and, by contrast, iron, iodine, potassium, and selenium DRIs were better complied by celiac men.

3.3. Food Consumption Frequency of Celiac Men

Figure 2 summarizes main food group consumption frequency. Cereal consumption data indicated that only 13% of celiac men fulfilled these food group recommendations, which means at least four servings per day (Figure 2). Moreover, almost half of them (44%) consumed a small or a very small amount of cereals (fewer than two servings) per day.

The vast majority of participants (84%) did not reach vegetable consumption recommendations (10 portions/week) [19]. One-third of celiac men did not consume the minimum recommended two servings of fruit daily. Furthermore, legume consumption was also low in 42% of participants, which means that they consumed less than two portions of pulses per week.

With regard to animal origin food consumption, almost half of the participants fulfilled the recommendations of dairy products, 2–3 servings per day, whereas 25% reported an excessive consumption, which means more than 4 dairy servings per day. Only 19% of celiac men achieved egg consumption recommended by the SENC, while 38% had an excessive consumption. The ingestion of fish and derivatives was sufficient in nearly half of celiac men and almost 20% of participants consumed it in excess. By contrast, meat consumption was excessive in the vast majority of the subjects (88%), which means that they ate more than 4–5 servings of meat per week.

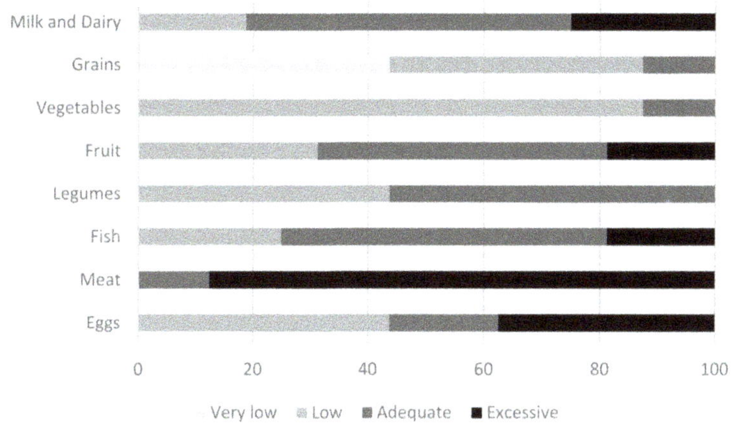

Figure 2. Compliance of food frequency consumption in celiac men by servings per day or week, according to the Spanish Society of Community Nutrition (SENC).

In relation to the foods considered for occasional consumption, it must be pointed out that celiac men followed the recommendations (data not shown). Participants used olive oil, which is rich in monounsaturated fatty acids, as their fat source, and discarded other lipid sources such as margarine or butter as their main lipid source for cooking.

Finally, the analysis of food frequency questionnaires in celiac men and celiac women revealed similar results. No differences were found in dairy products, grains, vegetables, fruits and meat consumption. However, when fish and egg consumption were evaluated, a tendency toward higher percentage of celiac men with excessive consumption of these foods was observed, compared to celiac women. Concretely, 19% of men consumed fish in excess vs. 6% of women ($p = 0.09$). Moreover, 37% of men consumed eggs in excess, whereas 17% of women did so ($p = 0.08$).

4. Discussion

Male participation in health promotion programs has usually been lower than that of women, probably due to their lower interest in health-related topics, among other reasons [4,5]. The studies in the literature comparing men and women's dietary habits provide different outcomes, attributable to differences in methodologies, population sizes, regional habits, and recommendations. Some studies described different patterns of deficiencies either in macro- or micronutrients between genders [24,25]. In the case of celiac disease, even though clinical trials have been published with both female and male participants, the recruited number of men is usually small. Thus, evidence about celiac men's body composition, diet quality, and eating pattern is rather scarce. The present study presents detailed energy and nutrient intake and dietary habits of a meaningful celiac male group, comparing them to a male control population and to celiac women from the same geographical region.

Obesity and overweight are rising among celiac patients, which is increasingly of concern to clinicians [11,26]. In this study, anthropometric data revealed that celiac men showed an alarming 38.1% of overweight and obesity, while 52% of participants showed an excessive fat mass. Nevertheless, this prevalence was lower than that observed in the control population [27,28]. These results were consistent with other studies, where celiac men registered similar BMI index values [8,29,30] which were also lower than those of the control populations [6,7,31,32].

Comparing these results with data from women (only 7.4% of overweight in celiac women), major gender differences were found. Accordingly, the prevalence of obesity and overweight in general population is greater for men [33–35]. These differences could, as stated before, be due to the lesser interest that men pay to health status and its care [4,5]. Nevertheless, it must be pointed out that in the case of celiac patients, most studies do not find gender differences in this parameter [8,29]. However, Tucker et al. (2012) [36] found that females were more likely to be obese, when BMI reaches values of 30 or above.

Even though energy intake of celiac men was similar to that of the control and to celiac men from other studies [8,20,29,30], our data revealed that 14% of celiac men consumed calories in excess, more than 120% of their energy expenditure, and 24% of them exceeded 110% of requirements. These results were not found in women, whose energy intake was suitable in 65% of the participants. All of the above explains the high percentage of obesity found among male participants from the present study. By contrast, 40% of the participants were under 80% of their energy expenditure, reflecting a possible underreporting, as found by others [29,37].

Celiac men showed imbalanced energy distribution, similarly to previous studies, but it must be pointed out that participants in this study consumed even fewer carbohydrates and more fat than those of earlier studies [29,30]. However, the macronutrient consumption of Spanish celiac women and the control population was similar to that observed in the male celiac group studied. Thus, it seems that imbalanced energy distribution is not GFD-related but could be associated to geographical dietary habits. Of these, low cereal and vegetable consumption and excessive meat intake, observed in both men and women [6], as well as in control men [38], could be the main contributors to the macronutrient imbalance.

With regard to dietary fat sources, SFA, MUFA and cholesterol were consumed in excess, although adequate fatty acid ratios were reached. These results were similar to those observed in control population, reinforcing the idea of this not being a GFD-related imbalance. The excessive consumption of meat (88% participants) and eggs (37%) could justify the results observed. However, the proportion of men eating excessive SFA and cholesterol was significantly greater than that of women. Although meat consumption did not differ between men and women, the excessive consumption of eggs among celiac men could impair these parameters. By contrast, intake of PUFAs was slightly lower in the male celiac population than in control men. However, 90% of celiac men participating showed adequate PUFA intake, more than women did. The higher fish consumption observed in men could be on the basis of this difference.

As far as fiber is concerned, celiac male consumption was low, similar to other studies conducted with celiac men and control population [8,20,29,30]. The low consumption of vegetables, legumes and grains could explain, at least in part, this outcome. However, fiber recommendations were more obeyed by celiac men than by celiac women, due to higher general food intake and thus greater amounts of plant origin foods.

The celiac population has been associated with an increased cardiovascular risk [39,40]. Although factors influencing the association between CD and cardiovascular disease could be related to the pathophysiology of CD, there is no doubt that the body composition and dietary pattern of celiac men described, with high intake of deleterious components, such as SFA, and low intake of protective ones, such as fiber, play an essential role.

As stated previously, micronutrients have also been a matter of concern for the celiac population. In our study, some differences in micronutrient mean intake arose between celiac men and their control. Vitamin E, niacin and magnesium was lower in celiac men than in control men and, by contrast, that of riboflavin, B6, zinc, potassium and selenium was higher, pointing to a different dietary pattern of this collective. While mean intakes provided some important information, it was necessary to analyze to what extent this population was below micronutrient recommendations, in order to identify possible deficiencies and health-risks.

The percentage of celiac men who complied with micronutrient DRI varied among nutrients, and also between genders. The most alarming deficiencies reported in this work for celiac men were those of vitamin D, vitamin E, and iodine, all of them with less than 50% of individuals fulfilling two thirds of DRI.

Wild et al. (2010) also reported vitamin D deficient intake in celiac men (no more than 20% of patients fulfilled the DRI) [8,29,30]. These data were also in accordance with the general population [8,20,29,30]. Vitamin E and iodine mean intakes were also low for both celiac and control men. In particular, vitamin E was even lower in celiacs, where only 48% reached the 67% of DRI. Iodine and vitamin E are not usually analyzed in GFD assessments, but considering their extremely low intake, specific nutritional advice, and probably supplementation, should be considered for the celiac male population.

In addition to the aforementioned important deficiencies, other micronutrients, such as folate and magnesium, were also below recommendations in celiac men (less than 80% achieved two-thirds of DRI). These data were in agreement with previous studies from the literature [8,30,37].

The comparison between celiac men and women in their adherence to vitamin and mineral recommendations revealed differences only in some mineral intakes. Less fulfilment of DRIs in women was reported for iron, iodine, potassium, and selenium, whereas magnesium intake was higher than that of men. This could be due to the lower energy intake of women [6], which could hinder the achievement of some mineral intakes. Iron was a special case, because men fulfilled totally the DRIs, but only 69% of women achieved 2/3, due to more demanding requirements of this mineral at some life stages for them. Considering the high prevalence of anemia in patients with CD, this is an important issue to be addressed in women.

In general, it can be stated that micronutrient deficiencies in celiac men were not directly related to a GFD, and were concerning for the entire population. Only magnesium and vitamin E intake appeared to be lower than the control, and below recommendations for both groups in the case of vitamin E. Folate, iodine and vitamin D intakes were the most worrying, giving the anemia, thyroid disease and osteopenia prevalence of this collective [41,42].

One of the most cited reasons for micronutrient deficiency in a GFD is gluten-free products (GFP) composition. In fact, gluten-containing grains and foods are a major source of micronutrients [43,44], and often GFP do not contain the same levels of micronutrients as their counterparts—e.g., thiamine, riboflavin, niacin, folate, vitamin D, calcium, or iron [10,45–48]. Instead of those GFP, higher gluten-free whole cereals (amaranth, sorghum, millet, etc.) and pseudocereals (quinoa, buckwheat, etc.) are more interesting, as they contain the fiber and micronutrients necessary to balance [11,49]. Nevertheless, fortification of gluten-free flours and GFP could be also of interest, but more research is necessary in order to correctly identify which nutrients are suitable for general fortification and which for personal supplementation.

For this purpose, all micronutrients should be addressed in the studies, and the micronutrient composition of GFP, which needs to be studied in depth, should be incorporated into the databases. Selenium, iodine and vitamin E intakes are scarcely analyzed in the literature, and they are still important to ensure the health status of celiac people.

The main limitation of the present study was that micronutrient intake coming from GFP was calculated according to the micronutrient content of their gluten-containing counterparts. Thus, data from the present work could represent an overestimation of the real consumption of vitamins and minerals. Moreover, people participating in this kind of studies are more concerned about health issues and self-caring, which could also have overestimated the results. Furthermore, the experimental design did not include a control group of men, and people with comorbidities were excluded from the study. Nevertheless, this is the first study where dietary habits of a cohort of Spanish celiac men were compared to those of the control population and to those of Spanish celiac women. It is worth noting that the sample size was higher than those used in other studies with celiac men.

In summary, inadequacies in terms of both, macro- and micronutrients, in celiac male diets are found. Some of them also appear in the diet of the control population, pointing to unsuitable habits of the entire population, but other changes are gender-specific and fewer GFD-dependent. Effective general recommendations for the global male population should be given, as well as specific advice for celiac people, principally regarding micronutrient intake. Greater consumption of gluten-free cereals or pseudocereals, vegetables, and legumes and less of that of meats should be recommended. Personalized dietary advice and long-term follow-up for celiac people, in particular for celiac men, could contribute towards preventing nutrient deficiencies related to dietary imbalance and to obtaining a better health status, lowering the risk of CD-related pathologies.

Author Contributions: T.G. and I.L. recruited the patients, performed anthropometric measurements and collected questionnaires. J.C.V. and L.C. designed the experiment. I.C. and A.L. performed the analysis of diet and food habits. V.N. and E.S. analyzed all data and contributed to statistical analysis. E.S., I.C., V.N. and A.L. wrote the manuscript.

Acknowledgments: Idoia Larretxi is a fellowship of the University of the Basque Country, UPV/EHU (Euskararen eta Etengabeko Prestakuntzaren arloko Errektoreordetza). This research was funded by University of the Basque Country (UPV/EHU) and Basque Government, grant numbers US12/10 and GV2008111042, respectively. We thank the participation of all patients, and the collaboration of "Asociación de Celiacos de Euskadi (EZE)", specifically that of Mireia Apraiz, Beatriz Zulueta, Nerea Segura, Estíbaliz Olabarri Elena Pérez-Estevez, Lissette Delgado, Aranzazu Sainz-Espiga, Sagrario Martínez and Lorea Martínez-Indart.

Conflicts of Interest: The authors declare that they have no conflict of interest.

References

1. Lionetti, E.; Catassi, C. New clues in celiac disease epidemiology, pathogenesis, clinical manifestations, and treatment. *Int. Rev. Immunol.* **2011**, *30*, 219–231. [CrossRef] [PubMed]
2. Peña, A.; Rodrigo, L. Epidemiology of celiac disease and non-celiac gluten-related disorders. In *Advances in the Understanding of Gluten Related Pathology and the Evolution of Gluten-Free Foods*; Arranz, E., Fernández-Bañares, F., Rosell, C., Rodrigo, L., Peña, A., Eds.; OmniaScience: Barcelona, Spain, 2015; pp. 27–73.
3. Catassi, C.; Gatti, S.; Fasano, A. The new epidemiology of celiac disease. *J. Pediatr. Gastroenterol. Nutr.* **2014**, *59 (Suppl. 1)* (Suppl. 1), S7–S9. [CrossRef]
4. Sharp, P.; Bottorff, J.L.; Hunt, K.; Oliffe, J.L.; Johnson, S.T.; Dudley, L.; Caperchione, C.M. Men's Perspectives of a Gender-Sensitized Health Promotion Program Targeting Healthy Eating, Active Living, and Social Connectedness. *Am. J. Men's Health* **2018**, 2157–2166. [CrossRef] [PubMed]
5. Galdas, P.M.; Cheater, F.; Marshall, P. Men and health help-seeking behaviour: Literature review. *J. Adv. Nurs.* **2005**, *49*, 616–623. [CrossRef] [PubMed]
6. Churruca, I.; Miranda, J.; Lasa, A.; Bustamante, M.; Larretxi, I.; Simon, E. Analysis of Body Composition and Food Habits of Spanish Celiac Women. *Nutrients* **2015**, *7*, 5515–5531. [CrossRef] [PubMed]
7. Bardella, M.T.; Fredella, C.; Prampolini, L.; Molteni, N.; Giunta, A.M.; Bianchi, P.A. Body composition and dietary intakes in adult celiac disease patients consuming a strict gluten-free diet. *Am. J. Clin. Nutr.* **2000**, *72*, 937–939. [CrossRef] [PubMed]
8. Martin, J.; Geisel, T.; Maresch, C.; Krieger, K.; Stein, J. Inadequate nutrient intake in patients with celiac disease: Results from a german dietary survey. *Digestion* **2013**, *87*, 240–246. [CrossRef] [PubMed]
9. Capristo, E.; Malandrino, N.; Farnetti, S.; Mingrone, G.; Leggio, L.; Addolorato, G.; Gasbarrini, G. Increased serum high-density lipoprotein-cholesterol concentration in celiac disease after gluten-free diet treatment correlates with body fat stores. *J. Clin. Gastroenterol.* **2009**, *43*, 946–949. [CrossRef] [PubMed]
10. Vici, G.; Belli, L.; Biondi, M.; Polzonetti, V. Gluten free diet and nutrient deficiencies: A review. *Clin. Nutr.* **2016**. [CrossRef] [PubMed]
11. Theethira, T.G.; Dennis, M. Celiac disease and the gluten-free diet: Consequences and recommendations for improvement. *Dig. Dis.* **2015**, *33*, 175–182. [CrossRef] [PubMed]
12. Phillips, C.M.; Kesse-Guyot, E.; McManus, R.; Hercberg, S.; Lairon, D.; Planells, R.; Roche, H.M. High dietary saturated fat intake accentuates obesity risk associated with the fat mass and obesity-associated gene in adults. *J. Nutr.* **2012**, *142*, 824–831. [CrossRef] [PubMed]
13. Slavin, J.L. Dietary fiber and body weight. *Nutrition* **2005**, *21*, 411–418. [CrossRef] [PubMed]
14. Capristo, E.; Mingrone, G.; Addolorato, G.; Greco, A.V.; Corazza, G.R.; Gasbarrini, G. Differences in metabolic variables between adult coeliac patients at diagnosis and patients on a gluten-free diet. *Scand. J. Gastroenterol.* **1997**, *32*, 1222–1229. [CrossRef] [PubMed]

15. Capristo, E.; Addolorato, G.; Mingrone, G.; De Gaetano, A.; Greco, A.V.; Tataranni, P.A.; Gasbarrini, G. Changes in body composition, substrate oxidation, and resting metabolic rate in adult celiac disease patients after a 1-y gluten-free diet treatment. *Am. J. Clin. Nutr.* **2000**, *72*, 76–81. [CrossRef] [PubMed]
16. Gallagher, D.; Heymsfield, S.B.; Heo, M.; Jebb, S.A.; Murgatroyd, P.R.; Sakamoto, Y. Healthy percentage body fat ranges: An approach for developing guidelines based on body mass index. *Am. J. Clin. Nutr.* **2000**, *72*, 694–701. [CrossRef] [PubMed]
17. Russolillo, G.; Marques, I. *Food Portion Sizes Album*; Imagen Comunicación Multimedia: Madrid, Spain, 2008; 186p.
18. FESNAD. Dietary reference intakes (DRI) for spanish population, 2010. *Actividad Dietética* **2010**, *14*, 196–197. [CrossRef]
19. Aranceta, J.; Serra-Majem, L. Dietary guidelines for the Spanish population. *Public Health Nutr.* **2001**, *4*, 1403–1408. [CrossRef] [PubMed]
20. AECOSAN, Agencia Española de Consumo, Seguridad Alimentaria y Nutrición. Spanish Population Dietary Intakes. National Health Survey (ENIDE). Available online: http://aesan.msssi.gob.es/AESAN/docs/docs/evaluacion_riesgos/estudios_evaluacion_nutricional/valoracion_nutricional_enide_macronutrientes.pdf (accessed on 8 June 2017).
21. SENC. Nutritional objectives for the Spanish population: Consensus from the Spanish Society of Community Nutrition. *Rev. Esp. Nutr. Com.* **2011**, *17*, 178–199.
22. Marshall, T.A.; Stumbo, P.J.; Warren, J.J.; Xie, X.J. Inadequate nutrient intakes are common and are associated with low diet variety in rural, community-dwelling elderly. *J. Nutr.* **2001**, *131*, 2192–2196. [CrossRef] [PubMed]
23. Roman-Vinas, B.; Ribas Barba, L.; Ngo, J.; Martinez-Gonzalez, M.A.; Wijnhoven, T.M.; Serra-Majem, L. Validity of dietary patterns to assess nutrient intake adequacy. *Br. J. Nutr.* **2009**, *101* (Suppl. 2), S12–S20. [CrossRef]
24. Arganini, C.; Saba, A.; Comitato, R.; Virgili, F.; Turrini, A. Gender Differences in Food Choice and Dietary Intake in Modern Western Societies. In *Public Health-Social and Behavioral Health*; Maddock, J., Ed.; InTech: Hampshire, UK, 2012; ISBN 978-953-51-0620-3. Available online: http://www.intechopen.com/books/public-health-social-and-behavioral-health/gender-differences-in-foodchoice-and-dietary-intake-in-modern-western-societies (accessed on 15 October 2018).
25. Rippin, H.L.; Hutchinson, J.; Jewell, J.; Breda, J.J.; Cade, J.E. Adult Nutrient Intakes from Current National Dietary Surveys of European Populations. *Nutrients* **2017**, *9*, 1288. [CrossRef] [PubMed]
26. Valletta, E.; Fornaro, M.; Cipolli, M.; Conte, S.; Bissolo, F.; Danchielli, C. Celiac disease and obesity: Need for nutritional follow-up after diagnosis. *Eur. J. Clin. Nutr.* **2010**, *64*, 1371–1372. [CrossRef] [PubMed]
27. Aranceta Bartrina, J.; Pérez Rodrigo, C. Inequality, health and nutrition in Spain: A regional view of the body mass index. *Nutr. Hosp.* **2018**, *35*, 142–149. [PubMed]
28. López-Sobaler, A.M.; Aparicio, A.; Aranceta-Bartrina, J.; Gil, Á.; González-Gross, M.; Serra-Majem, L.; Varela-Moreiras, G.; Ortega, R.M. Overweight and General and Abdominal Obesity in a Representative Sample of Spanish Adults: Findings from the ANIBES Study. *Biomed. Res. Int.* **2016**, *2016*, 8341487. [CrossRef] [PubMed]
29. Wild, D.; Robins, G.G.; Burley, V.J.; Howdle, P.D. Evidence of high sugar intake, and low fibre and mineral intake, in the gluten-free diet. *Aliment. Pharmacol. Ther.* **2010**, *32*, 573–581. [CrossRef] [PubMed]
30. Shepherd, S.J.; Gibson, P.R. Nutritional inadequacies of the gluten-free diet in both recently-diagnosed and long-term patients with coeliac disease. *J. Hum. Nutr. Diet.* **2013**, *26*, 349–358. [CrossRef] [PubMed]
31. Brambilla, P.; Picca, M.; Dilillo, D.; Meneghin, F.; Cravidi, C.; Tischer, M.C.; Vivaldo, T.; Bedogni, G.; Zuccotti, G.V. Changes of body mass index in celiac children on a gluten-free diet. *Nutr. Metab. Cardiovasc. Dis.* **2013**, *23*, 177–182. [CrossRef] [PubMed]
32. Larretxi, I.; Simon, E.; Benjumea, L.; Miranda, J.; Bustamante, M.A.; Lasa, A.; Eizaguirre, F.J.; Churruca, I. Gluten-free-rendered products contribute to imbalanced diets in children and adolescents with celiac disease. *Eur. J. Nutr.* **2018**. [CrossRef] [PubMed]
33. Peralta, M.; Ramos, M.; Lipert, A.; Martins, J.; Marques, A. Prevalence and trends of overweight and obesity in older adults from 10 European countries from 2005 to 2013. *Scand. J. Public Health* **2018**, *46*, 522–529. [CrossRef] [PubMed]
34. Rodríguez-Rodríguez, E.; López-Plaza, B.; López-Sobaler, A.M.; Ortega, R.M. Overweight and obesity among Spanish adults. *Nutr. Hosp.* **2011**, *26*, 355–363. [CrossRef] [PubMed]

35. Gutiérrez-Fisac, J.L.; Banegas Banegas, J.R.; Artalejo, F.R.; Regidor, E. Increasing prevalence of overweight and obesity among Spanish adults, 1987–1997. *Int. J. Obes. Relat. Metab. Disord.* **2000**, *24*, 1677–1682. [CrossRef] [PubMed]
36. Tucker, E.; Rostami, K.; Prabhakaran, S.; Al Dulaimi, D. Patients with coeliac disease are increasingly overweight or obese on presentation. *J. Gastrointest. Liver Dis.* **2012**, *21*, 11–15.
37. Hallert, C.; Grant, C.; Grehn, S.; Grännö, C.; Hultén, S.; Midhagen, G.; Ström, M.; Svensson, H.; Valdimarsson, T. Evidence of poor vitamin status in coeliac patients on a gluten-free diet for 10 years. *Aliment. Pharmacol. Ther.* **2002**, *16*, 1333–1339. [CrossRef] [PubMed]
38. De Batlle, J.; Gracia-Lavedan, E.; Romaguera, D.; Mendez, M.; Castaño-Vinyals, G.; Martín, V.; Aragonés, N.; Gómez-Acebo, I.; Olmedo-Requena, R.; Jimenez-Moleon, J.J.; et al. Meat intake, cooking methods and doneness and risk of colorectal tumours in the Spanish multicase-control study (MCC-Spain). *Eur. J. Nutr.* **2018**, *57*, 643–653. [CrossRef] [PubMed]
39. Emilsson, L.; Lebwohl, B.; Sundström, J.; Ludvigsson, J.F. Cardiovascular disease in patients with coeliac disease: A systematic review and meta-analysis. *Dig. Liver Dis.* **2015**, *47*, 847–852. [CrossRef] [PubMed]
40. Ciaccio, E.J.; Lewis, S.K.; Biviano, A.B.; Iyer, V.; Garan, H.; Green, P.H. Cardiovascular involvement in celiac disease. *World J. Cardiol.* **2017**, *9*, 652–666. [CrossRef] [PubMed]
41. Lucendo, A.J.; García-Manzanares, A. Bone mineral density in adult coeliac disease: An updated review. *Rev. Esp. Enferm. Dig.* **2013**, *105*, 154–162. [CrossRef] [PubMed]
42. Nijhawan, S.; Katiyar, P.; Nagaich, N.; Saradava, V.; Nijhawan, M.; Gupta, G.; Mathur, A.; Sharma, R.; Nepalia, S. Prevalence of associated disorders in Indian patients with celiac disease. *Indian J. Gastroenterol.* **2013**, *32*, 330–334. [CrossRef] [PubMed]
43. Whitton, C.; Nicholson, S.K.; Roberts, C.; Prynne, C.J.; Pot, G.K.; Olson, A.; Fitt, E.; Cole, D.; Teucher, B.; Bates, B.; et al. National Diet and Nutrition Survey: UK food consumption and nutrient intakes from the first year of the rolling programme and comparisons with previous surveys. *Br. J. Nutr.* **2011**, *106*, 1899–1914. [CrossRef] [PubMed]
44. Størsrud, S.; Hulthén, L.R.; Lenner, R.A. Beneficial effects of oats in the gluten-free diet of adults with special reference to nutrient status, symptoms and subjective experiences. *Br. J. Nutr.* **2003**, *90*, 101–107. [CrossRef] [PubMed]
45. Thompson, T. Thiamin, riboflavin, and niacin contents of the gluten-free diet: Is there cause for concern? *J. Am. Diet. Assoc.* **1999**, *99*, 858–862. [CrossRef]
46. Penagini, F.; Dilillo, D.; Meneghin, F.; Mameli, C.; Fabiano, V.; Zuccotti, G.V. Gluten-free diet in children: An approach to a nutritionally adequate and balanced diet. *Nutrients* **2013**, *5*, 4553–4565. [CrossRef] [PubMed]
47. Cornicelli, M.; Saba, M.; Machello, N.; Silano, M.; Neuhold, S. Nutritional composition of gluten-free food versus regular food sold in the Italian market. *Dig. Liver Dis.* **2018**. [CrossRef] [PubMed]
48. Kulai, T.; Rashid, M. Assessment of Nutritional Adequacy of Packaged Gluten-free Food Products. *Can. J. Diet. Pract Res.* **2014**, *75*, 186–190. [CrossRef] [PubMed]
49. Lee, A.R.; Ng, D.L.; Dave, E.; Ciaccio, E.J.; Green, P.H. The effect of substituting alternative grains in the diet on the nutritional profile of the gluten-free diet. *J. Hum. Nutr. Diet.* **2009**, *22*, 359–363. [CrossRef] [PubMed]

nutrients

MDPI

Review

Gluten-Free Diet and Its 'Cousins' in Irritable Bowel Syndrome

Anupam Rej [1] and David Surendran Sanders [1,2,*]

[1] Academic Unit of Gastroenterology, Royal Hallamshire Hospital, Sheffield Teaching Hospital NHS Foundation Trust, Sheffield S10 2JF, UK; anupam.rej@sth.nhs.uk

[2] Academic Unit of Gastroenterology, Department of Infection, Immunity and Cardiovascular Disease, University of Sheffield, Sheffield, S10 2RX, UK

* Correspondence: david.sanders@sth.nhs.uk; Tel.: +0114-226-1179

Received: 11 October 2018; Accepted: 8 November 2018; Published: 11 November 2018

Abstract: Functional disorders are common, with irritable bowel syndrome (IBS) being the commonest and most extensively evaluated functional bowel disorder. It is therefore paramount that effective therapies are available to treat this common condition. Diet appears to play a pivotal role in symptom generation in IBS, with a recent interest in the role of dietary therapies in IBS. Over the last decade, there has been a substantial increase in awareness of the gluten-free diet (GFD), with a recent focus of the role of a GFD in IBS. There appears to be emerging evidence for the use of a GFD in IBS, with studies demonstrating the induction of symptoms following gluten in patients with IBS. However, there are questions with regards to which components of wheat lead to symptom generation, as well as the effect of a GFD on nutritional status, gut microbiota and long-term outcomes. Further studies are required, although the design of dietary studies remain challenging. The implementation of a GFD should be performed by a dietitian with a specialist interest in IBS, which could be achieved via the delivery of group sessions.

Keywords: non-coeliac gluten sensitivity; gluten; wheat; low FODMAP diet; irritable bowel syndrome

1. Introduction

Functional disorders are common, with the Rome IV guidelines classifying these disorders into oesophageal, gastroduodenal, bowel, centrally mediated, anorectal, gallbladder, and sphincter of Oddi disorders [1]. The commonest and most extensively evaluated functional bowel disorder is irritable bowel syndrome (IBS), with a reported global pooled prevalence of 11 percent [2]. IBS can be classified into diarrhoea-predominant (IBS-D), constipation-predominant (IBS-C), mixed (IBS-M) and unclassified (IBS-U) [1]. The pathophysiology of IBS is not fully understood, but several pathophysiological mechanisms have been proposed, including visceral hypersensitivity, inflammation, increased intestinal mucosal permeability, and genetic and psychological factors [3,4]. The impact of IBS can lead to a significant impact on sufferers, with a reduced quality of life, increased time off work and greater utilisation of healthcare [5]. It is also associated with several other conditions such as depression, fibromyalgia, chronic fatigue disorder, and temporomandibular joint disorder [6]. As a result of this, it is paramount that there are effective treatments for this common condition.

Despite many individuals using medication for the treatment of functional disorders, up to two-thirds of individuals with functional disorders also use diet or dietary supplements as a therapy [7]. A large proportion of individuals with IBS note that they have dietary triggers, with up to two-thirds of individuals noting the induction of symptoms after ingestion of food [8–10]. As a result of this, there has been great interest in the role of dietary therapies in IBS, with a focus recently in a low fermentable oligo-, di-, and mono-saccharides and polyols (FODMAPs) diet, wheat free diet (WFD) and gluten-free diet (GFD).

There has been an increase in the awareness of the GFD over the last decade [11], with the gluten-free food industry continuing to rise, with more than $15 billion dollars spent in the USA in 2016 [12]. Whilst GFDs are known as the mainstay of treatment for people with an established diagnosis of coeliac disease [13], we will explore the emerging evidence for this dietary therapy in individuals with IBS.

2. Wheat Free Diet

Gluten is found in the endosperm of grass-related grains, including wheat, barley, and rye. In view of this, it is important to explore the role of a WFD in IBS as many individuals consuming a GFD maybe avoiding wheat.

Wheat avoidance is common, with a cross-sectional population survey in Australia reporting wheat avoidance in approximately 10% of individuals [14]. A significant proportion of individuals with IBS who reduce wheat consumption may have a wheat sensitivity. A large study [15], in which 920 patients with IBS who had a self-reduced wheat consumption, underwent an elimination diet for 4 weeks, subsequently followed by a double-blind placebo-controlled (DBPC) challenge. Out of these patients, 276 patients (30%) were suffering from a wheat sensitivity, as they were identified as being asymptomatic on an elimination diet, followed by symptoms during the DBPC challenge.

The same group evaluated the same cohort of patients in a prospective study [16], with a median follow up of 99 months in 200 patients. A total of 148 patients (74%) were still following a wheat free diet at follow up, and 127 patients (64%) were on a strict gluten-free diet. A total of 22 of these patients were randomised to the DBPC wheat re-challenge. A total of 20 of the 22 patients (91%) still reacted to wheat. This suggests that even in the long term, a subgroup of patients with IBS is likely to have a persistent sensitivity to wheat.

Confocal endomicroscopy has shown immediate and dramatic mucosal responses to wheat as an antigen [17]. Another study with 80 participants who reported symptoms related to wheat, demonstrated systemic immune activation and compromised intestinal epithelial barrier integrity in these individuals [18]. This may provide a morphological basis for wheat causing symptoms in individuals with IBS. There is currently little data known on the long-term risks of a wheat free diet in patients with IBS, with studies required to assess this.

3. Gluten-Free Diet

Many individuals note symptoms following the ingestion of gluten. This has led to the term of non-coeliac gluten sensitivity (NCGS), being described as early as the 1980s [19]. The mechanism of induction of symptoms in individuals is unclear, but it has been suggested that gluten proteins may be insufficiently degraded by gut proteases, which could lead to an innate immune response [20]. However, further research is required to elucidate the mechanism.

Gluten has been demonstrated to generate symptoms in individuals with IBS [21]. A DBPC trial in 34 patients with a diagnosis of IBS who had improved on a GFD were given either gluten or placebo in the form of two bread slices plus one muffin per day, with a GFD for up to 6-weeks. The study demonstrated worsening symptoms on the visual analogue scale (VAS) for overall symptoms ($p = 0.047$), pain ($p = 0.016$), bloating ($p = 0.016$), stool consistency ($p = 0.024$), and tiredness ($p = 0.001$) with gluten. The same group later performed a study demonstrating no effects of gluten in patients with NCGS and IBS [22], in contrast to their previous study. This double-blind crossover trial in 37 subjects with NCGS and IBS involved placing participants on a 2-week diet of reduced FODMAPs, followed by the random allocation to high-gluten (16 g gluten/day), low-gluten (2 g gluten/day and 14 g whey protein/day), or control (16 g whey protein/day) diets for 1 week, followed by a washout period of at least 2 weeks. The authors concluded that there were no dose-dependent effects of gluten on patients placed on a low FODMAP diet. However, the findings of this study may be explained by the study design and participants. As participants knew they were going to receive either high-gluten, low-gluten, or control, there may have been an anticipatory nocebo response which may have accounted for these findings. Secondly, participants at baseline had a high VAS, which may not be truly representative of this group.

There have also been other double-blind placebo-controlled trials evaluating the effect of gluten on IBS. A study in 148 patients with IBS involved commencing individuals on a GFD, followed by packages containing powdered gluten or gluten-free powder [23]. Symptomatic improvement was different in the gluten-containing group in comparison to the placebo group, with symptoms being controlled in 25.7% in the gluten-containing group, compared to 83.8% in the placebo group. Another DBPC trial in India [24] showed similar findings. A total of 60 patients with IBS completed this study, in which participants underwent a GFD for 4 weeks, followed by a re-challenge of placebo (gluten-free breads) or gluten (whole cereal breads). The study demonstrated that participants in the gluten intervention group scored higher in terms of abdominal pain, bloating, and tiredness ($p < 0.05$).

Randomised controlled trials (RCT) have demonstrated the benefit of a GFD. An RCT [25] in 45 patients with IBS-D, in which participants were allocated to either a 4 week trial of a GFD or gluten-containing diet, demonstrated an increase in bowel movements per day in those on a gluten-containing diet ($p = 0.04$). Interestingly, individuals taking a gluten-containing diet were noted to be associated with a higher small bowel permeability, with small bowel permeability greater in HLA DQ2/8 positive than negative patients ($p = 0.018$). A GFD was noted to have a greater effect of bowel movements per day in HLA DQ2/8 positive than negative patients ($p = 0.019$). It is, therefore, possible that gluten affects the bowel barrier function on IBS, with HLA DQ2/8 being a susceptible factor. A prospective study [26] in 41 patients also demonstrated a clinical response (reduction in IBS-Symptom Severity Score from 286 to 131, $p < 0.001$) in individuals with IBS-D placed on a 6 week GFD. Interestingly, from this study, 21 out of the 29 individuals (72%) in the study planned to continue this diet in the long term, with individuals noted to still be on the diet at a mean of 18 months.

The majority of patients taking a GFD in IBS appear to be adherent to the diet. A study [27] in 35 patients with IBS noted that in those individuals who responded to a GFD, 64% (7 out of 11 patients) were still adherent. This data are similar to patients with coeliac disease, where full adherence has been reported at 65 percent and partial adherence at 31 percent [28]. This may suggest the ease of implementation of a GFD in IBS. Additionally, the GFD is an exclusion diet, which is defined as the exclusion of one or two foods from the diet, in comparison to an elimination diet, which involves the removal of a selection of foods [29]. This may help with ease of implementation of the GFD in comparison to elimination diets, such as the low FODMAP diet. However, there have been no direct comparisons in the literature between the low FODMAP diet and GFD with regards to ease of implementation.

Individuals who maintain a GFD have the option of purchasing specialised gluten-free products. For individuals with coeliac disease consuming a GFD, it has been demonstrated that the majority of individuals purchase gluten-free products [30]. A study in the UK demonstrated that gluten-free foods were 4 times more expensive than non-gluten-free alternatives ($p < 0.0001$), with regular and quality supermarkets stocking a median of 22 items, in comparison to nil in budget supermarkets [31]. This may suggest that cost may limit the purchase of specialised gluten-products, especially for individuals from lower socioeconomic classes. However, it is important to note that alternatively there are naturally occurring foods free of gluten, which do not require the purchase of specialist products to maintain a GFD. Therefore, it is uncertain whether a GFD is more expensive to implement than a standard diet, and there is no literature to date on this in patients with IBS.

Recently a combination of the low FODMAP diet and GFD (LF-GFD) demonstrated benefit in patients with coeliac disease and co-existing functional symptoms [32]. This randomised double-blind study recruited patients with coeliac disease on a GFD for at least one year, with a negative plasma tissue transglutaminase (TTG) value with IBS symptoms fulfilling the Rome III criteria. A total of 50 participants were randomly allocated to an LF-GFD or GFD only. Participants received a structured dietary plan from a nutritionist for a 21-day period. A significant reduction in the VAS for abdominal pain was noted in the LF-GFD group versus the regular GFD group ($p < 0.01$). The general well-being increased in both groups, although a higher improvement was noted in the LF-GFD combination group ($p = 0.03$) [32]. Further studies are required to assess whether this could be an effective therapy for individuals with coeliac disease and IBS, as well as long-term studies being required.

4. Unanswered Questions

Despite the growing evidence for a GFD, a number of questions remain. Little is known about the potential effect of nutritional deficiencies in patients with IBS undergoing a GFD, with data being extrapolated from individuals on a GFD as a result of coeliac disease. A prospective validated 5-day food diary [33], in which 139 patients with coeliac disease were invited to fill, demonstrated similar intake of nutrients and energy to comparator populations, but a higher proportion of carbohydrate intake was obtained from non-milk extrinsic sugars and intakes of non-starch polysaccharides were low. Another study in 47 individuals with coeliac disease on a GFD, estimated three-day food records. Lower than recommended intakes of fibre and calcium in men and women was noted [34]. A GFD has been demonstrated to be poor in alimentary fibre, as well as micronutrient deficiencies being noted [35]. Whilst macronutrient and micronutrient deficiencies have been demonstrated on a GFD, these may not necessarily be a result of the GFD itself. It may be that the changes seen are reflective of overall community dietary habits and pre-existing individual eating habits, rather than the GFD alone [36,37]. For example, a cross-sectional population-based study in the UK [38] demonstrated that over 95% of men and women were not adherent to fibre recommendations. A significant reduction in energy intake has also been demonstrated in individuals following traditional dietary advice [39]. Additionally, it is unknown whether individuals with IBS will have the same macro- and micro-nutrient deficiencies as individuals on a GFD for coeliac disease, and this may differ on the level of gluten restriction implemented by individuals.

As can be seen, macro- and micronutrient deficiencies can occur with any diet, and this highlights the importance of dietetic involvement in the implementation of dietary therapies and is supported by other reviews [40,41]. It has been shown that whilst the vast majority of physicians gave patients advice about the improvement of diet or dietary habit for IBS [42], only a minority would recommend referral to a specialist dietitian [43]. The GFD for IBS should be implemented by a dietitian with a specialist interest in IBS, with physicians referring to dietitians for assessment. This is on the basis that the evidence base for dietary therapies for IBS has been derived from dietitian-led studies rather than physician-led dietary advice [41]. Whilst a GFD diet may be beneficial for some individuals with IBS, it is important that the most appropriate dietary therapy is identified by a dietitian through a detailed history involving the patient. This is important as there is evidence also for the use of a low FODMAP diet and WFD [44], with the NICE [45] and BDA [46] guidelines being recommended as first-line dietary therapies for IBS currently. The implementation of dietary therapies can also lead to the development of obsessive behaviours and orthorexia nervosa [47], highlighting the need for dietetic input to prevent this. Whilst a dietitian-led approach is advised, this is likely to lead to a strain on existing resources though, with the need for novel methods to increase efficiency if able. In IBS patients undergoing a low FODMAP diet ($n = 364$), dietitian-led group education has been demonstrated to be clinically effective [48], and this method could potentially be a cost-effective way to implement a GFD to patients with IBS. It is important to note, however, that there is little data evaluating group therapies versus one-to-one for a GFD in IBS to date.

Studies have explored the effect of the gut microbiota in individuals on a GFD in healthy individuals, as well as in individuals with coeliac disease [49–52]. A study in ten healthy individuals [52] using faecal samples assessed the effect of a GFD over 4 weeks on gut composition and microbiota. Bacterial populations regarded to be beneficial for health such as Bifidobacterium proportions were shown to decrease after the consumption of a GFD, raising potential concerns of a GFD. Additionally, Faecalibacterium prausnitzii proportions were shown to decrease after the consumption of a GFD in this study, with these bacteria known to be an important butyrate-producer in the colon, with butyrate being known as a key modulator of colonic health [53]. It has also been suggested that taxon-specific shifts as a result of the GFD may explain the benefits of a GFD seen in patients with IBS. A study [49] in 21 healthy individuals consuming a GFD over 4 weeks demonstrated stable inter-individual variation in the gut microbiota, with a shift of taxon-specific differences, most marked with Veillonellaceae. Veillonellaceae is considered to be a pro-inflammatory family of bacteria, and a decrease in its abundance on the GFD could be one of the mediators of the benefit observed in patients with IBS on a GFD. The GFD appears to affect species particularly involved in starch and carbohydrate metabolisms [49]. It is unclear whether this would occur in a population of IBS patients and, therefore, studies are required to assess this. Assessment of the effect of a GFD on the gut microbiota in both the short and long term is required in patients with IBS. Currently, the role of the GFD on the gut microbiota is unclear. The changes seen could be due to a GFD, or they could be due to other dietary alterations made whilst on a GFD. In the studies mentioned above [49,52], faecal flora was analysed. The faecal flora is highly organised and spatially organised [54], leading to an uneven distribution in stool samples [55], which suggests that faecal samples are unlikely to be truly representative of the gut microbiota. Sample sizes used in the studies have been small and individuals tend to be unique in terms of their gut microbiota [55]. It is also important to note that these studies focussed on the gut bacteriome, rather than the virome and mycobiome and, therefore, may not be truly representative of the entire microbiota. Further studies are required to explore the effect of the GFD on the microbiome, with the assessment of both short-term and long-term changes.

A recent systematic review and meta-analysis assessing the efficacy of a GFD in IBS [40] concluded that there was insufficient evidence to recommend a GFD to reduce IBS symptoms. Participants in the two studies [21,23] included in the review were intolerant of gluten in addition to IBS, which may suggest that these studies were not fully representative of the entire IBS population. As only two RCTs were deemed suitable for review, this led to a small sample size (n = 111), giving insufficient evidence for the reviewers to recommend this diet. However, as seen in Table 1, there have been a number of studies in addition to these assessing the role of the GFD in IBS [21,23–27,56–58]. It would be difficult to include all these studies in a meta-analysis as it would be difficult to combine the data from all these studies due to the heterogeneity of these studies. Studies assessing the GFD in IBS have used different methods of delivering a GFD, such as using feeding studies in some trials and dietary advice in others. In feeding studies, different doses of gluten have also been used. Different primary outcomes have been assessed, different population groups have been enrolled, as well as different study durations. As can be seen in Table 1, the studies have been performed in a wide variety of geographic locations which may lead to divergent results as different geographic locations may employ the GFD differently, which also may potentially have an impact on their resident gut microbiota [55]. The design of these studies is important as this may result in different outcomes. For example, the studies by Biesiekierski and colleagues [21,22], assessing the role of a GFD in IBS, led to different outcomes as mentioned earlier, which could be attributed to study design.

Studies have focussed on patient symptoms to determine response using validated questionnaires such as the IBS-SSS [59], rather than objective biomarkers. Currently, the evidence does not suggest one biomarker in IBS, but rather a panel of biomarkers [60]. Currently, even using a panel of biomarkers has a poor sensitivity and specificity and, therefore, has limited the use of biomarkers to assess response to dietary therapies in IBS [60,61]. Therefore, further research is required in this area before objective biomarkers can be used to assess response to therapies in IBS. It appears from Table 1 that there are several individual trials demonstrating the benefit of a GFD in IBS, demonstrating the growing evidence base for its use in IBS.

Table 1. The studies evaluating gluten and wheat in Irritable Bowel Syndrome.

Lead Author for Study	Year	Location	Study Design	Study Duration	Total Number of Participants in Study	Intervention	Outcome
Wahnschaffe [56]	2001	Germany	Prospective study	6 months	102 patients with IBS-D	Gluten-free diet	Improvement in stool frequency in HLA DQ2/DQ8 positive subjects
Biesiekierski [21]	2011	Australia	DBPC trial	6 weeks	34 patients with IBS symptomatically controlled on gluten-free diet	Placebo $n = 15$ Gluten $n = 19$	Worsening of overall symptoms on VAS ($p = 0.047$), as well as pain ($p = 0.016$), bloating ($p = 0.016$), stool consistency ($p = 0.024$) and tiredness ($p = 0.001$) following gluten introduction
Carroccio [15]	2012	Italy	Crossover DBPC trial	5 weeks	276 patients with IBS identified as having wheat sensitivity	All participants received wheat or xylose (placebo) capsules	Increase in overall symptoms following the introduction of wheat ($p < 0.0001$)
Vazquez-Roque [25]	2013	USA	Randomised controlled trial	4 weeks	45 patients with IBS-D	Gluten-containing diet $n = 22$ Gluten-free diet $n = 23$	More bowel movements per day on a gluten-containing diet ($p = 0.04$)
Biesiekierski [22]	2013	Australia	Crossover DBPC trial	2-week run in of low FODMAPs then 1 week of high-gluten, low gluten, or placebo for 1 week followed by 2-week washout period	37 patients with IBS and NCGS	All participants received high gluten, low gluten or placebo	No effect of gluten on GI symptoms
Di Sabatino [57]	2015	Italy	Crossover DBPC trial	5 weeks	59 patients with self-reported NCGS	Gluten $n = 30$ Placebo $n = 29$	Intake of gluten significantly increased overall symptoms compared to placebo ($p = 0.034$)
Shahbazkhani [23]	2015	Iran	DBPC trial	6 weeks	72 patients with IBS on GFD	Placebo $n = 37$ Gluten $n = 35$	Statistically significant worsening of symptoms in the gluten-containing group versus placebo ($p < 0.001$)
Aziz [26]	2016	UK	Prospective study	6 weeks	41 patients with IBS-D	All participants received GFD	Reduction in mean IBS Symptom Severity Score from 286 to 131 ($p < 0.001$)
Zanwar [24]	2016	India	DBPC trial	4 weeks	60 patients with IBS who responded to GFD	Placebo $n = 30$ Gluten $n = 30$	Worsening of symptoms following intake of gluten ($p < 0.05$)
Elli [58]	2016	Italy	Crossover DBPC trial	3-week run in of GFD, followed by randomisation to gluten or placebo for 1 week followed by 1 week washout period	140 patients with functional symptoms (77 patients with IBS)	Placebo $n = 48$ Gluten $n = 50$	14% of patients who responded to gluten withdrawal noted to have symptomatic relapse during gluten challenge
Barmeyer [27]	2017	Germany	Prospective study	12 months	35 patients with IBS-D/M	Gluten-free diet	34% of participants ($n = 12$) responded to GFD

DBPC: double-blind placebo-controlled; IBS: irritable bowel syndrome; VAS: visual analogue scale; IBS-D, diarrhoea-predominant IBS; NCGS: non-coeliac gluten sensitivity; GFD: gluten-free diet; FODMAPs: fermentable oligo-, di-, and mono-saccharides, and polyols.

There have been a relatively smaller number of patients recruited to studies assessing the GFD in IBS. This is likely to be an issue for dietary studies in general, with a lack of pharmaceutical support for dietary therapy trials in comparison to pharmaceutical trials, as well as IBS not being a priority area for research [40]. Significant challenges remain, with a lack of guidelines for dietary trials, unlike drug trials which are closely regulated [62]. Issues also remain with regards to blinding, for example, as the GFD is well known to the general public, with up to 5 percent of individuals taking a GFD on their own volition [63,64]. In addition, other challenges remain in designing dietary trials, including difficulties in manipulating the diet and the adherence and modification of dietary habits. It is also difficult to practically implement the findings from dietary trials to the real world [65].

It is unclear which component of wheat leads to symptom generation. Several components have been suggested as the causal agent, including gluten, alpha-amylase trypsin inhibitors (ATIs), wheat germ agglutinins (WGAs), and fructans, which are part of the low FODMAP diet [66]. Studies have been performed to try to elucidate the pathophysiological mechanisms of these components in symptom generation. Gluten has been demonstrated to alter bowel barrier functions in patients with IBS. The expression of tight junction proteins (ZO-1, occludin, and claudin-1) have been demonstrated to be significantly lower in the colonic mucosa of individuals on a gluten-containing diet, especially in individuals who are HLA DQ2/ 8 positive [25]. Tight junction proteins, claudin-2, 8 and 15, as well as myosin light chain kinase (MLCK)-myosin II regulatory light chain (MLC) pathway have been demonstrated to be important in intestinal physiology and barrier function, regulating paracellular permeability. A study [67] evaluating biopsies from 27 patients with IBS-D demonstrated alterations in MLC phosphorylation and claudin-15 and claudin-2 expression with gluten with intestinal permeability changes. This also could potentially explain permeability responses to gluten challenge in patients with IBS [67]. ATIs have been demonstrated to be strong induces of the innate immune responses, in vitro and in vivo, via the activation of the toll-like receptor 4, with the release of pro-inflammatory cytokines leading to intestinal inflammation [68]. WGA is the best-studied cereal grain lectin. When delivered in vitro, WGAs have been demonstrated to stimulate monocytes and macrophages, which have the ability to initiate and maintain inflammatory responses [69]. WGA has been demonstrated to affect enterocyte permeability in vitro. However, it is important to note that human data demonstrating WGA on inflammatory markers are lacking [69]. FODMAPs are short-chain carbohydrates which are rapidly fermentable and poorly absorbed, increasing the small bowel water content, passing unaltered into the colon, where they are rapidly fermented, generating gas and distention [70]. Similar physiological responses to FODMAPs has been demonstrated in both healthy individuals and patients with IBS, indicating that colonic hypersensitivity to distention in patients with IBS is likely to be the pathophysiological mechanism [71]. FODMAPs are considered to be beneficial to epithelial cell integrity and health [72].

A recent study has suggested that fructans rather than gluten are responsible for symptoms seen in patients with IBS. The study [73] in 59 individuals who had already self-instituted a GFD involved a double-blind crossover challenge, in which individuals were randomly assigned to diets containing fructans, placebo, and gluten for 7 days, followed by a minimum 7 day washout period. The overall gastrointestinal symptom rating scale (GSRS) score for participants consuming fructans was significantly higher than those consuming gluten ($p = 0.049$).

It is likely that there is a significant overlap between dietary therapies used in IBS including the GFD, WFD, and low FODMAP diet. They are likely to be 'dietary cousins', with each diet being needed to be tailored to the individual patient after a detailed assessment by a dietitian. There appears to be a spectrum of gluten-related disorders, as seen in Figure 1.

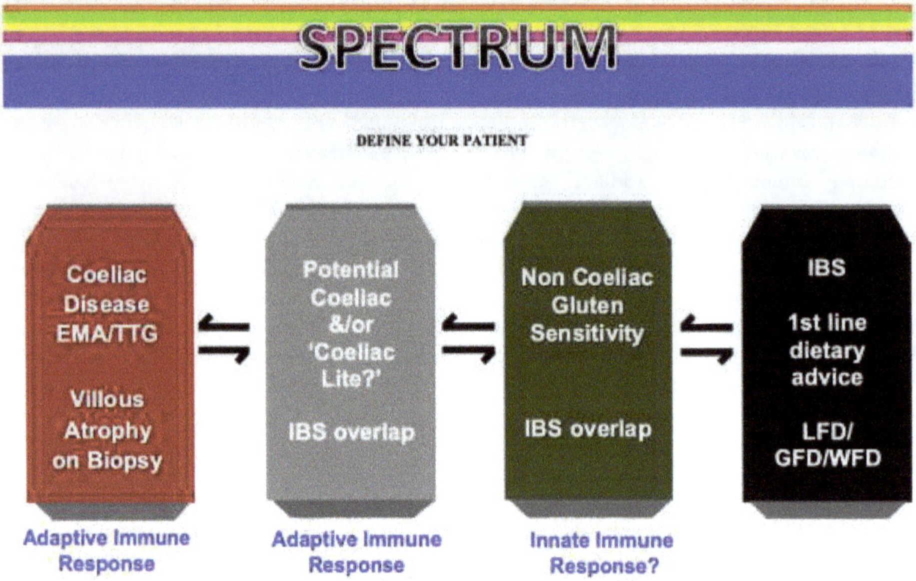

Figure 1. The spectrum of Gluten Related Disorders. EMA: endomysial antibodies; TTG: tissue transglutaminase; IBS: irritable bowel syndrome; LFD: low fermentable oligo-, di-, and mono-saccharides, and polyols diet; GFD: gluten-free diet; WFD; wheat-free diet.

It is important to note that there are several other dietary therapies which are being explored in patients with IBS. As the evidence is growing for gluten in generating symptoms in IBS, it is possible to hypothesise that other foods may also contain harmful molecules for patients with IBS. Some dietary therapies have focussed on diets with a primary focus on bioactive food molecules, such as the low capsaicin diet, low amine/histamine diet, and low food chemical diet [47]. Additionally, there are diets in addition to the low FODMAP diet focussing on the carbohydrates like the specific carbohydrate diet and paleo diet. Likewise, there are diets in addition to the GFD focussing on proteins, such as reduced resistant protein diet. However, to date, there is little evidence for the use of these diets in patients with IBS [47].

5. Conclusions

There appears to be emerging evidence for the use of a GFD in IBS. A number of unanswered questions remain, including the effect on the gut microbiota in both the short and long term, as well as the effect on short- and long-term nutritional adequacy. This dietary therapy should be implemented by a dietitian with a specialist interest in IBS, which could be done through group clinics, although research is required to validate this. There is likely to be an overlap with other dietary therapies such as the low FODMAP diet, with which component of wheat leading to the induction of symptoms still being unclear. Further research is required on the use of a GFD in IBS, but dietary studies are likely to be challenging, with blinding and funding being some of the issues.

Author Contributions: A.R. and D.S.S. wrote the initial manuscript and D.S.S. approved the final version.

Funding: This research received no external funding.

Conflicts of Interest: The authors declare no conflict of interest.

References

1. Schmulson, M.J.; Drossman, D.A. What Is New in Rome IV. *J. Neurogastroenterol. Motil.* **2017**, *23*, 151–163. [CrossRef] [PubMed]
2. Lovell, R.M.; Ford, A.C. Global prevalence of and risk factors for irritable bowel syndrome: A meta-analysis. *Clin. Gastroenterol. Hepatol.* **2012**, *10*, 712–721. [CrossRef] [PubMed]
3. Camilleri, M.; Lasch, K.; Zhou, W. Irritable bowel syndrome: Methods, mechanisms, and pathophysiology. The confluence of increased permeability, inflammation, and pain in irritable bowel syndrome. *AJP: Gastrointest. Liver Physiol.* **2012**, *303*, G775–G785. [CrossRef] [PubMed]
4. Portincasa, P.; Bonfrate, L.; De Bari, O.; Lembo, A.; Ballou, S. Irritable bowel syndrome and diet. *Gastroenterol. Rep. (Oxf)* **2017**, *5*, 11–19. [CrossRef] [PubMed]
5. Akehurst, R.L.; Brazier, J.E.; Mathers, N.; O'Keefe, C.; Kaltenthaler, E.; Morgan, A.; Platts, M.; Walters, S.J. Health-related quality of life and cost impact of irritable bowel syndrome in a uk primary care setting. *Pharm. Economics.* **2002**, *20*, 455–462. [CrossRef] [PubMed]
6. Whitehead, W.E.; Palsson, O.; Jones, K.R. Systematic review of the comorbidity of irritable bowel syndrome with other disorders: What are the causes and implications? *Gastroenterology* **2002**, *122*, 1140–1156. [CrossRef] [PubMed]
7. Lahner, E.; Bellentani, S.; Bastiani, R.D.; Tosetti, C.; Cicala, M.; Esposito, G.; Arullani, P.; Annibale, B. A survey of pharmacological and nonpharmacological treatment of functional gastrointestinal disorders. *States Eur. Gastroenterol. J.* **2013**, *1*, 385–393. [CrossRef] [PubMed]
8. Simrén, M.; Månsson, A.; Langkilde, A.M.; Svedlund, J.; Abrahamsson, H.; Bengtsson, U.; Björnsson, E.S. Food-related gastrointestinal symptoms in the irritable bowel syndrome. *Digestion* **2001**, *63*, 108–115. [CrossRef] [PubMed]
9. Monsbakken, K.W.; Vandvik, P.O.; Farup, P.G. Perceived food intolerance in subjects with irritable bowel syndrome—etiology, prevalence and consequences. *Eur. J. Clin. Nutr.* **2005**, *60*, 667–672. [CrossRef] [PubMed]
10. Böhn, L.; Störsrud, S.; Simrén, M. Nutrient intake in patients with irritable bowel syndrome compared with the general population. *Neurogastroenterol. Motil.* **2013**, *25*, 23–30. [CrossRef] [PubMed]
11. Aziz, I.; Karajeh, M.A.; Zilkha, J.; Tubman, E.; Fowles, C.; Sanders, D.S. Change in awareness of gluten-related disorders among chefs and the general public in the uk. *Eur. J. Gastroenterol. Hepatol.* **2014**, *26*, 1228–1233. [CrossRef] [PubMed]
12. Niland, B.; Cash, B.D. Health Benefits and Adverse Effects of a Gluten-Free Diet in Non-Celiac Disease Patients. *Gastroenterol. Hepatol.* **2018**, *14*, 82–91.
13. Lebwohl, B.; Sanders, D.S.; Green, P.H.R. Coeliac disease. *Lancet* **2018**, *391*, 70–81. [CrossRef]
14. Golley, S.; Corsini, N.; Topping, D.; Morell, M.; Mohr, P. Motivations for avoiding wheat consumption in australia: Results from a population survey. *Public Heal. Nutr.* **2014**, *18*, 490–499. [CrossRef] [PubMed]
15. Carroccio, A.; Mansueto, P.; Iacono, G.; Soresi, M.; D'Alcamo, A.; Cavataio, F.; Brusca, I.; Florena, A.M.; Ambrosiano, G.; Seidita, A.; et al. Non-celiac wheat sensitivity diagnosed by double-blind placebo-controlled challenge: Exploring a new clinical entity. *Am. J. Gastroenterol* **2012**, *107*, 1898–1906. [CrossRef] [PubMed]
16. Carroccio, A.; D'Alcamo, A.; Iacono, G.; Soresi, M.; Iacobucci, R.; Arini, A.; Geraci, G.; Cavataio, F.; La Biasca, F.; Florena, A.M.; et al. Persistence of Nonceliac Wheat Sensitivity, Based on Long-term Follow-up. *Gastroenterology* **2017**, *153*, 56–58. [CrossRef] [PubMed]
17. Fritscher-Ravens, A.; Schuppan, D.; Ellrichmann, M.; Schoch, S.; Röcken, C.; Brasch, J.; Bethge, J.; Böttner, M.; Klose, J.; Milla, P.J. Confocal endomicroscopy shows food-associated changes in the intestinal mucosa of patients with irritable bowel syndrome. *Gastroenterology* **2014**, *147*, 1012–1020. [CrossRef] [PubMed]
18. Uhde, M.; Ajamian, M.; Caio, G.; De Giorgio, R.; Indart, A.; Green, P.H.; Verna, E.C.; Volta, U.; Alaedini, A. Intestinal cell damage and systemic immune activation in individuals reporting sensitivity to wheat in the absence of coeliac disease. *Gut* **2016**, *65*, 1930–1937. [CrossRef] [PubMed]
19. Cooper, B.T.; Holmes, G.K.; Ferguson, R.; Thompson, R.A.; Allan, R.N.; Cooke, W.T. Gluten-sensitive diarrhea without evidence of celiac disease. *Gastroenterology* **1980**, *79*, 801–806. [PubMed]
20. Volta, U.; Pinto-Sanchez, M.I.; Boschetti, E.; Caio, G.; De Giorgio, R.; Verdu, E.F. Dietary Triggers in Irritable Bowel Syndrome: Is There a Role for Gluten? *J. Neurogastroenterol. Motil.* **2016**, *22*, 547–557. [CrossRef] [PubMed]

21. Biesiekierski, J.R.; Newnham, E.D.; Irving, P.M.; Barrett, J.S.; Haines, M.; Doecke, J.D.; Shepherd, S.J.; Muir, J.G.; Gibson, P.R. Gluten causes gastrointestinal symptoms in subjects without celiac disease: A double-blind randomized placebo-controlled trial. *Am. J. Gastroenterol.* **2011**, *106*, 508–514. [CrossRef] [PubMed]
22. Biesiekierski, J.R.; Peters, S.L.; Newnham, E.D.; Rosella, O.; Muir, J.G.; Gibson, P.R. No effects of gluten in patients with self-reported non-celiac gluten sensitivity after dietary reduction of fermentable, poorly absorbed, short-chain carbohydrates. *Gastroenterology* **2013**, *145*, 320–328. [CrossRef] [PubMed]
23. Shahbazkhani, B.; Sadeghi, A.; Malekzadeh, R.; Khatavi, F.; Etemadi, M.; Kalantri, E.; Rostami-Nejad, M.; Rostami, K. Non-celiac gluten sensitivity has narrowed the spectrum of irritable bowel syndrome: A double-blind randomized placebo-controlled trial. *Nutrients* **2015**, *7*, 4542–4554. [CrossRef] [PubMed]
24. Zanwar, V.G.; Pawar, S.V.; Gambhire, P.A.; Jain, S.S.; Surude, R.G.; Shah, V.B.; Contractor, Q.Q.; Rathi, P.M. Symptomatic improvement with gluten restriction in irritable bowel syndrome: A prospective, randomized, double blinded placebo controlled trial. *Intest. Res.* **2016**, *14*, 343–350. [CrossRef] [PubMed]
25. Vazquez–Roque, M.I.; Camilleri, M.; Smyrk, T.; Murray, J.A.; Marietta, E.; O'Neill, J.; Carlson, P.; Lamsam, J.; Janzow, D.; Eckert, D.; et al. A controlled trial of gluten-free diet in patients with irritable bowel syndrome-diarrhea: Effects on bowel frequency and intestinal function. *Gastroenterology* **2013**, *144*, 903–911. [CrossRef] [PubMed]
26. Aziz, I.; Trott, N.; Briggs, R.; North, J.R.; Hadjivassiliou, M.; Sanders, D.S. Efficacy of a gluten-free diet in subjects with irritable bowel syndrome-diarrhea unaware of their hla-dq2/8 genotype. *Clin. Gastroenterol. Hepatol.* **2016**, *14*, 696–703. [CrossRef] [PubMed]
27. Barmeyer, C.; Schumann, M.; Meyer, T.; Zielinski, C.; Zuberbier, T.; Siegmund, B.; Schulzke, J.-D.; Daum, S.; Ullrich, R. Long-term response to gluten-free diet as evidence for non-celiac wheat sensitivity in one third of patients with diarrhea-dominant and mixed-type irritable bowel syndrome. *Int. J. Color. Dis.* **2016**, *32*, 29–39. [CrossRef] [PubMed]
28. Barratt, S.M.; Leeds, J.S.; Sanders, D.S. Quality of life in Coeliac Disease is determined by perceived degree of difficulty adhering to a gluten-free diet, not the level of dietary adherence ultimately achieved. *J. Gastrointest. Liver Dis.* **2011**, *20*, 241–245.
29. McKenzie, Y.A.; Alder, A.; Anderson, W.; Wills, A.; Goddard, L.; Gulia, P.; Jankovich, E.; Mutch, P.; Reeves, L.B.; Singer, A.; et al. British dietetic association evidence-based guidelines for the dietary management of irritable bowel syndrome in adults. *J. Hum. Nutr. Diet.* **2012**, *25*, 260–274. [CrossRef] [PubMed]
30. Kinsey, L.; Burden, S.T.; Bannerman, E. A dietary survey to determine if patients with coeliac disease are meeting current healthy eating guidelines and how their diet compares to that of the british general population. *Eur. J. Clin. Nutr.* **2011**, *65*, 283. [CrossRef]
31. Burden, M.; Mooney, P.D.; Blanshard, R.J.; White, W.L.; Cambray-Deakin, D.R.; Sanders, D.S. Cost and availability of gluten-free food in the UK: In store and online. *Postgrad Med. J.* **2015**, *91*, 622–626. [CrossRef] [PubMed]
32. Roncoroni, L.; Bascuñán, K.A.; Doneda, L.; Scricciolo, A.; Lombardo, V.; Branchi, F.; Ferretti, F.; Dell'Osso, B.; Montanari, V.; Bardella, M.T.; et al. A Low FODMAP Gluten-Free Diet Improves Functional Gastrointestinal Disorders and Overall Mental Health of Celiac Disease Patients: A Randomized Controlled Trial. *Nutrients* **2018**, *10*, 1023. [CrossRef] [PubMed]
33. Wild, D.; Robins, G.G.; Burley, V.J.; Howdle, P.D. Evidence of high sugar intake, and low fibre and mineral intake, in the gluten-free diet. *Aliment. Pharmacol. Ther.* **2010**, *32*, 573–581. [CrossRef] [PubMed]
34. Thompson, T.; Dennis, M.; Higgins, L.A.; Lee, A.R.; Sharrett, M.K. Gluten-free diet survey: Are Americans with coeliac disease consuming recommended amounts of fibre, iron, calcium and grain foods? *J. Hum. Nutr. Diet.* **2005**, *18*, 163–169. [CrossRef] [PubMed]
35. Vici, G.; Belli, L.; Biondi, M.; Polzonetti, V. Gluten free diet and nutrient deficiencies: A review. *Clin. Nutr.* **2016**, *35*, 1236–1241. [CrossRef] [PubMed]
36. Shepherd, S.J.; Gibson, P.R. Nutritional inadequacies of the gluten-free diet in both recently-diagnosed and long-term patients with coeliac disease. *J. Hum. Nutr. Diet.* **2012**, *26*, 349–358. [CrossRef] [PubMed]
37. El Khoury, D.; Balfour-Ducharme, S.; Joye, I.J. A Review on the Gluten-Free Diet: Technological and Nutritional Challenges. *Nutrients* **2018**, *10*, 1410. [CrossRef] [PubMed]

38. Bennett, E.; Peters, S.A.E.; Woodward, M. Sex differences in macronutrient intake and adherence to dietary recommendations: Findings from the UK Biobank. *BMJ Open* **2018**, *8*, e020017. [CrossRef] [PubMed]
39. Böhn, L.; Störsrud, S.; Liljebo, T.; Collin, L.; Lindfors, P.; Törnblom, H.; Simrén, M. Diet low in fodmaps reduces symptoms of irritable bowel syndrome as well as traditional dietary advice: A randomized controlled trial. *Gastroenterology* **2015**, *149*, 1399–1407. [CrossRef] [PubMed]
40. Lonshteyn, M.; Chandar, A.; Falck-Ytter, Y. Su2061 large effects of a low fodmaps diet in patients with irritable bowel syndrome: A systematic review and meta-analysis. *Gastroenterology* **2014**, *146*, S535–S536. [CrossRef]
41. O'Keeffe, M.; Lomer, M.C. Who should deliver the low FODMAP diet and what educational methods are optimal: A review. *J. Gastroenterol Hepatol* **2017**, *32* (Suppl. 1), 23–26. [CrossRef] [PubMed]
42. Miura, S.; Sugano, K.; Kinoshita, Y.; Fock, K.M.; Goh, K.L.; Gibson, P. Diagnosis and treatment of functional gastrointestinal disorders in the asia-pacific region: A survey of current practices. *J. Gastroenterol. Hepatol.* **2011**, *26*, 2–11. [CrossRef] [PubMed]
43. Lenhart, A.; Ferch, C.; Shaw, M.; Chey, W.D. Use of Dietary Management in Irritable Bowel Syndrome: Results of a Survey of Over 1500 United States Gastroenterologists. *J. Neurogastroenterol. Motil.* **2018**, *24*, 437–451. [CrossRef] [PubMed]
44. Rej, A.; Avery, A.; Ford, A.C.; Holdoway, A.; Kurien, M.; McKenzie, Y.; Thompson, J.; Trott, N.; Whelan, K.; Williams, M.; Sanders, D.S. Clinical application of dietary therapies in irritable bowel syndrome. *J. Gastrointest. Liver Dis.* **2018**, *27*, 307–316. [CrossRef]
45. National Institute for Health and Clinical Excellence. Irritable Bowel Syndrome in Adults: Diagnosis and Management. Clinical Guideline [CG61]. 2008. Available online: https://www.nice.org.uk/guidance/cg61 (accessed on 8 October 2018).
46. McKenzie, Y.A.; Bowyer, R.K.; Leach, H.; Gulia, P.; Horobin, J.; O'Sullivan, N.A.; Pettitt, C.; Reeves, L.B.; Seamark, L.; Williams, M.; et al. British dietetic association systematic review and evidence-based practice guidelines for the dietary management of irritable bowel syndrome in adults (2016 update). *J. Hum. Nutr. Diet.* **2016**, *29*, 549–575. [CrossRef] [PubMed]
47. Tuck, C.J.; Vanner, S.J. Dietary therapies for functional bowel symptoms: Recent advances, challenges, and future directions. *Neurogastroenterol. Motil.* **2018**, *30*. [CrossRef] [PubMed]
48. Whigham, L.; Joyce, T.; Harper, G.; Irving, P.M.; Staudacher, H.M.; Whelan, K.; Lomer, M.C.E. Clinical effectiveness and economic costs of group versus one-to-one education for short-chain fermentable carbohydrate restriction (low fodmap diet) in the management of irritable bowel syndrome. *J. Hum. Nutr. Diet.* **2015**, *28*, 687–696. [CrossRef] [PubMed]
49. Bonder, M.J.; Tigchelaar, E.F.; Cai, X.; Trynka, G.; Cenit, M.C.; Hrdlickova, B.; Zhong, H.; Vatanen, T.; Gevers, D.; Wijmenga, C.; et al. The influence of a short-term gluten-free diet on the human gut microbiome. *Genome Med.* **2016**, *8*. [CrossRef] [PubMed]
50. De Palma, G.; Nadal, I.; Medina, M.; Donat, E.; Ribes-Koninckx, C.; Calabuig, M.; Sanz, Y. Intestinal dysbiosis and reduced immunoglobulin-coated bacteria associated with coeliac disease in children. *BMC Microbiol.* **2010**, *10*, 63. [CrossRef] [PubMed]
51. Schippa, S.; Iebba, V.; Barbato, M.; Di Nardo, G.; Totino, V.; Checchi, M.P.; Longhi, C.; Maiella, G.; Cucchiara, S.; Conte, M.P. A distinctive 'microbial signature' in celiac pediatric patients. *BMC Microbiol* **2010**, *10*, 175. [CrossRef] [PubMed]
52. De Palma, G.; Nadal, I.; Collado, M.C.; Sanz, Y. Effects of a gluten-free diet on gut microbiota and immune function in healthy adult human subjects. *Br. J. Nutr.* **2009**, *102*, 1154–1160. [CrossRef] [PubMed]
53. Ferreira-Halder, C.V.; Faria, A.V.S.; Andrade, S.S. Action and function of Faecalibacterium prausnitzii in health and disease. *Best Pract. Res. Clin. Gastroenterol.* **2017**, *31*, 643–648. [CrossRef] [PubMed]
54. Swidsinski, A.; Loening-Baucke, V.; Vaneechoutte, M.; Doerffel, Y. Active crohn's disease and ulcerative colitis can be specifically diagnosed and monitored based on the biostructure of the fecal flora. *Inflamm. Bowel. Dis.* **2008**, *14*, 147–161. [CrossRef] [PubMed]
55. Garcia-Mazcorro, J.F.; Noratto, G.; Remes-Troche, J.M. The Effect of Gluten-Free Diet on Health and the Gut Microbiota Cannot Be Extrapolated from One Population to Others. *Nutrients* **2018**, *10*, 1421. [CrossRef] [PubMed]
56. Wahnschaffe, U.; Ullrich, R.; Riecken, E.O.; Schulzke, J.D. Celiac disease-like abnormalities in a subgroup of patients with irritable bowel syndrome. *Gastroenterology* **2001**, *121*, 1329–1338. [CrossRef] [PubMed]

57. Di Sabatino, A.; Volta, U.; Salvatore, C.; Biancheri, P.; Caio, G.; De Giorgio, R.; Di Stefano, M.; Corazza, G.R. Small amounts of gluten in subjects with suspected nonceliac gluten sensitivity: A randomized, double-blind, placebo-controlled, cross-over trial. *Clin. Gastroenterol. Hepatol.* **2015**, *13*, 1604–1612. [CrossRef] [PubMed]
58. Elli, L.; Tomba, C.; Branchi, F.; Roncoroni, L.; Lombardo, V.; Bardella, M.T.; Ferretti, F.; Conte, D.; Valiante, F.; Fini, L.; et al. Evidence for the Presence of Non-Celiac Gluten Sensitivity in Patients with Functional Gastrointestinal Symptoms: Results from a Multicenter Randomized Double-Blind Placebo-Controlled Gluten Challenge. *Nutrients* **2016**, *8*, 84. [CrossRef] [PubMed]
59. Francis, C.Y.; Morris, J.; Whorwell, P.J. The irritable bowel severity scoring system: A simple method of monitoring irritable bowel syndrome and its progress. *Aliment. Pharmacol. Ther.* **1997**, *11*, 395–402. [CrossRef] [PubMed]
60. Chira, A.; Dumitrascu, D.L. Serum biomarkers for irritable bowel syndrome. *Clujul. Med.* **2015**, *88*, 258–264. [CrossRef] [PubMed]
61. Kim, J.H.; Lin, E.; Pimentel, M. Biomarkers of Irritable Bowel Syndrome. *J. Neurogastroenterol. Motil.* **2017**, *23*, 20–26. [CrossRef] [PubMed]
62. Staudacher, H.M.; Irving, P.M.; Lomer, M.C.E.; Whelan, K. The challenges of control groups, placebos and blinding in clinical trials of dietary interventions. *Proc. Nutr. Soc.* **2017**, *76*, 628. [CrossRef] [PubMed]
63. Aziz, I.; Lewis, N.R.; Hadjivassiliou, M.; Winfield, S.N.; Rugg, N.; Kelsall, A.; Newrick, L.; Sanders, D.S. A uk study assessing the population prevalence of self-reported gluten sensitivity and referral characteristics to secondary care. *Eur. J. Gastroenterol. Hepatol.* **2014**, *26*, 33–39. [CrossRef] [PubMed]
64. Tanpowpong, P.; Ingham, T.R.; Lampshire, P.K.; Kirchberg, F.F.; Epton, M.J.; Crane, J.; Carmargo, C.A. Coeliac disease and gluten avoidance in New Zealand children. *Arch. Dis. Child.* **2012**, *97*, 12–16. [CrossRef] [PubMed]
65. Yao, C.K.; Gibson, P.R.; Shepherd, S.J. Design of clinical trials evaluating dietary interventions in patients with functional gastrointestinal disorders. *Am. J. Gastroenterol.* **2013**, *108*, 748–758. [CrossRef] [PubMed]
66. Aziz, I.; Hadjivassiliou, M.; Sanders, D.S. The spectrum of noncoeliac gluten sensitivity. *Nat. Rev. Gastroenterol. Hepatol.* **2015**, *12*, 516–526. [CrossRef] [PubMed]
67. Wu, R.L.; Vazquez-Roque, M.I.; Carlson, P.; Burton, D.; Grover, M.; Camilleri, M.; Turner, J.R. Gluten-induced symptoms in diarrhea-predominant irritable bowel syndrome are associated with increased myosin light chain kinase activity and claudin-15 expression. *Lab. Invest.* **2017**, *97*, 14–23. [CrossRef] [PubMed]
68. Junker, Y.; Zeissig, S.; Kim, S.-J.; Barisani, D.; Wieser, H.; Leffler, D.A.; Zevallos, V.; Libermann, T.A.; Dillon, S.; Freitag, T.L.; et al. Wheat amylase trypsin inhibitors drive intestinal inflammation via activation of toll-like receptor 4. *J. Exp. Med.* **2012**, *209*, 2395–2408. [CrossRef] [PubMed]
69. De Punder, K.; Pruimboom, L. The dietary intake of wheat and other cereal grains and their role in inflammation. *Nutrients* **2013**, *5*, 771–787. [CrossRef] [PubMed]
70. Spiller, R. How do FODMAPs work? *J. Gastroenterol. Hepatol.* **2017**, *32* (Suppl. 1), 36–39. [CrossRef] [PubMed]
71. Major, G.; Pritchard, S.; Murray, K.; Alappadan, J.P.; Hoad, C.L.; Marciani, L.; Gowland, P.; Spiller, R. Colon, Hypersensitivity to Distension, Rather Than Excessive Gas Production, Produces Carbohydrate-Related Symptoms in Individuals With Irritable Bowel Syndrome. *Gastroenterology* **2017**, *152*, 124–133. [CrossRef] [PubMed]
72. Catassi, C.; Alaedini, A.; Bojarski, C.; Bonaz, B.; Bouma, G.; Carroccio, A.; Castillejo, G.; De Magistris, L.; Dieterich, W.; Di Liberto, D.; et al. The Overlapping Area of Non-Celiac Gluten Sensitivity (NCGS) and Wheat-Sensitive Irritable Bowel Syndrome (IBS). *Nutrients* **2017**, *9*, 1268. [CrossRef] [PubMed]
73. Skodje, G.I.; Sarna, V.K.; Minelle, I.H.; Rolfsen, K.L.; Muir, J.G.; Gibson, P.R.; Veierod, M.B.; Henricksen, C.; Lendin, K.E.A. Fructan, Rather Than Gluten, Induces Symptoms in Patients With Self-reported Non-celiac Gluten Sensitivity. *Gastroenterology* **2017**, *154*, 529–539. [CrossRef] [PubMed]

nutrients

Review

Possible Prevention of Diabetes with a Gluten-Free Diet

Martin Haupt-Jorgensen *, Laurits J. Holm, Knud Josefsen † and Karsten Buschard †

The Bartholin Institute, Ole Maaløes Vej 5, Rigshospitalet, 2200 Copenhagen, Denmark; laurits.juulskov.holm@regionh.dk (L.J.H.); knud@eln.dk (K.J.); buschard@dadlnet.dk (K.B.)

* Correspondence: Martin.Haupt-Joergensen@regionh.dk; Tel.: +45-3545-5717

† These authors shared senior authorship.

Received: 15 October 2018; Accepted: 7 November 2018; Published: 13 November 2018

Abstract: Gluten seems a potentially important determinant in type 1 diabetes (T1D) and type 2 diabetes (T2D). Intake of gluten, a major component of wheat, rye, and barley, affects the microbiota and increases the intestinal permeability. Moreover, studies have demonstrated that gluten peptides, after crossing the intestinal barrier, lead to a more inflammatory milieu. Gluten peptides enter the pancreas where they affect the morphology and might induce beta-cell stress by enhancing glucose- and palmitate-stimulated insulin secretion. Interestingly, animal studies and a human study have demonstrated that a gluten-free (GF) diet during pregnancy reduces the risk of T1D. Evidence regarding the role of a GF diet in T2D is less clear. Some studies have linked intake of a GF diet to reduced obesity and T2D and suggested a role in reducing leptin- and insulin-resistance and increasing beta-cell volume. The current knowledge indicates that gluten, among many environmental factors, may be an aetiopathogenic factors for development of T1D and T2D. However, human intervention trials are needed to confirm this and the proposed mechanisms.

Keywords: beta cell; beta-cell stress; celiac disease; gluten-free diet; high-fat diet-induced obesity; intestinal permeability; islet of Langerhans; NOD mouse; type 1 diabetes; type 2 diabetes

1. Gluten

During the recent years, there has been a tremendous increase in the number of GF products available with the promise of diverse health benefits. The incidence of celiac disease (CD) was estimated to be 33.6 per 10,000 person-years in a recent retrospective cohort study from the United Kingdom [1]. Non-celiac gluten sensitivity is thought to be more common, although the precise number is unknown [2–5]. Consumption of gluten is believed to affect many aspects of human health and is hypothesised to contribute to the diabetes pandemic, in which the number of people suffering from diabetes have quadrupled since 1980 to an estimated 422 million in 2014 [6]. Gluten entered our diet about 10,000 years ago in Mesopotamia when our ancestors began eating cereals. Today cereals are an essential food source around the world and more than 50% of the worlds daily caloric intake is derived from consumption of cereals [7].

Wheat, rye, and barley contain high amounts of gluten in their endosperm storage tissue. Chemically, gluten is classified as a prolamin, containing monomeric gliadins and polymeric glutenins. Glutenins can be subdivided into low and high molecular weight proteins while gliadins are divided into α-, γ-, and ω-gliadins [8]. The major amino acid constituents of gluten are proline, glutamine, and hydrophobic amino acids [9], which make gluten resistant to complete degradation by gastric, pancreatic, and brush-border enzymes [10,11]. α-gliadin contains some of the most toxic peptides in gluten, as evidenced by in vitro studies, and their effect has been mapped to specific domains in the structure [12]. The effect of the peptides are diverse and include gut-permeating [13], cytokine-releasing [14], and cytotoxic [15] effects. The 33-mer from α-gliadin is the most immunogenic gluten peptide discovered so far, as it contains three overlapping T cell epitopes [16], and processing by APCs is not required before T cell presentation [17]. The 33-mer is resistant to degradation by intestinal peptidases [18,19] and was recently identified in all of the modern and old cultivars of wheat and spelt analysed [20].

2. Gluten and T1D

T1D is initiated when autoreactive T cells destroy the insulin-producing beta cells in the pancreas leading to hypoinsulinaemia, and hyperglycaemia; however, the aetiology and pathogenesis are still not fully understood. T1D is classified as a multifactorial disease in which the genetic background, as well as environmental factors, are important determinants. Approximately 50% of the genetic risk of the disease is explained by the HLA class II region [21], and the haplotypes HLA-DR3-DQ2 and HLA-DR4-DQ8 are the most important individual genetic risk factors known [22].

In the period from 1990–1999, the average annual increase in the incidence of T1D was 2.8% in children aged ≤14 years [23]. Another epidemiological study predicted that the incidence would double between 2005 and 2020 in European children below five years of age [24].

A key question is why the incidence of T1D is increasing now when gluten was introduced 10,000 years ago. Among many possible reasons, such as an increased exposure to other diabetogenic environmental factors, a recent study in non-obese diabetic (NOD) mice, an animal model of autoimmune diabetes, found that modern wheat sources are more diabetogenic that old wheat sources [25].

2.1. *The Role of Environmental Factors*

Environmental factors are important in the pathogenesis of T1D. First, the incidence of T1D has been rising globally at a pace that cannot be explained by genetic drift [23,24]. Second, increasing incidence has been observed in population groups that have migrated from regions with low incidence of T1D to regions with high incidence [26]. Third, a six-fold gradient in the incidence of T1D is observed between Russian Karelia and Finland, although the frequency of the high-risk HLA-DQ genotypes is equal in the two populations [27], and similar gradients between neighbouring countries are also known [23]. Fourth, monozygotic twins are most often discordant for T1D [28,29]. Fifth, T1D develops in less than 10% of subjects with HLA-conferred risk genotypes [30], although all risk genotypes are most likely not identified yet.

Many environmental factors have been associated with increased susceptibility to T1D, including physiological stress, vaccines, toxins, cow milk [31], and dietary gluten. Evidence for a viral aetiology has grown during the recent years [32–35] exemplified by the Diabetes virus detection (DiViD) study that demonstrated low-grade enterovirus infection in islets from the majority of the newly diagnosed T1D patients investigated but not in any of the non-diabetic controls [36]. In this regard, the hygiene hypothesis is central, stating that children who are exposed to microorganisms will develop strong immunity against these, which will dampen the harmful effects from them, but also protect the child from T1D [37].

Thus, T1D is a multifactorial disease where many environmental factors are likely to contribute to the pathogenesis, including gluten.

2.2. *GF Diet, Early Evidence and Timing*

Early studies in NOD mice [38] and biobreeding (BB) rats [39], which are animal models for autoimmune diabetes, suggested that cereals might have a role in the aetiopathogenesis of T1D. Later, a study in NOD mice demonstrated that a lifelong GF diet compared to a gluten-containing standard (STD) diet reduced the incidence of autoimmune diabetes from 64% to 15%, although insulitis score was not significantly reduced [40], and subsequent studies in NOD mice demonstrated similar results [41,42]. In a more recent study in NOD mice, we showed that the incidence of autoimmune diabetes could be reduced even further, to 8%, together with reduced insulitis in offspring, by keeping the mothers on a GF diet exclusively during pregnancy [43]. Similar, but smaller effects on incidence and insulitis in NOD mouse offspring were demonstrated by keeping the mice GF in utero and in early postnatal life [44]. The GF diets used it these studies had the gluten protein replaced with other proteins (meat, casein, or egg white) while keeping an equal content relative to the STD diets of protein, fat, and components that may influence the risk of diabetes such as milk and soybean [40,43]. Although the major difference between the GF and STD diets was gluten, small differences were present between other dietary components. Human evidence for the existence of an early time-window for the introduction of gluten and tolerance induction includes the BABYDIAB and Diabetes and Autoimmunity Study in the Young (DAISY) cohort studies. These studies showed that the risk of islet autoimmunity increased if gluten was introduced before the age of three months compared with receiving only breast milk during this period [45] or first exposure to gluten between age four and six months [46], after adjustment for covariates. Moreover, it was shown that breastfeeding during the introduction of gluten was associated with decreased risk of islet autoimmunity in children at high risk of T1D [46]. Recently, we published a study based on the Danish National Birth Cohort, which demonstrated that maternal ingestion of low versus high amounts of gluten during pregnancy reduced the risk (2-fold) of T1D in their children, after adjustment of covariates [47]. Other cohort studies showed no association between intake of GF diet during pregnancy and T1D, again after adjustment of covariates [48,49]. In two Danish studies, a GF diet was administered to children after T1D diagnosis and the children showed improvements in disease parameters including prolonged partial remission periods and reduced HBA1c compared to control children with T1D matched by diabetes duration and age [50,51]. Another study investigated how children at increased risk of T1D responded to six months of GF diet followed by six months of gluten-containing diet (diets were not matched for carbohydrate content etc.) [52]. Following the GF diet, the children showed improved glucose tolerance and insulin sensitivity (non-significant) but unchanged titres of islet autoantibodies. Following the months of the gluten-containing diet, the study reported a decreased insulin sensitivity. Hence, a GF diet may have a preserving effect on beta-cell function on older children with T1D.

In summary, the studies suggest that a GF diet may have the potential to reduce the risk of T1D. Interestingly, a GF diet seems to be most effective when applied in utero, and timing of the introduction of gluten is apparently critical. Moreover, a few studies indicate that a GF diet, when applied to older children with T1D, may preserve the beta cells to some extent.

2.3. GF Diet and the Intestine

The intestinal microbiota seems to play an important role in the pathogenesis of T1D but causality is still unclear. Patients with T1D have an increased intestinal permeability [53–56] and show a decrease in bacteria that maintain the intestinal permeability [57,58]. Perturbation of the intestinal microbiota in childhood is thought to disturb the developing immune system and may thus be a pathogenic factor [59,60]. NOD mice fed a GF versus a STD diet had overall fewer bacteria as well as fewer aerobic and microaerobic bacteria in caecum [41]. In a similar study, NOD mice on a GF diet showed decreased *Bifidobacterium*, *Tanerella* and *Barnesiella* species and increased *Akkermansia* species in faeces [42]. A GF diet during pregnancy and early postnatal life has been demonstrated to induce pronounced differences in the intestinal microbiota of NOD mouse mothers and offspring, including increased numbers of bacteria from the phylae *Akkermansia*, *Proteobacteria*, and *TM7* [44]. The mucin-degrading *Akkermansia* is of special interest in T1D. For example, NOD mice treated with vancomycin from an early age had increased proportions of *Akkermansia* and reduced incidence of autoimmune diabetes [61]. In addition to the association to T1D, *Akkermansia* species reversed the increased intestinal permeability in Apolipoprotein E (Apoe)−/− mice and decreased the entry of lipopolysaccharide (LPS) into the circulation [62]. Interestingly, a study in children from the BABYDIET study showed that *Bacteroides*-dominated children were more likely to develop islet autoantibodies and had decreased potential to butyrate production compared to *Akkermansia*-dominated children [63]. Short-chain fatty acids (SCFAs) are produced by bacteria during breakdown of dietary fibre and include butyrate, acetate, and propionate. Butyrate and acetate diminish the intestinal permeability [64,65], and butyrate can boost the number and function of regulatory T cells (Tregs) [65,66], which are known to suppress inflammatory responses. Acetate can reduce the proportion of autoreactive T cells [65].

Thus, a GF diet may improve the intestinal microbiota and permeability (Figure 1), but more studies are needed in order to gain knowledge about mechanisms and causality.

2.4. GF Ddiet and the Immune System

We and others have conducted a range of animal studies, which suggest that a GF diet modulates the innate and adaptive immune system (Table 1).

Table 1. An overview of some of the effects that a gluten-free (GF) diet has on the immune system in animal models of type 1 diabetes (T1D).

Immunological Effects of a GF versus a STD Diet in Utero in NOD Mice	References
↑M2 macrophage gene expression in intestine.	[44]
↓DC ($CD11b^+CD11c^+$) numbers in PLN, MLN and spleen.	[44]
↓TH1 cell ($IFNG^+CD4^+$) numbers in spleen.	[67]
↓TH17 (*RORGT*) gene expression in colon.	[43]
↓gdTCR cell ($IL22^+gdTCR^+$) numbers in spleen.	[67]
↑Treg cell ($FOXP3^+CD4^+$) numbers in PLN.	[44]
↑T cell ($\alpha4\beta7^+CD4^+/CD8^+$) numbers in PLN.	[44]
↓proinflammatory cytokine gene expression in intestine.	[44]
↓T cells ($gdTCR^+$, $CD4^+$, $CD8^+$ and $FOXP3^+$) inflammatory cytokine profile in spleen, PLN, MLN and ILN.	[67]
Immunological Effects of a GF versus a STD Diet Postnatally in Animal Models of T1D	**References**
↓NK cell (activated) ($NKG2D^+NKp46^+/DX5^+$) numbers in PLN (BALB/c mice) and spleen (NOD mice).	[68,69]
↓DC ($CD11b^+CD11c^+$) numbers in PLN and MLN (BALB/c mice).	[69]
↓DC ($CD11b^+CD11c^+$) numbers in colon (NOD mice).	[70]
↓DC (activated) ($CD40^+/CCR7^+/MHCII^+$ on $CD11c^+$) numbers in different lymphoid organs (BALB/c mice).	[69]
↑DC (tolerogenic) ($CD103^+CD11b^+$) numbers in PLN (BALB/c mice).	[69]
↓TH cell ($CD4^+$) numbers in colon (NOD mice).	[70]
↓TH1 cell ($IFNG^+CD4^+$) numbers in MLN (BB rats).	[71]
↓TH17 cell ($IL17^+CD4^+$) numbers in PLN (BALB/c mice).	[72]
↓TH17 cell ($IL17^+CD4^+$) numbers in colon (NOD mice).	[70]
↓T cell ($CD3^+$) proinflammatory profile (BALB/c mice).	[73]
↓CTL (activated) ($NKG2D^+CD8^+$) numbers in PLN (NOD mice).	[69]

↑: increased; ↓: decreased.

A GF diet reduced the natural killer (NK) cell activity in pancreatic lymph nodes (PLNs) from Bagg albino (BALB/c) mice and in spleen from NOD mice compared to mice on a STD diet [68]. Another study in NOD mice confirmed this observation in spleen and found reduced activity of cytotoxic T lymphocytes (CTLs) in PLN [69]. Besides NK cells, macrophages from mice have been shown to produce proinflammatory cytokines (interleukin (IL)6, IL12 and tumor necrosis factor alpha (TNFA), among others) upon gliadin stimulation [74]. Dendritic cells (DCs) may also be affected by a GF diet, as the diet reduced the proportions in thePLN and mesenteric lymph node (MLN) and increased the proportions of tolerogenic DCs in PLN in BALB/c mice [69]. This study also found downregulation of DC activation markers in lymphoid organs from the GF mice. This is supported by a study showing that gliadin stimulation of bone marrow-derived DCs from BALB/c mice resulted in maturation of the cells, as seen by evaluation of activation markers and chemokines (keratinocyte-derived cytokine (KC) and macrophage inflammatory protein 2 (MIP-2)) [75]. Moreover, gliadin stimulation may increase the expression of toll-like receptor (TLR)4, 7, 8 and interferon alpha (IFNA) in DCs of DQ8 transgenic mice [76]. As for the adaptive immune system, we have shown that a GF diet reduced the proportion of T helper (TH)17 cells in PLN of BALB/c mice [72] and dampened the inflammatory profile of T cells [73]. A wheat-free versus a wheat-based diet has been shown to reduce the proportion of TH1 cells in MLN from young diabetes-prone BB rats [71]. Three studies in NOD mice found that a GF diet during pregnancy alleviated T1D in the offspring and that the mechanisms were likely to involve changes in the immune system. The first study showed that the intestines from the offspring exposed to the GF diet in utero had an increased gene expression of immunosuppressive M2 macrophages and reduced expression of proinflammatory cytokines [44]. This study also showed that the GF diet increased the proportion of Tregs in PLN and decreased the proportion of DCs in PLN, MLN, and spleen in the offspring. Moreover, the traffic of T cells between PLN and the gut-associated lymphoid tissue (GALT) was increased. Recently, we demonstrated that a GF diet during pregnancy reduced the expression of interferon gamma (IFNG) in TH cells and IL22 in gamma delta T receptor (gdTCR)$^+$ T cells from spleen of NOD mouse offspring [67]. This is of interest because IFNG [77] and IL22 [78] might have a role in T1D. Furthermore, we demonstrated a reduced inflammatory profile in subpopulations of T cells from lymphoid organs of offspring exposed to a GF diet in utero [67]. In another study, we observed that the gene expression of TH17 cells was reduced in colon from NOD mice exposed to a GF diet in utero [43]. These results were confirmed in NOD mice fed an anti-diabetogenic diet compared to a wheat-based diet from a young age [70]. The mice showed reduced numbers of TH17 cells, besides reduced numbers of activated TH cells and DCs and reduced incidence of autoimmune diabetes. Taken together, a GF diet has a dampening effect on the innate and adaptive immune system, as evidenced in different animal models (Table 1).

Human evidence of the effect of gluten on the immune system is more limited. Early evidence includes a study from 1987 demonstrating increased titres of anti-gliadin antibodies at the onset of T1D in 54% of patients with no signs of CD and in none of the healthy controls [79]. Moreover, a study in children with T1D and no CD showed that rectal gluten application resulted in an increased percentage of epithelium and lamina propria CD3$^+$ and gdTCR$^+$ cells in 26% of the patients compared to approximately 15% of the healthy controls [80], indicating that some T1D patients have an abnormal mucosal immune response towards gluten. In another study, 47% of the included patients with T1D and no CD and none of the healthy controls displayed increased proliferation of peripheral blood mononuclear cells (PBMCs) after stimulation with wheat polypeptides, and the cytokine response was a proinflammatory TH1/TH17 [81]. On the other hand, CD4$^+$ cells from children with pre-T1D and multiple islet autoantibodies compared to healthy controls showed decreased proliferative responses after gliadin stimulation [82]. DCs may be affected by gluten as well. This is shown in a study where gliadin stimulation of monocyte-derived DCs from healthy donors resulted in increased expression of maturation markers (CD80, CD83, CD86, and HLA-DR molecules), increased production of chemokines and cytokines (TNFA, IL6, IL8, IL10 among others), increased capacity to stimulate proliferation of allogeneic T cells, as well as reduced endocytic activity [83].

Thus, the studies suggest that a GF diet reduces inflammation in the intestines and pancreas, involving many cell types of the immune system (Figure 1).

2.5. GF Diet, Risk of T1D and CD

CD is a chronic autoimmune disease that results in inflammation of the intestinal submucosa and destruction of the intestinal epithelium. The following clinical signs are typically observed: increased numbers of intraepithelial lymphocytes, villus atrophy, and crypt hyperplasia. The treatment consists of a strict GF diet and if not initiated it will lead to undernourishment. The pathogenesis is thought to start with binding of gliadin to the chemokine receptor CXCR3 on enterocytes, which results in increased intestinal permeability by myeloid differentiation primary response 88 (MyD88)-dependent zonulin release and crossing of the lamina propria by gliadin [13]. At this site, tissue transglutaminase (tTG) deamidates glutamine residues in gliadin to glutamate, which mediates high affinity of gliadin to HLA-DQ2/DQ8 on APCs and thus activation of CD4$^+$ T cells specific for gliadin [84,85]. Next, production of proinflammatory cytokines and activation of CD8$^+$ T cells specific for gliadin are thought to further worsen the damage to the intestine [86].

Interestingly, human studies indicate that T1D and CD are comorbid diseases and they share the genetically predisposing haplotypes HLA-DQ2/DQ8. The risk of developing other autoimmune diseases is increased for patients with CD, in particular for those diagnosed early (<16 years of age [87]) (<18 years of age [1]). The prevalence of CD is 5–10% in patients with T1D [88–92]; however, the risk is lower in patients compliant to a GF diet [87]. The majority of NOD mice [93] and 12% of patients with

T1D are seropositive for anti-tTG [94]. In addition, NOD mice on a STD versus a GF diet have reduced villus height and increased infiltration of intraepithelial lymphocytes (enteropathy) [95], and human subjects exhibit signs of enteropathy already from the pre-diabetic stage [54]. Jejunal biopsies from children with T1D versus healthy controls were stimulated with gliadin [96]. The result was increased proportions in lamina propria of intraepithelial T cells and increased expression of CD25$^+$ (IL2RA), CD80$^+$ (co-stimulatory), intracellular adhesion molecule 1 (ICAM-1), and crypt HLA-DR. Thus, NOD mice and patients with T1D exhibit signs of CD, which underlines that the two diseases are associated and indicates that gluten may be a common environmental factor. This is supported by a study in NOD mice, which showed that a GF versus a STD diet decreased intraepithelial infiltration of T cells, expression of IFNG, enteropathy and incidence of autoimmune diabetes [95]. Moreover, we recently published a study showing that young NOD mice exposed to a GF versus a STD diet in utero had persistently reduced titres of anti-tTG in serum together with increased villus-to-crypt (V:C) ratios (improved enteropathy) [67], indicating that a GF diet during pregnancy may not only ameliorate T1D but also dampen the symptoms of CD in the offspring.

Hence, studies in animals and humans with T1D indicate that a GF diet may reduce the signs of CD and that the prenatal period may be of special importance (Figure 1).

2.6. Mucosal Tolerance Induction by Gliadin

A study showed that BB rats fed wheat gluten neonatally versus at weaning were protected from autoimmune diabetes [97]. It was later demonstrated that NOD mice exposed to a diet with a three times higher content of gluten compared to a normal diet in utero and the rest of their lives were protected from autoimmune diabetes to the same extent as those on a GF diet [98]. The authors proposed that the high amount of gluten might result in mucosal tolerance or unresponsiveness, which was also seen in a human monocyte cell line regarding LPS in high doses and long exposure times [99]. More recently, administration of gliadin intranasally to four-week-old NOD mice was shown to decrease the incidence of autoimmune diabetes and insulitis and increase the numbers of gdTCR$^+$ cells and forkhead box P3 (FOXP3)$^+$CD4$^+$ Tregs in mucosal lymphoid organs [100]. Intestinal gdTCR$^+$ cells are important for the induction of peripheral Tregs and during induction of mucosal tolerance they seem to have a central role in maintenance of tolerance [101]. Tregs are functionally deficient in patients with T1D [102]. The hypothesis on mucosal tolerance induction against gluten is backed by an exploratory registry-based case-control study that we conducted, which demonstrated that occupation with grain crops, i.e., by bakers, was associated with lower incidence of T1D [103]. We speculated that the lower incidence among workers occupied with grain crops was due to nasal mucosal exposure to gluten during work and hence tolerance induction.

These studies show that a possible strategy in the prevention of T1D may be induction of mucosal tolerance against gluten, but human intervention studies are needed to confirm this.

2.7. GF Diet and the Beta Cell

From studies in NOD, C57BL/6 (B6), and BALB/c mice, we demonstrated that gliadin peptides cross the intestinal barrier after oral gavage and thereafter localise to the pancreas and to a smaller extent the islets [104]. The ability of gluten peptides to cross the intestinal barrier has been independently confirmed [105]. Gliadin does also seem to cross the intestinal barrier in humans, evidenced by observations of gliadin in breast milk and serum from healthy mothers [106]. Gluten peptides are likely in close contact with the beta cells because of the high degree of vascularisation in islets [107]. In vitro studies on INS-1E insulinoma cells and isolated rat islets showed that gliadin increased glucose-stimulated insulin-secretion (GSIS) by closing ATP-dependent K-channels [108]. This could be part of the pathogenesis of T1D by means of gliadin-mediated beta-cell hyperactivity and thus increased expression of islet antigens and autoimmunity [109]. A gluten-containing STD versus a GF diet is known to increase insulitis in animal models of T1D [39,40,43,44,67], and inflammatory cell-stress increases the expression and enzyme activity of tTG [110]. tTG has been shown to induce posttranslational modifications of human islet antigens and thereby increase the affinity to HLA-DQ [111]. Thus, it is likely that a GF diet reduces the tTG activity in islets and reduce insulitis. Interestingly, NOD mice exposed to a GF diet exclusively in utero had increased numbers of islets throughout the prediabetic phase, besides reduced insulitis and autoimmune diabetes incidence [67]. The finding is in agreement with an older study in BB rats, which were fed a diet based on hydrolysed casein versus a diet based on cereals from early life [39]. The rats had increased total islet area and numbers, together with lower insulitis and autoimmune diabetes incidence.

Altogether, it is likely that a GF diet reduces beta-cell stress and this may result in increased numbers of islets, besides reduced insulitis and autoimmune diabetes incidence, an effect that has also been observed when the diet was applied in utero (Figure 1).

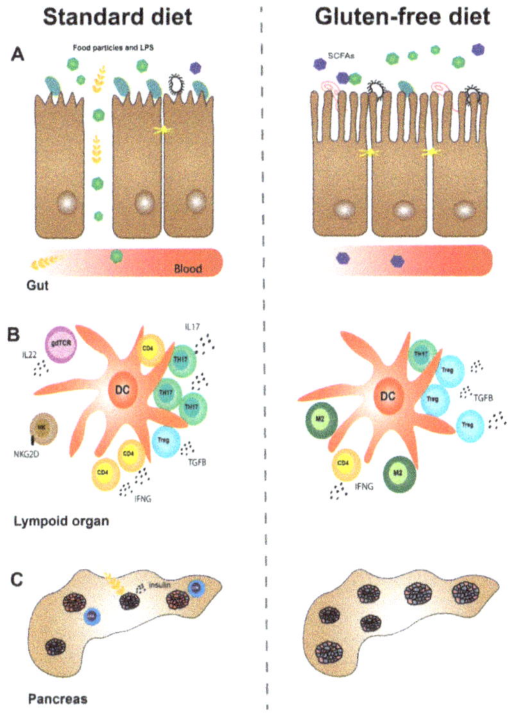

Figure 1. Gluten free (GF) diet and the development of type 1 diabetes (T1D)—a hypothesis. (**A**) A GF diet decreases the intestinal permeability and increases the villus-to-crypt (V:C) ratio, thereby preventing food particles such as gliadin peptides from crossing the intestinal barrier and reacting the pancreas. A GF diet increases the number of *Akkermansia* bacteria, among other changes, and the amount of short-chain fatty acids (SCFAs) such as butyrate. (**B**) A GF diet modulates the innate and adaptive immune system resulting in reduced interferon gamma (IFNG) secretion from CD4$^+$ T helper (TH) cells, reduced interleukin (IL)22 secretion from gamma delta T cell receptor (gdTCR)$^+$ T cells, and lower numbers of activated (NKG2D$^+$) natural killer (NK) cells, among other things. TH17 cell numbers are reduced and immunosuppressant M2 macrophage numbers and forkhead box P3 (FOXP3)$^+$ regulatory T cell (Treg) numbers are increased. (**C**) A GF diet reduces beta-cell stress by reducing the insulin secretion. This may preserve the number of islets, reduce insulitis, and ameliorate T1D.

3. Gluten and T2D

T2D is associated with obesity and the incidence is expected to increase between 2010 and 2030 [112]. Overall, T2D is a result of insulin resistance and beta-cell dysfunction [113]. Although insulin resistance is often present in obese subjects, their beta cells initially compensate by increasing the insulin production [114] and mass [115]. Eventually beta-cell dysfunction occurs, resulting in hyperglycaemia and diabetes [116]. As for T1D and CD, genetic susceptibility genes are important disease determinants in T2D, and so far studies have found over 40 associated genes, although only a few of them have been verified in several patients and laboratories including peroxisome proliferator activated receptor gamma (*PPARG*), ATP binding cassette subfamily C member 8 (*ABCC8*), and potassium voltage-gated channel subfamily J member 11 (*KCNJ11*) [117].

3.1. The Role of Environmental Factors

The rising incidence [6,112] and the observation that monozygotic twins are often discordant for T2D [29,118,119] indicates that environmental factors, besides genetic susceptibility genes, are important for the development of T2D. Obesity, a result of imbalance between energy intake and expenditure because of excess intake of food and insufficient physical activity [120], most likely plays a causal role in the pathogenesis of T2D [121]. According to the thrifty gene hypothesis, genes that were advantageous for accumulation of adipose tissue during times of caloric excess in the previous hunter/gatherer period might explain the present rise in the incidence of T2D in populations with caloric excess [122]. The intrauterine environment may be of special importance, in which pesticides [123], hormonal agents, patterns of feeding and undernutrition are potential determinants [120]. In this context, the thrifty phenotype hypothesis should be mentioned. It suggests that poor foetal and early postnatal nutrition leads to insulin resistance and beta-cell dysfunction in the adult, which, in combination with the effects from ageing and obesity, manifests in T2D [124].

3.2. GF Diet, Leptin Resistance and the Link to Obesity

Leptin resistance is likely involved in the pathogenesis of obesity and thus T2D [125,126]. Leptin resistance has been hypothesised to be the result of insufficient genetic adaptation to a cereal-based diet [127], as humans began consuming cereals only 10,000 years ago. The hypothesis was tested in piglets receiving a palaeolithic diet, i.e., a diet containing nuts, vegetables etc., versus a cereal-based diet from the age of 2–17 months [128]. Following this period, the palaeolithic piglets showed reduced body weight, subcutaneous fat thickness, and pancreatic lymphocyte numbers but increased insulin sensitivity. Interestingly, clinically relevant concentrations of trypsin- and pepsin-digested wheat gluten was demonstrated to hinder the binding between leptin and its receptor, indicating that gluten could be linked to leptin resistance and obesity [125].

3.3. GF Diet and the Intestine

Obesity and T2D are associated with intestinal dysbiosis [129]. Obese subjects have changes in the intestinal microbiota (↑phylum *Firmicutes* and ↓phylum *Bacteroides*) [130], which, as seen in mice, increase the capacity of the microbiota to harvest energy and increase fat stores [131]. A large study in T2D patients showed a reduced abundance of bacteria (*Roseburia*, among others) capable of producing the SCFA butyrate [132]. SCFAs have been demonstrated to prevent high-fat (HF) diet-induced obesity in B6 mice [133] and studies in Caco-2 epithelial cells showed that butyrate may decrease intestinal permeability [64], which is increased in T2D patients [134,135]. Interestingly, gliadin stimulation of intestinal tissue from mice and humans increased the permeability [13], and studies in different mouse strains found that oral gavage of gluten peptides resulted in accumulation in extraintestinal organs [104,105]. Regarding the intestinal permeability, B6 mice fed a gluten-free high-fat (GF-HF) diet versus a gluten-containing HF diet showed improved intestinal barrier function [136]. Moreover, the GF-HF mice showed changes in the intestinal microbiota (↑genus *Lactobacillus* and ↓genera *Clostridium XI*, *Coriobacteriaceae* and *Dorea*) associated with improved health [137–140]. Moreover, the abundance of *Akkermansia* species was reduced in GF-HF versus HF mice, which is puzzling for several reasons. First, increased intestinal permeability and leakage of LPS to the circulation may be reversed by the bacterial species *Akkermansia muciniphila*, as shown in Apoe−/− mice [62]. Second, B6 mice receiving oral gavage of the bacterium showed reduced HF diet-induced metabolic disorders i.e., metabolic endotoxaemia, adipose tissue inflammation, insulin resistance, and fat mass gain [141]. Third, *Akkermansia muciniphila* is found in lower abundance in intestines of pre-T2D patients compared with healthy controls [142].

Studies in mice show that the early onset of HF diet-induced hyperglycaemia is associated with increased leakage of LPS and gram-negative bacteria from the intestine to the adipose tissue, which is thought to continuously fuel metabolic bacteraemia and endotoxaemia [143], and may contribute to low-grade inflammation, insulin resistance, beta-cell dysfunction, and, thus, T2D. This is relevant because intake of gluten seems to both increase the intestinal permeability and lead to a disease-associated intestinal microbiota. The intake of gluten could therefore contribute to T2D by the above-mentioned mechanism.

Thus, studies in mouse models of T2D indicate that a GF diet may improve the intestinal barrier function and lead to a healthier microbiota, both of which could alleviate the disease by reducing passage of inflammatory gluten peptides, bacterial products etc. (Figure 2).

3.4. GF Diet, the Beta Cell and Adipose Tissue

Signalling through the pattern-recognition receptor TLR4, which is expressed on most cell types [144], has been associated with insulin resistance [145] and beta-cell dysfunction in T2D [146]. This is relevant because gliadin may activate signalling through this receptor [147]. Thus, gliadin may induce insulin resistance and beta-cell dysfunction through TLR4 and possibly also through other innate immune receptors. Moreover, we have demonstrated that gliadin peptides affect the beta cells directly, as the peptides increase GSIS in rat islets and INS-1E cells and potentiate the fatty acid-stimulated insulin secretion in INS-1E cells [108].

These studies imply that a GF diet may alleviate insulin resistance as well as beta-cell stress and dysfunction in T2D (Figure 2). However, the results need further confirmation.

3.5. GF Diet, the Immune System, Obesity and T2D

We have shown that intravenous injections with enzymatically degraded gluten increase the body weight of NOD mice [108]. Likewise, rats fed a casein-based versus a gluten-based diet for two weeks had reduced liver lipogenesis [148]. Moreover, B6 mice fed a GF-HF versus a HF diet for eight weeks had reduced concentrations in serum of the proinflammatory adipokines leptin and resistin and increased concentrations of the anti-inflammatory adipokine adiponectin, together with reduced body weight, epididymal fat stores, fasting glucose, and insulin [149]. This indicated that gluten could directly contribute to obesity and hence T2D. The improved glucose homeostasis in the GF-HF mice was thought to involve a reduced inflammatory profile leading to increased expression of *PPARG*, an important regulator of lipid metabolism, and thus increased expression of adiponectin and glucose transporter 4 (*GLUT-4*) i.e., improved insulin sensitivity [149]. Similar observations were seen in another study in B6 mice fed a GF diet [105], both in normal and HF settings. The study also showed that increased thermogenesis and energy expenditure were behind the observed effects. We showed that long-term feeding of B6 mice with a GF-HF versus a HF diet increased the beta-cell volume and improved the glucose tolerance [150], which we believe could be a result of beta-cell rest, as we have shown that gluten potentiates the fatty acid-stimulated insulin secretion [108]. Not all animal studies have been able to demonstrate these anti-obesity and anti-diabetes effects from a GF diet. As an example, Apo−/− mice were fed a GF diet in utero and until 16 weeks of age, but no effect was observed on body weight, glucose tolerance, insulin levels, and plasma lipids; however, a transient change was seen in the intestinal microbiota [151]. Thus, the effects of a GF diet on obesity and T2D have been tested only in a few animal studies, some of which indicate that a GF diet may have the potential to reduce obesity and T2D (Figure 2).

In a randomised, crossover study, T2D patients were fasted and received a test meal differing in the protein sources whey, casein, cod, and gluten [152]. After eight hours, the patients from the gluten-group showed increased incremental area under the curve (AUC) for plasma glucose compared to patients from the other groups. Moreover, the patients eating gluten showed increased incremental AUC for fatty acids and triglycerides compared to patients receiving whey. The national health and nutrition examination survey (NHANES) study, which consists of a number of cross-sectional surveys carried out every second year, demonstrated higher high-density lipoprotein (HDL), smaller waist circumference and self-reported weight loss in persons on a GF diet [153]. Further human evidence includes a study in children with autism spectrum disorder on a GF casein-free diet versus a regular diet for three months, showing lower body weight and body mass index [154]. A recent prospective cohort study from the USA based on the Nurses' Health Study I and II and the Health Professionals Follow-Up Study found an inverse association between intake of gluten and risk of T2D [155]. The analyses were adjusted for relevant covariates such as fibre and folic acid, which are often low in a GF diet, and the association was slightly weakened after adjustment of cereal fibre. Excluding gluten from the diet will mediate exclusion of other potential anti-diabetogenic factors; hence, this study is not conclusive and should be followed up with an intervention study. In summary, a few intervention studies have shown that a GF diet may alleviate obesity and T2D in humans (Figure 2). On the other hand, a recent prospective cohort study report that a GF diet is associated with T2D. Thus, larger intervention studies clarifying the effect of a GF diet on T2D patients are needed.

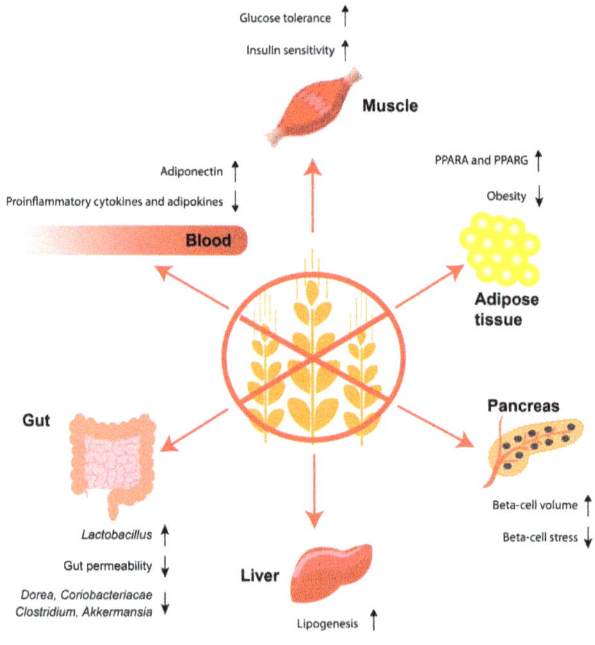

Figure 2. Gluten-free (GF) diet and the development of type 2 diabetes (T2D)—a hypothesis. A GF diet decreases intestinal permeability thereby preventing food particles such a gliadin from crossing the intestinal barrier and reaching the adipose tissue and pancreas. A GF diet increases the proportion of *Lactobacillus* and decreases the proportion of *Akkermansia*, *Dorea*, *Clostridium*, and *Coriobacteriacae*. In the blood, a GF diet decreases the level of proinflammatory cytokines and adipokines and increases the anti-inflammatory adiponectin. A GF diet reduces obesity and improves the regulation of lipid metabolism by upregulating peroxisome proliferator activator receptor alpha (PPARA) and peroxisome proliferator activator receptor gamma (PPARG) in adipose tissue. This, in turn, leads to increased insulin sensitivity and improved glucose tolerance, which is further improved by reduced beta-cell stress and increased beta-cell volume.

4. Conclusions

In this review, we looked at the role of dietary gluten as a contributing factor in the aetiopathogenesis of T1D and T2D. Gluten has multiple effects in the body starting in the intestine where it affects the composition of the microbiota, may induce enteropathy in T1D, and increases the intestinal permeability, all of which seem to improve with a GF diet. In animals, gluten has been found to cross the intestinal barrier together with LPS among other substances and may accumulate in different tissues including islets and adipose tissue. In animal beta cells, gluten peptides induce insulin secretion, an effect that is potentiated by palmitate, suggesting that gluten peptides may induce beta cell-stress, -dysfunction, -loss, and autoimmunity, and thus contribute to both T1D and T2D. Moreover, gluten peptides may also contribute to leptin- and insulin resistance, regarding obesity and T2D. Primarily animal studies have shown that a GF diet dampens the innate and adaptive immune system leading to a less inflammatory profile. In T1D, the timing of gluten introduction to children is most likely critical, and the efficiency of gluten exclusion during pregnancy, combined with early introduction of gluten postnatally, should be investigated as a prevention strategy in an intervention study. Interestingly, animal studies suggest that a GF diet in utero may also reduce the risk of CD and report changes in the pancreas morphology including increased numbers of islets. Postnatally, a GF diet remains an interesting therapeutic option for the prevention and treatment of T1D, but more human intervention studies must be carried out. Mucosal tolerance induction of gluten is another potential strategy in reducing the risk of T1D but this also needs further exploration.

In T2D, the evidence for an alleviating effect of a GF diet is more uncertain especially regarding the few human studies that have been conducted, although animal studies report improvements of both obesity and T2D. A GF diet is typically low in fibres and other antidiabetogenic nutrients, and studies investigating the long-term effects on obesity and T2D of gluten specifically are therefore needed.

Author Contributions: Conceptualisation, M.H.-J.; writing—original draft preparation, M.H.-J.; writing—review and editing, M.H.-J., L.J.H., K.J. and K.B.; visualisation, M.H.-J. and L.J.H.; funding acquisition, K.B.

Funding: This article was supported by Kirsten and Freddy Johansen's foundation.

Conflicts of Interest: The authors declare no conflict of interest.

Abbreviations

ABCC8	ATP binding cassette subfamily C member 8
Apoe	Apolipoprotein E
AUC	Area under the curve
BALB/c	Bagg albino
BB	Biobreeding
B6	C57BL/6
CCR7	CC-chemokine receptor 7
CD	Celiac disease
CTL	Cytotoxic T lymphocyte
DAISY	Diabetes autoimmunity study in the young
DC	Dendritic cell
DiViD	Diabetes virus detection study
FOXP3	Forkhead box P3
GALT	Gut-associated lymphoid tissue
gdTCR	Gamma delta T cell receptor
GF	Gluten-free
GF-HF	Gluten-free high-fat
GLUT-4	Glucose transporter 4
GSIS	Glucose-stimulated insulin secretion
HDL	High-density lipoprotein
HF	High-fat

ICAM-1	Intercellular adhesion molecule 1
IFNA	Interferon alpha
IFNG	Interferon gamma
IL	Interleukin
ILN	Inguinal lymph node
KC	Keratinocyte-derived cytokine
KCNJ11	Potassium voltage-gated channel subfamily J member 11
LPS	Lipopolysaccharide
MIP-2	Macrophage inflammatory protein 2
MLN	Mesenteric lymph node
MyD88	Myeloid differentiation primary response 88
NHANES	National health and nutrition examination survey
NK	Natural killer
NOD	Non-obese diabetic
PBMC	Peripheral blood mononuclear cell
PLN	Pancreatic lymph node
PPARA	Peroxisome proliferator activated receptor alpha
PPARG	Peroxisome proliferator activated receptor gamma
RORGT	Retinoid orphan receptor gamma t
SCFA	Short-chain fatty acid
STD	Standard
TH	T helper
TLR	Toll-like receptor
TNFA	Tumor necrosis factor alpha
Treg	Regulatory T cell
tTG	Tissue transglutaminase
T1D	Type 1 diabetes
T2D	Type 2 diabetes
V:C	Villus-to-crypt

References

1. Vajravelu, M.E.; Keren, R.; Weber, D.R.; Verma, R.; De Leon, D.D.; Denburg, M.R. Incidence and Risk of Celiac Disease after Type 1 Diabetes: A Population-Based Cohort Study Using the Health Improvement Network Database. *Pediatr. Diabetes* **2018**. [CrossRef] [PubMed]
2. Fasano, A.; Berti, I.; Gerarduzzi, T.; Not, T.; Colletti, R.B.; Drago, S.; Elitsur, Y.; Green, P.H.; Guandalini, S.; Hill, I.D.; et al. Prevalence of celiac disease in at-risk and not-at-risk groups in the United States: A large multicenter study. *Arch. Intern. Med.* **2003**, *163*, 286–292. [CrossRef] [PubMed]
3. West, J.; Logan, R.F.; Hill, P.G.; Lloyd, A.; Lewis, S.; Hubbard, R.; Reader, R.; Holmes, G.K.; Khaw, K.T. Seroprevalence, correlates, and characteristics of undetected coeliac disease in England. *Gut* **2003**, *52*, 960–965. [CrossRef] [PubMed]
4. Maki, M.; Mustalahti, K.; Kokkonen, J.; Kulmala, P.; Haapalahti, M.; Karttunen, T.; Ilonen, J.; Laurila, K.; Dahlbom, I.; Hansson, T.; et al. Prevalence of Celiac disease among children in Finland. *N. Engl. J. Med.* **2003**, *348*, 2517–2524. [CrossRef] [PubMed]
5. Leonard, M.M.; Sapone, A.; Catassi, C.; Fasano, A. Celiac Disease and Nonceliac Gluten Sensitivity: A Review. *JAMA* **2017**, *318*, 647–656. [CrossRef] [PubMed]
6. NCD Risk Factor Collaboration (NCD-RisC). Worldwide trends in diabetes since 1980: A pooled analysis of 751 population-based studies with 4.4 million participants. *Lancet* **2016**, *387*, 1513–1530. [CrossRef]
7. Awika, J.M. Major cereal grains production and use around the world. *Adv. Cereal Sci. Implic. Food Process. Health Promot.* **2011**, *1089*, 1–13.
8. Shewry, P.R.; Halford, N.G. Cereal seed storage proteins: Structures, properties and role in grain utilization. *J. Exp. Bot.* **2002**, *53*, 947–958. [CrossRef] [PubMed]

9. Stern, M.; Ciclitira, P.J.; Van Eckert, R.; Feighery, C.; Janssen, F.W.; Mendez, E.; Mothes, T.; Troncone, R.; Wieser, H. Analysis and clinical effects of gluten in coeliac disease. *Eur. J. Gastroenterol. Hepatol.* **2001**, *13*, 741–747. [CrossRef] [PubMed]
10. Piper, J.L.; Gray, G.M.; Khosla, C. Effect of prolyl endopeptidase on digestive-resistant gliadin peptides in vivo. *J. Pharmacol. Exp. Ther.* **2004**, *311*, 213–219. [CrossRef] [PubMed]
11. Hausch, F.; Shan, L.; Santiago, N.A.; Gray, G.M.; Khosla, C. Intestinal digestive resistance of immunodominant gliadin peptides. *Am. J. Physiol. Gastrointest. Liver Physiol.* **2002**, *283*. [CrossRef] [PubMed]
12. Fasano, A. Zonulin and its regulation of intestinal barrier function: The biological door to inflammation, autoimmunity, and cancer. *Physiol. Rev.* **2011**, *91*, 151–175. [CrossRef] [PubMed]
13. Lammers, K.M.; Lu, R.; Brownley, J.; Lu, B.; Gerard, C.; Thomas, K.; Rallabhandi, P.; Shea-Donohue, T.; Tamiz, A.; Alkan, S.; et al. Gliadin induces an increase in intestinal permeability and zonulin release by binding to the chemokine receptor CXCR3. *Gastroenterology* **2008**, *135*, 194–204.e3. [CrossRef] [PubMed]
14. Lammers, K.M.; Khandelwal, S.; Chaudhry, F.; Kryszak, D.; Puppa, E.L.; Casolaro, V.; Fasano, A. Identification of a novel immunomodulatory gliadin peptide that causes interleukin-8 release in a chemokine receptor CXCR3-dependent manner only in patients with coeliac disease. *Immunology* **2011**, *132*, 432–440. [CrossRef] [PubMed]
15. Maiuri, L.; Troncone, R.; Mayer, M.; Coletta, S.; Picarelli, A.; De Vincenzi, M.; Pavone, V.; Auricchio, S. In vitro activities of A-gliadin-related synthetic peptides: Damaging effect on the atrophic coeliac mucosa and activation of mucosal immune response in the treated coeliac mucosa. *Scand. J. Gastroenterol.* **1996**, *31*, 247–253. [CrossRef] [PubMed]
16. Sollid, L.M.; Qiao, S.W.; Anderson, R.P.; Gianfrani, C.; Koning, F. Nomenclature and listing of celiac disease relevant gluten T-cell epitopes restricted by HLA-DQ molecules. *Immunogenetics* **2012**, *64*, 455–460. [CrossRef] [PubMed]
17. Qiao, S.W.; Bergseng, E.; Molberg, O.; Xia, J.; Fleckenstein, B.; Khosla, C.; Sollid, L.M. Antigen presentation to celiac lesion-derived T cells of a 33-mer gliadin peptide naturally formed by gastrointestinal digestion. *J. Immunol.* **2004**, *173*, 1757–1762. [CrossRef] [PubMed]
18. Shan, L.; Molberg, O.; Parrot, I.; Hausch, F.; Filiz, F.; Gray, G.M.; Sollid, L.M.; Khosla, C. Structural basis for gluten intolerance in celiac sprue. *Science* **2002**, *297*, 2275–2279. [CrossRef] [PubMed]
19. Shan, L.; Qiao, S.W.; Arentz-Hansen, H.; Molberg, O.; Gray, G.M.; Sollid, L.M.; Khosla, C. Identification and analysis of multivalent proteolytically resistant peptides from gluten: Implications for celiac sprue. *J. Proteome Res.* **2005**, *4*, 1732–1741. [CrossRef] [PubMed]
20. Schalk, K.; Lang, C.; Wieser, H.; Koehler, P.; Scherf, K.A. Quantitation of the immunodominant 33-mer peptide from alpha-gliadin in wheat flours by liquid chromatography tandem mass spectrometry. *Sci. Rep.* **2017**, *7*, 45092. [CrossRef] [PubMed]
21. Clayton, D.G. Prediction and interaction in complex disease genetics: Experience in type 1 diabetes. *PLOS Genet.* **2009**, *5*, e1000540. [CrossRef] [PubMed]
22. Pociot, F.; Lernmark, A. Genetic risk factors for type 1 diabetes. *Lancet* **2016**, *387*, 2331–2339. [CrossRef]
23. Group, D.P. Incidence and trends of childhood Type 1 diabetes worldwide 1990–1999. *Diabet. Med.* **2006**, *23*, 857–866. [CrossRef] [PubMed]
24. Patterson, C.C.; Dahlquist, G.G.; Gyurus, E.; Green, A.; Soltesz, G.; Group, E.S. Incidence trends for childhood type 1 diabetes in Europe during 1989–2003 and predicted new cases 2005–20: A multicentre prospective registration study. *Lancet* **2009**, *373*, 2027–2033. [CrossRef]
25. Gorelick, J.; Yarmolinsky, L.; Budovsky, A.; Khalfin, B.; Klein, J.D.; Pinchasov, Y.; Bushuev, M.A.; Rudchenko, T.; Ben-Shabat, S. The Impact of Diet Wheat Source on the Onset of Type 1 Diabetes Mellitus-Lessons Learned from the Non-Obese Diabetic (NOD) Mouse Model. *Nutrients* **2017**, *9*. [CrossRef] [PubMed]
26. Bodansky, H.J.; Staines, A.; Stephenson, C.; Haigh, D.; Cartwright, R. Evidence for an environmental effect in the aetiology of insulin dependent diabetes in a transmigratory population. *BMJ* **1992**, *304*, 1020–1022. [CrossRef] [PubMed]
27. Kondrashova, A.; Reunanen, A.; Romanov, A.; Karvonen, A.; Viskari, H.; Vesikari, T.; Ilonen, J.; Knip, M.; Hyoty, H. A six-fold gradient in the incidence of type 1 diabetes at the eastern border of Finland. *Ann. Med.* **2005**, *37*, 67–72. [CrossRef] [PubMed]
28. Kyvik, K.O.; Green, A.; Beck-Nielsen, H. Concordance rates of insulin dependent diabetes mellitus: A population based study of young Danish twins. *BMJ* **1995**, *311*, 913–917. [CrossRef] [PubMed]

29. Kaprio, J.; Tuomilehto, J.; Koskenvuo, M.; Romanov, K.; Reunanen, A.; Eriksson, J.; Stengard, J.; Kesaniemi, Y.A. Concordance for type 1 (insulin-dependent) and type 2 (non-insulin-dependent) diabetes mellitus in a population-based cohort of twins in Finland. *Diabetologia* **1992**, *35*, 1060–1067. [CrossRef] [PubMed]
30. Knip, M.; Veijola, R.; Virtanen, S.M.; Hyoty, H.; Vaarala, O.; Akerblom, H.K. Environmental triggers and determinants of type 1 diabetes. *Diabetes* **2005**, *54*, S125–S136. [CrossRef] [PubMed]
31. Atkinson, M.A.; Eisenbarth, G.S. Type 1 diabetes: New perspectives on disease pathogenesis and treatment. *Lancet* **2001**, *358*, 221–229. [CrossRef]
32. Stene, L.C.; Oikarinen, S.; Hyoty, H.; Barriga, K.J.; Norris, J.M.; Klingensmith, G.; Hutton, J.C.; Erlich, H.A.; Eisenbarth, G.S.; Rewers, M. Enterovirus infection and progression from islet autoimmunity to type 1 diabetes: The Diabetes and Autoimmunity Study in the Young (DAISY). *Diabetes* **2010**, *59*, 3174–3180. [CrossRef] [PubMed]
33. Oikarinen, S.; Martiskainen, M.; Tauriainen, S.; Huhtala, H.; Ilonen, J.; Veijola, R.; Simell, O.; Knip, M.; Hyoty, H. Enterovirus RNA in blood is linked to the development of type 1 diabetes. *Diabetes* **2011**, *60*, 276–279. [CrossRef] [PubMed]
34. Buschard, K.; Hastrup, N.; Rygaard, J. Virus-induced diabetes mellitus in mice and the thymus-dependent immune system. *Diabetologia* **1983**, *24*, 42–46. [CrossRef] [PubMed]
35. Dotta, F.; Censini, S.; van Halteren, A.G.; Marselli, L.; Masini, M.; Dionisi, S.; Mosca, F.; Boggi, U.; Muda, A.O.; Del Prato, S.; et al. Coxsackie B4 virus infection of beta cells and natural killer cell insulitis in recent-onset type 1 diabetic patients. *Proc. Natl. Acad. Sci. USA* **2007**, *104*, 5115–5120. [CrossRef] [PubMed]
36. Krogvold, L.; Edwin, B.; Buanes, T.; Frisk, G.; Skog, O.; Anagandula, M.; Korsgren, O.; Undlien, D.; Eike, M.C.; Richardson, S.J.; et al. Detection of a low-grade enteroviral infection in the islets of langerhans of living patients newly diagnosed with type 1 diabetes. *Diabetes* **2015**, *64*, 1682–1687. [CrossRef] [PubMed]
37. Hober, D.; Sauter, P. Pathogenesis of type 1 diabetes mellitus: Interplay between enterovirus and host. *Nat. Rev. Endocrinol.* **2010**, *6*, 279–289. [CrossRef] [PubMed]
38. Hoorfar, J.; Buschard, K.; Dagnaes-Hansen, F. Prophylactic nutritional modification of the incidence of diabetes in autoimmune non-obese diabetic (NOD) mice. *Br. J. Nutr.* **1993**, *69*, 597–607. [CrossRef] [PubMed]
39. Scott, F.W. Food-induced type 1 diabetes in the BB rat. *Diabetes Metab. Rev.* **1996**, *12*, 341–359. [CrossRef]
40. Funda, D.P.; Kaas, A.; Bock, T.; Tlaskalova-Hogenova, H.; Buschard, K. Gluten-free diet prevents diabetes in NOD mice. *Diabetes Metab. Res. Rev.* **1999**, *15*, 323–327. [CrossRef]
41. Hansen, A.K.; Ling, F.; Kaas, A.; Funda, D.P.; Farlov, H.; Buschard, K. Diabetes preventive gluten-free diet decreases the number of caecal bacteria in non-obese diabetic mice. *Diabetes Metab. Res. Rev.* **2006**, *22*, 220–225. [CrossRef] [PubMed]
42. Marietta, E.V.; Gomez, A.M.; Yeoman, C.; Tilahun, A.Y.; Clark, C.R.; Luckey, D.H.; Murray, J.A.; White, B.A.; Kudva, Y.C.; Rajagopalan, G. Low incidence of spontaneous type 1 diabetes in non-obese diabetic mice raised on gluten-free diets is associated with changes in the intestinal microbiome. *PLoS ONE* **2013**, *8*, e78687. [CrossRef] [PubMed]
43. Antvorskov, J.C.; Josefsen, K.; Haupt-Jorgensen, M.; Fundova, P.; Funda, D.P.; Buschard, K. Gluten-Free Diet Only during Pregnancy Efficiently Prevents Diabetes in NOD Mouse Offspring. *J. Diabetes Res.* **2016**, *2016*, 3047574. [CrossRef] [PubMed]
44. Hansen, C.H.; Krych, L.; Buschard, K.; Metzdorff, S.B.; Nellemann, C.; Hansen, L.H.; Nielsen, D.S.; Frokiaer, H.; Skov, S.; Hansen, A.K. A maternal gluten-free diet reduces inflammation and diabetes incidence in the offspring of NOD mice. *Diabetes* **2014**, *63*, 2821–2832. [CrossRef] [PubMed]
45. Ziegler, A.G.; Schmid, S.; Huber, D.; Hummel, M.; Bonifacio, E. Early infant feeding and risk of developing type 1 diabetes-associated autoantibodies. *JAMA* **2003**, *290*, 1721–1728. [CrossRef] [PubMed]
46. Norris, J.M.; Barriga, K.; Klingensmith, G.; Hoffman, M.; Eisenbarth, G.S.; Erlich, H.A.; Rewers, M. Timing of initial cereal exposure in infancy and risk of islet autoimmunity. *JAMA* **2003**, *290*, 1713–1720. [CrossRef] [PubMed]
47. Antvorskov, J.C.; Halldorsson, T.I.; Josefsen, K.; Svensson, J.; Granstrom, C.; Roep, B.O.; Olesen, T.H.; Hrolfsdottir, L.; Buschard, K.; Olsen, S.F. Association between maternal gluten intake and type 1 diabetes in offspring: National prospective cohort study in Denmark. *BMJ* **2018**, *362*, k3547. [CrossRef] [PubMed]
48. Lamb, M.M.; Myers, M.A.; Barriga, K.; Zimmet, P.Z.; Rewers, M.; Norris, J.M. Maternal diet during pregnancy and islet autoimmunity in offspring. *Pediatr. Diabetes* **2008**, *9*, 135–141. [CrossRef] [PubMed]

49. Virtanen, S.M.; Uusitalo, L.; Kenward, M.G.; Nevalainen, J.; Uusitalo, U.; Kronberg-Kippila, C.; Ovaskainen, M.L.; Arkkola, T.; Niinisto, S.; Hakulinen, T.; et al. Maternal food consumption during pregnancy and risk of advanced beta-cell autoimmunity in the offspring. *Pediatr. Diabetes* **2011**, *12*, 95–99. [CrossRef] [PubMed]
50. Sildorf, S.M.; Fredheim, S.; Svensson, J.; Buschard, K. Remission without insulin therapy on gluten-free diet in a 6-year old boy with type 1 diabetes mellitus. *BMJ Case Rep.* **2012**, *2012*. [CrossRef] [PubMed]
51. Svensson, J.; Sildorf, S.M.; Pipper, C.B.; Kyvsgaard, J.N.; Bojstrup, J.; Pociot, F.M.; Mortensen, H.B.; Buschard, K. Potential beneficial effects of a gluten-free diet in newly diagnosed children with type 1 diabetes: A pilot study. *Springerplus* **2016**, *5*, 994. [CrossRef] [PubMed]
52. Pastore, M.R.; Bazzigaluppi, E.; Belloni, C.; Arcovio, C.; Bonifacio, E.; Bosi, E. Six months of gluten-free diet do not influence autoantibody titers, but improve insulin secretion in subjects at high risk for type 1 diabetes. *J. Clin. Endocrinol. Metab.* **2003**, *88*, 162–165. [CrossRef] [PubMed]
53. Mooradian, A.D.; Morley, J.E.; Levine, A.S.; Prigge, W.F.; Gebhard, R.L. Abnormal intestinal permeability to sugars in diabetes mellitus. *Diabetologia* **1986**, *29*, 221–224. [CrossRef] [PubMed]
54. Bosi, E.; Molteni, L.; Radaelli, M.G.; Folini, L.; Fermo, I.; Bazzigaluppi, E.; Piemonti, L.; Pastore, M.R.; Paroni, R. Increased intestinal permeability precedes clinical onset of type 1 diabetes. *Diabetologia* **2006**, *49*, 2824–2827. [CrossRef] [PubMed]
55. Carratu, R.; Secondulfo, M.; de Magistris, L.; Iafusco, D.; Urio, A.; Carbone, M.G.; Pontoni, G.; Carteni, M.; Prisco, F. Altered intestinal permeability to mannitol in diabetes mellitus type I. *J. Pediatr. Gastroenterol. Nutr.* **1999**, *28*, 264–269. [CrossRef] [PubMed]
56. Sapone, A.; De Magistris, L.; Pietzak, M.; Clemente, M.G.; Tripathi, A.; Cucca, F.; Lampis, R.; Kryszak, D.; Carteni, M.; Generoso, M.; et al. Zonulin upregulation is associated with increased gut permeability in subjects with type 1 diabetes and their relatives. *Diabetes* **2006**, *55*, 1443–1449. [CrossRef] [PubMed]
57. Murri, M.; Leiva, I.; Gomez-Zumaquero, J.M.; Tinahones, F.J.; Cardona, F.; Soriguer, F.; Queipo-Ortuno, M.I. Gut microbiota in children with type 1 diabetes differs from that in healthy children: A case-control study. *BMC Med.* **2013**, *11*, 46. [CrossRef] [PubMed]
58. De Goffau, M.C.; Fuentes, S.; Dan den Bogert, B.; Honkanen, H.; De Vos, W.M.; Welling, G.W.; Hyoty, H.; Harmsen, H.J. Aberrant gut microbiota composition at the onset of type 1 diabetes in young children. *Diabetologia* **2014**, *57*, 1569–1577. [CrossRef] [PubMed]
59. Vangay, P.; Ward, T.; Gerber, J.S.; Knights, D. Antibiotics, pediatric dysbiosis, and disease. *Cell Host Microbe* **2015**, *17*, 553–564. [CrossRef] [PubMed]
60. Vaarala, O. Gut microbiota and type 1 diabetes. *Rev. Diabet. Stud.* **2012**, *9*, 251–259. [CrossRef] [PubMed]
61. Hansen, C.H.; Krych, L.; Nielsen, D.S.; Vogensen, F.K.; Hansen, L.H.; Sorensen, S.J.; Buschard, K.; Hansen, A.K. Early life treatment with vancomycin propagates Akkermansia muciniphila and reduces diabetes incidence in the NOD mouse. *Diabetologia* **2012**, *55*, 2285–2294. [CrossRef] [PubMed]
62. Li, J.; Lin, S.; Vanhoutte, P.M.; Woo, C.W.; Xu, A. Akkermansia Muciniphila Protects Against Atherosclerosis by Preventing Metabolic Endotoxemia-Induced Inflammation in Apoe−/−Mice. *Circulation* **2016**, *133*, 2434–2446. [CrossRef] [PubMed]
63. Endesfelder, D.; Engel, M.; Davis-Richardson, A.G.; Ardissone, A.N.; Achenbach, P.; Hummel, S.; Winkler, C.; Atkinson, M.; Schatz, D.; Triplett, E.; et al. Towards a functional hypothesis relating anti-islet cell autoimmunity to the dietary impact on microbial communities and butyrate production. *Microbiome* **2016**, *4*, 17. [CrossRef] [PubMed]
64. Ohata, A.; Usami, M.; Miyoshi, M. Short-chain fatty acids alter tight junction permeability in intestinal monolayer cells via lipoxygenase activation. *Nutrition* **2005**, *21*, 838–847. [CrossRef] [PubMed]
65. Marino, E.; Richards, J.L.; McLeod, K.H.; Stanley, D.; Yap, Y.A.; Knight, J.; McKenzie, C.; Kranich, J.; Oliveira, A.C.; Rossello, F.J.; et al. Gut microbial metabolites limit the frequency of autoimmune T cells and protect against type 1 diabetes. *Nat. Immunol.* **2017**, *18*, 552–562. [CrossRef] [PubMed]
66. Furusawa, Y.; Obata, Y.; Fukuda, S.; Endo, T.A.; Nakato, G.; Takahashi, D.; Nakanishi, Y.; Uetake, C.; Kato, K.; Kato, T.; et al. Commensal microbe-derived butyrate induces the differentiation of colonic regulatory T. cells. *Nature* **2013**, *504*, 446–450. [CrossRef] [PubMed]
67. Haupt-Jorgensen, M.; Larsen, J.; Josefsen, K.; Jorgensen, T.Z.; Antvorskov, J.C.; Hansen, A.K.; Buschard, K. Gluten-free diet during pregnancy alleviates signs of diabetes and celiac disease in NOD mouse offspring. *Diabetes Metab. Res. Rev.* **2018**, *34*, e2987. [CrossRef] [PubMed]

68. Larsen, J.; Dall, M.; Antvorskov, J.C.; Weile, C.; Engkilde, K.; Josefsen, K.; Buschard, K. Dietary gluten increases natural killer cell cytotoxicity and cytokine secretion. *Eur. J. Immunol.* **2014**, *44*, 3056–3067. [CrossRef] [PubMed]
69. Larsen, J.; Weile, C.; Antvorskov, J.C.; Engkilde, K.; Nielsen, S.M.; Josefsen, K.; Buschard, K. Effect of dietary gluten on dendritic cells and innate immune subsets in BALB/c and NOD mice. *PLoS ONE* **2015**, *10*, e0118618. [CrossRef] [PubMed]
70. Alam, C.; Valkonen, S.; Palagani, V.; Jalava, J.; Eerola, E.; Hanninen, A. Inflammatory tendencies and overproduction of IL-17 in the colon of young NOD mice are counteracted with diet change. *Diabetes* **2010**, *59*, 2237–2246. [CrossRef] [PubMed]
71. Chakir, H.; Lefebvre, D.E.; Wang, H.; Caraher, E.; Scott, F.W. Wheat protein-induced proinflammatory T helper 1 bias in mesenteric lymph nodes of young diabetes-prone rats. *Diabetologia* **2005**, *48*, 1576–1584. [CrossRef] [PubMed]
72. Antvorskov, J.C.; Fundova, P.; Buschard, K.; Funda, D.P. Impact of dietary gluten on regulatory T cells and Th17 cells in BALB/c mice. *PLoS ONE* **2012**, *7*, e33315. [CrossRef] [PubMed]
73. Antvorskov, J.C.; Fundova, P.; Buschard, K.; Funda, D.P. Dietary gluten alters the balance of pro-inflammatory and anti-inflammatory cytokines in T cells of BALB/c mice. *Immunology* **2013**, *138*, 23–33. [CrossRef] [PubMed]
74. Thomas, K.E.; Sapone, A.; Fasano, A.; Vogel, S.N. Gliadin stimulation of murine macrophage inflammatory gene expression and intestinal permeability are MyD88-dependent: Role of the innate immune response in Celiac disease. *J. Immunol.* **2006**, *176*, 2512–2521. [CrossRef] [PubMed]
75. Nikulina, M.; Habich, C.; Flohe, S.B.; Scott, F.W.; Kolb, H. Wheat gluten causes dendritic cell maturation and chemokine secretion. *J. Immunol.* **2004**, *173*, 1925–1933. [CrossRef] [PubMed]
76. Ciccocioppo, R.; Rossi, M.; Pesce, I.; Ricci, G.; Millimaggi, D.; Maurano, F.; Corazza, G.R. Effects of gliadin stimulation on bone marrow-derived dendritic cells from HLA-DQ8 transgenic MICE. *Dig. Liver Dis.* **2008**, *40*, 927–935. [CrossRef] [PubMed]
77. Healey, D.; Ozegbe, P.; Arden, S.; Chandler, P.; Hutton, J.; Cooke, A. In vivo activity and in vitro specificity of CD4+ Th1 and Th2 cells derived from the spleens of diabetic NOD mice. *J. Clin. Investig.* **1995**, *95*, 2979–2985. [CrossRef] [PubMed]
78. Yang, X.; Zheng, S.G. Interleukin-22: A likely target for treatment of autoimmune diseases. *Autoimmun. Rev.* **2014**, *13*, 615–620. [CrossRef] [PubMed]
79. Catassi, C.; Guerrieri, A.; Bartolotta, E.; Coppa, G.V.; Giorgi, P.L. Antigliadin antibodies at onset of diabetes in children. *Lancet* **1987**, *2*, 158. [CrossRef]
80. Troncone, R.; Franzese, A.; Mazzarella, G.; Paparo, F.; Auricchio, R.; Coto, I.; Mayer, M.; Greco, L. Gluten sensitivity in a subset of children with insulin dependent diabetes mellitus. *Am. J. Gastroenterol.* **2003**, *98*, 590–595. [CrossRef] [PubMed]
81. Mojibian, M.; Chakir, H.; Lefebvre, D.E.; Crookshank, J.A.; Sonier, B.; Keely, E.; Scott, F.W. Diabetes-specific HLA-DR-restricted proinflammatory T-cell response to wheat polypeptides in tissue transglutaminase antibody-negative patients with type 1 diabetes. *Diabetes* **2009**, *58*, 1789–1796. [CrossRef] [PubMed]
82. Hamari, S.; Kirveskoski, T.; Glumoff, V.; Kulmala, P.; Simell, O.; Knip, M.; Ilonen, J.; Veijola, R. CD4(+) T-cell proliferation responses to wheat polypeptide stimulation in children at different stages of type 1 diabetes autoimmunity. *Pediatr. Diabetes* **2015**, *16*, 177–188. [CrossRef] [PubMed]
83. Palova-Jelinkova, L.; Rozkova, D.; Pecharova, B.; Bartova, J.; Sediva, A.; Tlaskalova-Hogenova, H.; Spisek, R.; Tuckova, L. Gliadin fragments induce phenotypic and functional maturation of human dendritic cells. *J. Immunol.* **2005**, *175*, 7038–7045. [CrossRef] [PubMed]
84. Molberg, O.; McAdam, S.; Lundin, K.E.; Kristiansen, C.; Arentz-Hansen, H.; Kett, K.; Sollid, L.M. T cells from celiac disease lesions recognize gliadin epitopes deamidated in situ by endogenous tissue transglutaminase. *Eur. J. Immunol.* **2001**, *31*, 1317–1323. [CrossRef]
85. Molberg, O.; McAdam, S.N.; Korner, R.; Quarsten, H.; Kristiansen, C.; Madsen, L.; Fugger, L.; Scott, H.; Noren, O.; Roepstorff, P.; et al. Tissue transglutaminase selectively modifies gliadin peptides that are recognized by gut-derived T cells in celiac disease. *Nat. Med.* **1998**, *4*, 713–717. [CrossRef] [PubMed]
86. Serena, G.; Camhi, S.; Sturgeon, C.; Yan, S.; Fasano, A. The Role of Gluten in Celiac Disease and Type 1 Diabetes. *Nutrients* **2015**, *7*, 7143–7162. [CrossRef] [PubMed]

87. Cosnes, J.; Cellier, C.; Viola, S.; Colombel, J.F.; Michaud, L.; Sarles, J.; Hugot, J.P.; Ginies, J.L.; Dabadie, A.; Mouterde, O.; et al. Incidence of autoimmune diseases in celiac disease: Protective effect of the gluten-free diet. *Clin. Gastroenterol. Hepatol.* **2008**, *6*, 753–758. [CrossRef] [PubMed]
88. Barera, G.; Bonfanti, R.; Viscardi, M.; Bazzigaluppi, E.; Calori, G.; Meschi, F.; Bianchi, C.; Chiumello, G. Occurrence of celiac disease after onset of type 1 diabetes: A 6-year prospective longitudinal study. *Pediatrics* **2002**, *109*, 833–838. [CrossRef] [PubMed]
89. Hansen, D.; Bennedbaek, F.N.; Hansen, L.K.; Hoier-Madsen, M.; Hegedu, L.S.; Jacobsen, B.B.; Husby, S. High prevalence of coeliac disease in Danish children with type I. diabetes mellitus. *Acta. Paediatr.* **2001**, *90*, 1238–1243. [CrossRef] [PubMed]
90. Aktay, A.N.; Lee, P.C.; Kumar, V.; Parton, E.; Wyatt, D.T.; Werlin, S.L. The prevalence and clinical characteristics of celiac disease in juvenile diabetes in Wisconsin. *J. Pediatr. Gastroenterol. Nutr.* **2001**, *33*, 462–465. [CrossRef] [PubMed]
91. Not, T.; Tommasini, A.; Tonini, G.; Buratti, E.; Pocecco, M.; Tortul, C.; Valussi, M.; Crichiutti, G.; Berti, I.; Trevisiol, C.; et al. Undiagnosed coeliac disease and risk of autoimmune disorders in subjects with Type, I. diabetes mellitus. *Diabetologia* **2001**, *44*, 151–155. [CrossRef] [PubMed]
92. Carlsson, A.K.; Axelsson, I.E.; Borulf, S.K.; Bredberg, A.C.; Lindberg, B.A.; Sjoberg, K.G.; Ivarsson, S.A. Prevalence of IgA-antiendomysium and IgA-antigliadin autoantibodies at diagnosis of insulin-dependent diabetes mellitus in Swedish children and adolescents. *Pediatrics* **1999**, *103*, 1248–1252. [CrossRef] [PubMed]
93. Sblattero, D.; Maurano, F.; Mazzarella, G.; Rossi, M.; Auricchio, S.; Florian, F.; Ziberna, F.; Tommasini, A.; Not, T.; Ventura, A.; et al. Characterization of the anti-tissue transglutaminase antibody response in nonobese diabetic mice. *J. Immunol.* **2005**, *174*, 5830–5836. [CrossRef] [PubMed]
94. Burbelo, P.D.; Lebovitz, E.E.; Bren, K.E.; Bayat, A.; Paviol, S.; Wenzlau, J.M.; Barriga, K.J.; Rewers, M.; Harlan, D.M.; Iadarola, M.J. Extrapancreatic autoantibody profiles in type I. diabetes. *PLoS ONE* **2012**, *7*, e45216. [CrossRef] [PubMed]
95. Maurano, F.; Mazzarella, G.; Luongo, D.; Stefanile, R.; D'Arienzo, R.; Rossi, M.; Auricchio, S.; Troncone, R. Small intestinal enteropathy in non-obese diabetic mice fed a diet containing wheat. *Diabetologia* **2005**, *48*, 931–937. [CrossRef] [PubMed]
96. Auricchio, R.; Paparo, F.; Maglio, M.; Franzese, A.; Lombardi, F.; Valerio, G.; Nardone, G.; Percopo, S.; Greco, L.; Troncone, R. In vitro-deranged intestinal immune response to gliadin in type 1 diabetes. *Diabetes* **2004**, *53*, 1680–1683. [CrossRef] [PubMed]
97. Scott, F.W.; Rowsell, P.; Wang, G.S.; Burghardt, K.; Kolb, H.; Flohe, S. Oral exposure to diabetes-promoting food or immunomodulators in neonates alters gut cytokines and diabetes. *Diabetes* **2002**, *51*, 73–78. [CrossRef] [PubMed]
98. Funda, D.P.; Kaas, A.; Tlaskalova-Hogenova, H.; Buschard, K. Gluten-free but also gluten-enriched (gluten+) diet prevent diabetes in NOD mice; the gluten enigma in type 1 diabetes. *Diabetes Metab. Res. Rev.* **2008**, *24*, 59–63. [CrossRef] [PubMed]
99. Labeta, M.O.; Durieux, J.J.; Spagnoli, G.; Fernandez, N.; Wijdenes, J.; Herrmann, R. CD14 and tolerance to lipopolysaccharide: Biochemical and functional analysis. *Immunology* **1993**, *80*, 415–423. [PubMed]
100. Funda, D.P.; Fundova, P.; Hansen, A.K.; Buschard, K. Prevention or early cure of type 1 diabetes by intranasal administration of gliadin in NOD mice. *PLoS ONE* **2014**, *9*, e94530. [CrossRef] [PubMed]
101. Locke, N.R.; Stankovic, S.; Funda, D.P.; Harrison, L.C. TCR gamma delta intraepithelial lymphocytes are required for self-tolerance. *J. Immunol.* **2006**, *176*, 6553–6559. [CrossRef] [PubMed]
102. Lindley, S.; Dayan, C.M.; Bishop, A.; Roep, B.O.; Peakman, M.; Tree, T.I. Defective suppressor function in CD4(+) CD25(+) T-cells from patients with type 1 diabetes. *Diabetes* **2005**, *54*, 92–99. [CrossRef] [PubMed]
103. Haupt-Jorgensen, M.; Nielsen, E.; Engkilde, K.; Lerche, M.; Larsen, J.; Buschard, K. Occupation with grain crops is associated with lower type 1 diabetes incidence: Registry-based case-control study. *PLoS ONE* **2017**, *12*, e0181143. [CrossRef] [PubMed]
104. Bruun, S.W.; Josefsen, K.; Tanassi, J.T.; Marek, A.; Pedersen, M.H.; Sidenius, U.; Haupt-Jorgensen, M.; Antvorskov, J.C.; Larsen, J.; Heegaard, N.H.; et al. Large Gliadin Peptides Detected in the Pancreas of NOD and Healthy Mice following Oral Administration. *J. Diabetes Res.* **2016**, *2016*, 2424306. [CrossRef] [PubMed]

105. Freire, R.H.; Fernandes, L.R.; Silva, R.B.; Coelho, B.S.; de Araujo, L.P.; Ribeiro, L.S.; Andrade, J.M.; Lima, P.M.; Araujo, R.S.; Santos, S.H.; et al. Wheat gluten intake increases weight gain and adiposity associated with reduced thermogenesis and energy expenditure in an animal model of obesity. *Int. J. Obes.* **2016**, *40*, 479–486. [CrossRef] [PubMed]
106. Chirdo, F.G.; Rumbo, M.; Anon, M.C.; Fossati, C.A. Presence of high levels of non-degraded gliadin in breast milk from healthy mothers. *Scand. J. Gastroenterol.* **1998**, *33*, 1186–1192. [PubMed]
107. In't Veld, P.; Marichal, M. Microscopic anatomy of the human islet of Langerhans. *Adv. Exp. Med. Biol.* **2010**, *654*, 1–19. [CrossRef] [PubMed]
108. Dall, M.; Calloe, K.; Haupt-Jorgensen, M.; Larsen, J.; Schmitt, N.; Josefsen, K.; Buschard, K. Gliadin fragments and a specific gliadin 33-mer peptide close KATP channels and induce insulin secretion in INS-1E cells and rat islets of langerhans. *PLoS ONE* **2013**, *8*, e66474. [CrossRef] [PubMed]
109. Aaen, K.; Rygaard, J.; Josefsen, K.; Petersen, H.; Brogren, C.H.; Horn, T.; Buschard, K. Dependence of antigen expression on functional state of beta-cells. *Diabetes* **1990**, *39*, 697–701. [CrossRef] [PubMed]
110. Ientile, R.; Caccamo, D.; Griffin, M. Tissue transglutaminase and the stress response. *Amino Acids* **2007**, *33*, 385–394. [CrossRef] [PubMed]
111. Van Lummel, M.; Duinkerken, G.; van Veelen, P.A.; De Ru, A.; Cordfunke, R.; Zaldumbide, A.; Gomez-Tourino, I.; Arif, S.; Peakman, M.; Drijfhout, J.W.; et al. Posttranslational modification of HLA-DQ binding islet autoantigens in type 1 diabetes. *Diabetes* **2014**, *63*, 237–247. [CrossRef] [PubMed]
112. Shaw, J.E.; Sicree, R.A.; Zimmet, P.Z. Global estimates of the prevalence of diabetes for 2010 and 2030. *Diabetes Res. Clin. Pract.* **2010**, *87*, 4–14. [CrossRef] [PubMed]
113. Leahy, J.L. Natural history of beta-cell dysfunction in NIDDM. *Diabetes Care* **1990**, *13*, 992–1010. [CrossRef] [PubMed]
114. Perley, M.; Kipnis, D.M. Plasma insulin responses to glucose and tolbutamide of normal weight and obese diabetic and nondiabetic subjects. *Diabetes* **1966**, *15*, 867–874. [CrossRef] [PubMed]
115. Kloppel, G.; Lohr, M.; Habich, K.; Oberholzer, M.; Heitz, P.U. Islet pathology and the pathogenesis of type 1 and type 2 diabetes mellitus revisited. *Surv. Synth. Pathol. Res.* **1985**, *4*, 110–125. [PubMed]
116. Kahn, S.E. Clinical review 135: The importance of beta-cell failure in the development and progression of type 2 diabetes. *J. Clin. Endocrinol. Metab.* **2001**, *86*, 4047–4058. [CrossRef] [PubMed]
117. Florez, J.C.; Hirschhorn, J.; Altshuler, D. The inherited basis of diabetes mellitus: Implications for the genetic analysis of complex traits. *Annu. Rev. Genomics Hum. Genet.* **2003**, *4*, 257–291. [CrossRef] [PubMed]
118. Poulsen, P.; Kyvik, K.O.; Vaag, A.; Beck-Nielsen, H. Heritability of type II (non-insulin-dependent) diabetes mellitus and abnormal glucose tolerance–a population-based twin study. *Diabetologia* **1999**, *42*, 139–145. [CrossRef] [PubMed]
119. Diabetes mellitus in twins: A cooperative study in Japan. Committee on Diabetic Twins, Japan Diabetes Society. *Diabetes Res. Clin. Pract.* **1988**, *5*, 271–280. [CrossRef]
120. Romao, I.; Roth, J. Genetic and environmental interactions in obesity and type 2 diabetes. *J. Am. Diet. Assoc.* **2008**, *108*, S24–S28. [CrossRef] [PubMed]
121. Alberti, G.; Zimmet, P.; Shaw, J.; Bloomgarden, Z.; Kaufman, F.; Silink, M. Type 2 diabetes in the young: The evolving epidemic: The international diabetes federation consensus workshop. *Diabetes Care* **2004**, *27*, 1798–1811. [CrossRef] [PubMed]
122. Neel, J.V. Diabetes mellitus: A 'thrifty' genotype rendered detrimental by 'progress'? *Am. J. Hum. Genet.* **1962**, *14*, 353–362. [PubMed]
123. Tinggaard, J.; Wohlfahrt-Veje, C.; Husby, S.; Christiansen, L.; Skakkebaek, N.E.; Jensen, T.K.; Grandjean, P.; Main, K.M.; Andersen, H.R. Prenatal pesticide exposure and PON1 genotype associated with adolescent body fat distribution evaluated by dual X-ray absorptiometry (DXA). *Andrology* **2016**, *4*, 735–744. [CrossRef] [PubMed]
124. Hales, C.N.; Barker, D.J. Type 2 (non-insulin-dependent) diabetes mellitus: The thrifty phenotype hypothesis. *Diabetologia* **1992**, *35*, 595–601. [CrossRef] [PubMed]
125. Jonsson, T.; Memon, A.A.; Sundquist, K.; Sundquist, J.; Olsson, S.; Nalla, A.; Bauer, M.; Linse, S. Digested wheat gluten inhibits binding between leptin and its receptor. *BMC Biochem.* **2015**, *16*, 3. [CrossRef] [PubMed]
126. Pan, H.; Guo, J.; Su, Z. Advances in understanding the interrelations between leptin resistance and obesity. *Physiol. Behav.* **2014**, *130*, 157–169. [CrossRef] [PubMed]

127. Jonsson, T.; Olsson, S.; Ahren, B.; Bog-Hansen, T.C.; Dole, A.; Lindeberg, S. Agrarian diet and diseases of affluence–do evolutionary novel dietary lectins cause leptin resistance? *BMC Endocr. Disord.* **2005**, *5*, 10. [CrossRef] [PubMed]
128. Jonsson, T.; Ahren, B.; Pacini, G.; Sundler, F.; Wierup, N.; Steen, S.; Sjoberg, T.; Ugander, M.; Frostegard, J.; Goransson, L.; et al. A Paleolithic diet confers higher insulin sensitivity, lower C-reactive protein and lower blood pressure than a cereal-based diet in domestic pigs. *Nutr. Metab.* **2006**, *3*, 39. [CrossRef] [PubMed]
129. Tilg, H.; Moschen, A.R. Microbiota and diabetes: An evolving relationship. *Gut* **2014**, *63*, 1513–1521. [CrossRef] [PubMed]
130. Ley, R.E.; Turnbaugh, P.J.; Klein, S.; Gordon, J.I. Microbial ecology: Human gut microbes associated with obesity. *Nature* **2006**, *444*, 1022–1023. [CrossRef] [PubMed]
131. Turnbaugh, P.J.; Ley, R.E.; Mahowald, M.A.; Magrini, V.; Mardis, E.R.; Gordon, J.I. An obesity-associated gut microbiome with increased capacity for energy harvest. *Nature* **2006**, *444*, 1027–1031. [CrossRef] [PubMed]
132. Karlsson, F.H.; Tremaroli, V.; Nookaew, I.; Bergstrom, G.; Behre, C.J.; Fagerberg, B.; Nielsen, J.; Backhed, F. Gut metagenome in European women with normal, impaired and diabetic glucose control. *Nature* **2013**, *498*, 99–103. [CrossRef] [PubMed]
133. Lu, Y.; Fan, C.; Li, P.; Lu, Y.; Chang, X.; Qi, K. Short Chain Fatty Acids Prevent High-fat-diet-induced Obesity in Mice by Regulating G Protein-coupled Receptors and Gut Microbiota. *Sci. Rep.* **2016**, *6*, 37589. [CrossRef] [PubMed]
134. Horton, F.; Wright, J.; Smith, L.; Hinton, P.J.; Robertson, M.D. Increased intestinal permeability to oral chromium (51 Cr) -EDTA in human Type 2 diabetes. *Diabet. Med.* **2014**, *31*, 559–563. [CrossRef] [PubMed]
135. Cox, A.J.; Zhang, P.; Bowden, D.W.; Devereaux, B.; Davoren, P.M.; Cripps, A.W.; West, N.P. Increased intestinal permeability as a risk factor for type 2 diabetes. *Diabetes Metab.* **2017**, *43*, 163–166. [CrossRef] [PubMed]
136. Zhang, L.; Andersen, D.; Roager, H.M.; Bahl, M.I.; Hansen, C.H.; Danneskiold-Samsoe, N.B.; Kristiansen, K.; Radulescu, I.D.; Sina, C.; Frandsen, H.L.; et al. Effects of Gliadin consumption on the Intestinal Microbiota and Metabolic Homeostasis in Mice Fed a High-fat Diet. *Sci. Rep.* **2017**, *7*, 44613. [CrossRef] [PubMed]
137. Rajilic-Stojanovic, M.; De Vos, W.M. The first 1000 cultured species of the human gastrointestinal microbiota. *FEMS Microbiol. Rev.* **2014**, *38*, 996–1047. [CrossRef] [PubMed]
138. Clavel, T.; Desmarchelier, C.; Haller, D.; Gerard, P.; Rohn, S.; Lepage, P.; Daniel, H. Intestinal microbiota in metabolic diseases: From bacterial community structure and functions to species of pathophysiological relevance. *Gut Microbes* **2014**, *5*, 544–551. [CrossRef] [PubMed]
139. Saulnier, D.M.; Riehle, K.; Mistretta, T.A.; Diaz, M.A.; Mandal, D.; Raza, S.; Weidler, E.M.; Qin, X.; Coarfa, C.; Milosavljevic, A.; et al. Gastrointestinal microbiome signatures of pediatric patients with irritable bowel syndrome. *Gastroenterology* **2011**, *141*, 1782–1791. [CrossRef] [PubMed]
140. Rajilic-Stojanovic, M.; Biagi, E.; Heilig, H.G.; Kajander, K.; Kekkonen, R.A.; Tims, S.; de Vos, W.M. Global and deep molecular analysis of microbiota signatures in fecal samples from patients with irritable bowel syndrome. *Gastroenterology* **2011**, *141*, 1792–1801. [CrossRef] [PubMed]
141. Everard, A.; Belzer, C.; Geurts, L.; Ouwerkerk, J.P.; Druart, C.; Bindels, L.B.; Guiot, Y.; Derrien, M.; Muccioli, G.G.; Delzenne, N.M.; et al. Cross-talk between Akkermansia muciniphila and intestinal epithelium controls diet-induced obesity. *Proc. Natl. Acad. Sci. USA* **2013**, *110*, 9066–9071. [CrossRef] [PubMed]
142. Zhang, X.; Shen, D.; Fang, Z.; Jie, Z.; Qiu, X.; Zhang, C.; Chen, Y.; Ji, L. Human gut microbiota changes reveal the progression of glucose intolerance. *PLoS ONE* **2013**, *8*, e71108. [CrossRef] [PubMed]
143. Amar, J.; Chabo, C.; Waget, A.; Klopp, P.; Vachoux, C.; Bermudez-Humaran, L.G.; Smirnova, N.; Berge, M.; Sulpice, T.; Lahtinen, S.; et al. Intestinal mucosal adherence and translocation of commensal bacteria at the early onset of type 2 diabetes: Molecular mechanisms and probiotic treatment. *EMBO Mol. Med.* **2011**, *3*, 559–572. [CrossRef] [PubMed]
144. Fagerberg, L.; Hallstrom, B.M.; Oksvold, P.; Kampf, C.; Djureinovic, D.; Odeberg, J.; Habuka, M.; Tahmasebpoor, S.; Danielsson, A.; Edlund, K.; et al. Analysis of the human tissue-specific expression by genome-wide integration of transcriptomics and antibody-based proteomics. *Mol. Cell. Proteom.* **2014**, *13*, 397–406. [CrossRef] [PubMed]
145. Shi, H.; Kokoeva, M.V.; Inouye, K.; Tzameli, I.; Yin, H.; Flier, J.S. TLR4 links innate immunity and fatty acid-induced insulin resistance. *J. Clin. Investig.* **2006**, *116*, 3015–3025. [CrossRef] [PubMed]

146. Ladefoged, M.; Buschard, K.; Hansen, A.M. Increased expression of toll-like receptor 4 and inflammatory cytokines, interleukin-6 in particular, in islets from a mouse model of obesity and type 2 diabetes. *APMIS* **2013**, *121*, 531–538. [CrossRef] [PubMed]
147. Palova-Jelinkova, L.; Danova, K.; Drasarova, H.; Dvorak, M.; Funda, D.P.; Fundova, P.; Kotrbova-Kozak, A.; Cerna, M.; Kamanova, J.; Martin, S.F.; et al. Pepsin digest of wheat gliadin fraction increases production of IL-1beta via TLR4/MyD88/TRIF/MAPK/NF-kappaB signaling pathway and an NLRP3 inflammasome activation. *PLoS ONE* **2013**, *8*, e62426. [CrossRef] [PubMed]
148. Mokady, S.; Einav, P. Effect of dietary wheat gluten in lipid metabolism in growing rats. *Nutr. Metab.* **1978**, *22*, 181–189. [CrossRef] [PubMed]
149. Soares, F.L.; de Oliveira Matoso, R.; Teixeira, L.G.; Menezes, Z.; Pereira, S.S.; Alves, A.C.; Batista, N.V.; De Faria, A.M.; Cara, D.C.; Ferreira, A.V.; et al. Gluten-free diet reduces adiposity, inflammation and insulin resistance associated with the induction of PPAR-alpha and PPAR-gamma expression. *J. Nutr. Biochem.* **2013**, *24*, 1105–1111. [CrossRef] [PubMed]
150. Haupt-Jorgensen, M.; Buschard, K.; Hansen, A.K.; Josefsen, K.; Antvorskov, J.C. Gluten-free diet increases beta-cell volume and improves glucose tolerance in an animal model of type 2 diabetes. *Diabetes Metab. Res. Rev.* **2016**, *32*, 675–684. [CrossRef] [PubMed]
151. Rune, I.; Rolin, B.; Larsen, C.; Nielsen, D.S.; Kanter, J.E.; Bornfeldt, K.E.; Lykkesfeldt, J.; Buschard, K.; Kirk, R.K.; Christoffersen, B.; et al. Modulating the Gut Microbiota Improves Glucose Tolerance, Lipoprotein Profile and Atherosclerotic Plaque Development in ApoE-Deficient Mice. *PLoS ONE* **2016**, *11*, e0146439. [CrossRef] [PubMed]
152. Mortensen, L.S.; Hartvigsen, M.L.; Brader, L.J.; Astrup, A.; Schrezenmeir, J.; Holst, J.J.; Thomsen, C.; Hermansen, K. Differential effects of protein quality on postprandial lipemia in response to a fat-rich meal in type 2 diabetes: Comparison of whey, casein, gluten, and cod protein. *Am. J. Clin. Nutr.* **2009**, *90*, 41–48. [CrossRef] [PubMed]
153. Kim, H.S.; Demyen, M.F.; Mathew, J.; Kothari, N.; Feurdean, M.; Ahlawat, S.K. Obesity, Metabolic Syndrome, and Cardiovascular Risk in Gluten-Free Followers Without Celiac Disease in the United States: Results from the National Health and Nutrition Examination Survey 2009–2014. *Dig. Dis. Sci.* **2017**. [CrossRef] [PubMed]
154. Mari-Bauset, S.; Llopis-Gonzalez, A.; Zazpe, I.; Mari-Sanchis, A.; Suarez-Varela, M.M. Nutritional Impact of a Gluten-Free Casein-Free Diet in Children with Autism Spectrum Disorder. *J. Autism. Dev. Disord.* **2016**, *46*, 673–684. [CrossRef] [PubMed]
155. Zong, G.; Lebwohl, B.; Hu, F.B.; Sampson, L.; Dougherty, L.W.; Willett, W.C.; Chan, A.T.; Sun, Q. Gluten intake and risk of type 2 diabetes in three large prospective cohort studies of US men and women. *Diabetologia* **2018**, *61*, 2164–2173. [CrossRef] [PubMed]

nutrients

MDPI

Article

A Retrospective Study on Dietary FODMAP Intake in Celiac Patients Following a Gluten-Free Diet

Leda Roncoroni [1,2,*], Luca Elli [1], Luisa Doneda [2], Karla A. Bascuñán [1,3], Maurizio Vecchi [4,5], Federico Morreale [6], Alice Scricciolo [1], Vincenza Lombardo [1] and Nicoletta Pellegrini [6]

1 Center for Prevention and Diagnosis of Celiac Disease, Gastroenterology and Endoscopy Unit, Fondazione IRCCS Ca' Granda, Ospedale Maggiore Policlinico, 20122 Milan, Italy; lucelli@yahoo.it (L.E.); kbascunan@med.uchile.cl (K.A.B.); scricciolo.alice@gmail.com (A.S.); vicky.l@hotmail.it (V.L.)

2 Department of Biomedical, Surgical and Dental Sciences, University of Milan, 20131 Milan, Italy; luisa.doneda@unimi.it

3 Department of Nutrition, University of Chile, 8380453 Santiago, Chile

4 Department of Pathophysiology and Transplantation, University of Milan, 20122 Milan, Italy; maurizio.vecchi@policlinico.mi.it

5 Gastroenterology and Endoscopic Unit, Fondazione IRCCS Ca' Granda, Ospedale Maggiore Policlinico, 20122 Milan, Italy

6 Human Nutrition Unit, Department of Food and Drug, University of Parma, 43121 Parma, Italy; morreale.federico@gmail.com (F.M.); nicoletta.pellegrini@unipr.it (N.P.)

* Correspondence: leda.roncoroni@unimi.it; Tel.: +39-02-5503-3384

Received: 13 October 2018; Accepted: 12 November 2018; Published: 15 November 2018

Abstract: Our aim was to evaluate the intake of foods containing fermentable oligo/di/mono-saccharides and polyols (FODMAP) as a possible factor that induces gastrointestinal symptoms in treated celiac disease (CD) patients. We collected seven-day weighed food records for 104 CD patients and 91 healthy volunteers. All evaluated food items were from sources with high and low content of FODMAP, which were divided into cereals and sweets, sweeteners and soft drinks, fruits, dried fruits, and vegetables. Nutrient intake was calculated using the food database of the European Institute of Oncology. The symptoms reported were assessed by a Rome IV Irritable bowel syndrome (IBS) diagnostic questionnaire and by specific questions for the evaluation of functional gastrointestinal disorders (FGIDs). The 12% of CD patients met IBS symptoms criteria as opposed to 6% of controls ($p = 0.09$) and 27% of patients reported FGIDs symptoms vs. 22% of healthy controls ($p = 0.42$). The intake by CD patients was significantly higher than healthy volunteers for: sweeteners and sugars with low content of FODMAP ($p = 0.0007$), fruits, dried fruits, and vegetables high in FODMAP ($p = 0.003$) and low in FODMAP ($p = 0.04$) when compared to controls. CD patients had a lower intake of cereals and sweets with a high content of FODMAP ($p = 0.00001$). Healthy volunteers consumed significantly higher alcoholic beverages and fats high in FODMAP (both $p < 0.044$). The mean daily intake of other food categories did not differ between both groups. Even though CD patients had a low intake of gluten-free cereals high in FODMAP, they still consumed a significant amount of fruits and vegetables high in FODMAP. The clinical effect of a concomitant gluten-free diet and low-FODMAP diet should be prospectively evaluated as a supportive therapy in CD patients.

Keywords: FODMAP intake; celiac disease; irritable bowel syndrome; gluten-free diet; gastrointestinal symptoms

1. Introduction

Celiac disease (CD) is a chronic autoimmune enteropathy triggered by dietary exposure to gluten and is characterized by villous atrophy. CD is considered the most common chronic enteropathy in Western countries with an estimated prevalence ranging from 0.5 to 1% [1,2]. An altered T cell mediated immune response triggered by gluten has a central role in the pathogenesis of CD. Genetic predisposition plays a key role in the development of CD and the presence of the HLA DQ2 and/or DQ8 haplotypes is a necessary (but not sufficient) factor [3,4]. CD patients may present with gastrointestinal symptoms, extra-intestinal symptoms, or no symptoms at all. The classical clinical symptoms include diarrhea, steatorrhea, and weight loss due to malabsorption [5].

Gluten is a complex of high molecular-weight proteins found in the endosperm of grass-borne grains including wheat, barley, and rye [6]. The treatment of CD is the withdrawal of gluten from the diet (i.e., a gluten-free diet, GFD), which usually silences symptoms and normalizes serological and histological signatures. CD is considered a lifelong disorder and, if left untreated, is associated with increased morbidity and mortality [7,8]. Despite the strict adherence to a GFD, there is a group of CD patients who keep suffering from functional gastrointestinal disorders (FGIDs) [9]. FGIDs include irritable bowel syndrome (IBS) and non-specific gastrointestinal symptoms (pain, diarrhea, bloating, nausea, vomiting). IBS is currently identified to be a global problem with a prevalence of 11%, which specifically affects women as compared to men (14.0% vs. 8.9%, respectively) [10,11]. IBS is characterized by a multiplicity of clinical symptoms such as abdominal pain, bloating, and changes in bowel habits including constipation and/or diarrhea. It also compromises the patients' abilities and quality of life, which implicates an increase in healthcare provision costs, use of drugs, and absence/leave from work [12].

The criteria for diagnosing gastrointestinal disorders have been revised by the Rome Foundation in their latest update (Rome IV, 2016). The pathogenesis of IBS is multi-factorial and may be connected to visceral hyper-sensitivity, alterations of the gut-brain axis and the microbiota, post infectious consequences, and environmental and genetic factors [13]. IBS can be suspected in patients suffering from persistent abdominal pain associated with more than one condition: defecation, change in the frequency of defecation, and change of stool form [14]. Moreover, IBS can be classified as IBS-C (predominant constipation), IBS-D (predominant diarrhea), and IBS-M (mixed) [15]. Nowadays medication (antispasmodics, bulking agents, probiotics, laxatives, or anti-depressants), diet, and lifestyle adjustments have been the main therapeutic options for IBS [16].

In recent years, data supporting that the dietary restriction of fermentable oligo/di/mono-saccharides and polyols (FODMAP) for the management of IBS symptoms have emerged [17–19]. Studies evaluating a low-FODMAP diet in patients with IBS have consistently shown symptomatic benefits in the majority of patients [20]. However, one study that compared the diet commonly used in these patients vs. a low-FODMAP diet failed to demonstrate differences in the improvement of the symptomatology [21]. The use of the low-FODMAP diet has been evaluated in other digestive pathologies with contradictory results. Pedersen et al. showed some degree of improvement in functional gut symptoms of patients with inflammatory bowel disease (IBD) [22] while Cox et al. showed exacerbated functional gastrointestinal symptoms in patients with IBD [23]. On the other hand, Testa et al. were able to demonstrate that a low-FODMAP diet could be one option to counteract abdominal symptoms in patients with IBS, non-active IBD, or CD on a GFD, which improves their quality of life [24].

The main dietary sources of FODMAP include fructose in honey, apples, and pears, fructans in wheat, rye, onion, and garlic, galactans in cabbage and legumes, lactose in milk and dairy products, and polyols including sorbitol and mannitol in stone fruits, mushrooms, and artificial sweeteners [25]. Among FODMAP, fructans and galacto-oligosaccharides are considered prebiotics. Prebiotics are non-digestible selectively fermented dietary fibers that promote the growth of positive bacterial genera in the gastrointestinal tract. Prebiotics such as inulin-type provides health benefits to the host [26]. These non-digestible food ingredients are also extensively employed in the food industry [27]. The main feature of these carbohydrates is their poor absorption in the small bowel. This is due to different reasons including reduced or absent digestive enzymes or by their slow transport across the intestinal mucosa. Undigested and unabsorbed FODMAP have the peculiarity to be highly osmotic and rapidly fermented by bacteria in the gut, which causes distension, bloating, cramping, and diarrhea, which are all symptoms found in IBS [28]. Moreover, high concentrations of FODMAP in the ileum and proximal colon exert osmotic pressure, which draws greater amounts of water into the lumen [29]. Fermentation as produced by short-chain FODMAP intensifies the luminal H_2 and CH_4 production and causes pain in the lumen. This gas production can be measured with a breath test, which shows an increase between 0–5 h after the ingestion of FODMAP [30]. As proposed mechanisms, it has been recently shown as a link between FODMAP and inflammation induction in vivo [31]. Zhou et al. [32] reported that a high-FODMAP diet could increase the serum lipopolysaccharide level and intestinal inflammation together with visceral hypersensitivity. On the contrary, a diet low in FODMAP could reduce LPS levels and the inflammatory status.

Nowadays, it is of great interest to evaluate if persistent gastrointestinal symptoms in celiac patients, classified as FGIDs and IBS, can be provoked by the ingestion of FODMAP. We aimed to evaluate the intake of foods containing FODMAP in a group of patients with CD compared with the intake of healthy volunteers.

2. Materials and Methods

2.1. Patients

The participants were recruited among patients referred to the Center of Prevention and Diagnosis of Celiac Disease Fondazione IRCCS Ca' Granda Ospedale Maggiore Policlinico, Milan, Italy. All the subjects were recruited between October 2012 and August 2014 and the data were collected during the same period. Over that time, during their annual medical examination, the patients were screened for their adherence to GFD by using the celiac diet adherence test (CDAT) [33].

The enrolment process of CD patients and healthy individuals has been previously described [34,35]. All patients included in the study fulfilled the Rome IV questionnaire criteria for IBS, functional dyspepsia, and functional bloating [15]. In detail, each patient was asked if they have had recurrent abdominal pain arising for at least 6 months and being present at least once a week in the last 3 months, which is associated with changes in the stool's volume and consistency. The presence of diarrhea and/or constipation associated with abdominal pain was confirmed in case of presence of IBS. They were also asked for the presence of dyspepsia and/or any other functional symptoms such as bloating (for FGIDs). The exclusion criteria were: CD diagnosis less than two years, the presence of metabolic or chronic disease (e.g., diabetes mellitus, Crohn's Disease, cardiovascular and neuro-vascular disease, cancer, neuro-degenerative disease, and rheumatoid arthritis), pregnancy or lactation, vegetarianism, or veganism. A group of healthy volunteers was recruited among students, researchers, and professors of the Universities of Parma, Parma, and University of the Studies, Milan. For healthy volunteers, CD was excluded by means of serological tests (anti-tissue transglutaminase IgA). Exclusion criteria for the healthy participants were the same as for the CD patients except for the diagnosis of CD.

The final sample included 104 celiac patients and 91 healthy controls. All the participants who agreed to participate signed a written informed consent and were enrolled in the study. The local Ethics Committee for Human Research of the City of Milan approved the protocol. The study was registered at ClinicalTrials.gov (ID NCT01975155).

2.2. Dietary Records

The total food and beverage consumption was assessed by using a food diary filled in daily for a total of seven days, which was previously described [36]. The participants were trained on how to record all of the food consumed by a nutritionist. The participants were asked to send their completed seven-day weighed food record to the Department of Food and Drugs of the University of Parma. A nutritionist reviewed the diaries and, in case of any error or omission, the participants were contacted by phone to clarify the issues.

The nutrient intake was calculated by using a Microsoft Access application (version 2003, Microsoft Corp, Redmond, WA, USA) linked to the European Institute of Oncology's food database, which covered the nutrient composition of 900+ Italian foods [37], integrated with the nutrient composition of 60 gluten-free foods available in the Italian market [38]. When a food recorded in a participant's seven-day weighed food record could not be found in the database, an alternative food was appropriately chosen based on similarities in energy and nutrient composition. The output consisted of the mean daily intake of energy and food items for each individual.

Food items of interest for the FODMAP intake evaluation were grouped into the following food categories (a summary of food sources of FODMAP, as reported in the literature, is provided in Table 1): pasta, bread (including crackers and salty snacks), other cereals (including corn, quinoa, buckwheat, and rice), fruits, vegetables and legumes, sweeteners (honey, saccharin, fructose, barley malt syrup), and sweets (including biscuits, sweet snacks, breakfast cereals, ice cream, candies, and chocolate), dried fruits, oil and fats, dairy products (including milk, yogurt, cream, cheese), soft drinks, juices, coffee/tea, and alcoholic beverages [18]. The categories of foods high and low in FODMAP content were also grouped in larger or macro-categories: cereals and sweets, sweeteners and soft drinks, fruits, dried fruits, and vegetables. For each individual, the mean daily intake of each food macro-category, i.e., low and high-FODMAP contents, was calculated.

Table 1. Foods with high and low amounts of FODMAP †.

Food Category	High in FODMAP	Low in FODMAP
Alcoholic beverages	Sweet wine, rum, vodka, whiskey	Beer, red wine, rosè wine, white wine, sparkling wine, gin
Cereals	Wheat, barley, rye, bran, whole wheat flour, spelt, Kamut® (Khorasan wheat)	Quinoa, rice, buckwheat, pearl millet, corn, gluten-free flour, bulgur, sourdough spelt bread, cornflakes, puffed rice
Sweets	Apricot jam, peach jam, blackberry jam, plum jam, milk chocolate	Strawberry jam, peanut butter, lactose-free ice cream, gluten-free sweets
Sweeteners	Honey, saccharin, fructose, malt syrup	Aspartame, sucrose, sugar, brown sugar
Fruit	Apple, apricot, avocado, ripe banana, blackberry, litchi, mango, white peach, yellow peach, pear, persimmon, pomegranate, blackcurrant, cranberry, plum, watermelon, cherry	Banana, blueberry, strawberry, raspberry, melon, white melon, kiwi, orange, mandarin orange, red grapes, black grapes, green grapes, lemon, coconut, pineapple, loquat, papaya, prickly pear, passion fruit, grapefruit
Dried fruit	Raisin, dried date, apple, apricot, fig, mango, pear, plum, cashew nut, pistachio	Hazelnut, pine nut, walnut, flax seed, sunflower seed, dried banana, coconut, dried cranberry, dried coconut
Fats	Butter, margarine, cream, lard	Olive oil, extra-virgin olive oil, sunflower oil, almond oil, peanut oil, linseed oil, sesame oil, rice oil, palm oil, coconut oil, colza oil, soybean oil
Dairy products	Milk, yogurt, fresh cheese, semi-aged cheese, aged cheese	Lactose-free milk, lactose-free yogurt, lactose-free cheese, feta, cottage cheese, Parmesan
Soft drinks	Apple juice, orange juice, apricot juice, pear juice, peach juice, pomegranate juice	Pineapple juice, lemon juice, cranberry juice, vegetables juice, orange fresh-squeezed juice
Vegetables	Red radicchio, green radicchio, artichoke, asparagus, cauliflower, red cabbage, green cabbage, sauerkraut, pea, snow pea, mushroom, garlic, leek, onion, Jerusalem artichoke, bean, white bean, lupine bean, broad bean (Vicia fabai), chickpea, broccoli, beet	Pepper, carrot, eggplant, zucchini, potato, sweet potato, tomato, lettuce, fennel, fennel leaves, spinach, chard, radish, green bean, turnip, chicory, rocket, stick, watercress, endive, valerian, olive, sweet corn, chestnut, pumpkin flower, cucumber, chives, chili pepper, ginger, Brussels cabbage, soy sprout, bean sprout, healing herb, okra, truffle, green alga, celery, pumpkin

† Examples of foods classified as having the high and low amount of FODMAP. FODMAP: fermentable oligo/di/mono-saccharides and polyols.

2.3. Statistical Analysis

Data were accordingly described as mean ± SD or median (with interquartile range), according to variables' distribution (evaluated by the Shapiro-Wilk test). The Pearson chi-square test was used to compare the number of individuals reporting IBS and FGIDs in between both studied groups. The daily nutrient intake data of energy, water, and FODMAP-containing foods were computed and tabulated. To reduce the effect of implausible extreme values on the analysis, we checked that the ratio of total energy intake determined from the food record to the basal metabolic rate (determined by the Harris-Benedict equation) of each participant was not in the first or the last percentile of the distribution. The dietary data were compared between the control patients and the celiac disease patients by using the independent sample Student's t-test or the Wilcoxon rank-sum test. STATA® v. 13.1 (StataCorp, College Station, TX, USA) was used in all the analyses. Statistical significance was set at a 5% α-level.

3. Results

Patients

Patients in the CD group were older ($p = 0.0002$) and there was a higher percentage of females in both groups (82.7% and 68.1% of CD patients and controls, respectively). Both groups were comparable regarding their mean BMI (22.4 ± 3.3 and 22.2 ± 3.0 for the CD and control group, respectively) and daily energy intake (2054.8 kcal (397.3) and 2044.7 kcal (329.3)), respectively. When analyzing the prevalence of gastrointestinal symptoms in both groups, we found out that 12% of CD patients suffered from IBS when compared with 6% of the controls ($p = 0.09$) while 27% of CD patients suffered from FGIDs symptoms (5.77% functional dyspepsia, 10.58% functional bloating) against 22% of controls ($p = 0.42$). Approximately 10.5% of CD patients did not suffer from either IBS, functional dyspepsia, or functional bloating (Figure 1).

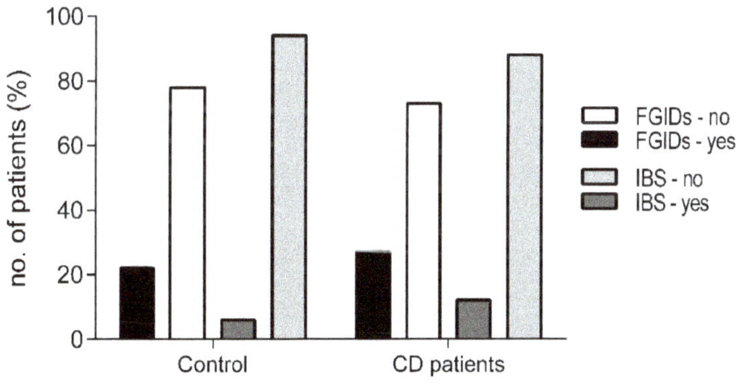

Figure 1. Presence of gastrointestinal symptoms. Data are shown as a percentage of individuals reporting IBS and FGIDs symptoms between both studied groups. IBS: Irritable bowel syndrome, FGIDs: Functional gastrointestinal disorders, CD: Celiac disease.

Regarding the dietary intake, a slightly higher total food intake was observed in the CD group, but the energy and water intake were similar between both groups (Table 2). A higher intake of foods with high FODMAP content was observed in the controls ($p < 0.001$) while a higher intake of foods with low FODMAP content was observed in CD patients ($p < 0.001$).

Table 2. Daily dietary intake of celiac patients and healthy controls.

Dietary Intake	Healthy Controls (n = 91)	Celiac Patients (n = 104)	p Value †
Food intake, g/day	1569.5 ± 337.0	1656.5 ± 284.2	0.05 ‡
Energy intake, kcal/day	2054.8 (397.3)	2044.7 (329.3)	0.68
Water intake, mL/day	742.8 (400.0)	647.1 (452.6)	0.52
High-FODMAP, g/day	681.4 (261.0)	457.4 (208.4)	0.00001
Low-FODMAP, g/day	835.1 (364.8)	1119.6 (366.9)	0.00001
High-FODMAP, %	45 (10)	28 (10)	0.00001
Low-FODMAP, %	54 (10)	71 (10)	0.00001

Data as median values (IQR) unless otherwise is indicated. a data as mean ± SD. † p value for the Wilcoxon rank-sum test unless otherwise is indicated. ‡ p value for the t-test for two independent groups.

The analysis of FODMAP-containing food intake according to food categories is shown in Tables 3 and 4. The consumption of high-FODMAP foods was higher in the control group with the exception of fruits, which was higher in the CD group. In turn, low-FODMAP food consumption was greater in the CD group. A larger amount of high-FODMAP cereals (p = 0.0001), high-FODMAP sweets (p = 0.0001), high-FODMAP alcoholic beverages (p = 0.0001), and high-FODMAP fats (p = 0.0447) was observed in the control group when compared to celiac patients. Instead, the CD group consumed significantly higher amount of cereals with low FODMAP content (p = 0.0001), low-FODMAP sweets (p = 0.0001), low-FODMAP sweeteners (p = 0.0099), fruit both high and low in FODMAPs (respectively p = 0.001 and p = 0.0158), and low-FODMAP juices (p = 0.0228). The mean daily intake of the other food categories did not differ between the two groups (Table 3).

Table 3. Daily intake of food categories containing low and high amounts of FODMAP by celiac patients and healthy controls.

Food Categories (g/day)	Healthy Controls		Celiac Patients		p Value *	p Value **
	High FODMAP	Low FODMAP	High FODMAP	Low FODMAP		
Alcoholic beverages, g/day	5.7 (57.1)	21.4 (64.2)	0 (5.7)	6.7 (61.1)	0.0001	0.22
Cereals, g/day	228.0 (61.1)	171 (30.7)	0 (0)	222.7 (95.1)	0.0001	0.0001
Sweets, g/day	22.8 (32.1)	2.1 (11.4)	2.8 (9.1)	35.7 (51.6)	0.0001	0.0001
Sweeteners, g/day	0 (1.6)	6.4 (8.8)	0 (1.2)	8.2 (11.7)	0.49	0.0099
Fruits, g/day	45.7 (108.7)	85.7 (115.7)	100.4 (126.8)	116.4 (128.0)	0.001	0.0158
Dried fruits, g/day	0 (0.2)	0 (2.1)	0 (0)	0.5 (4.1)	0.53	0.28
Fats, g/day	3.3 (6.7)	25.7 (14.4)	2.4 (5.6)	26.0 (13.6)	0.0447	0.25
Dairy, g/day	188.6 (211.4)	7.4 (16.4)	196.2 (184.2)	7.5 (17.6)	0.61	0.85
Juices, g/day	1.4 (47.1)	0 (2.8)	25.7 (67.8)	0.7 (34.2)	0.49	0.0228
Vegetables, g/day	55.0 (87.4)	236.2 (146.4)	73.1 (85.8)	245.8 (139.6)	0.21	0.60

Data as median values (IQR). * p value for comparisons between groups regarding high-FODMAP foods. ** p value for comparisons between groups regarding low-FODMAP foods.

When the foods containing FODMAP were grouped into large categories (i.e., cereals and sweets, sweeteners and sugars, fruits, dried fruits, and vegetables), a higher consumption of cereals and sweets with high FODMAP content was present in the control group (p = 0.00001) while CD patients showed significantly higher consumption of fruits, dried fruits, and vegetables with high FODMAP content (p = 0.003). In addition, other large categories of foods with low FODMAP content were significantly more consumed by the CD patients as compared to the control group (Table 4). Lastly, no correlation between FODMAP intake and gastrointestinal symptoms was found.

Table 4. Daily intake of grouped food categories containing low and high amounts of FODMAP by celiac patients and healthy controls.

Food Categories	Healthy Controls (n = 91)		Celiac Patients (n = 104)		p Value *	p Value **
	High FODMAP	Low FODMAP	High FODMAP	Low FODMAP		
Cereals & sweets, g/day	253.7 (74.2)	28.6 (37.4)	3.6 (11.4)	265.8 (103.4)	0.00001	0.00001
Sweeteners & sugar, g/day	14.2 (47.1)	9.0 (14.4)	28.6 (73.6)	15.4 (38.5)	0.64	0.0007
Fruits, dried fruits & vegetables, g/day	135.0 (185.2)	360.7 (175.2)	181.3 (126.0)	399.8 (232.1)	0.003	0.04

Data as median values (IQR). * p value for comparisons between groups regarding high-FODMAP foods. ** p value for comparisons between groups regarding low-FODMAP foods.

4. Discussion

This is the first time that a classification is made in relation to food consumption, according to the amount of FODMAP in patients with CD. In our study, 12% of CD patients met the Rome IV symptom criteria and 27% suffered from FGIDs symptoms. The data available confirms that the prevalence of IBS-type symptoms among the group of celiac patients is higher than that in a group of control subjects [39]. While it was true, CD patients showed a low intake of high FODMAP cereals, which reflects treatment with a GFD. We observed that the intake of high FODMAP fruits in this group could in some way be associated with the higher percentage of CD patients reporting IBS and FGIDs symptoms as compared to controls [40].

When CD is diagnosed, there is usually the assumption that gastrointestinal symptoms will resolve once gluten is eliminated from the diet. Instead, it has been demonstrated that some celiac patients carry on suffering of gastrointestinal symptoms one year after diagnosis even with their correct adherence to GFD and normalization of serum tTG levels [9]. Such a finding also includes the fact that celiac patients do not report great quality-of-life scores as compared to those of the healthy population [41]. Therefore, the hypothesis that only mucosal inflammation may have a sensitizing effect or predispose to IBS-type symptoms is not the only way to run. The diet can play a pivotal role in the induction of IBS symptoms [42] especially FODMAP [43]. IBS is a common syndrome characterized by abdominal discomfort or pain and is associated with altered bowel habits [14]. Currently, once major organic gastrointestinal disorders have been excluded, specialists focus on the possible link between an "IBS" clinical picture and molecules such as α-amylase/trypsin inhibitors (resistance molecules contained in cereals to fend off pests and parasites) or dietary habits such as the intake of lactose, dietary nickel, poorly absorbed, and short-chain carbohydrates (i.e., FODMAP). FODMAP are contained in different types of cereals such as wheat, barley, rye, and derived products and sweets and sweeteners such as honey, saccharin, and fructose. There are two other categories that contain high levels of FODMAP including several types of fruits/dried fruit (such as apple, apricot, peach, pear, watermelon, and plum) and vegetables (such as artichoke, asparagus, cauliflower, onion, garlic, and beans). In addition, dairy products are given attention for their high FODMAP content (lactose): milk, yogurt, fresh cheese, semi-aged cheese, and aged cheese. At present, no data is available about FODMAP intake in CD patients [44,45].

In our study, a group of celiac patients was compared with a group of healthy subjects with regard to their intake of FODMAP through foods containing different (low and high) levels of them. We recorded all the foods and beverages consumed during a week and then consumed foods that were classified as being high or low in FODMAP content. We used such an approach since the direct measurement of FODMAP content by means of reliable analytical methods in common foods is unavailable yet. As expected, CD patients had a lower intake of cereals and sweets containing high FODMAP levels (including the gluten-containing grains forbidden to celiac patients) as compared to healthy volunteers. Conversely, patients had a higher intake of low FODMAP cereals including cereals allowed in GFD such as rice, corn, and pseudo cereals. Interestingly, a significantly higher intake of fruits (both high and low in FODMAP) was found in the CD patients. Moreover, when all vegetable foods, i.e., fruits, dried fruits, and vegetables were grouped together, we observed a significantly high intake of both categories in CD patients when compared to healthy volunteers. This suggests a greater level of attention about a healthy diet paid by CD patients than controls. However, since cereals contain fructans, fruit and vegetables are two food categories with a high content of FODMAP. This high intake of fruits rich in FODMAP might partly explain the tendency to a higher number of CD patients reporting IBS and FGIDs symptoms when compared to controls. When comparing sweeteners intake, both groups had a comparable low intake of high-FODMAP foods. This suggests that fructose as a sweetener was not commonly used by all the volunteers. In fact, only 12 out of 91 controls and 11 out of 104 CD patients made use of it (data not shown). By contrast, CD patients consumed more low-FODMAP sweeteners such as sugar and aspartame than controls. Lastly, the results suggest that patients with CD did not exclude or limit dairy products with a high content of FODMAP, which shows a pattern similar to that of the control group. Of note, milk and its derivatives provide important nutrients due to its content of vitamins, minerals, and macronutrients essential for the growth, development, and maintenance of tissues [46]. On the other hand, the benefits of the fatty component of dairy products have been demonstrated and elicit a greater bioavailability of high-value nutrients and also show anti-inflammatory properties [47–49]. The presumed anti-inflammatory benefits described in dairy products could potentially be the reason, at least in part, why some CD patients can tolerate them despite the secondary lactose intolerance described in some of them.

Currently, little is known about the level of FODMAP intake in different population groups. Nevertheless, it is of great interest to confirm a potential relationship between specific dietary carbohydrates and gastrointestinal symptoms [25]. FODMAP have been reported as triggers of gastrointestinal symptoms in IBS, Crohn's disease, and ulcerative colitis with the hypothesis being that the rapid fermentation and passage of FODMAP through the gastrointestinal tract leads to an increase in intestinal permeability [50]. Particularly in IBD patients who have superimposed IBS, the luminal distension (caused by the fermentation of FODMAP by bacteria in the distal small and proximal large bowel) can cause gastrointestinal symptoms such as bloating, distension, cramping, and diarrhea [51]. There are few antecedents on the long-term effectiveness, acceptability, and nutrient adequacy of a diet with low FODMAP content. Studies have evaluated retrospectively and prospectively changes in the gastrointestinal symptomatology [52–54] while long-term nutritional characteristics of a diet with low FODMAP content had not been studied. O'Keeffe et al. [55] evaluated the long-term impact of the low FODMAP diet on clinical response, nutritional adequacy, dietary acceptability, and quality of life related to foods. The authors concluded that the education provided in relation to a diet with low FODMAP content is effective in the management of IBS by allowing the maintenance of a nutritionally adequate diet among patients. However, one unintended consequence associated with FODMAP restriction is its impact on the gut microbiota. Probiotic supplementation with Bifidobacterium is associated with a reduction in IBS symptoms but the low FODMAP diet markedly reduces luminal Bifidobacterium concentration [56]. It is likely that both interventions can be successful in specific groups of patients [30]. In this sense, Staudacher et al. [19] showed that a low-FODMAP diet was associated with adequate relief of symptoms in patients with IBS when compared to the placebo and concomitant administration with probiotics (Bifidobacterium) could be administered to restore these bacteria in patients on a low-FODMAP diet.

For the first time, this study evaluated the intake of low or high-FODMAP foods in CD patients affected by IBS and FGIDs symptoms. As limitations, we would like to mention that our results were obtained through food diaries in a seven-day period, which is a period of time that is short and does not allow conclusions about the long-term impact of this dietary pattern. Even though the recording period is short, the participants accurately reported and weighed all the consumed food and beverages. Moreover, in a previous publication on almost the same participants, we compared this tool to a food frequency questionnaire and demonstrated that the two tools were correlated especially in terms of food groups [34]. The study of the diet during a longer period of time could provide relevant knowledge regarding dietary characteristics in patients with CD. Because of the explorative nature of our study, we could not find any causative relationship between the intake of FODMAP-rich foods and the presence of gastrointestinal symptoms in our patients. However, the clinical effect of a GFD together with low-FODMAP diet should be prospectively evaluated as a supportive therapy for CD patients. In this sense, our group has recently reported that a GFD associated with a low-FODMAP content is beneficial as a supportive therapy for a group of CD patients with persistent gastrointestinal symptoms [57]. When consolidated data on the FODMAP content of foods become available, it will allow the investigation of specific FODMAP groups among oligosaccharides, disaccharides, monosaccharides, and polyols that are more consumed by CD patients than by controls.

ClinicalTrials.gov, ref. no. NCT01975155.

Author Contributions: Conceptualization, L.R., K.A.B., L.E., and N.P. Methodology, L.R., K.A.B., and L.D. Investigation, L.R., A.S., V.L., and L.E. Data Curation, K.A.B. and F.M. Formal analysis, K.A.B. Writing-Original Draft Preparation, L.R. and K.A.B. Writing-Review & Editing, L.R., K.A.B., L.D., L.E., V.L., A.S., and M.V. Funding Acquisition, L.E.

Funding: Fondazione IRCCS Ca' Granda and through grants from the Italian Ministry of Health and Lumbardy's Regional Government Authority (Ministero della Salute and Regione Lombardia, call no. 2011-02348234).

Acknowledgments: We thank Marcello Hinxman-Allegri for the English language revision and editing of the manuscript.

Conflicts of Interest: The authors declare no conflict of interest.

References

1. Rubio-Tapia, A.; Murray, J.A. Celiac disease. *Curr. Opin. Gastroenterol.* **2010**, *26*, 116–122. [CrossRef] [PubMed]
2. Van Berge-Henegouwen, G.P.; Mulder, C.J.J. Pioneer in the gluten free diet: Willem-Karel Dicke 1905–1962, over 50 years of gluten free diet. *Gut* **1993**, *34*, 1473–1475. [CrossRef] [PubMed]
3. Bardella, M.T.; Elli, L.; Velio, P.; Fredella, C.; Prampolini, L.; Cesana, B. Silent Celiac Disease Is Frequent in the Siblings of Newly Diagnosed Celiac Patients. *Digestion* **2007**, *75*, 182–187. [CrossRef] [PubMed]
4. Megiorni, F.; Mora, B.; Bonamico, M.; Barbato, M.; Montuori, M.; Viola, F.; Trabace, S.; Mazzilli, M.C. HLA-DQ and susceptibility to celiac disease: Evidence for gender differences and parent-of-origin effects. *Am. J. Gastroenterol.* **2008**, *103*, 997–1003. [CrossRef] [PubMed]
5. Gujral, N.; Freeman, H.J.; Thomson, A.B.R. Celiac disease: Prevalence, diagnosis, pathogenesis and treatment. *World J. Gastroenterol.* **2012**, *18*, 6036–6059. [CrossRef] [PubMed]
6. Tosi, P.; Gritsch, C.S.; He, J.; Shewry, P.R. Distribution of gluten proteins in bread wheat (*Triticum aestivum*) grain. *Ann. Bot.* **2011**, *108*, 23–35. [CrossRef] [PubMed]
7. Corrao, G.; Corazza, G.R.; Bagnardi, V.; Brusco, G.; Ciacci, C.; Cottone, M.; Sategna Guidetti, C.; Usai, P.; Cesari, P.; Pelli, M.A.; et al. Mortality in patients with coeliac disease and their relatives: A cohort study. *Lancet* **2001**, *358*, 356–361. [CrossRef]
8. Mäki, M.; Collin, P. Coeliac Disease. *Lancet* **1997**, *349*, 1755–1759. [CrossRef]
9. Silvester, J.A.; Graff, L.A.; Rigaux, L.; Bernstein, C.N.; Leffler, D.A.; Kelly, C.P.; Walker, J.R.; Duerksen, D.R. Symptoms of Functional Intestinal Disorders Are Common in Patients with Celiac Disease Following Transition to a Gluten-Free Diet. *Dig. Dis. Sci.* **2017**, *62*, 2449–2454. [CrossRef] [PubMed]
10. Stern, E.K.; Brenner, D.M. Gut Microbiota-Based Therapies for Irritable Bowel Syndrome. *Clin. Transl. Gastroenterol.* **2018**, *9*, e134. [CrossRef] [PubMed]
11. Lovell, R.M.; Ford, A.C. Global Prevalence of and Risk Factors for Irritable Bowel Syndrome: A Meta-analysis. *Clin. Gastroenterol. Hepatol.* **2012**, *10*, 712–721. [CrossRef] [PubMed]
12. Longstreth, G.; Thompson, W.G.; Chey, W.; Houghton, L.; Mearin, F.; Spiller, R. Functional bowel disorders. *Gastroenterology* **2006**, *130*, 1480–1491. [CrossRef] [PubMed]
13. Quigley, E. The Gut-Brain Axis and the Microbiome: Clues to Pathophysiology and Opportunities for Novel Management Strategies in Irritable Bowel Syndrome (IBS). *J. Clin. Med.* **2018**, *7*, 6. [CrossRef] [PubMed]

14. Oswiecimska, J.; Szymlak, A.; Roczniak, W.; Girczys-Poledniok, K.; Kwiecien, J. New insights into the pathogenesis and treatment of irritable bowel syndrome. *Adv. Med. Sci.* **2017**, *62*, 17–30. [CrossRef] [PubMed]
15. Drossman, D.A. Functional gastrointestinal disorders: History, pathophysiology, clinical features, and Rome IV. *Gastroenterology* **2016**, *150*, 1262–1279. [CrossRef] [PubMed]
16. Fass, R.; Longstreth, G.F.; Pimentel, M.; Fullerton, S.; Russak, S.M.; Chiou, C.F.; Reyes, E.; Crane, P.; Eisen, G.; McCarberg, B.; et al. Evidence- and consensus-based practice guidelines for the diagnosis of irritable bowel syndrome. *Arch. Intern. Med.* **2001**, *161*, 2081–2088. [CrossRef] [PubMed]
17. Halmos, E.P.; Power, V.A.; Shepherd, S.J.; Gibson, P.R.; Muir, J.G. A diet low in FODMAPs reduces symptoms of irritable bowel syndrome. *Gastroenterology* **2014**, *146*, 67–75. [CrossRef] [PubMed]
18. Gibson, P.R.; Shepherd, S.J. Evidence-based dietary management of functional gastrointestinal symptoms: The FODMAP approach. *J. Gastroenterol. Hepatol.* **2010**, *25*, 252–258. [CrossRef] [PubMed]
19. Staudacher, H.M.; Lomer, M.C.E.; Farquharson, F.M.; Louis, P.; Fava, F.; Franciosi, E.; Scholz, M.; Tuohy, K.M.; Lindsay, J.O.; Irving, P.M.; et al. A Diet Low in FODMAPs Reduces Symptoms in Patients with Irritable Bowel Syndrome and a Probiotic Restores Bifidobacterium Species: A Randomized Controlled Trial. *Gastroenterology* **2017**, *153*, 936–947. [CrossRef] [PubMed]
20. Nanayakkara, W.S.; Skidmore, P.M.; O'Brien, L.; Wilkinson, T.J.; Gearry, R.B. Efficacy of the low FODMAP diet for treating irritable bowel syndrome: The evidence to date. *Clin. Exp. Gastroenterol.* **2016**, *9*, 131–142. [PubMed]
21. Böhn, L.; Störsrud, S.; Liljebo, T.; Collin, L.; Lindfors, P.; Törnblom, H.; Simrén, M. Diet Low in FODMAPs Reduces Symptoms of Irritable Bowel Syndrome as Well as Traditional Dietary Advice: A Randomized Controlled Trial. *Gastroenterology* **2015**, *149*, 1399–1407. [CrossRef] [PubMed]
22. Pedersen, N.; Ankersen, D.V.; Felding, M.; Wachmann, H.; Végh, Z.; Molzen, L.; Burisch, J.; Andersen, J.R.; Munkholm, P. Low-FODMAP diet reduces irritable bowel symptoms in patients with inflammatory bowel disease. *World J. Gastroenterol.* **2017**, *23*, 3356–3366. [CrossRef] [PubMed]
23. Cox, S.R.; Prince, A.C.; Myers, C.E.; Irving, P.M.; Lindsay, J.O.; Lomer, M.C.; Whelan, K. Fermentable carbohydrates (FODMAPs) exacerbate functional gastrointestinal symptoms in patients with inflammatory bowel disease: A randomised, double-blind, placebo-controlled, cross-over, re-challenge trial. *J. Crohn's Colitis* **2017**, *11*, 1420–1429. [CrossRef] [PubMed]
24. Testa, A.; Imperatore, N.; Rispo, A.; Rea, M.; Tortora, R.; Nardone, O.M.; Lucci, L.; Accarino, G.; Caporaso, N.; Castiglione, F. Beyond Irritable Bowel Syndrome: The Efficacy of the Low Fodmap Diet for Improving Symptoms in Inflammatory Bowel Diseases and Celiac Disease. *Dig. Dis.* **2018**, *36*, 271–280. [CrossRef] [PubMed]
25. Barrett, J.S.; Gibson, P.R. Development and Validation of a Comprehensive Semi-Quantitative Food Frequency Questionnaire that Includes FODMAP Intake and Glycemic Index. *J. Am. Diet. Assoc.* **2010**, *110*, 1469–1476. [CrossRef] [PubMed]
26. Wilson, B.; Whelan, K. Prebiotic inulin-type fructans and galacto-oligosaccharides: Definition, specificity, function, and application in gastrointestinal disorders. *J. Gastroenterol. Hepatol.* **2017**, *32*, 64–68. [CrossRef] [PubMed]
27. Patel, S.; Goyal, A. The current trends and future perspectives of prebiotics research: A review. *3 Biotech* **2012**, *2*, 115–125. [CrossRef]
28. Marcason, W. What Is the FODMAP Diet? *J. Acad. Nutr. Diet.* **2012**, *112*, 1696. [CrossRef] [PubMed]
29. Dugum, M.; Barco, K.; Garg, S. Managing irritable bowel syndrome: The low-FODMAP diet. *Cleve. Clin. J. Med.* **2016**, *83*, 655–662. [CrossRef] [PubMed]
30. Staudacher, H.M.; Irving, P.M.; Lomer, M.C.E.; Whelan, K. Mechanisms and efficacy of dietary FODMAP restriction in IBS. *Nat. Rev. Gastroenterol. Hepatol.* **2014**, *11*, 256–266. [CrossRef] [PubMed]
31. Dickson, I. High FODMAP diet induces LPS-derived intestinal inflammation and visceral hypersensitivity. *Nat. Rev. Gastroenterol. Amp. Hepatol.* **2018**, *15*, 68. [CrossRef] [PubMed]
32. Zhou, S.Y.; Gillilland, M.; Wu, X.; Leelasinjaroen, P.; Zhang, G.; Zhou, H.; Ye, B.; Lu, Y.; Owyang, C. FODMAP diet modulates visceral nociception by lipopolysaccharide-mediated intestinal inflammation and barrier dysfunction. *J. Clin. Investig.* **2018**, *128*, 267–280. [CrossRef] [PubMed]

33. Leffler, D.A.; Dennis, M.; Edwards George, J.B.; Jamma, S.; Magge, S.; Cook, E.F.; Schuppan, D.; Kelly, C.P. A Simple Validated Gluten-Free Diet Adherence Survey for Adults With Celiac Disease. *Clin. Gastroenterol. Hepatol.* **2009**, *7*, 530–536. [CrossRef] [PubMed]
34. Mazzeo, T.; Roncoroni, L.; Lombardo, V.; Tomba, C.; Elli, L.; Sieri, S.; Grioni, S.; Bardella, M.T.; Agostoni, C.; Doneda, L.; et al. Evaluation of a Modified Italian European Prospective Investigation into Cancer and Nutrition Food Frequency Questionnaire for Individuals with Celiac Disease. *J. Acad. Nutr. Diet.* **2016**, *116*, 1810–1816. [CrossRef] [PubMed]
35. Morreale, F.; Agnoli, C.; Roncoroni, L.; Sieri, S.; Lombardo, V.; Mazzeo, T.; Elli, L.; Bardella, M.T.; Agostoni, C.; Doneda, L.; et al. Are the dietary habits of treated individuals with celiac disease adherent to a Mediterranean diet? *Nutr. Metab. Cardiovasc. Dis.* **2018**, *28*, 1148–1154. [CrossRef] [PubMed]
36. Dall'Asta, C.; Scarlato, A.P.; Galaverna, G.; Brighenti, F.; Pellegrini, N. Dietary exposure to fumonisins and evaluation of nutrient intake in a group of adult celiac patients on a gluten-free diet. *Mol. Nutr. Food Res.* **2012**, *56*, 632–640. [CrossRef] [PubMed]
37. European Institute of Oncology Food Composition Database for Epidemiological Studies in Italy. 2008. Available online: http://www.bda-ieo.it/ (accessed on 19 November 2017).
38. Mazzeo, T.; Cauzzi, S.; Brighenti, F.; Pellegrini, N. The development of a composition database of gluten-free products. *Public Health Nutr.* **2015**, *18*, 1353–1357. [CrossRef] [PubMed]
39. Barratt, S.M.; Leeds, J.S.; Robinson, K.; Shah, P.J.; Lobo, A.J.; McAlindon, M.E.; Sanders, D.S. Reflux and irritable bowel syndrome are negative predictors of quality of life in coeliac disease and inflammatory bowel disease. *Eur. J. Gastroenterol. Hepatol.* **2011**, *23*, 159–165. [CrossRef] [PubMed]
40. Sainsbury, A.; Sanders, D.S.; Ford, A.C. Prevalence of irritable bowel syndrome-type symptoms in patients with celiac disease: A meta-analysis. *Clin. Gastroenterol. Hepatol.* **2013**, *11*, 359–365. [CrossRef] [PubMed]
41. O'Leary, C.; Wieneke, P.; Buckley, S.; O'Regan, P.; Cronin, C.C.; Quigley, E.M.M.; Shanahan, F. Celiac disease and irritable bowel-type symptoms. *Am. J. Gastroenterol.* **2002**, *97*, 1463–1467. [CrossRef] [PubMed]
42. Hayes, P.; Corish, C.; O'Mahony, E.; Quigley, E.M.M. A dietary survey of patients with irritable bowel syndrome. *J. Hum. Nutr. Diet.* **2014**, *27*, 36–47. [CrossRef] [PubMed]
43. De Giorgio, R.; Volta, U.; Gibson, P.R. Sensitivity to wheat, gluten and FODMAPs in IBS: Facts or fiction? *Gut* **2016**, *65*, 169–178. [CrossRef] [PubMed]
44. Varney, J.; Barrett, J.; Scarlata, K.; Catsos, P.; Gibson, P.R.; Muir, J.G. FODMAPs: Food composition, defining cutoff values and international application. *J. Gastroenterol. Hepatol.* **2017**, *32*, 53–61. [CrossRef] [PubMed]
45. Tuck, C.; Ly, E.; Bogatyrev, A.; Costetsou, I.; Gibson, P.; Barrett, J.; Muir, J. Fermentable short chain carbohydrate (FODMAP) content of common plant-based foods and processed foods suitable for vegetarian- and vegan-based eating patterns. *J. Hum. Nutr. Diet.* **2018**, *31*, 422–435. [CrossRef] [PubMed]
46. Lordan, R.; Tsoupras, A.; Mitra, B.; Zabetakis, I. Dairy Fats and Cardiovascular Disease: Do We Really Need to Be Concerned? *Foods* **2018**, *7*, 29. [CrossRef] [PubMed]
47. Lordan, R.; Zabetakis, I. Invited review: The anti-inflammatory properties of dairy lipids. *J. Dairy Sci.* **2017**, *100*, 4197–4212. [CrossRef] [PubMed]
48. Lordan, R.; Tsoupras, A.; Zabetakis, I. Phospholipids of animal and marine origin: Structure, function, and anti-inflammatory properties. *Molecules* **2017**, *22*, 1964. [CrossRef] [PubMed]
49. Bordoni, A.; Danesi, F.; Dardevet, D.; Dupont, D.; Fernandez, A.S.; Gille, D.; Nunes dos Santos, C.; Pinto, P.; Re, R.; Rémond, D.; et al. Dairy products and inflammation: A review of the clinical evidence. *Crit. Rev. Food Sci. Nutr.* **2017**, *57*, 2497–2525. [CrossRef] [PubMed]
50. Gearry, R.B.; Irving, P.M.; Barrett, J.S.; Nathan, D.M.; Shepherd, S.J.; Gibson, P.R. Reduction of dietary poorly absorbed short-chain carbohydrates (FODMAPs) improves abdominal symptoms in patients with inflammatory bowel disease-a pilot study. *J. Crohn's Colitis* **2009**, *3*, 8–14. [CrossRef] [PubMed]
51. Knight-Sepulveda, K.; Kais, S.; Santaolalla, R.; Abreu, M.T. Diet and Inflammatory Bowel Disease. *Gastroenterol. Hepatol.* **2015**, *11*, 511–520.
52. Shepherd, S.J.; Gibson, P.R. Fructose Malabsorption and Symptoms of Irritable Bowel Syndrome: Guidelines for Effective Dietary Management. *J. Am. Diet. Assoc.* **2006**, *106*, 1631–1639. [CrossRef] [PubMed]
53. Maagaard, L.; Ankersen, D.V.; Vegh, Z.; Burisch, J.; Jensen, L.; Pedersen, N.; Munkholm, P. Follow-up of patients with functional bowel symptoms treated with a low FODMAP diet. *World J. Gastroenterol.* **2016**, *22*, 4009–4019. [CrossRef] [PubMed]

54. De Roest, R.H.; Dobbs, B.R.; Chapman, B.A.; Batman, B.; O'Brien, L.A.; Leeper, J.A.; Hebblethwaite, C.R.; Gearry, R.B. The low FODMAP diet improves gastrointestinal symptoms in patients with irritable bowel syndrome: A prospective study. *Int. J. Clin. Pract.* **2013**, *67*, 895–903. [CrossRef] [PubMed]
55. O'Keeffe, M.; Jansen, C.; Martin, L.; Williams, M.; Seamark, L.; Staudacher, H.M.; Irving, P.M.; Whelan, K.; Lomer, M.C. Long-term impact of the low-FODMAP diet on gastrointestinal symptoms, dietary intake, patient acceptability, and healthcare utilization in irritable bowel syndrome. *Neurogastroenterol. Motil.* **2018**. [CrossRef] [PubMed]
56. Staudacher, H.M.; Whelan, K. Altered gastrointestinal microbiota in irritable bowel syndrome and its modification by diet: Probiotics, prebiotics and the low FODMAP diet. *Proc. Nutr. Soc.* **2016**, *75*, 306–318. [CrossRef] [PubMed]
57. Roncoroni, L.; Bascuñán, K.A.; Doneda, L.; Scricciolo, A.; Lombardo, V.; Branchi, F.; Ferretti, F.; Dell'osso, B.; Montanari, V.; Bardella, M.T.; et al. A low FODMAP gluten-free diet improves functional gastrointestinal disorders and overall mental health of celiac disease patients: A randomized controlled trial. *Nutrients* **2018**, *10*, 1023. [CrossRef] [PubMed]

nutrients

MDPI

Review

Descriptive Study of the Different Tools Used to Evaluate the Adherence to a Gluten-Free Diet in Celiac Disease Patients

Luis Rodrigo *, Isabel Pérez-Martinez, Eugenia Lauret-Braña and Adolfo Suárez-González

Gastroenterology Unit, Hospital Universitario Central de Asturias (HUCA), CSIC, Avda. de Roma s/n, 33011 Oviedo, Spain; ipermar_79@hotmail.com (I.P.-M.); meugelb@hotmail.com (E.L.-B.); adolfo.suarez@hcabuenes.es (A.S.-G.)

* Correspondence: lrodrigosaez@gmail.com; Tel.: +34-985-23-44-16

Received: 15 October 2018; Accepted: 14 November 2018; Published: 16 November 2018

Abstract: Celiac disease (CD) is a genetically conditioned autoimmune process that appears in susceptible people. It can affect people of any age, and slightly predominates in females. It has a fairly homogenous global distribution, with an average prevalence of 1–2%, the frequency having increased in recent decades. The only effective treatment is a strict and permanent gluten-free diet (GFD), although the level of compliance is poor, at about 50% of cases. To monitor the effectiveness of the GFD, several procedures involving various approaches are employed: (a) Periodic visits by expert Nutritionists; (b) Clinical follow-up; (c) Serological time controls of specific antibodies; (d) Serial endoscopies with collection of duodenal biopsies; (e) Use of structured questionnaires; and (f) Determination of gluten peptides derived from gluten in faeces and/or urine. All of these procedures are useful when applied, alone or in combination, depending on the cases. Some patients will only need to consult to their doctors, while others will require a multidisciplinary approach to assess their compliance with the GFD. In children, normalization of duodenal mucosa was achieved in 95% of cases within two years, while it is more delayed in adults, whose mucosa take longer time (3–5 years) to heal completely.

Keywords: celiac disease; gluten-free diet; effectiveness; adherence; nutritionists; clinic; serology; duodenal biopsies; structured questionnaires; peptides derived from gluten in faeces and urine

1. Introduction

Celiac disease (CD) is defined as a systemic autoimmune process that appears as a consequence of a permanent intolerance to gluten and that affects genetically predisposed people. It is widely, although unevenly, distributed throughout the world, affecting all ethnicities, with an average prevalence of 1–2% in the general population, its frequency having increased notably in recent years [1].

A gluten-free diet (GFD), followed strictly and permanently throughout life, is the only currently available treatment that successfully controls most cases of this disease. It is remarkably effective in the vast majority of cases, producing a significant clinical improvement not only in digestive symptoms, but also in the extra-intestinal symptoms associated with CD, causing its progressive disappearance, and the associated slow and sustained decrease in intestinal lesions [2,3].

Permanent adherence to a GFD is difficult, and largely unnoticed but repeated transgressions, as well as frequent contaminations may occur, all of which delay patient recovery in some way. This was confirmed in a meta-analysis published in 2018 [3]. If the transgressions are frequent, various types of associated long-term complications may appear, including a variety of malignancies [4].

Physicians involved in the management of CD should insist strongly to their patients that compliance with the GFD is fundamental and is the cornerstone of the success of this treatment.

They need to explain this concept convincingly to the patients, as well as the main features of the GFD, with the greatest possible clarity and simplicity at the time of diagnosis.

It has not yet been well established which person or doctor who should carry out the follow-up to confirm the adherence to the GFD: it could be the gastroenterologist, the primary care physician, or an expert dietician [5]. Clinical control by family physicians and gastroenterologists is considered to be very similar, in the sense of them being able to achieve high rates of adherence to GFD [6].

The available evidence indicates that consulting with a dietician can be useful, especially when gluten contamination is suspected. However, joint monitoring by a dietician and a doctor may not be better, than the control that either one can offer separately [7]. The final decision will depend, not only on the availability of an expert dietician in different centres, but also on the collaboration that exists between the gastroenterology services and primary care physicians.

Patient associations or support groups can provide help with trying to achieve proper compliance with the diet. These associations offer detailed information about the importance of a strict GFD and answer all questions related to the characteristics of gluten-free foods and different recipes. They also organize regular meetings, during which patients can share information about CD with other patients and thereby improve compliance with their diet [8].

In general, it is reckoned that fewer than 50% of patients, mainly those from the adult celiac population, manage to keep strictly to a GFD. Generally, better dietary adherence is achieved (in 90–95% of cases, on average in the paediatric population, or in those people whose disease is diagnosed in early childhood [9].

There are clear differences in the prevalence of CD between Caucasians and South East Asian people, that may be due to different reasons, such as socioeconomic status, healthcare facilities, associated infections, presence of villous atrophy and others, and the adherence to GFD in general is irregular, but if it were strict, it would possibly be similar in both ethnicities, but for the moment, there are scarce information for this.

The main objective of the present study is to review the usefulness of the diverse available methods to use in different clinical situations and phases of CD evolution following a GFD, pointing out its strengths and weak points, in order to facilitate its selection, both in children and adults.

2. Control of the Follow-Up of the GFD

Compliance with the GFD can be evaluated through different approaches, and various health professionals, may participate or collaborate to carry this out, in line with the following study procedures:

1. Periodic control visits by an expert dietician
2. Regular consultations with a gastroenterologist/family doctor
3. Structured specific questionnaires
4. Regular control of serum antibody titres for CD
5. Serial endoscopies with duodenal biopsies
6. Determination of derived peptides from gluten, in faeces/urine

2.1. *Periodic Interviews Conducted by Dieticiass*

The dieticians are the health professionals best placed to assess the degree of compliance with the GFD. They should try to participate and collaborate actively in the follow-up of celiac patients, whenever possible maintaining a close collaboration with nutritionists and gastroenterologists, ideally carrying out their task during the same visit and, as far as is practicable, simultaneously in the same consulting room.

However, many patients tend to have consultations only with their gastroenterologist or family doctor, and these are also effective at achieving strict adherence to the GFD. On the other hand, patients with more complex needs will require a multidisciplinary approach, including various medical specialists, to assess their associated diseases and their compliance with the GFD.

2.2. Evolutionary Clinical Follow-up

The disappearance or improvement of symptoms, might not seem a very accurate method, although an indicative one, for trying to evaluate adherence to the GFD during a consultation with the doctor. This evaluation can be done either by the gastroenterologist who diagnosed the patient, or by the family doctor who controls their evolution, facilitating their outpatient visits, reducing the number trips to the hospital and generally shortening the wait.

The lack of improvement with the GFD, or the persistence of symptoms, are generally related to irregular, or poor dietary compliance, or, clearly, with continued gluten consumption, specially in adolescents [10]. The main cause, in addition to any frequent transgressions, is the inadvertent intake of gluten. This is mainly due to "cross-contamination", which arises from eating at a table with other people who eat bread or other wheat products and who often inadvertently drop small fragments of foods that have been contaminated with flour residues during their preparation or handling, etc. It may also be due to the "hidden gluten" that is present in some products that are not adequately labelled [11,12]. People with a basic elementary education and/or with little understanding of how to follow a GFD, or who have little motivation, often believe that they are following the diet strictly, although in practice, they are frequently making mistakes [13].

The follow-up and control visits serve to assess the improvement in the initial symptoms and to collect evidence of new ones. On many occasions at the time of diagnosis there is an overlap of the patient's discomfort with the symptoms of irritable bowel, which, naturally, do not improve with the implementation of a GFD, unlike the case in many celiac patients [14]. The persistence of previous symptoms, or the appearance of new ones, may be related to CD itself, to a complication that has arisen, or to the presence of a new, associated disease.

A series of alarm symptoms have been described, such as the rapid deterioration in the general state of health, accompanied by striking weight loss, the presence of high fever, serious diarrhoea, or signs of intestinal obstruction, all of which require an exhaustive clinical and analytical study to be carried out in search of important associated complications, such as an evolution towards refractory forms of the disease, or the development of a primary intestinal T-cell lymphoma [15–17].

CD usually presents a broad spectrum of related symptoms, not only digestive, but also extra-intestinal. It has a clear predominance in females compared with men, with an average ratio of 2:1 in most series described. It is more prevalent in adults than in children. Children are more likely to exhibit typical symptoms along with a higher frequency of villous atrophy (VA) and higher antibody titres related to tissue Trans Glutaminase (tTG) than in adults. Delay in diagnosis is also less in children than in adults in general. Curiously, this pattern is more evident in children under three years of age, and the differences between all other age groups decrease, or disappear with age, such that adolescents behave like adults in all the aspects discussed [18].

Children may have reduced bone mass at the time of diagnosis. However, they are more likely than adults to achieve a full recovery of their bone mass, 6–12 months after the starting on their GFD. Generally, it is not necessary to perform bone mineral density (BMD) explorations in paediatric patients who have been newly diagnosed with CD without complications. It is recommended to monitor the weight and height of children regularly, at every visit, in order to evaluate them properly, and to try to help them attain normal growth and skeletal development [19].

The main cause of a drop in BMD in CD patients is probably vitamin D deficiency, but it may arise for other reasons. However, the risk of fractures in patients with CD is not very high, and the predictive value of the systematic performance of BMD is not sufficient to identify individuals at high risk of fractures. It seems reasonable to measure BMD periodically in adult patients with CD, especially in those with a high risk of osteoporosis, such as in post-menopausal women, men older than 55 years, and people known to have osteopenia prior to the diagnosis of CD [20]. Further studies are needed to establish the true efficacy and cost-effectiveness of the periodic performance of BMD, in all adult patients with CD at the time of diagnosis, and to identify the frequency of follow-up with which this exploration should be carried out [21].

Autoimmune diseases are frequently associated with CD and can appear at any time during the follow-up, especially in adults, with a clear predominance in females. Physicians should be aware of the possible related autoimmune diseases and other illnesses associated with CD, so they can detect them systematically and early during follow-up visits [22].

CD is associated with many various diseases with which it often shares a genetic base. Type 1 Diabetes Mellitus (T1DM), is one disease, which occurs particularly frequently in children. Many of them present it in a silent or oligo-symptomatic way, for which reason, it is recommended to perform an annual follow-up screening for the presence of associated CD in children with T1DM, since its average prevalence is high, occurring in 5–10% of juvenile diabetic patients [23]. T1DM is diagnosed in 90% of patients before CD is confirmed [24]. Patients with T1DM and symptoms associated with CD, show clear clinical improvement overall when they follow a GFD. Increases in the rate of growth and in haemoglobin levels are often observed in these children. There is an improvement in control of diabetes mellitus, as confirmed by the reduction in the frequency of hypoglycaemic episodes and the reduced daily need for insulin [25–27].

There is also an increased risk of developing non-Hodgkin lymphoma in individuals with relatives affected with CD. The same may be said about the presence of various associated neurological diseases, above all cerebellar ataxia [28,29].

It is highly recommended and mandatory to carry out screening studies for CD in first and second grade relatives, especially if they present clinical symptoms. The index case must be informed about this family risk and its implementation is recommended for all first-and second-degree relatives [30,31].

The periodic determination of a series of laboratory tests is very important, in order to be able to detect the presence of nutritional deficiencies and the development of diseases and associated complications. The basic laboratory tests that should be done at each visit include, amongst others, a CBC with leukocyte formula, blood glucose, cholesterol and triglycerides, measurements of levels of iron, transferrin, ferritin, vitamin B12, folates, calcium, alkaline phosphatase, and liver function tests.

Likewise, the serum levels of thyroid stimulating hormone (TSH), anti-thyroid antibodies and levels of dihydroxy—vitamin D should be determined' in case they exhibit an associated deficiency. This will be complemented with the determination of the antibody titre against deamidated gliadin peptides (DGPs) of the IgA type and/or the tTG, also of the IgA type, and occasionally by determining the endomysial antibodies (EMAs) [31].

Women of childbearing age must be checked regularly by their gynaecologist, especially those presenting menstrual disorders, infertility problems, or those who have a history of recurrent miscarriages [32].

Hypersplenism can affect more than a third of adult patients with CD, but it is not a complication in paediatric patients. The incidence of hyposplenism is correlated with the duration of pre-exposure to gluten and is higher in concomitant autoimmune disorders and premalignant conditions. Based on these associated factors, the function of the spleen can be determined in a select group of adult patients with CD and a previous history of associated major infections or episodes of thromboembolism [33].

The count of red blood cells with small surface irregularities (marks or notches) is a useful diagnostic tool, involving a precise, quantitative and low-cost method. The conjugated protein vaccines should be administered to patients with significant hyposplenism, defined as more than 10% of erythrocytes with irregularities on their surface or fewer than 10% of IgM memory type B cells [34].

2.3. Structured Questionnaires

Structured short questionnaires are used as an alternative to consultations with a dietician to obtain a rapid assessment of the adherence to the GFD. It is easy to complete this type of questionnaire in the patient's usual clinic. The responses are highly correlated with antibody levels and the presence of VA in duodenal biopsies and useful for monitoring. In general, questionnaires are easy to administer and often complement each other. They not only assess the quality of life, in a general or specific way, but also are able to estimate the changes occurring after the follow-up of the GFD. However, all of them must be validated in different countries and diverse clinical contexts before they can be applied and come into general use. Leffler et al. have developed a simple questionnaire to assess adherence to GFD in adults with CD. It consists of seven structured questions about compliance and is scored on a Likert scale from 1 to 5, so that summing the values obtained gives an overall score from 7 to 35. Values less than 13 are considered to show good compliance, while those over 17, represent intermediate or low adherence. It is easily applied and is a very useful tool that can be included as part of the monitoring of adult patients, but not of children. This scoring system is known as "CDAT score" from (Coeliac Dietary Adherence Test) [35].

2.4. Periodic Evaluation of Serum Antibody Levels

Levels of antibodies circulating in the blood, which are usually used to diagnose CD, including DGPs and tTG, are related to the levels of gluten consumed. It is expected, therefore, that there will be a decrease in their titres a few weeks or months after a strict GFD is initiated. The sustained or sporadic consumption of foods containing gluten increases these values and thereby the persistence of high levels of gluten-related antibodies, suggests a lack of adherence to GFD [36].

Periodic serological tests for PDGs DGP and/or tTG may be useful for controlling the degree of compliance with a GFD [37]. However, the normalization of antibody titres cannot identify the existence of small dietary transgressions, so its use is limited to indicating a lack of compliance, but is of no value for evaluating whether there is strict adherence to the GFD.

The diagnostic security of the various commercial kits used is lower in clinical practice than the values reported in the medical literature in general, especially in the patients with mild VA or those with patchy lesions.

A collaborative multinational study revealed a high variability in levels of tTG, which is very striking with respect to diagnostic sensitivity (ranging from 69% to 93%), and somewhat less in terms of specificity (from 96% to 100%), among the 20 participating laboratories. This once again demonstrates the need for better standardization of the various techniques available for determining the tTG antibodies [38–41].

CD is often diagnosed in adults even when the values of positive antibody are very low (5–10% according to various series), or even zero, especially in cases that present with lymphocytic enteritis but not VA. The serology of such cases is entirely without value for monitoring because the levels of antibodies present at the start of the GFD are normal [42–44].

This does not usually occur in children, who, in most cases, have very high titres. Levels of tTG more than 10 times the normal value indicate the existence of significant VA. In these cases it is not considered necessary to perform duodenal biopsies in order to confirm the diagnosis of CD, as recommended in the new criteria drawn up by experts of the European Society of Paediatric Gastroenterology, Hepatology, and Nutrition (ESPGHAN), which were published in 2012 [45].

Subsequent follow-up studies have confirmed the safety and efficacy of this diagnostic strategy for children. It is recommended following a diagnosis based on raised levels of tTG, if it is confirmed by a positive determination of EMA in a second blood sample, and the presence of at least one symptom indicative of CD. This could avoid unnecessary risks and the costs related to endoscopy in at least 50% of the children worldwide who present with CD. Carrying out genetic studies to determine related HLA-II markers (HLA-DQ2 and DQ8) is not essential for obtaining a safe diagnosis [46].

The evaluation of antibody titres in these cases is a good, and indeed the only currently available method of monitoring. It is recommended that titres be measured every six months. Most children presenting with CD exhibit a gradual, progressive and continuous decrease in titres over time, their values becoming normalized within 1–2 years of starting the GFD.

2.5. Periodic Endoscopic Controls with Taking of Duodenal Biopsies

CD exhibits marked differences in children and adults, not only at the time of diagnosis, but also in the degree of response to the GFD and in their histological recovery. These are clearly higher in children (95% on average) than in adults (50%) after two years of monitoring [43,44].

Examining the histology of the small intestine continues to be the best procedure for evaluating with certainty the healing of the intestinal mucosa. Complete recovery from VA confirms that the GFD has been followed strictly and effectively, independently of the evolution of the serological titers of the antibodies, or of the symptoms that the patients present. Intestinal biopsies taken during follow-up are important in adults who have persistent VA, even in the absence of symptoms and with negative serology [47].

Adult patients are usually less symptomatic than children, most of them exhibiting atypical forms of the disease. For this reason, clinical-based monitoring is not usually of much value. Changes in serology are also not very marked, so the best way of assessing the effectiveness of the GFD is to perform periodic duodenal biopsies. These are not needed for children, because, in most cases, they achieve complete mucosal recovery earlier than do adults [48].

The guidelines published by the American College of Gastroenterology (ACG) include the recommendation to perform follow-up duodenal biopsies in adults, two years after the start of the GFD, in order to assess mucosal healing. However, its implementation is not recommended as a routine procedure for children [2]. Clinical guides published by the British Society of Gastroenterology are less demanding and suggest that there is little evidence to determine whether the clinical results differ significantly depending on the result of repeated biopsies. In the absence of results of a cost-benefit analysis of repeated biopsies and the lack of prospective studies in this regard, they postulate that follow-up biopsies are not generally necessary for asymptomatic patients who are successfully following a GFD and for whom there are no data to suggest an increased risk of developing VA-related complications [49].

One of the benefits of carrying out repeated biopsies in adult patients with CD is the ability to separate patients into two groups: those whose mucosa recovers completely and who can be monitored with less strict controls, and those with persistent VA, who require more frequent clinical control. It is clear that the persistence of VA is generally associated with a higher frequency of complications related to CD and adverse medium- and long-term outcomes.

Even patients who have persistent mild forms of lymphocytic enteropathy (Marsh I type or duodenal lymphocytosis) while following a GFD can also present nutritional deficiencies or complications. It takes 2–5 years for the mucosa of adult celiac patients with AV in their biopsies to recover. Therefore, the control biopsies can be programmed for adult patients over that period, taking into account that it is better to carry them out after the third or fourth year after initiation of the GFD to avoid too many unnecessary repetitions [50].

Mucosal recovery is defined, from the histological point of view, as the reestablishment of the normal height of the intestinal villi, taken as a ratio of villus height to crypt depth of at least 3:1 according to what is observed when comparing with non-celiac subjects. Monitoring the intra-epithelial lymphocyte count was not considered appropriate, because it is not exclusively related to gluten consumption, since it can also have other causes [51].

Usually the comparative evaluation of duodenal biopsies of the same patient, is mainly focused on the finding of the presence of an architectural damage (mainly VA). These parameters have been summarised following the Marsh-Oberhuber (MO) classification [52] and strongly influence to the gastroenterologists in their clinical/therapeutic decisions, especially when the histological pattern is unmodified [53].

Elli et al. reported the results of an interesting study including two different methods of comparing duodenal biopsies. One was the classical MO score and the second one compared the areas covered by each MO grade and expressed as percentages, the final grade being calculated from the analysis of ten power fields per duodenal biopsy. They studied 69 patients (17 males 52 females, age at diagnosis

36 ± 15 years) who underwent repeated duodenal biopsies. According to the classical MO scale, 32 patients (46%) did not present VA during one year follow-up, while 37 (54%) showed VA, among whom, 26 improved the grade of severity and 11 retained the same one. Of these latter, according to the second method, eight patients were considered improved, two showed a worsened duodenal damage and only one remained unchanged; the evaluation changed in 91% of cases. The authors suggest that the use of the second method provides a good additional information about the progression/regression of the mucosal damage, especially in unmodified cases following the GFD [54].

In 2010, Rubio-Tapia et al. described the results of a retrospective follow-up study with repeated biopsies in a large series of 241 adult patients with CD and VA at diagnosis. They reported that mucosal recovery in their patients was 34% (95% CI: 27–40%) at two years and 66% (95% CI: 58–74%) at five years. However, most of the patients (82%) presented a clinical improvement that was not significantly correlated with the recovery of the mucosa ($p = 0.7$), unlike the serological response, which did have a significant association ($p = 0.01$) In the same study, poor compliance with the GFD ($p < 0.01$), the presence of a severe CAD diagnosis, defined by the intensity of diarrhoea and weight loss ($p < 0.001$), and complete VA at the start ($p < 0.001$), were significantly correlated with a lack or delay of mucosal recovery. There was a nearly significant association between the disappearance of VA and a reduction in all-cause mortality (hazard ratio (HR) = 0.13, 95% CI: 0.02–1.06, $p = 0.06$), adjusted for age and sex. The authors recommended that most adults with CD should be followed up by endoscopy and periodic biopsies [55].

In another study, conducted by Lebwohl et al., published in 2013, the authors tried to establish whether there is an association between the presence of AV and increased mortality. They studied a series of 7648 patients with CD for a mean follow-up time of 11.5 years. A total of 3317 (43%) of them had persistent atrophy. There were 606 deaths (8%) in the entire series. Patients with persistent VA had no greater risk of mortality than those with normal mucosa (HR = 1.01; 95% CI: 0.86–1.19). This pattern was the same for children and adults, including patients older than 50 years of age. However, follow-up biopsies are useful for confirming diagnoses or in cases of refractory CD [56]. A description of the different published studies evaluating the adherence of the GFD and its impact on the duodenal mucosal healing and the survival in relation to persistence of VA is shown (Table 1).

Table 1. Summary of studies looking to GFD adherence and efficacy using various procedures.

Author, [Ref] City, Country Publication year	Number Type of pts.	Time of Follow-up	Study Procedures	Final Results
Dewar [16] London, England 2012	112 CD adults Non-responders to a GFD (NRCD)	18 months	Dietician Duod. Biopsies Colon biopsies H2-breath test	12, No CD 45%, not strict adherence GFD 11 MC; 9 SBBO; 9 RCD
Leffler [35] Boston, USA 2009	200 CD adults On GFD	Cohort evaluation	Dietician CDAT 7-item questionnaire Serology (tTG)	CDAT is easy to use and seems to be superior to periodic tTG determinations
Nachman [36] Buenos Aires, Argentina 2011	53 CD adults On GFD	At 1 and 4 years	Serum evaluation of tTG and DGP Compl. cut-offs	AUC at 1 year (0.64–0.72) AUC at 4 years (0.58–0.78)
Lebwohl [47] New York, USA 2014	7648 CD pts 3317 with VA 28 Swedish Pathology Departments	From 1969 to 2008 years Comparison of biopsies 2–5 years	Control of different predictor variables in VA persistent	VA is commoner in males (OR = 1.43)
Sharkey [48] Cambridge, England 2013	595 CD pts Paired biopsies in 391 cases Persistent VA in 47%	Retrospective study from database of only one hospital	Serum tTG sensitivity and VA persistent	Serology is a poor surrogate marker for the evaluation of mucosal recovery

Table 1. *Cont.*

Author, [Ref] City, Country Publication year	Number Type of pts.	Time of Follow-up	Study Procedures	Final Results
Rubio-Tapia [55] Mayo Clinic, Minnesota, USA 2010	381 CD adults with biopsy proven CD	At 2 and 5 years	Clinical records Serological response Repeated biopsies VA persistent	Mucosal recovery was 34% (27–40%) at 2 years and 66% (58–74%) at 5 years (95% CI)
Lebwohl [56] New York, USA 2014	7648 CD pts 3317 with VA (43%)	Mean 11.5 years	Cox-regression Evaluating the mortality 606 pts (8%) in VA persistent	Persistent VA is not associated with increased mortality in CD

CD: celiac disease; GFD: gluten free diet; NRCD: non-responders to GFD; MC: microscopic colitis; SBBO: small bowel bacterial overgrowth; RCD: refractory celiac disease; CDAT: celiac dietary adherence test; tTG: tissue trans-glutaminase; DGP: deamidated gliadin peptides; Compl.: compliance; AUC: area under the curve; pts: patients; VA: villous atrophy.

The endoscopic capsule does not play any role in the follow-up of mucosal lesions in CD, since it does not allow biopsy samples to be taken. However, it is of use for detecting complications, especially when the appearance of an intestinal lymphoma or haemorrhages of unknown origin is suspected [57].

2.6. Determination of Peptides Derived from Gluten in Feces and Urine

Although the importance of controlling the follow-up of the GFD for effectiveness is clearly accepted by everyone, there are currently no unanimously accepted clinical guidelines that guarantee the results, nor are there adequate procedures to assess the adherence of the patients to the diet, and the transgressions that occasionally occur. Serological tests are very sensitive and specific to a diagnosis, but their effectiveness decreases with follow-up and they are not able to provide an adequate evaluation. It is difficult to ensure that repeated endoscopies are conducted, since they are inconvenient and invasive tests, so their application in practice is complicated. Recently, immunogenic gluten peptides (IGPs) have been identified that can be determined from faeces and urine. These have been proposed as simple, non-invasive markers, to be measured when frequent transgressions and/or contamination of the GFD are suspected. Their determination is simple and represents a new tool with which to determine compliance with the GFD objectively, at any time during the follow-up of patients with CD who are receiving treatment [58].

Several prospective studies have been carried out that have confirmed the efficacy of the determination of IGP in faeces. In a Spanish study of 188 patients with CD who were on a GFD, Comino et al. found that 56 patients (29.8%) had high levels of IGPs in their faeces, and that there were significant associations with age (39.2% over 13 years) and gender (a predominance of males in this evaluation). However, they found no correlation with antibody levels, or with the responses to the dietary questionnaires administered [59].

The determination of levels of IGPs in urine has been equally useful and simple as a way of monitoring the adherence of patients to the GFD. A highly effective lateral flow technique is used to detect the presence of the monoclonal antibody G12, which is the most immunogenic within the group of IGPs. This same procedure can be applied to the determination of the gluten content in food and in some beverages, such as beer [60,61].

3. Refractory Celiac Disease

Refractory celiac disease (RCD) is defined as the presence of persistent or recurrent symptoms of CD, accompanied by signs of malabsorption, with continued VA, despite the patient following a strict GFD for more than one year, in the absence of other complications, such as intestinal lymphoma. It is rare, affecting 1–2% of adult patients with CD and is divided into two categories: type I and type II [62,63].

In type I RCD, the lymphocyte infiltration of the mucosa of the small intestine is similar to that found in patients with CD before treatment with the GFD. In contrast, in type 2 RCD, the CD3 (+) intraepithelial lymphocytes present an abnormal immunophenotype, with a lack of expression of surface cells with CD8 (+) markers and that also feature oligoclonal or monoclonal type growth.

Their differences are not only immunophenotypic, but also involve their clinical behaviour, their response to medical treatment, and their prognosis. Type 1 RCD is the more frequent (60–80% of cases), and it responds better to treatment and has a better prognosis, while type 2 is the opposite, responding poorly to various treatments, being associated with a high frequency of intestinal lymphoma, and with greater mortality [64–66].

In a recent study of 57 patients who presented with RCD, in which immunosuppressive treatments had failed in more than half of the cases, oral treatment with budesonide in open capsules, dissolving their contents in apple juice at a dose of three 3-mg capsules per day, produced significant clinical improvement in 93% of cases, and histological improvement in 89% of cases, of both types [67].

Follow-up of both types of RCD should be frequent and complete, multidisciplinary, and based mainly on the findings of duodenal biopsies. These should be performed at regular intervals and with general examinations to rule out associated complications.

4. Indicative Timetable for Conducting the Evaluations

Once the diagnosis of CD has been confirmed and the treatment with GFD explained in depth by the gastroenterologist and the nutritionist, it is recommended to draw up a schedule of periodic review visits every six months during the first year, to evaluate the overall response to the GFD. This will be done from the clinical point of view, as well as from an analytical and serological perspective. In principle, it is not considered necessary to repeat the duodenal biopsies during the first year because, with a few exceptions, they are of little use.

After the first year, if the symptoms persist, the antibody titres remain elevated or if poor adherence to the GFD is confirmed, the possibility that the patient has RCD may be considered, in which case the surveillance and controls should be increased, applying the specific protocols of each hospital or the currently available clinical guidelines.

If this eventuality has been ruled out, and it is considered worthwhile to evaluate mucosal healing in adult patients, a control endoscopy can be arranged, with a biopsy taken after the third year of follow-up. In children, it is not considered necessary to perform provocation tests or duodenal control biopsies.

5. Conclusions

In clinical practice, CD that presents with digestive and/or extra-intestinal symptoms, but can also be oligo-symptomatic or occur in a silent way, is usually suspected from the finding of a positive serology and is confirmed by performing duodenal biopsies.

The effectiveness of compliance with the GSD by celiac patients can be monitored by a nutritionist or dietician through the repeated administration of questionnaires. However, these are not always available in all centres.

It must also be principally clinical, when the disappearance of the symptoms is evident, a significant improvement having been achieved. However, this is not sufficient for the other cases. Serological controls are only effective when the basal levels of the related antibodies are very high, but they are not useful when changes are small.

Carrying out periodic duodenal biopsies is useful but has the disadvantage of being an invasive procedure and, like serology, is more useful in cases with significant VA and that are not associated with clinical improvement or serological changes.

Finally, determination of the IGPs in isolated samples of faeces or urine has proved useful for controlling transgressions of the GFD.

However, some of these processes must be employed in order to monitor and encourage patient compliance and to rule out possible any associated shortcomings and/or the appearance of new complications.

Author Contributions: All the authors contributed equally and substantially to the work. All of them fully reviewed the final version of the manuscript.

Funding: This research received no external funding.

Conflicts of Interest: The authors declare no conflict of interest.

References

1. Lohl, S.; Mustalahti, K.; Kaukinen, K.; Laurila, K.; Collin, P.; Rissanen, H.; Lohi, O.; Bravi, E.; Gasparin, M.; Reunanen, A.; et al. Increasing prevalence of coeliac disease over time. *Aliment. Pharmacol. Ther.* **2007**, *26*, 1217–1225.
2. Rubio-Tapia, A.; Hill, I.D.; Kelly, C.P.; Calderwood, A.H.; Murray, J.A.; American College of Gastroenterology. ACG Clinical Guidelines: Diagnosis and management of celiac disease. *Am. J. Gastroenterol.* **2013**, *108*, 656–676. [PubMed]
3. Hall, N.J.; Rubin, G.; Charnock, A. Systematic review: Adherence to a gluten-free diet in adult patients with coeliac disease. *Aliment. Pharmacol. Ther.* **2009**, *30*, 315–330. [CrossRef] [PubMed]
4. Syage, J.A.; Kelly, C.P.; Dickson, M.A.; Ramirez, A.C.; Leon, F.; Dominguez, R.; Sealey-Voyksner, J.A. Determination of gluten consumption in celiac disease patients on a gluten-free diet. *Am. J. Clin. Nutr.* **2018**, *107*, 201–207. [CrossRef] [PubMed]
5. Han, Y.; Chen, W.; Li, P.; Ye, J. Association between coeliac disease and risk of any malignancy and gastrointestinal malignancy: A meta-analysis. *Medicine* **2015**, *94*, e1612. [CrossRef] [PubMed]
6. Haines, M.L.; Anderson, R.P.; Gibson, P.R. Systematic review: The evidence base for long-term management of coeliac disease. *Aliment. Pharmacol. Ther.* **2008**, *28*, 1042–1066. [CrossRef] [PubMed]
7. Kurppa, K.; Lauronen, O.; Collin, P.; Ukkola, A.; Laurila, K.; Huhtal, H.; Mäki, M.; Kaukinen, K. Factors associated with dietary adherence in celiac disease: A nationwide study. *Digestion* **2012**, *86*, 309–314. [CrossRef] [PubMed]
8. Simpson, S.; Thompson, T. Nutrition assessment in celiac disease. *Gastrointest. Endosc. Clin. N. Am.* **2012**, *22*, 797–809. [CrossRef] [PubMed]
9. Penagini, F.; Dilillo, D.; Meneghin, F.; Mameli, C.; Fabiano, V.; Zuccotti, G.V. Gluten-free diet in children: An approach to a nutritionally adequate and balanced diet. *Nutrients* **2013**, *5*, 4553–4565. [CrossRef] [PubMed]
10. Hogberg, L.; Grodzinsky, E.; Stenhammar, L. Better dietary compliance in patients with coeliac disease diagnosed in early childhood. *Scand. J. Gastroenterol.* **2003**, *38*, 751–754. [PubMed]
11. Rodrigues, M.; Yonamine, G.H.; Fernandes Satiro, C.A. Rate and determinant of non-adherence to a gluten-free diet and nutritional assessment in children and adolescents with celiac disease in a tertiary Brazilian referal center: A cross-sectional and retrospective study. *BMC Gastroenterol.* **2018**, *18*, 15.
12. See, J.A.; Kaukinen, K.; Makharia, G.K.; Gibson, P.R.; Murray, J.A. Practical insights into gluten-free diets. *Nat. Rev. Gastroenterol. Hepatol.* **2015**, *12*, 580–591. [CrossRef] [PubMed]
13. Rostom, A.; Murray, J.A.; Kagnoff, M.F.; American Gastroenterological Association (AGA) Institute. Technical review on the diagnosis and management of celiac disease. *Gastroenterology* **2006**, *131*, 1981–2002. [CrossRef] [PubMed]
14. Sapone, A.; Bai, J.C.; Ciacci, C.; Dolinsek, J.; Verde, P.H.; Hadjivassiliou, M.; Kaukinen, K.; Rostami, K.; Sanders, D.S.; Schumann, M.; et al. Spectrum of gluten-related disorders: consensus on new nomenclature and classification. *BMC. Med.* **2012**, *10*, 13. [CrossRef] [PubMed]
15. Makharia, A.; Catassi, C.; Makharia, G.K. The overlap between irritable bowel syndrome and non-celiac gluten sensitivity: A clinical dilemma. *Nutrients* **2015**, *7*, 10417–10426. [CrossRef] [PubMed]
16. Dewar, D.H.; Donnelly, S.C.; McLaughlin, S.D.; Johnson, M.W.; Ellis, H.J.; Ciclitira, P.J. Celiac disease: Management of persistent symptoms in patients on a gluten-free diet. *World J. Gastroenterol.* **2012**, *18*, 1348–1356. [CrossRef] [PubMed]

17. Wierdsma, N.J.; Nijeboer, P.; de van der Schueren, M.A.; Berkenpas, M.; van Bodegraven, A.A.; Mulder, C.J. Refractory celiac disease and EATL patients show severe malnutrition and malabsorption at diagnosis. *Clin. Nutr.* **2016**, *35*, 685–691. [CrossRef] [PubMed]
18. Malamut, G.; Cellier, C. Complications of coeliac disease. *Best Pract. Res. Clin. Gastroenterol.* **2015**, *29*, 451–458. [CrossRef] [PubMed]
19. Vivas, S.; Ruiz de Morales, J.M.; Fernández, M.; Hernando, M.; Herrero, B.; Casqueiro, J.; Gutierrez, S. Age-related clinical, serological and histopathological features of celiac disease. *Am. J. Gastroenterol.* **2008**, *103*, 2360–2365. [CrossRef] [PubMed]
20. Ribes-Koninckx, C.; Mearin, M.L.; Korponay-Szabo, I.R.; Shamir, R.; Husby, S.; Ventura, A.; Branski, D.; Catassi, C.; Koletzko, S.; Mäki, M.; et al. Coeliac disease diagnosis: ESPGHAN 1990 criteria or need for a change? Results of a questionnaire. *J. Pediatr. Gastroenterol. Nutr.* **2012**, *54*, 15–19. [CrossRef] [PubMed]
21. Lewis, N.R.; Scott, B.B. Should patients with coeliac disease have their bone mineral density measured? *Eur. J. Gastroenterol. Hepatol.* **2005**, *17*, 1065–1070. [CrossRef] [PubMed]
22. West, J.; Logan, R.F.; Card, T.R.; Smith, C.; Hubbard, R. Fracture risk in people with celiac disease: A population-based cohort study. *Gastroenterology* **2003**, *125*, 429–436. [CrossRef]
23. Lauret, E.; Rodrigo, L. Celiac disease and autoimmune-associated conditions. *Biomed. Res. Int.* **2013**, *2013*, 127589. [CrossRef] [PubMed]
24. Larsson, K.; Carlsson, A.; Cederwall, E.; Jönsson, E.; Neiderud, J.; Jonsson, B.; Lemmark, A.; Ivarsson, S.A.; Skâne Study Group. Annual screening detects celiac disease in children with type 1 diabetes. *Pediatr. Diabetes* **2008**, *9*, 354–359. [CrossRef] [PubMed]
25. Koletzko, S.; Burgin-Wolff, A.; Koletzko, B.; Knapp, M.; Burger, W.; Grüneklee, D.; Herz, G.; Ruch, W.; Thon, A.; Wendel, U.; et al. Prevalence of coeliac disease in diabetic children and adolescents. A multicentre study. *Eur. J. Pediatr.* **1988**, *148*, 113–117. [CrossRef] [PubMed]
26. Lorini, R.; Scaramuzza, A.; Vitali, L.; d'Annunzio, G.; Avanzini, M.A.; De Giacomo, C.; Severi, F. Clinical aspects of coeliac disease in children with insulin-dependent diabetes mellitus. *J. Pediatr. Endocrinol. Metab.* **1996**, *9*, 101–111. [CrossRef] [PubMed]
27. Westman, E.; Ambler, G.R.; Royle, M.; Peat, J.; Chan, A. Children with coeliac disease and insulin dependent diabetes mellitus-growth, diabetes control and dietary intake. *J. Pediatr. Endocrinol. Metab.* **1999**, *12*, 433–442. [CrossRef] [PubMed]
28. Gao, Y.; Kristinsson, S.Y.; Goldin, L.R.; Björkholm, M.; Caporaso, N.E.; Landgren, O. Increased risk for non-Hodgkin lymphoma in individuals with celiac disease and a potential familial association. *Gastroenterology* **2009**, *136*, 91–98. [CrossRef] [PubMed]
29. Hadjivassiliou, M.; Aeschlimann, P.; Strigun, A.; Sanders, D.S.; Woodrofe, N.; Aeschlimann, D. Autoantibodies in gluten ataxia recognize a novel neuronal transglutaminase. *Ann. Neurol.* **2008**, *64*, 332–343. [CrossRef] [PubMed]
30. Vaquero, L.; Caminero, A.; Nunez, A.; Hernando, M.; Iglesias, C.; Casqueiro, J.; Vivas, S. Coeliac disease screening in first-degree relatives on the basis of biopsy and genetic risk. *Eur. J. Gastroenterol. Hepatol.* **2014**, *26*, 263–267. [CrossRef] [PubMed]
31. Singh, P.; Arora, S.; Lai, S.; Strand, T.A.; Makharia, G.K. Risk of celiac disease in the first- and second-degree relatives of patients with celiac disease: A systematic review and meta-analysis. *Am. J. Gastroenterol.* **2015**, *110*, 1539–1548. [CrossRef] [PubMed]
32. Casella, G.; Orfanotti, G.; Giacomantonio, L.; Bella, C.D.; Crisafulli, V.; Villanacci, V.; Baldini, V. Celiac disease and obstetrical-gynecological contribution. *Gastroenterol. Hepatol. Bed Bench* **2016**, *9*, 241–249. [PubMed]
33. Di Sabatino, A.; Brunetti, L.; Carnevale Maffe, G.; Giuffrida, P.; Corazza, G.R. Is it worth investigating splenic function in patients with celiac disease? *World J. Gastroenterol.* **2013**, *19*, 2313–2318. [CrossRef] [PubMed]
34. Thomas, H.J.; Wotton, C.J.; Yeates, D.; Ahmad, T.; Jewell, D.P.; Goldacre, M.J. Pneumococcal infection in patients with coeliac disease. *Eur. J. Gastroenterol. Hepatol.* **2008**, *20*, 624–628. [CrossRef] [PubMed]
35. Leffler, D.A.; Dennis, M.; Edwards George, J.B.; Jamma, S.; Magge, S.; Cook, E.F.; Schuppan, D.; Kekky, C.P. A simple validated gluten-free diet adherence survey for adults with Celiac Disease. *Clin. Gastroenterol. Hepatol.* **2009**, *7*, 530–536. [CrossRef] [PubMed]
36. Nachman, F.; Sugai, E.; Vazquez, H.; Gonzalez, A.; Andrenacci, P.; Niveloni, S.; Mazure, R.; Smecuol, E.; Moreno, M.L.; Hwang, H.J.; et al. Serological tests for celiac disease as indicators of long-term compliance with the gluten-free diet. *Eur. J. Gastroenterol. Hepatol.* **2011**, *23*, 473–480. [CrossRef] [PubMed]

37. Rodrigo, L. Celiac disease. *World J. Gastroenterol.* **2006**, *12*, 6585–6593. [CrossRef] [PubMed]
38. Lewis, N.R.; Scott, B.B. Meta-analysis: Deamidated gliadin peptide antibody and tissue transglutaminase antibody compared as screening tests for coeliac disease. *Aliment. Pharmacol. Ther.* **2010**, *31*, 73–81. [CrossRef] [PubMed]
39. Naiyer, A.J.; Hernandez, L.; Ciaccio, E.J.; Papadakis, K.; Manavalan, J.S.; Baghat, G.; Green, P.H. Comparison of commercially available serologic kits for the detection of celiac disease. *J. Clin. Gastroenterol.* **2009**, *43*, 225–232. [CrossRef] [PubMed]
40. Kowalski, K.; Mulak, A.; Jasinska, M.; Paradowski, L. Diagnostic challenges in celiac disease. *Adv. Clin. Exp. Med.* **2017**, *26*, 729–737.
41. Li, M.; Yu, L.; Tiberti, C.; Bonamico, M.; Taki, I.; Miao, D.; Murray, J.A.; Rewers, M.J.; Hoffenberg, E.J.; Agardh, D.; et al. A report on the International Transglutaminase Autoantibody Workshop for Celiac Disease. *Am. J. Gastroenterol.* **2009**, *104*, 154–163. [CrossRef] [PubMed]
42. Aziz, I.; Peerally, M.F.; Barnes, J.H.; Kandasamy, V.; Whiteley, J.C.; Partridge, D.; Vergani, P.; Cross, S.S.; Green, P.H.; Sanders, D.S. The clinical and phenotypical assessment of seronegative villous atrophy; a prospective UK centre experience evaluating 200 adult cases over a 15-year period (2000–2015). *Gut* **2017**, *66*, 1563–1572. [CrossRef] [PubMed]
43. Vivas, S.; Vaquero, L.; Rodriguez-Martin, L.; Caminero, A. Age-related differences in celiac disease: Specific characteristics of adult presentation. *World J. Gastrointest. Pharmacol. Ther.* **2015**, *6*, 207–212. [CrossRef] [PubMed]
44. Ciccocioppo, R.; Kruzliak, P.; Cangemi, G.C.; Pohanka, M.; Betti, E.; Lauret, E.; Rodrigo, L. The spectrum of differences between childhood and adulthood celiac disease. *Nutrients* **2015**, *7*, 8733–8751. [CrossRef] [PubMed]
45. Husby, S.; Koletzko, S.; Korponay-Szabó, I.R.; Mearin, M.L.; Phillips, A.; Shamir, R.; Troncone, R.; Giersiepen, K.; Branski, D.; Catassi, C.; et al. European society for pediatric gastroenterology, hepatology, and nutrition guidelines, for the diagnosis of coeliac disease. *J. Pediatr. Gastroenterol. Nutr.* **2012**, *54*, 136–160. [CrossRef] [PubMed]
46. Werkstetter, K.J.; Korponay-Szabó, I.R.; Popp, A.; Villanacci, V.; Salemme, M.; Heilig, G.; Lillevang, S.T.; Mearin, M.L.; Ribes-Koninckx, C.; Thomas, A.; et al. Accuracy in diagnosis of celiac disease without biopsies in clinical practice. *Gastroenterology* **2017**, *153*, 924–935. [CrossRef] [PubMed]
47. Lebwohl, B.; Murray, J.A.; Rubio-Tapia, A.; Green, P.H.; Ludvigsson, J.F. Predictors of persistent villous atrophy in coeliac disease: A population-based study. *Aliment. Pharmacol. Ther.* **2014**, *39*, 488–495. [CrossRef] [PubMed]
48. Sharkey, L.M.; Corbett, G.; Currie, E.; Lee, J.; Sweeney, N.; Woodward, J.M. Optimising delivery of care in coeliac disease. Comparison of the benefits of repeat biopsy and serological follow-up. *Aliment. Pharmacol. Ther.* **2013**, *38*, 1278–1291. [CrossRef] [PubMed]
49. Ludvigsson, J.F.; Bai, J.C.; Biagi, F.; Card, T.R.; Ciacci, C.; Ciclitira, P.; Green, P.H.; Hadjivassiliou, M.; Holdoway, A.; van Heel, D.A.; et al. Diagnosis and management of adult coeliac disease: Guidelines from the British society of gastroenterology. *Gut* **2014**, *63*, 1210–1228. [CrossRef] [PubMed]
50. Rosinach, M.; Esteve, M.; Gonzalez, C.; Temino, R.; Marine, M.; Monzon, H.; Sainz, E.; Loras, C.; Espinós, J.C.; Forné, M.; et al. Lymphocytic duodenosis: Aetiology and long-term response to specific treatment. *Dig. Liver Dis.* **2012**, *44*, 643–648. [CrossRef] [PubMed]
51. Corazza, G.R.; Villanacci, V.; Zambelli, C.; Milione, M.; Luinetti, O.; Vindigni, C.; Chioda, C.; Albarello, L.; Bertolini, D.; Donato, F. Comparison of the interobserver reproducibility with different histologic criteria used in celiac disease. *Clin. Gastroenterol. Hepatol.* **2007**, *5*, 838–843. [CrossRef] [PubMed]
52. Oberhüber, G.; Granditsh, G.; Vogelsang, H. The histopathology of coeliac disease: Time for a standardized report scheme for pathologists. *Eur. J. Gastroenterol. Hepatol.* **1999**, *11*, 1185–1194. [CrossRef] [PubMed]
53. Al-toma, A.; Verbeek, W.H.; Mulder, C.J. The management of complicated celiac disease. *Dig. Dis.* **2007**, *25*, 230–236. [CrossRef] [PubMed]
54. Elli, L.; Zini, E.; Tomba, C.; Bardella, M.T.; Bisari, S.; Conte, D.; Runza, L.; Roncoroni, L.; Ferrero, S. Histological evaluation of duodenal biopsies from coeliac patients: The need for different grading criteria during follow-up. *BMC. Gastroenterology* **2015**, *15*, 133. [CrossRef] [PubMed]

55. Rubio-Tapia, A.; Rahim, M.W.; See, J.A.; Lahr, B.D.; Wu, T.T.; Murray, J.A. Mucosal recovery and mortality in adults with celiac disease after treatment with a gluten-free-diet. *Am. J. Gastroenterol.* **2010**, *105*, 1412–1420. [CrossRef] [PubMed]
56. Lebwohl, B.; Granath, F.; Ekbom, A.; Montgomery, S.M.; Murray, J.A.; Rubio-Tapia, A.; Green, P.H.; Ludvigsson, J.F. Mucosal healing and mortality in coeliac disease. *Aliment. Pharmacol. Ther.* **2013**, *37*, 332–339. [CrossRef] [PubMed]
57. Chetcuti Zammit, S.; Sanders, D.S.; Sidhu, R. Capsule endoscopy for patients with coeliac disease. *Expert Rev. Gastroenterol. Hepatol.* **2018**, *12*, 779–790. [CrossRef] [PubMed]
58. Moreno, M.L.; Rodríguez-Herrera, A.; Sousa, C.; Comino, I. Biomarkers to monitor gluten-free diet compliance in celiac patients. *Nutrients* **2017**, *9*, 46. [CrossRef] [PubMed]
59. Comino, I.; Fernández-Bañares, F.; Esteve, M.; Ortigosa, L.; Castillejo, G.; Fambuena, B.; Ribes-Koninckx, C.; Sierra, C.; Rodríguez-Herrera, A.; Salazar, J.C.; et al. Fecal gluten peptides reveal limitations of serological tests and food questionnaires for monitoring gluten-free diet in celiac disease patients. *Am. J. Gastroenterol.* **2016**, *111*, 1456–1465. [CrossRef] [PubMed]
60. Moreno, M.L.; Cebolla, A.; Muñoz-Suano, A.; Carrillo-Carrion, C.; Comino, I.; Pizarro, A.; León, F.; Rodríguez-Herrera, A.; Sousa, C. Detection of gluten immunogenic peptides in the urine of patients with coeliac disease reveals transgressions in the gluten-free diet and incomplete mucosal healing. *Gut* **2017**, *66*, 250–257. [CrossRef] [PubMed]
61. Real, A.; Comino, I.; Moreno, M.L.; López-Casado, M.A.; Lorite, P.; Torres, M.I.; Cebolla, A.; Sousa, C. Identification and in vitro reactivity of celiac immunoactive peptides in an apparent gluten-free beer. *PLoS ONE* **2014**, *9*, e100917. [CrossRef] [PubMed]
62. Roshan, B.; Leffler, D.A.; Jamma, S.; Dennis, M.; Sheth, S.; Falchuk, S.; Najarian, R.; Goldsmith, J.; Tariq, S.; Schuppan, D.; et al. The incidence and clinical spectrum of refractory celiac disease in a North American referral center. *Am. J. Gastroenterol.* **2011**, *106*, 923–928. [CrossRef] [PubMed]
63. Malamut, G.; Afchain, P.; Verkarre, V.; Lecomte, T.; Amiot, A.; Damotte, D.; Bouhnik, Y.; Colombel, J.F.; Delchier, J.C.; Allez, M.; et al. Presentation and long-term follow-up of refractory celiac disease: Comparison of type I with type II. *Gastroenterology* **2009**, *136*, 81–90. [CrossRef] [PubMed]
64. Hussein, S.; Gindin, T.; Lagana, S.M.; Arguelles-Grande, C.; Krishnareddy, S.; Alobeid, B.; Lewis, S.K.; Mansukhani, M.M.; Green, P.H.R.; Bhagat, G. Clonal T cell receptor gene rearrangements in coeliac disease: implications for diagnosing refractory coeliac disease. *J. Clin. Pathol.* **2018**, *71*, 825–831. [CrossRef] [PubMed]
65. Nijeboer, P.; van Wanrooij, R.; van Gils, T.; Wierdsma, N.J.; Tack, G.J.; Witte, B.I.; Bontkes, H.J.; Visser, O.; Mulder, C.; Bouma, G. Lymphoma development and survival in refractory coeliac disease type II: Histological response as prognostic factor. *United Eur. Gastroenterol. J.* **2017**, *5*, 208–217. [CrossRef] [PubMed]
66. Rubio-Tapia, A.; Malamut, G.; Verbeek, W.H.; van Wanrooij, R.L.; Leffler, D.A.; Niveloni, S.I.; Arguelles-Grande, C.; Lahr, B.D.; Zinsmeister, A.R.; Murray, J.A. Creation of a model to predict survival in patients with refractory coeliac disease using a multinational registry. *Aliment. Pharmacol. Ther.* **2016**, *44*, 704–714. [CrossRef] [PubMed]
67. Mukewar, S.S.; Sharma, A.; Rubio-Tapia, A.; Wu, T.T.; Jabri, B.; Murray, J.A. Open-capsule budesonide for refractory celiac disease. *Am. J. Gastroenterol.* **2017**, *112*, 959–967. [CrossRef] [PubMed]

nutrients

MDPI

Review

Gluten-Free Diet in Celiac Disease—Forever and for All?

Alice Itzlinger [1], Federica Branchi [1], Luca Elli [2] and Michael Schumann [1,*]

[1] Division of Gastroenterology, Infectious Diseases and Rheumatology, Campus Benjamin Franklin, Charité Universitätsmedizin Berlin, 12203 Berlin, Germany; alice.itzlinger@charite.de (A.I.); federica.branchi@charite.de (F.B.)

[2] Center for the Prevention and Diagnosis of Celiac Disease, Fondazione IRCCS Ca' Granda Ospedale Maggiore Policlinico, 20122 Milan, Italy; luca.elli@policlinico.mi.it

* Correspondence: michael.schumann@charite.de; Tel.: +49-(0)30-450514536

Received: 16 October 2018; Accepted: 15 November 2018; Published: 18 November 2018

Abstract: The gluten-free diet is the only effective treatment available for celiac disease. However, it is difficult to adhere to and a closer look on the diet's implementation and indications reveals several ambiguities: Not only is there controversy on the threshold of gluten that can be tolerated in the frame of a strict gluten-free diet, but it is also unclear whether the gluten-free diet is an appropriate treatment in patient subgroups with asymptomatic or potential celiac disease. Reports from a number of research groups suggest that a certain proportion of patients may effectively develop tolerance to gluten and thus become suitable for gluten reintroduction over time. In this review, we set out to create an overview about the current state of research as regards the definition of a strict gluten-free diet in terms of the gluten thresholds considered tolerable and the indication for a gluten-free diet in the absence of histological abnormalities or symptoms. Furthermore, we discuss the concept that a gluten-free diet must be followed for life by all patients.

Keywords: gluten; adherence; serology; villous atrophy; mucosal recovery; threshold

1. Introduction

Celiac disease (CD) is an autoimmune disorder triggered by the ingestion of gluten. As a consequence of dietary exposure to gluten, genetically susceptible individuals develop autoimmune reactions resulting in histological changes in the small intestine. These are characterized by duodenal villous atrophy and intraepithelial lymphocytosis (IEL), leading to malabsorption and gastrointestinal as well as extraintestinal symptoms [1]. The clinical presentation of CD is diverse, with a considerable number of patients being asymptomatic. The classical form of CD is characterized by an overt malabsorption syndrome that features chronic diarrhea, steatorrhea, weight loss, and failure to thrive in children. Gastrointestinal symptoms as well as extraintestinal symptoms such as fatigue, osteopenia, iron deficiency, anemia and neurological/psychological disorders such as depression may be present [1,2]. On the other hand, in the non-classical form of CD patients present only one or few gastrointestinal or extraintestinal symptoms [2]. Table 1 shows the characteristics of different clinical presentations.

Table 1. The spectrum of clinical presentations of celiac disease.

Clinical Features	Celiac Disease			
	Classical	Non-Classical	Asymptomatic	Potential
Malabsorption syndrome diarrhea, steatorrhea, weight loss/growth failure, with or without anemia	+	−	−	−
Gastrointestinal symptoms abdominal pain, bloating, constipation	+/−	+/−	−	−
Extraintestinal manifestations fatigue, osteopenia/osteoporosis, iron deficiency, neurological disorders	+/−	+/−	−	−
Serology (tTG/EMA)	+	+	+	+
Histological alterations (Marsh)	+	+	+	−

tTG, anti-transglutaminase antibodies; EMA, anti-endomysial antibodies.

A lifelong gluten-free diet (GFD) has long been considered the only effective treatment for CD. Strict adherence to a GFD has been shown to lead to partial—if not complete—healing of the duodenal mucosa along with resolution of symptoms and signs of malabsorption [2]. It has been observed that mucosal recovery takes more time and is more frequently incomplete in adults than in children [3,4]. There remain, however, open issues regarding not only the tolerable threshold of gluten ingestion but also the appropriateness of a lifelong indication to GFD, particularly in patients with subclinical and potential CD. Considering the impact on the patients' quality of life posed by a restrictive GFD [5,6], its necessity should be reviewed carefully when prescribing it.

First of all, the natural course of CD is not as clearly understood as one might think. It is still unclear if a strict GFD needs to be followed throughout the whole life in all patients or if tolerance may develop in certain patients. While the GFD generally leads to clinical improvement, mucosal abnormalities may persist, but do not add up to functional malabsorption as clinical symptoms decline. Rubio-Tapia et al. observed mucosal recovery in about 35% two years after starting a GFD and in about 66% after five years; however, 82% improved clinically. In line with these findings, clinical improvement of symptoms was not a reliable marker of mucosal recovery ($p = 0.7$) [7]. On the other hand, cases of patients who—in many cases on their own—interrupt the GFD and remain symptom-free have been reported in some studies [8].

Furthermore, while there are strong data supporting the benefits of a GFD in patients with symptomatic CD or CD irrespective of symptomatology, the outcome of GFD within the subgroups of asymptomatic and potential CD is mostly unclear. In these patients, the response to GFD can neither be measured in terms of symptom relief—nor in terms of mucosal healing for potential CD. For this reason, the issue of the actual role of the GFD in the prevention of CD-related complications (e.g., refractory disease, intestinal lymphoma) and other immune disorders should be addressed. In view of the scattered data on the risk of CD-related complications in these patient groups, the prescription of a GFD needs to be critically debated.

The aim of this article is to critically review existing literature data on the therapeutic and prognostic role of the GFD in CD in order to give an overview about the current clinical indications for the GFD and future perspectives for celiac patients.

2. Methods

A comprehensive literature search was carried out on PubMed to identify peer-reviewed articles on GFD in CD published until August 2018. Search strategies included the following key words: celiac disease, gluten-free diet, adherence, autoimmune disorders, gluten re-challenge, gluten tolerance, gluten contamination, celiac disease complications, lymphoproliferative disorders, and enteropathy-associated T-cell lymphoma. A manual search was also carried out on the bibliographies of the identified articles. The most relevant original research articles in the English language, including randomized controlled trials and observational studies (prospective and retrospective) were selected by the authors and are discussed in the following sections.

3. Gluten-Free Diet: How Strict Should It Be?

Current guidelines suggest that the GFD should be strict, with complete avoidance of gluten containing products and attention to cross-contaminations [2].

Gluten contamination, even within the frame of a strict GFD, cannot be entirely avoided: Plenty of products contain hidden gluten, such as sausages, soups, soy sauce and ice cream. But even in gluten-free-labeled products there are traces of gluten. This is mostly due to cross-contamination with gluten-containing products that are processed or stored in the same place [9]. The term "gluten-free" thus generally refers to an amount of gluten that is thought to be harmless and does not imply total absence of gluten. In fact, the amount of gluten deriving solely from cross-contamination in a supposedly GFD may range from 5 to 50 mg per day [10,11]. The level of gluten content in food products is expressed as parts per million (ppm, corresponding to mg/kg). Gibert et al., collected consumption data of gluten-free products by CD patients in order to estimate the average gluten exposure of celiac patients who follow a GFD. Taking into account different dietary habits in European countries (Norway, Germany, Italy, Spain) they concluded that a limit of 20 ppm for products naturally gluten-free and 100 ppm for products rendered gluten-free would be acceptable [12]. According to the current guidelines of the European Commission a commercially sold product may be called "gluten-free" if it contains less than 20 ppm gluten (20mg/kg) [13].

Several studies have tried to establish a safe threshold of daily gluten intake, as summarized in Table 2. A prospective, multicenter, placebo-controlled, double-blind, randomized gluten challenge trial by Catassi et al., found that the chronic ingestion of small amounts of gliadin leads to a dose-dependent relapse in symptoms: children diagnosed with CD who had followed a GFD for at least three months were given small amounts of gluten for a period of four weeks [14]. Patients who had received 100 mg gliadin/day (= about 200 mg of gluten or the equivalent of 2–5 g wheat flour) displayed minimal morphometric changes in the jejunal histology. Patients who had ingested 500 mg gliadin per day showed significantly more histological abnormalities. Additionally, some patients became positive to antibodies again and experienced a symptom relapse. These results support the findings of a previous study by Ciclitira et al., who found no changes in mucosal histology after the infusion of 10 mg gliadin, minimal changes after 100 mg of gliadin and significant changes after an additional 500 mg of gliadin [15].

A further prospective, double blind, placebo-controlled trial by Catassi et al., analyzed the effects of daily ingestion of 0, 10, or 50 mg gluten for 90 days [9]. While the villous height to crypt depth ratio of the placebo group raised by 9%, no difference was found in the 10 mg group and a −20% was found in the group receiving 50 mg gluten/day. The IEL count did not differ significantly between the three groups. Catassi et al., concluded that the ingestion of contaminating gluten should be kept lower than 50 mg/day in the treatment of CD [9,16].

Table 2. Relevant original studies evaluating the safe daily gluten threshold for celiac disease patients (adapted from Akobeng et al. [17]). CD: celiac disease; GFD: gluten-free diet; IEL: intraepithelial lymphocytosis; RCT: Randomized Controlled Trial.

Study	Methods	Participants	Diet	Aim of the Study	Results/Conclusion
Catassi 2007 [9]	RCT from Italy	39 adults with CD on GFD for >2 years	90 days, - 50 mg gluten/day ($n = 13$) - 10 mg gluten/day ($n = 13$) - 50 mg placebo/day ($n = 13$)	To evaluate the safe threshold of ingestion of contaminating gluten	Ingestion of contaminating gluten should be lower than 50 mg/day
Collin 2004 [10]	Cross-sectional study from Finland	76 adults, 16 children with CD on GFD for 1–10 years	Median 2 years - naturally GFD ($n = 28$) - wheat starch-based GFD ($n = 64$)	To establish a limit for residual gluten in gluten-free products	Threshold should be lower than 100 mg/day
Peräaho 2003 [18]	RCT from Finland	57 adults with newly diagnosed, untreated CD	1 year - wheat-starch-based-GFD ($n = 28$) - natural GFD ($n = 29$)	To evaluate the difference between a wheat starch-based GFD and natural GFD	No histological/clinical differences between the two groups
Lohiniemi 2000 [19]	Cross-sectional study from Finland	58 adults with CD, 110 healthy controls	Patients on wheat starch-based GFD	To evaluate the effect of wheat-starch based GFD on clinical symptoms	Wheat starch-based gluten-free products are suitable for CD patients
Selby 1999 [20]	Cross-sectional study from Australia	89 adults with CD	- Codex GFD (<500 ppm) ($n = 39$) - GFD < 30 mg ($n = 50$)	To evaluate the effect of gluten traces in GFD	No histological differences between the groups
Catassi 1993 [14]	Randomized controlled trial from Italy	20 children with CD on GFD	4 weeks - 100 mg gliadin/day ≈ 200 mg gluten/day ($n = 10$) - 500 mg gliadin/day ≈ 1 g gluten/day ($n = 10$)	To evaluate the effects of chronic ingestion of gliadin	Histological deterioration and increase in IEL count in both groups, clinical relapse in 30% of 1 g-group

Two systematic reviews aimed to determine the safe maximum gluten intake. Hischenhuber et al., suggested that the maximum daily gluten intake should lie between 10 and 100 mg [11]. Akobeng and Thomas included thirteen studies and similarly found that the amount of tolerable gluten varied widely between the studies, ranging from patients who tolerated an average of 34–36 mg gluten per day to others who developed symptoms and/or histological abnormalities when consuming 10 mg gluten per day [17]. The results of these systematic reviews show that there is no single definitive threshold for gluten intake but that a daily intake of <10 mg is unlikely to cause mucosal abnormalities (see also Table 2).

More Than A Strict Gluten-Free Diet

Several research groups have observed that in a considerable portion of patients complying to a presumed strict GFD, complete mucosal recovery and/or resolution of symptom do not occur [5,19–22]. These results led to questions regarding the efficacy of the GFD in obtaining histological remission.

The first step in patients with signs of non-responsive CD should be the evaluation of the GFD by a trained dietitian to unveil possible unwitting intake of gluten. However, current methods and questionnaires still rely on the patients' subjective assertions and not able to accurately measure dietary compliance [23]. A relatively new method to monitor GFD compliance is the detection of gluten immunogenic peptides that can be found in the urine and feces after gluten consumption. This offers an objective method to assess the dietary adherence and has shown to be very sensitive [24–26].

While most patients tolerate trace gluten under the 20 ppm threshold, a subgroup might react even more sensitively. It has therefore been suggested that a more-than-strict GFD regimen has the potential to induce mucosal recovery in these patients [27]. The Gluten Contamination Elimination Diet (GCED) is a diet that was developed to remove even minute amount of gluten from the diet, consisting of a more restrictive dietary regimen focusing on the use of naturally gluten-free products rather than processed gluten-free food [27–29].

Hollon et al., identified 17 patients not responsive to GFD. Before starting the GCED, all subjects were assessed by a dietitian who excluded hidden gluten ingestion. After completing the GCED for 3–6 months, 82% responded to the GCED and became asymptomatic [28].

Zanini et al., investigated if complete mucosal recovery can be achieved by adopting this restrictive diet or, alternatively, after a prolonged time of GFD [29]. In this small study, after three months of GCED, no changes in villous height and crypt depth were observed as compared to two years of GFD. Only a slight, though significant decrease in IELs and T-cells with a distinctive T-cell receptor (TCR) on their surface, so called TCRγδ+ cells, was found. The study suggested that the intraepithelial lymphocytosis persisting in CD patients during GFD cannot completely be eliminated even on a GCED and is furthermore independent of the duration of adherence to a standard GFD. Whether gluten contamination is unavoidable despite GCED, or a three-month period of GCED was too short, could not be clarified by the study, possibly also due to the small sample size [29]. Given the scarce data, there is insufficient evidence to recommend a gluten contamination elimination diet on a routine basis in patients with CD. However, it should be considered in patients who are not responsive to traditional GFD.

4. Does the Gluten-free Diet Prevent the Development of Autoimmune Diseases and of Celiac Disease Complications?

4.1. Diet and Autoimmune Diseases

Patients with CD are at increased risk for various autoimmune disorders, particularly diabetes mellitus type I and autoimmune thyroiditis but also autoimmune hepatitis, rheumatoid arthritis and Sjögren's syndrome among others [30–32]. The same applies vice versa: Patients with autoimmune diseases have a significantly higher prevalence of CD than the healthy population—a Norwegian study found that around 5% patients with type 1 diabetes also have celiac disease [30]. The association between CD and other autoimmune conditions is presumably caused by a common genetic background (the presence of predisposing human leucocyte antigen (HLA) class II haplotypes), but the direct role of gluten exposure in the development of associated autoimmune conditions is still a matter of debate [33].

There are a number of contradictory studies concerning the association between the development of an additional autoimmune disorder and the duration of gluten exposure. Initially, it was hypothesized that strict adherence to GFD could prevent the development of further autoimmune diseases in patients with celiac disease. A cross-sectional study by Ventura et al., in 1999 showed an association between the prevalence of autoimmune disorders in CD patients and the age at diagnosis of CD, suggesting that duration of exposure to gluten might be a predictor of the development of other autoimmune conditions [34]. However, more recent studies tend to argue against a connection: A study by Sategna et al., found no correlation between the duration of exposure to gluten and the prevalence of autoimmune diseases [35]. Similar results were shown in a Finnish study in 2005 [31] as well as by a follow-up study by the same group [36].

All in all, current data allow for the assumption that the GFD has no definite role in the prevention of development of other autoimmune conditions.

4.2. Diet and Celiac Disease Complications

In children, early detection and treatment of celiac disease are of utmost importance to prevent complications such as poor growth, decreased bone mineral density, and enamel defects which can be irreversible [37,38]. But even for adults, a diagnostic delay is associated with decreased quality of life, more days of sickness, and frequent use of medicines and health care services [39]. The GFD is an effective tool against gastrointestinal and extraintestinal manifestations as well as complications such as malabsorption and osteoporosis [39–41].

Another complication is refractory CD which is defined as the persistence of clinical signs of CD, as well as villous atrophy, despite adherence to a strict GFD for at least 12 months [1]. Of the two subtypes of refractory CD, type II is associated with a worse prognosis in view of the high risk of development of malignancy. The enteropathy-associated T-cell lymphoma (EATL) is a lymphoproliferative disorder that typically develops in the setting of refractory CD. This is a rare type of T-cell lymphoma that arises from intraepithelial T-cells in the small intestine. A higher risk for developing other malignancies, including small bowel adenocarcinoma, has been reported in the setting of CD, but the underlying pathogenesis is still unclear [42–46].

Given the poor prognosis and limited therapeutic options available for type II refractory CD and EATL, research focused on both early diagnosis and identification of risk factors. The role of the GFD for the prevention of EATL development is controversial. From a pathophysiological point of view, EATL develops from aberrant intestinal lymphocytes that proliferate clonally independently of gluten exposure—a longer exposure to gluten, and thus a prolonged immune activation in the intestinal mucosa, may in fact contribute to create a favorable environment to the development and proliferation of aberrant lymphocytes [47]. However, the natural history of CD and the actual prognostic effect of the GFD are difficult to investigate and mainly based on retrospective data analysis.

Observational studies investigating the association between undiagnosed CD and mortality risk showed contradicting results, possibly also due to difficulty of differentiating between undiagnosed asymptomatic CD from mono-/oligosymptomatic or symptomatic CD based on medical record and patients reports. Rubio-Tapia et al., reported an up to 4-fold increased mortality rate in undiagnosed CD during 45 years of follow up, suggesting both a possible role of gluten exposure in the development of malignancies and the necessity of very long follow-ups in order to investigate this area [42]. Similarly, a German study showed an excess in mortality, particularly due to cancer, in patients with elevated transglutaminase antibody levels [43]. On the other hand, population-based study like that by Lohi et al., could not find an excess of mortality in unrecognized CD, though reporting a tendency to die from lymphoproliferative disorders, stroke and respiratory diseases [48]. In a case-control study published in 2011, Olén et al., assessed the characteristics of CD patients with particular attention to their diet compliance and compared it with the risk of developing malignant lymphoma [49]. They could not find an association between the development of lymphoma and non-compliance to GFD even though they could not entirely exclude a moderate effect. A study by Biagi et al., suggested the amount of exposure to gluten to be a relevant risk factor for developing malignancies such as EATL [50]. This hypothesis was based on an indirect link: the authors observed that reported mortality rates in CD patients were higher in Southern than in Northern Europe and correlated with the gluten content of the typical diet of each country. Hence, it was presumed that the amount of dietary gluten ingested (before and after diagnosis) was responsible for a higher incidence of complications and higher mortality.

Given the ambiguity that exists, we cannot exclude a causal association between duration and amount of gluten consumption and the development of refractory celiac disease (RCD) and malignancies. It therefore remains essential to advise and stress the importance of a strict GFD to patients with celiac disease. Further research and in particular prospective studies about the aforementioned linkage are needed in order to clarify the role of gluten exposure in this setting.

5. Gluten-Free Diet in Potential Celiac Disease

Potential CD is characterized by positive endomysium and/or anti-transglutaminase antibodies and a normal intestinal histology [1]. It is important to emphasize the distinct difference between potential and asymptomatic celiac disease. While all other forms of celiac disease are characterized by intestinal mucosal abnormalities, patients with potential celiac disease do, by definition, not display any histological abnormalities. Individuals with potential CD are often identified as a result of screening or incidental findings on routine examinations (e.g., screening of first-degree relatives or after diagnosis of related autoimmune diseases). The question arises whether individuals with potential CD benefit from a GFD or if the GFD results in a social and economic burden and a risk of malnutrition devoid of health benefits for this subgroup of patients.

First of all, it must be pointed out that individuals with potential CD may not always be completely asymptomatic and a GFD could be of benefit even in the absence of histologically evident mucosal changes [51,52]. Moreover, the adequacy of histology sampling has to be reviewed before classifying a patient with positive serology as potential CD, since at least four duodenal biopsies (according to some guidelines even six biopsies) are required to ensure an adequate diagnosis and some subjects may show histological changes only in the duodenal bulb [2,53,54]. It is a matter of debate if a reference pathologist should be consulted in contradictory cases. This claim is substantiated by data revealing a high interobserver variability in histopathology [55–57].

Kurppa et al., studied the effects of a GFD in screening-detected asymptomatic patients with CD [51]. They included also 40 patients positive to IgA-anti-endomysium antibodies that were at risk for CD (potential CD), who were randomized to either group A following a GFD or group B continuing a normal diet for a year. Despite the fact that all subjects prior to the study described themselves as "asymptomatic", only group A improved significantly on the Gastrointestinal Symptoms Rating Scale. However, social functioning was impaired by the GFD. The authors concluded that even apparently asymptomatic patients with positive antibodies benefit from a GFD.

In another study, Mandile et al., evaluated the effect of GFD on clinical symptoms and mucosal histology in children with potential CD [58]. After one year on GFD no significant differences were observed in terms of Marsh grade, lamina propria CD25+ cells, CD3+ and $\gamma\delta$+ intraepithelial lymphocytes density and intestinal anti-TG2 deposits. However, about half of the patients reported improved clinical symptoms. A similar result was observed by Volta et al. [52]. Patients with potential CD that showed symptoms improved clinically by following a GFD.

On the other hand, it is interesting to assess the question how many patients with positive CD serology and normal histology will eventually develop CD characteristic celiac histology. Biagi et al., found only 35% to have developed a flat mucosa in the course of their disease. However, 29% of those with a normal histology decided to switch onto a GFD early on in the course, making it impossible to judge on their further natural course [59]. Interestingly, a reversal of CD serology has also been observed, especially in children [60]. Auricchio et al., studied 210 children with potential CD of which 175 were left on a gluten-containing diet [61]. Antibodies and clinical symptoms were checked twice a year and a small bowel biopsy was taken every second year. They found that 37% of the subjects showed fluctuation and 20% normalization of antibody production over the years, most of them (67%) without ever displaying mucosal damage during 9 years of follow-up. They concluded that a GFD might not always be necessary for individuals with potential CD. Volta et al., after collecting data from 77 adult patients from CD, proposed to prescribe a GFD only to clinically symptomatic patients with potential CD due to the observed improvement of symptoms after gluten withdrawal [52]. In asymptomatic patients who remained on a gluten-containing diet, progression to overt CD could merely be observed in 1 of 16 patients during a 5-years follow up. A possible rational approach in view of available data is shown in Figure 1.

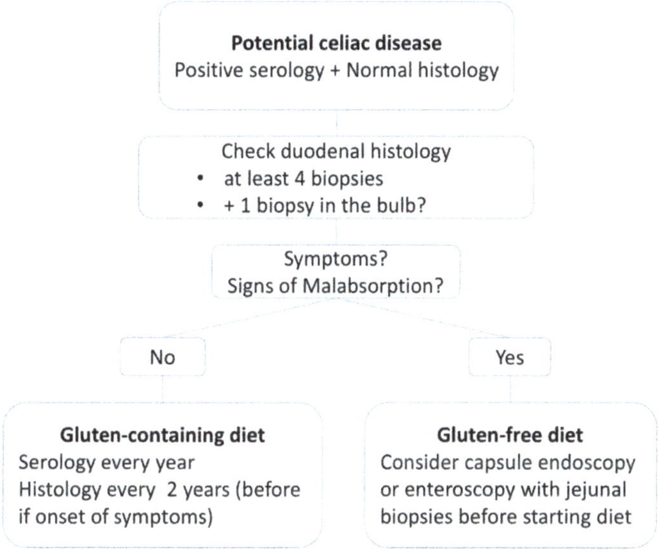

Figure 1. Rational approach to patients with potential CD.

6. Is There A Way Towards Gluten Reintroduction in Celiac Disease?

In recent years, there has been active debate on whether the GFD should be continued lifelong in all celiac patients. Data on the natural history of CD suggest that an excess of mortality, possibly derived from lymphoproliferative disorders, may be subsequent to higher/longer exposure to dietary gluten [7,33,51,62]: On this basis, the GFD should be continued indefinitely not only to prevent clinical relapse and malabsorption, but also to prevent complications.

Nevertheless, there are a number of studies published during the last 30 years that showed proof for the existence of a "latent" form of CD, where symptoms and histologic changes disappear in the course of disease despite consumption of a GFD. As early as 1989, a Finnish study tried to evaluate the possibility of development of gluten tolerance in children: 38 post pubertal children with CD were rebiopsied before a gluten challenge was carried out [63]. Eleven percent did not relapse (clinically and histologically) after 2 years, indicating a possible recovery from CD in this small subgroup.

Matysiak-Budnik et al., in 2007 conducted a retrospective analysis of clinical symptoms, mucosal recovery and laboratory findings of patients diagnosed with CD in childhood who, despite diagnosis, did not follow a GFD but resumed a normal diet and remained clinically silent [64]. They found that about a fifth of CD patients developed long-term latency (normal duodenal histology) after gluten reintroduction. Patients who remained clinically silent but displayed histological abnormalities were at increased risk for osteoporosis. The authors therefore concluded that a GFD is advisable in patients with asymptomatic CD, but that a subgroup of celiac patients may actually become gluten tolerant over time. However, tolerance could be transient and therefore demands regular follow-up. In fact, two "gluten-tolerant" patients actually showed clinical and mucosal relapse during the follow up.

Hopman et al., performed a follow-up with 77 patients who had been diagnosed with CD for over ten years [65]. Gluten consumption, symptoms, bone mineral density and antibodies were examined. Two thirds adhered to GFD, 15% were partially compliant and 23% followed a regular gluten-containing diet. Interestingly, biopsies revealed a normal mucosal histology in four of eight patients on gluten-containing diet and in all patients who were partially compliant. The authors concluded that development of tolerance to gluten was possible in some patients with CD. They suggest a regular follow-up to determine if this tolerance is permanent or not.

Although poor adherence to the GFD is the major predictor of persistence of mucosal lesions at follow-up histology, a recent study by Norsa et al., showed no excess in mortality among celiac patients with a long history of CD with poor or no adherence to the GFD, also reporting a proportion of patients of almost 30% with no relapse of villous atrophy despite chronic voluntary gluten ingestion [8].

Who Could Benefit Most from Gluten Reintroduction?

Screening-detected CD patients are a subgroup of patients that experience more difficulty accepting the diagnosis and permanent dietary restriction since its justification, in the absence of symptoms, is less evident than in symptomatic patients that experience immediate improvement in health when adhering to GFD [66]. They report a decreased perception of health on a GFD [6] and may feel less motivated to adhere to the diet than symptomatic patients [67]. Accordingly, a recent study published in August 2018 studied the long-term health and treatment outcomes in screening-detected CD patients [66]. At a median of 18.5 years after diagnosis, 236 patients completed follow-up questionnaires. With regard to clinical symptoms and quality of life, the screening-detected subgroup showed more anxiety and lower general well-being than CD patients that had been diagnosed due to clinical suspicion. In this group of patients, the GFD is recommended in order to avoid long-term consequences of malabsorption. Moreover, epidemiological data on the excess mortality of CD complications linked to gluten exposure have been questioned [8,48].

In other words, considering the reported proportion—20–30% of CD patients able to develop a gluten tolerance over time and the limited risk of developing osteoporosis and complications over a short time of histological relapse of villous atrophy—it needs to be questioned whether a gluten reintroduction (or "re-challenge") under careful follow-up could be a rational therapeutic option in patients with asymptomatic celiac disease. As follow-up, lifelong assessments including histology would be needed, in order to detect a possible relapse and worsening of mucosal histology. More research is needed before this option can be implemented into the clinical routine, however.

7. Conclusions and Future Perspectives

In patients affected by CD, the GFD ensures improvement of clinical symptoms and signs of malabsorption in the vast majority of cases. Despite extensive research aimed at developing alternative therapies for CD, the GFD remains the only effective treatment available to date [68]. However, it is not easy to follow and may result in a psychological and social burden for patients [5,6]. For this reason, the GFD should be prescribed only once CD diagnosis has been established by means of serology and duodenal histology.

In potential CD, the diet should be reserved to subjects reporting symptoms, while those asymptomatic can be maintained on a gluten-containing diet but should be followed up on a regular basis.

In patients with symptomatic CD, the diet should be followed strictly in view of the risk for complications such as osteoporosis and other consequences of malabsorption. Gluten exposure neither appears to be linked to the onset of other autoimmune disorders nor has an increased risk for malignancies been shown in asymptomatic CD so far. The current literature available, however, does not provide enough evidence to safely recommend a gluten-containing regimen in asymptomatic CD. More research on this topic is needed before introducing a gluten re-challenge for asymptomatic CD patients into the clinical routine.

The natural history of CD on a gluten-containing diet is still far from understood: It is unclear whether the large group of patients with mild or asymptomatic CD is indeed at risk of developing long-term-complications such as EATL. Further studies aimed at investigating the effects of gluten reintroduction in CD are required to identify the subgroup of patients that may develop gluten tolerance over time, without increasing the risk for CD related complications.

Author Contributions: Conceptualization, F.B., A.I., M.S. and L.E.; Methodology, A.I. and F.B.; Software, A.I.; Validation, A.I., F.B., M.S. and L.E.; Formal Analysis, A.I., F.B. and M.S.; Investigation, A.I. and F.B.; Resources, A.I., F.B., M.S. and L.E.; Data Curation, A.I. and F.B.; Writing—Original Draft Preparation, A.I. and F.B.; Writing—Review & Editing, A.I, F.B, M.S and L.E.; Visualization, A.I. and F.B.; Supervision, M.S.; Project Administration, F.B., M.S. and L.E.

Funding: FB received funding from the ECCO (European Crohn´s and Colitis Organization) fellowship program. MS was funded by the Clinical Scientist program and received funding by the DFG GRK 2318 and DFG TRR241 collaborative research center.

Conflicts of Interest: The authors declare no conflict of interest.

References

1. Ludvigsson, J.F.; Leffler, D.A.; Bai, J.C.; Biagi, F.; Fasano, A.; Green, P.H.R.; Hadjivassiliou, M.; Kaukinen, K.; Kelly, C.P.; Leonard, J.N.; et al. The Oslo definitions for coeliac disease and related terms. *Gut* **2013**, *62*, 43–52. [CrossRef] [PubMed]
2. Ludvigsson, J.F.; Bai, J.C.; Biagi, F.; Card, T.R.; Ciacci, C.; Ciclitira, P.J.; Green, P.H.R.; Hadjivassiliou, M.; Holdoway, A.; van Heel, D.A.; et al. Diagnosis and management of adult coeliac disease: Guidelines from the British Society of Gastroenterology. *Gut* **2014**. [CrossRef] [PubMed]
3. Husby, S.; Koletzko, S.; Korponay-Szabó, I.R.; Mearin, M.L.; Phillips, A.; Shamir, R.; Troncone, R.; Giersiepen, K.; Branski, D.; Catassi, C.; et al. ESPGHAN Working Group on Coeliac Disease Diagnosis; ESPGHAN Gastroenterology Committee; European Society for Pediatric Gastroenterology, Hepatology, and Nutrition European Society for Pediatric Gastroenterology, Hepatology, and Nutrition guidelines for the diagnosis of coeliac disease. *J. Pediatr. Gastroenterol. Nutr.* **2012**, *54*, 136–160. [CrossRef] [PubMed]
4. Ciccocioppo, R.; Kruzliak, P.; Cangemi, G.C.; Pohanka, M.; Betti, E.; Lauret, E.; Rodrigo, L. The Spectrum of Differences between Childhood and Adulthood Celiac Disease. *Nutrients* **2015**, *7*, 8733–8751. [CrossRef] [PubMed]
5. Barratt, S.M.; Leeds, J.S.; Sanders, D.S. Quality of life in Coeliac Disease is determined by perceived degree of difficulty adhering to a gluten-free diet, not the level of dietary adherence ultimately achieved. *J. Gastrointest. Liver Dis.* **2011**, *20*, 241–245.
6. Ukkola, A.; Mäki, M.; Kurppa, K.; Collin, P.; Huhtala, H.; Kekkonen, L.; Kaukinen, K. Diet improves perception of health and well-being in symptomatic, but not asymptomatic, patients with celiac disease. *Clin. Gastroenterol. Hepatol. Off. Clin. Pract. J. Am. Gastroenterol. Assoc.* **2011**, *9*, 118–123. [CrossRef] [PubMed]
7. Rubio-Tapia, A.; Rahim, M.W.; See, J.A.; Lahr, B.D.; Wu, T.-T.; Murray, J.A. Mucosal recovery and mortality in adults with celiac disease after treatment with a gluten-free diet. *Am. J. Gastroenterol.* **2010**, *105*, 1412–1420. [CrossRef] [PubMed]
8. Norsa, L.; Branchi, F.; Bravo, M.; Ferretti, F.; Roncoroni, L.; Somalvico, F.; Conte, D.; Bardella, M.T.; Fabiano, S.; Barigelletti, G.; et al. Celiac Disease 30 Years After Diagnosis: Struggling With Gluten-free Adherence or Gaining Gluten Tolerance? *J. Pediatr. Gastroenterol. Nutr.* **2018**, *67*, 361–366. [CrossRef] [PubMed]
9. Catassi, C.; Fabiani, E.; Iacono, G.; D'Agate, C.; Francavilla, R.; Biagi, F.; Volta, U.; Accomando, S.; Picarelli, A.; De Vitis, I.; et al. A prospective, double-blind, placebo-controlled trial to establish a safe gluten threshold for patients with celiac disease. *Am. J. Clin. Nutr.* **2007**, *85*, 160–166. [CrossRef] [PubMed]

10. Collin, P.; Thorell, L.; Kaukinen, K.; Mäki, M. The safe threshold for gluten contamination in gluten-free products. Can trace amounts be accepted in the treatment of coeliac disease? *Aliment. Pharmacol. Ther.* **2004**, *19*, 1277–1283. [CrossRef] [PubMed]
11. Hischenhuber, C.; Crevel, R.; Jarry, B.; Mäki, M.; Moneret-Vautrin, D.A.; Romano, A.; Troncone, R.; Ward, R. Review article: Safe amounts of gluten for patients with wheat allergy or coeliac disease. *Aliment. Pharmacol. Ther.* **2006**, *23*, 559–575. [CrossRef] [PubMed]
12. Gibert, A.; Espadaler, M.; Angel Canela, M.; Sánchez, A.; Vaqué, C.; Rafecas, M. Consumption of gluten-free products: Should the threshold value for trace amounts of gluten be at 20, 100 or 200 p.p.m.? *Eur. J. Gastroenterol. Hepatol.* **2006**, *18*, 1187–1195. [CrossRef] [PubMed]
13. Commission Implementing Regulation (EU) No 828/2014 of 30 July 2014 on the Requirements for the Provision of Information to Consumers on the Absence or Reduced Presence of Gluten in Food Text with EEA Relevance. Available online: https://eur-lex.europa.eu/legal-content/EN/TXT/?uri=CELEX%3A32014R0828 (accessed on 16 October 2018).
14. Catassi, C.; Rossini, M.; Rätsch, I.M.; Bearzi, I.; Santinelli, A.; Castagnani, R.; Pisani, E.; Coppa, G.V.; Giorgi, P.L. Dose dependent effects of protracted ingestion of small amounts of gliadin in coeliac disease children: A clinical and jejunal morphometric study. *Gut* **1993**, *34*, 1515–1519. [CrossRef] [PubMed]
15. Ciclitira, P.J.; Evans, D.J.; Fagg, N.L.; Lennox, E.S.; Dowling, R.H. Clinical testing of gliadin fractions in coeliac patients. *Clin. Sci.* **1984**, *66*, 357–364. [CrossRef] [PubMed]
16. Collin, P.; Mäki, M.; Kaukinen, K. Safe gluten threshold for patients with celiac disease: Some patients are more tolerant than others. *Am. J. Clin. Nutr.* **2007**, *86*, 260. [CrossRef] [PubMed]
17. Akobeng, A.K.; Thomas, A.G. Systematic review: Tolerable amount of gluten for people with coeliac disease. *Aliment. Pharmacol. Ther.* **2008**, *27*, 1044–1052. [CrossRef] [PubMed]
18. Peräaho, M.; Kaukinen, K.; Paasikivi, K.; Sievänen, H.; Lohiniemi, S.; Mäki, M.; Collin, P. Wheat-starch-based gluten-free products in the treatment of newly detected coeliac disease: Prospective and randomized study. *Aliment. Pharmacol. Ther.* **2003**, *17*, 587–594. [CrossRef] [PubMed]
19. Lohiniemi, S.; Mäki, M.; Kaukinen, K.; Laippala, P.; Collin, P. Gastrointestinal symptoms rating scale in coeliac disease patients on wheat starch-based gluten-free diets. *Scand. J. Gastroenterol.* **2000**, *35*, 947–949. [PubMed]
20. Selby, W.S.; Painter, D.; Collins, A.; Faulkner-Hogg, K.B.; Loblay, R.H. Persistent mucosal abnormalities in coeliac disease are not related to the ingestion of trace amounts of gluten. *Scand. J. Gastroenterol.* **1999**, *34*, 909–914. [PubMed]
21. Ciacci, C.; Cirillo, M.; Cavallaro, R.; Mazzacca, G. Long-term follow-up of celiac adults on gluten-free diet: Prevalence and correlates of intestinal damage. *Digestion* **2002**, *66*, 178–185. [CrossRef] [PubMed]
22. Mahadev, S.; Murray, J.A.; Wu, T.-T.; Chandan, V.S.; Torbenson, M.S.; Kelly, C.P.; Maki, M.; Green, P.H.R.; Adelman, D.; Lebwohl, B. Factors associated with villus atrophy in symptomatic coeliac disease patients on a gluten-free diet. *Aliment. Pharmacol. Ther.* **2017**, *45*, 1084–1093. [CrossRef] [PubMed]
23. Biagi, F.; Andrealli, A.; Bianchi, P.I.; Marchese, A.; Klersy, C.; Corazza, G.R. A gluten-free diet score to evaluate dietary compliance in patients with coeliac disease. *Br. J. Nutr.* **2009**, *102*, 882–887. [CrossRef] [PubMed]
24. De Lourdes Moreno, M.; Cebolla, Á.; Muñoz-Suano, A.; Carrillo-Carrion, C.; Comino, I.; Pizarro, Á.; León, F.; Rodríguez-Herrera, A.; Sousa, C. Detection of gluten immunogenic peptides in the urine of patients with coeliac disease reveals transgressions in the gluten-free diet and incomplete mucosal healing. *Gut* **2017**, *66*, 250–257. [CrossRef] [PubMed]
25. Moreno Amador, M.L.; Rodríguez-Herrera, A.; Sousa, C.; Comino, I. Biomarkers to Monitor Gluten-Free Diet Compliance in Celiac Patients. *Nutrients* **2017**, *9*. [CrossRef] [PubMed]
26. Comino, I.; Fernández-Bañares, F.; Esteve, M.; Ortigosa, L.; Castillejo, G.; Fambuena, B.; Ribes-Koninckx, C.; Sierra, C.; Rodríguez-Herrera, A.; Salazar, J.C.; et al. Fecal Gluten Peptides Reveal Limitations of Serological Tests and Food Questionnaires for Monitoring Gluten-Free Diet in Celiac Disease Patients. *Am. J. Gastroenterol.* **2016**, *111*, 1456–1465. [CrossRef] [PubMed]
27. Leonard, M.M.; Cureton, P.; Fasano, A. Indications and Use of the Gluten Contamination Elimination Diet for Patients with Non-Responsive Celiac Disease. *Nutrients* **2017**, *9*. [CrossRef] [PubMed]

28. Hollon, J.R.; Cureton, P.A.; Martin, M.L.; Puppa, E.L.L.; Fasano, A. Trace gluten contamination may play a role in mucosal and clinical recovery in a subgroup of diet-adherent non-responsive celiac disease patients. *BMC Gastroenterol.* **2013**, *13*, 40. [CrossRef] [PubMed]
29. Zanini, B.; Marullo, M.; Villanacci, V.; Salemme, M.; Lanzarotto, F.; Ricci, C.; Lanzini, A. Persistent Intraepithelial Lymphocytosis in Celiac Patients Adhering to Gluten-Free Diet Is Not Abolished Despite a Gluten Contamination Elimination Diet. *Nutrients* **2016**, *8*. [CrossRef] [PubMed]
30. Elfström, P.; Sundström, J.; Ludvigsson, J.F. Systematic review with meta-analysis: Associations between coeliac disease and type 1 diabetes. *Aliment. Pharmacol. Ther.* **2014**, *40*, 1123–1132. [CrossRef] [PubMed]
31. Viljamaa, M.; Kaukinen, K.; Huhtala, H.; Kyrönpalo, S.; Rasmussen, M.; Collin, P. Coeliac disease, autoimmune diseases and gluten exposure. *Scand. J. Gastroenterol.* **2005**, *40*, 437–443. [CrossRef] [PubMed]
32. Hadithi, M.; de Boer, H.; Meijer, J.W.R.; Willekens, F.; Kerckhaert, J.A.; Heijmans, R.; Peña, A.S.; Stehouwer, C.D.A.; Mulder, C.J.J. Coeliac disease in Dutch patients with Hashimoto's thyroiditis and vice versa. *World J. Gastroenterol.* **2007**, *13*, 1715–1722. [CrossRef] [PubMed]
33. Diamanti, A.; Capriati, T.; Bizzarri, C.; Ferretti, F.; Ancinelli, M.; Romano, F.; Perilli, A.; Laureti, F.; Locatelli, M. Autoimmune diseases and celiac disease which came first: Genotype or gluten? *Expert Rev. Clin. Immunol.* **2016**, *12*, 67–77. [CrossRef] [PubMed]
34. Ventura, A.; Magazzù, G.; Greco, L. Duration of exposure to gluten and risk for autoimmune disorders in patients with celiac disease. SIGEP Study Group for Autoimmune Disorders in Celiac Disease. *Gastroenterology* **1999**, *117*, 297–303. [CrossRef] [PubMed]
35. Sategna Guidetti, C.; Solerio, E.; Scaglione, N.; Aimo, G.; Mengozzi, G. Duration of gluten exposure in adult coeliac disease does not correlate with the risk for autoimmune disorders. *Gut* **2001**, *49*, 502–505. [CrossRef] [PubMed]
36. Metso, S.; Hyytiä-Ilmonen, H.; Kaukinen, K.; Huhtala, H.; Jaatinen, P.; Salmi, J.; Taurio, J.; Collin, P. Gluten-free diet and autoimmune thyroiditis in patients with celiac disease. A prospective controlled study. *Scand. J. Gastroenterol.* **2012**, *47*, 43–48. [CrossRef] [PubMed]
37. Mustalahti, K.; Collin, P.; Sievänen, H.; Salmi, J.; Mäki, M. Osteopenia in patients with clinically silent coeliac disease warrants screening. *Lancet Lond. Engl.* **1999**, *354*, 744–745. [CrossRef]
38. Majorana, A.; Bardellini, E.; Ravelli, A.; Plebani, A.; Polimeni, A.; Campus, G. Implications of gluten exposure period, CD clinical forms, and HLA typing in the association between celiac disease and dental enamel defects in children. A case-control study. *Int. J. Paediatr. Dent.* **2010**, *20*, 119–124. [CrossRef] [PubMed]
39. Fuchs, V.; Kurppa, K.; Huhtala, H.; Mäki, M.; Kekkonen, L.; Kaukinen, K. Delayed celiac disease diagnosis predisposes to reduced quality of life and incremental use of health care services and medicines: A prospective nationwide study. *United Eur. Gastroenterol. J.* **2018**, *6*, 567–575. [CrossRef] [PubMed]
40. Pantaleoni, S.; Luchino, M.; Adriani, A.; Pellicano, R.; Stradella, D.; Ribaldone, D.G.; Sapone, N.; Isaia, G.C.; Di Stefano, M.; Astegiano, M. Bone mineral density at diagnosis of celiac disease and after 1 year of gluten free diet. *Sci. World J.* **2014**, *2014*, 173082. [CrossRef] [PubMed]
41. Laurikka, P.; Salmi, T.; Collin, P.; Huhtala, H.; Mäki, M.; Kaukinen, K.; Kurppa, K. Gastrointestinal Symptoms in Celiac Disease Patients on a Long-Term Gluten-Free Diet. *Nutrients* **2016**, *8*. [CrossRef] [PubMed]
42. Rubio-Tapia, A.; Kyle, R.A.; Kaplan, E.L.; Johnson, D.R.; Page, W.; Erdtmann, F.; Brantner, T.L.; Kim, W.R.; Phelps, T.K.; Lahr, B.D.; et al. Increased prevalence and mortality in undiagnosed celiac disease. *Gastroenterology* **2009**, *137*, 88–93. [CrossRef] [PubMed]
43. Metzger, M.-H.; Heier, M.; Mäki, M.; Bravi, E.; Schneider, A.; Löwel, H.; Illig, T.; Schuppan, D.; Wichmann, H.-E. Mortality excess in individuals with elevated IgA anti-transglutaminase antibodies: The KORA/MONICA Augsburg cohort study 1989-1998. *Eur. J. Epidemiol.* **2006**, *21*, 359–365. [CrossRef] [PubMed]
44. Catassi, C.; Fabiani, E.; Corrao, G.; Barbato, M.; De Renzo, A.; Carella, A.M.; Gabrielli, A.; Leoni, P.; Carroccio, A.; Baldassarre, M.; et al. Italian Working Group on Coeliac Disease and Non-Hodgkin's-Lymphoma Risk of non-Hodgkin lymphoma in celiac disease. *JAMA* **2002**, *287*, 1413–1419. [CrossRef] [PubMed]
45. Logan, R.F.; Rifkind, E.A.; Turner, I.D.; Ferguson, A. Mortality in celiac disease. *Gastroenterology* **1989**, *97*, 265–271. [CrossRef]
46. West, J.; Logan, R.F.A.; Smith, C.J.; Hubbard, R.B.; Card, T.R. Malignancy and mortality in people with coeliac disease: Population based cohort study. *BMJ* **2004**, *329*, 716–719. [CrossRef] [PubMed]

47. Chander, U.; Leeman-Neill, R.J.; Bhagat, G. Pathogenesis of Enteropathy-Associated T Cell Lymphoma. *Curr. Hematol. Malig. Rep.* **2018**, *13*, 308–317. [CrossRef] [PubMed]
48. Lohi, S.; Mäki, M.; Rissanen, H.; Knekt, P.; Reunanen, A.; Kaukinen, K. Prognosis of unrecognized coeliac disease as regards mortality: A population-based cohort study. *Ann. Med.* **2009**, *41*, 508–515. [CrossRef] [PubMed]
49. Olén, O.; Askling, J.; Ludvigsson, J.F.; Hildebrand, H.; Ekbom, A.; Smedby, K.E. Coeliac disease characteristics, compliance to a gluten free diet and risk of lymphoma by subtype. *Dig. Liver Dis.* **2011**, *43*, 862–868. [CrossRef] [PubMed]
50. Biagi, F.; Corazza, G.R. Mortality in celiac disease. *Nat. Rev. Gastroenterol. Hepatol.* **2010**, *7*, 158–162. [CrossRef] [PubMed]
51. Kurppa, K.; Paavola, A.; Collin, P.; Sievänen, H.; Laurila, K.; Huhtala, H.; Saavalainen, P.; Mäki, M.; Kaukinen, K. Benefits of a gluten-free diet for asymptomatic patients with serologic markers of celiac disease. *Gastroenterology* **2014**, *147*, 610–617. [CrossRef] [PubMed]
52. Volta, U.; Caio, G.; Giancola, F.; Rhoden, K.J.; Ruggeri, E.; Boschetti, E.; Stanghellini, V.; Giorgio, R.D. Features and Progression of Potential Celiac Disease in Adults. *Clin. Gastroenterol. Hepatol.* **2016**, *14*, 686–693. [CrossRef] [PubMed]
53. Lebwohl, B.; Kapel, R.C.; Neugut, A.I.; Green, P.H.R.; Genta, R.M. Adherence to biopsy guidelines increases celiac disease diagnosis. *Gastrointest. Endosc.* **2011**, *74*, 103–109. [CrossRef] [PubMed]
54. Gonzalez, S.; Gupta, A.; Cheng, J.; Tennyson, C.; Lewis, S.K.; Bhagat, G.; Green, P.H.R. Prospective study of the role of duodenal bulb biopsies in the diagnosis of celiac disease. *Gastrointest. Endosc.* **2010**, *72*, 758–765. [CrossRef] [PubMed]
55. Villanacci, V.; Lorenzi, L.; Donato, F.; Auricchio, R.; Dziechciarz, P.; Gyimesi, J.; Koletzko, S.; Mišak, Z.; Laguna, V.M.; Polanco, I.; et al. Histopathological evaluation of duodenal biopsy in the PreventCD project. An observational interobserver agreement study. *APMIS Acta Pathol. Microbiol. Immunol. Scand.* **2018**, *126*, 208–214. [CrossRef] [PubMed]
56. Corazza, G.R.; Villanacci, V.; Zambelli, C.; Milione, M.; Luinetti, O.; Vindigni, C.; Chioda, C.; Albarello, L.; Bartolini, D.; Donato, F. Comparison of the interobserver reproducibility with different histologic criteria used in celiac disease. *Clin. Gastroenterol. Hepatol. Off. Clin. Pract. J. Am. Gastroenterol. Assoc.* **2007**, *5*, 838–843. [CrossRef] [PubMed]
57. Taavela, J.; Koskinen, O.; Huhtala, H.; Lähdeaho, M.-L.; Popp, A.; Laurila, K.; Collin, P.; Kaukinen, K.; Kurppa, K.; Mäki, M. Validation of morphometric analyses of small-intestinal biopsy readouts in celiac disease. *PLoS ONE* **2013**, *8*, e76163. [CrossRef] [PubMed]
58. Mandile, R.; Discepolo, V.; Scapaticci, S.; Del Vecchio, M.R.; Maglio, M.A.; Greco, L.; Troncone, R.; Auricchio, R. The Effect of Gluten-free Diet on Clinical Symptoms and the Intestinal Mucosa of Patients With Potential Celiac Disease. *J. Pediatr. Gastroenterol. Nutr.* **2018**, *66*, 654–656. [CrossRef] [PubMed]
59. Biagi, F.; Trotta, L.; Alfano, C.; Balduzzi, D.; Staffieri, V.; Bianchi, P.I.; Marchese, A.; Vattiato, C.; Zilli, A.; Luinetti, O.; et al. Prevalence and natural history of potential celiac disease in adult patients. *Scand. J. Gastroenterol.* **2013**, *48*, 537–542. [CrossRef] [PubMed]
60. Lionetti, E.; Castellaneta, S.; Pulvirenti, A.; Tonutti, E.; Francavilla, R.; Fasano, A.; Catassi, C. Italian Working Group of Weaning and Celiac Disease Risk Prevalence and natural history of potential celiac disease in at-family-risk infants prospectively investigated from birth. *J. Pediatr.* **2012**, *161*, 908–914. [CrossRef] [PubMed]
61. Auricchio, R.; Tosco, A.; Piccolo, E.; Galatola, M.; Izzo, V.; Maglio, M.; Paparo, F.; Troncone, R.; Greco, L. Potential celiac children: 9-year follow-up on a gluten-containing diet. *Am. J. Gastroenterol.* **2014**, *109*, 913–921. [CrossRef] [PubMed]
62. Elli, L.; Discepolo, V.; Bardella, M.T.; Guandalini, S. Does gluten intake influence the development of celiac disease-associated complications? *J. Clin. Gastroenterol.* **2014**, *48*, 13–20. [CrossRef] [PubMed]
63. Mäki, M.; Lähdeaho, M.L.; Hällström, O.; Viander, M.; Visakorpi, J.K. Postpubertal gluten challenge in coeliac disease. *Arch. Dis. Child.* **1989**, *64*, 1604–1607. [CrossRef] [PubMed]
64. Matysiak-Budnik, T.; Malamut, G.; de Serre, N.P.-M.; Grosdidier, E.; Seguier, S.; Brousse, N.; Caillat-Zucman, S.; Cerf-Bensussan, N.; Schmitz, J.; Cellier, C. Long-term follow-up of 61 coeliac patients diagnosed in childhood: Evolution toward latency is possible on a normal diet. *Gut* **2007**, *56*, 1379–1386. [CrossRef] [PubMed]

65. Hopman, E.G.D.; von Blomberg, M.E.; Batstra, M.R.; Morreau, H.; Dekker, F.W.; Koning, F.; Lamers, C.B.H.W.; Mearin, M.L. Gluten tolerance in adult patients with celiac disease 20 years after diagnosis? *Eur. J. Gastroenterol. Hepatol.* **2008**, *20*, 423–429. [CrossRef] [PubMed]
66. Kivelä, L.; Popp, A.; Arvola, T.; Huhtala, H.; Kaukinen, K.; Kurppa, K. Long-term health and treatment outcomes in adult coeliac disease patients diagnosed by screening in childhood. *United Eur. Gastroenterol. J.* **2018**, *6*, 1022–1031. [CrossRef] [PubMed]
67. O'Leary, C.; Wieneke, P.; Healy, M.; Cronin, C.; O'Regan, P.; Shanahan, F. Celiac disease and the transition from childhood to adulthood: A 28-year follow-up. *Am. J. Gastroenterol.* **2004**, *99*, 2437–2441. [CrossRef] [PubMed]
68. Wungjiranirun, M.; Kelly, C.P.; Leffler, D.A. Current Status of Celiac Disease Drug Development. *Am. J. Gastroenterol.* **2016**, *111*, 779–786. [CrossRef] [PubMed]

nutrients

MDPI

Article

The Relationship between Body Composition and a Gluten Free Diet in Children with Celiac Disease

Paweł Więch [1,*], Zdzisława Chmiel [1], Dariusz Bazaliński [1], Izabela Sałacińska [1], Anna Bartosiewicz [1], Artur Mazur [2], Bartosz Korczowski [2], Monika Binkowska-Bury [1] and Mariusz Dąbrowski [1,3]

1 Institute of Nursing and Health Sciences, Faculty of Medicine, University of Rzeszów, 35959 Rzeszów, Poland; zchmiel77@gmail.com (Z.C.); darek.bazalinski@wp.pl (D.B.); izabela.salacinska@wp.pl (I.S.); ania.bartosiewicz@gmail.com (A.B.); mbinkowskabury@gmail.com (M.B.-B.); mariusz.dabrowski58@gmail.com (M.D.)

2 Pediatric Department, Clinical Provincial Hospital No. 2 in Rzeszów, Faculty of Medicine, University of Rzeszów, 35301 Rzeszów, Poland; drmazur@poczta.onet.pl (A.M.); korczowski@op.pl (B.K.)

3 Diabetic Outpatient Clinic, Medical Center "Beta-Med" Rzeszów, 35073 Rzeszów, Poland

* Correspondence: p.k.wiech@gmail.com; Tel.: +48-66-719-2696

Received: 14 October 2018; Accepted: 17 November 2018; Published: 21 November 2018

Abstract: The primary and proven therapy, in cases of celiac disease (CD), is a rigorous gluten-free diet (GFD). However, there are reports of its negative effects in the form of nutritional deficiencies, obesity, and adverse changes in body composition. The study aimed to assess the impact of a GFD on the body composition of children with CD. In a case-controlled study ($n = 41$; mean age 10.81 y; SD = 3.96) children with CD, in various stages of treatment, underwent medical assessment. The control group consisted of healthy children and adolescents, strictly matched for gender and age in a 1:1 case-control manner. More than half of the examined children ($n = 26$) followed a GFD. CD children had significantly higher mean values of the fat free mass (FFM% = 80.68 vs. 76.66, $p = 0.015$), and total body water (TBW% = 65.22 vs. 60.47, $p = 0.012$), and lower mean values of the fat mass (FM% = 19.32 vs. 23.34, $p = 0.015$). Children who were on a GFD presented slightly higher, but not statistically significant, mean values of FM and FFM, than children who did not follow dietary recommendations (FM [kg] = 7.48 vs. 5.24, $p = 0.064$; FM% = 20.81 vs. 16.73, $p = 0.087$; FFM [kg] = 28.19 vs. 22.62, $p = 0.110$). After minimum one year of a GFD, CD children showed significantly higher values of FFM [kg] ($p = 0.001$), muscle mass (MM) [kg] ($p < 0.001$), TBW [L] ($p < 0.001$) and body cell mass (BCM) [kg] ($p < 0.001$). Furthermore, CD children who were on a GFD presented a significantly higher increase in weight ($p = 0.034$) and body mass index (BMI) ($p = 0.021$). The children adhering to a GFD demonstrate a tendency towards higher indices of selected body composition components.

Keywords: celiac disease; body composition; gluten free diet; children

1. Introduction

Celiac disease (CD) is a diet-dependent disease and one of the most common food intolerances in Europe posing significant health-related problems [1]. The disease may manifest itself at any age, yet it is frequently diagnosed in children up to 5 years of age, three in four cases being identified in female subjects. It is estimated that for each case diagnosed, there are 5 undetected cases [2], which is partly linked to the high prevalence of subclinical CD [3]. The expected global prevalence of CD is in the range from 0.2% to 5.6% [4]. In Europe, the relevant rate generally varies from 0.5% to 1% (in some countries reaching the level of 3%), and in Poland CD affects approximately 0.8% of the whole population. In the age group of 2.5–15 years, the condition affects 1 in 80 to 1 in 300 children [5,6].

CD is a life-long autoimmune enteropathy due to gluten sensitivity [7]. In CD patients the ingestion of gluten leads to an enteropathy with an impairment of the mucosal surface and abnormal absorption of nutrients [8]. In the case of patients with diagnosed CD, basic therapy involves the life-long adherence to a gluten free diet (GFD). The diet is designed to eliminate any type of food, drink or even medication containing wheat, rye or barley [9,10]. Early diagnosis and treatment make it possible to prevent numerous complications and to effectively eliminate physical and mental development impairments in children with this condition. Compliance with dietary recommendations closely correlates with symptom relief, improved condition of the mucous membrane, and consequently the patient's improved nutritional status. Some studies confirm the effectiveness of a GFD in patients with celiac disease [9,11], yet other researchers argue that the use of this diet alone may contribute to nutritional deficiencies or to excessive body mass [12–14]. Therefore, systematic monitoring of both the nutritional status and body composition appears to be an important part of the therapy in CD [15,16]. The monitoring of dietary compliance is associated with a high chance of healing intestinal lesions and correction of specific body compositional abnormalities, expressed by normalizing fat mass, muscle mass, and bone mass. [16–18]. The changes in lean body mass take longer and, probably, are related more to improvement in the inflammatory state than to changes in absorption of food intake [16].

In practice, body composition assessment can be based on measurements of skin fold thickness, and methods of bioelectrical impedance (BIA) and dual-energy X-ray absorptiometry (DXA) [19–21]. Currently, there are no studies assessing body composition in children with CD. The scarcity of documentation describing body composition in patients with CD, representing varied age groups (at the time of the diagnosis, and during the nutritional therapy), provides for ambiguous evidence and leads to a difficulty in the ability to make comparisons [22,23]. The lack of unanimity of opinion in this regard suggests a need for further research and analyses, in particular, related to children and adolescents. Given the above, the present study was designed to assess the effects of a GFD in the body composition in children with CD.

2. Materials and Methods

2.1. Ethics

The study was approved by the institutional Bioethics Committee at the University of Rzeszów (Resolution No. 5/02/2012) and by all appropriate administrative bodies. The study was conducted in accordance with ethical standards laid down in an appropriate version of the Declaration of Helsinki and in Polish national regulations. The study was conducted according to the Strengthening the Reporting of Observational Studies in Epidemiology (STROBE) criteria.

2.2. Subjects

The study involved 41 children and adolescents (20 girls, 48.7%) with celiac disease receiving inpatient treatment at the Clinical Department of Pediatrics with the Pediatric Neurology Unit, at the Clinical Regional Hospital No. 2 in Rzeszów. The study group consisted of patients with newly diagnosed CD and subjects at different stages of treatment.

The inclusion criteria were as follows: diagnosed celiac disease, age 4 to 18 years, no other autoimmune or chronic diseases affecting height, weight or nutritional status, as well as written informed consent, signed by parents or legal guardians, and by the adolescents over 16 years of age.

The control group consisted of the same number of children and adolescents attending primary, middle, and secondary schools in urban and rural areas. Inclusion criteria were the same as for the study group with the exception for CD diagnosis. The healthy participants and those with CD were strictly matched for age (the nearest birth date) and gender in a 1:1 case-control manner. Figure 1 presents the recruitment process for the study group and the controls, while Table 1 shows the characteristics of the groups.

Detailed information concerning the children with CD, namely the diagnosis, the course and treatment of the disease, and comorbidities, was retrieved from their medical records. In addition, laboratory tests (level of IgA class anti-tissue transglutaminase antibodies TTG, level of IgA anti-endomysium antibodies EmA, and level of IgA class anti-deamidated gliadin-analog antibodies, GAF-3X) and endoscopy were performed to ensure CD diagnosis and to assess the intestinal mucosa status at the time of the diagnosis according to the Marsh scale, modified by Oberhuber [24]. These assessments were supplemented by a medical history of eating habits, based on a questionnaire about the frequency of usual intake of basic product groups during the week.

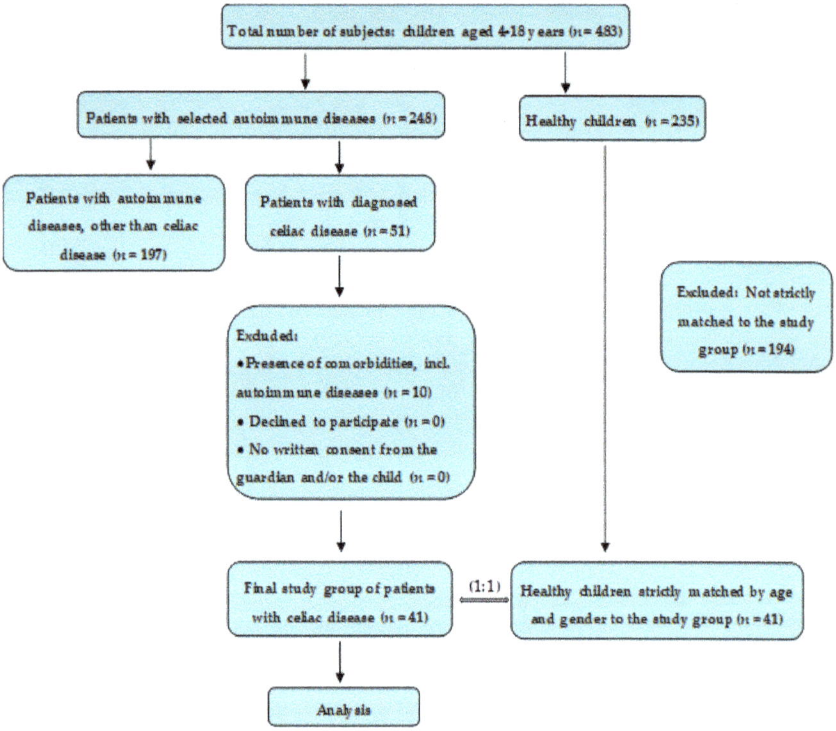

Figure 1. Flow chart demonstrating study participants selection.

Table 1. Anthropometric parameters of the study and control groups. Significant differences in bold.

Parameter	Celiac Disease (N = 41)		Control (N = 41)		*p Value*
	Mean	**SD**	**Mean**	**SD**	
Age, years	10.81	3.96	10.63	4.01	0.989
Gender, n					
Male	21	n/a	21	n/a	1.000
Female	20	n/a	20	n/a	
Weight, kg	33.59	13.79	39.70	15.25	**0.046** *
Height, cm	137.62	21.68	144.20	19.63	0.167
BMI, kg/m^2	16.94	2.65	18.29	3.49	0.089

* indicate significant values ($p < 0.05$); BMI-body mass index; SD-standard deviation; n/a—not applicable.

2.3. Assessments

All the adolescents were assessed for height and weight, and their body mass index (BMI) was calculated. Subsequently, BIA was performed with AKERN BIA-101 analyser (Akern SRL, Pontassieve, Florence, Italy) to examine their body composition and nutritional status. The measurements were performed between 7:00 a.m. and noon, on an empty stomach, in the supine position, with abducted upper (30°) and lower (45°) limbs, following at least a 5-min rest.

A tetrapolar electrode arrangement was applied with the contralateral recording mode. The amplitude of the measured current was 800 μA, sinusoidal, 50 kHz. To ensure the results were reliable and reproducible, two measurements were performed, one after another. Disposable electrodes were placed on the dorsal surface of the right arm (above the wrist) and the right leg (on the ankle). All measurements were performed according to guidelines described by other authors [25–27]. Dedicated software (Bodygram1_31 from AKERN, Pontassieve, Florence, Italy) was used to perform analyses of the results. The BIA took into account: fat mass (FM), fat free mass (FFM), muscle mass (MM) (kg and %), total body water (TBW), intra- and extra-cellular water (ICW and ECW) (litres and %), body cell mass (BCM) (kg and %) and body cell mass index (BCMI). Additionally, phase angle (PA) was calculated, based on resistance and reactance.

2.4. Statistical Analysis

Statistical analysis was performed using the Statistical Software for the Social Sciences SPSS Statistics 20 (IBM Software Group, San Francisco, CA, USA). For this purpose, parametric and non-parametric tests of significance were applied. Normality of the distributions of the quantitative variables was verified with the Kolmogorov–Smirnov test. Homogeneity of variances was then examined with the Levene's test, and equivalence of variables distributions was verified using the χ^2 test. If the conditions for application of parametric tests were fulfilled, it was possible to use the t-test for independent samples, one-way analysis of variance (ANOVA) or Pearson's correlation. A *p*-value below 0.05 was considered statistically significant.

3. Results

Body composition parameters were significantly different between the CD and control groups. CD children had significantly higher mean values of the fat-free mass and total body water, and lower mean values of the fat mass (Table 2).

Table 2. Results of BIA in the study and control groups.

Parameter	Celiac Disease (N = 41)		Control (N = 41)		*p Value*
	Mean	SD	Mean	SD	
FM, kg	6.66	4.19	9.47	5.15	**0.007** *
FFM, kg	26.15	10.72	30.24	11.57	0.098
MM, kg	17.17	7.45	19.55	8.10	0.168
TBW, L	22.71	10.96	23.73	8.72	0.312
ECW, L	9.33	3.47	10.28	3.73	0.246
ICW, L	12.35	4.86	13.55	5.16	0.170
BCM, kg	13.89	6.11	15.85	6.64	0.164
FM%	19.32	7.36	23.34	7.36	**0.015** *
FFM%	80.68	7.36	76.66	7.36	**0.015** *
MM%	50.72	5.98	48.94	5.62	0.168
TBW%	65.22	8.94	60.47	7.66	**0.012** *
ECW%	43.86	5.18	43.82	3.59	0.981
ICW%	56.14	5.18	56.18	3.59	0.981
BCM%	50.66	3.96	51.62	3.73	0.373
BCMI	6.91	1.28	7.22	1.50	0.322
PA	5.45	0.67	5.63	0.69	0.241

SD—standard deviation; FM—fat mass; FFM–fat free mass; MM—muscle mass; TBW–total body water; ECW—extracellular water; ICW—intracellular water; BCM—body cell mass; BCMI—body cell mass index; PA—phase angle; * Bold characters indicate significant values ($p < 0.05$).

Among children with CD participants who were non-compliant to GFD presented apparently lower mean values of FM (kg) and also FM% and FFM%, than children who did follow dietary recommendations, but the difference did not reach the level of statistical significance (Table 3).

Table 3. Anthropometric parameters and bioelectrical impedance (BIA) results among patients following and non-compliant to gluten free diet.

Parameter	Compliant to GFD (*N* = 26)		Non-Compliant to GFD (*N* = 15)		*p Value*
	Mean	SD	Mean	SD	
Age, years	11.00	4.10	10.47	3.82	0.683
Gender, n					
Male	11	n/a	10	n/a	0.239
Female	15	n/a	5	n/a	
Disease duration, months	74.23	58.10	26.07	40.93	**0.002** *
Marsh scale					
IIIA	4	n/a	3	n/a	0.584
IIIB	9	n/a	7	n/a	
IIIC	13	n/a	5	n/a	
Weight, kg	35.67	14.07	29.99	12.96	0.208
Height, cm	141.02	21.73	131.73	21.00	0.190
BMI	17.22	2.55	16.45	2.84	0.272
FM	7.48	4.24	5.24	3.82	0.064
FFM	28.19	11.01	22.62	9.53	0.110
MM	17.95	7.63	15.83	7.17	0.388
TBW	22.49	8.00	23.08	15.12	0.675
ECW	9.65	3.56	8.76	3.35	0.434
ICW	12.91	4.67	11.37	5.18	0.457
BCM	14.52	6.26	12.79	5.89	0.390
FM%	20.81	6.60	16.73	8.10	0.087
FFM%	79.19	6.60	83.27	8.10	0.087
MM%	49.88	5.60	52.17	6.52	0.241
TBW%	63.89	8.69	67.52	9.19	0.214
ECW%	43.27	4.15	44.88	6.64	0.345
ICW%	56.73	4.15	55.12	6.64	0.345
BCM%	50.80	3.18	50.41	5.17	0.745
BCMI	6.91	1.16	6.90	1.50	0.978
PA	5.47	0.58	5.43	0.83	0.862

GFD—gluten-free diet; SD—standard deviation; FM—fat mass; FFM—fat free mass; MM—muscle mass; TBW—total body water; ECW—extracellular water; ICW—intracellular water; BCM—body cell mass; BCMI—body cell mass index; PA—phase angle; * Bold characters indicate significant values ($p < 0.05$); n/a—not applicable.

In a subset of 22 children and adolescents with CD, we performed a follow-up examination after a mean of 17.2 months. In this analysis children with CD demonstrated, as could be expected, significant weight, height and (borderline) BMI gain higher values of fat free mass, muscle mass, total body water (extracellular and intracellular), body cell mass and body cell mass index, while fat mass in kg did not increase significantly. None of these parameters expressed as a percentage of body composition has changed significantly during follow-up (Table 4).

Table 4. Anthropometric parameters and BIA results among 22 patients (14 boys) followed for mean 17.2 months.

Parameter	Baseline (*N* = 22)		Follow-Up (*N* = 22)		*p Value*
	Mean	SD	Mean	SD	
Age, years	10.05	4.08	11.41	4.08	**<0.001** *
Disease duration, months	63.68	67.61	80.86	68.14	**<0.001** *
Weight, kg	32.40	15.68	36.01	14.08	**<0.001** *
Height, cm	134.50	24.62	142.14	23.14	**<0.001** *
BMI, kg/m^2	16.81	2.76	17.07	2.09	**0.046** *
FM, kg	7.20	4.62	7.42	3.75	0.101
FFM, kg	25.20	12.17	28.59	11.91	**0.001** *
MM, kg	16.05	8.45	18.33	8.24	**<0.001** *
TBW, L	20.16	9.25	22.81	9.02	**<0.001** *
ECW, L	8.63	3.89	9.83	3.95	**0.003** *
ICW, L	11.63	5.61	12.98	5.28	**<0.001** *
BCM, kg	12.99	6.93	14.85	6.74	**<0.001** *
FM%	22.05	6.50	21.17	6.94	0.972
FFM%	77.95	6.50	78.83	6.94	0.972
MM%	48.78	5.76	49.96	5.76	0.167
TBW%	62.66	8.50	63.39	9.00	0.455
ECW%	43.79	5.03	43.56	4.40	0.788
ICW%	56.21	5.03	56.44	4.40	0.788
BCM%	50.40	3.58	51.13	3.19	0.102
BCMI	6.60	1.26	6.88	1.12	**0.005** *
PA	5.40	0.64	5.54	0.61	0.121

SD—standard deviation; FM—fat mass; FFM—fat free mass; MM—muscle mass; TBW—total body water; ECW—extracellular water; ICW—intracellular water; BCM—body cell mass; BCMI—body cell mass index; PA—phase angle; * Bold characters indicate significant values ($p < 0.05$).

Children and adolescents with CD who were non-compliant to GFD presented lower weight increase, and fall in BMI which was significantly different compared to group compliant to GFD. In addition, fat mass decreased, but the difference with participants who followed GFD did not achieve the level of statistical significance (Table 5).

Table 5. Differences in anthropometric parameters and body composition between 17 patients compliant and 5 patients non-compliant to gluten-free diet during follow-up.

Parameter	Compliant to GFD (*N* = 17)		Non-Compliant to GFD (*N* = 5)		*p Value*
	Mean	SD	Mean	SD	
Weight increase, kg	4.16	6.65	1.74	0.40	**0.034** *
Height increase, cm	8.12	5.47	6.00	3.37	0.426
BMI increase, kg/m^2	0.47	2.13	-0.44	0.78	**0.021** *
FM increase, kg	0.47	3.66	-0.64	2.06	0.078
FFM increase, kg	3.69	4.90	2.38	2.39	0.308
MM increase, kg	2.51	3.26	1.48	1.86	0.182
TBW increase, L	2.45	3.21	3.34	3.47	0.597
ECW increase, L	1.37	2.04	0.64	0.60	0.209
ICW increase, L	0.96	1.45	2.70	2.92	0.610
BCM increase, kg	2.05	2.64	1.22	1.57	0.240
BCMI increase	0.31	0.72	0.20	0.53	0.289
PA increase	0.14	0.41	0.12	0.40	0.919

GFD—gluten-free diet; SD—standard deviation; FM—fat mass; FFM—fat free mass; MM—muscle mass; TBW—total body water; ECW—extracellular water; ICW—intracellular water; BCM—body cell mass; BCMI—body cell mass index; PA—phase angle; * Bold characters indicate significant values ($p < 0.05$).

4. Discussion

In the present case-controlled study, we observed that selected body composition parameters (fat mass, fat free mass, muscle mass, total, intracellular and extracellular body water, and body cell mass) and nutritional indicators (body mass index and body cell mass index) in children with CD are significantly different than in healthy controls. Reports related to changes in body composition, in adults and in children, both at the stage of diagnosis and during treatment, are limited and ambiguous. They depend on a number of variables, such as the age at the time of diagnosis, the disease progression, duration of impairments associated with malabsorption syndrome, methods of body composition assessment, as well as the degree of compliance to dietary guidelines.

The results of the present study showed that children with CD had significantly lower mean values of the FM expressed both in kg and as percentage of body mass (p = 0.007 and p = 0.015, respectively), and higher mean percentage values of the FFM (p = 0.015), and TBW (p = 0.012). Our results provide evidence that children with CD have lower energy reserves reflected as a lower total body fat mass, which may result in reduced immunity, a potential higher risk of malnutrition and faster dynamics of body components changes due to existing malnutrition. Furthermore, our results show, that children who were at baseline compliant to GFD presented apparently higher, but not statistically significant, mean values of FM and FFM (both in kg and in %), than children who did not follow dietary recommendations. The described differences in body composition components were close to the level of statistical significance despite the relatively low number of children in each group. After mean 17.2 months of follow-up, children with CD, as could be expected, demonstrated a significant increase of FFM, MM, TBW, BCM, and BCMI expressed in kg or L. However, the percentage of body mass components did not change significantly. Within this group children who did not follow strictly GFD presented lower weight gain and even decrease in BMI which was significantly different compared to the children compliant to GFD (p = 0.034 and p = 0.021, respectively). In addition, changes in fat mass tended to be different between compliant and non-compliant groups, which did not achieve statistical significance due to a very small number of children in each group. This indicates lower energy reserves and increased the potential risk of malnutrition in case of exacerbation of the disease in children not following GFD. Some studies report no significant changes in the specific components of body composition after a GFD is introduced [28], or, in fact, describe a decrease in fat-free components coinciding with stable fat mass one year after gluten withdrawal [19]. Other studies, including long-term research, provide evidence that after a GFD is introduced, the majority of the components of body composition are stable [17,18], sometimes with a slightly higher increase in FM than in FFM [29].

Our findings support suggestions made by other authors who agree that the earlier the diet is introduced, the faster it is possible to reverse abnormalities in body composition [18]. Important and constructive opinions regarding the necessity of the strict adherence to a GFD are voiced by studies which show that children, who fail to follow the recommendations, are found to have a significantly lower bone mineral density, which leads to a risk of osteoporosis in adulthood [30,31].

Another important, yet controversial issue, is the effect of a GFD in anthropometric parameters, in particular, the value of weight and BMI. Dyspepsia and malabsorption associated with progressing CD lead to malnutrition in quantitative and qualitative terms [32,33], which results, e.g., in both delayed growth and puberty [34]. Due to this, until recently, these patients were identified exclusively with low BMI. Currently, we know that over time CD may be accompanied by normal as well as excessive body mass, or even by obesity [35–37], because a GFD may contain both a high energy and high fat load [32]. The effects of a GFD, related to BMI vary greatly. Numerous studies show that the strict GFD results in normalization of BMI in initially underweight children and adults [28,35,38,39], and leads to significantly improved and faster growth and development in children, if the disease is diagnosed and treated early [40]. Conversely, in individuals with excessive body mass, at the time of CD diagnosis, BMI tends to decrease after the diet is introduced [39]. One should keep in mind that CD is a very heterogeneous disease, and the occurrence of the diagnosis among obese patients is no more surprising [37]. Our findings could be highly influenced by the duration of the disease and adherence to the GFD.

Based on current research it should be emphasized that adherence to a GFD is of critical importance in the treatment of CD and the further prevention of related complications. However, in order to achieve satisfying results, it is necessary to ensure the consistent monitoring of dietary restrictions, in combination with a systematic assessment of the patient's nutritional status and body composition. Despite this, most patients with CD respond to a GFD, approximately 20% of them have persistent or recurrent symptoms. Following a GFD can be difficult for patients with CD and understanding the barriers/challenges experienced by patients in maintaining a GFD is essential for compliance [41]. There is also evidence suggesting that adherence to GFD is not enough, particularly in adolescent patients [42,43]. Our studies present 36.5% (15/41) non-compliant patients and our findings are similar to UK cross-sectional study in a group of patients with CD recruited from two London children's hospitals. The high number of noncompliant participants 35.3% (36/102) indicates that maintaining GFD is difficult for practical and social reasons [44]. There are many studies evaluating not only the number of patients who do not follow the GFD but also analyzing the reasons for this noncompliance and their consequences for the quality of life [45]. Furthermore, a poorly balanced GFD may lead to deficiencies and, consequently, nutritional imbalance, which is particularly important in the case of children as it adversely affects growth, development, and physical activity. By monitoring the diet and by applying the simple methods to assess anthropometric parameters and indices, as well as body composition, it is possible to quickly identify and adequately correct any effects of nutritional errors, such as selective deficiencies of nutrients, as well as obesity, and to prevent health-related consequences.

Our study is obviously not free from several limitations. Despite our best efforts and inclusion in our study of as many participants as was possible, the relatively low number of study participants is the most important limitation. It did not allow us to find other significant differences between study and control groups as well as between participants with CD following and not-following GFD. Because assessment of important markers of nutritional status (albumin and/or pre-albumin level) was not done in all the children, we were not able to analyze the association of these variables with body composition components. Searching for such relationships would be an intriguing implication for further research. We also did not perform serology markers assessment at the follow-up visit. It would be interesting to analyze its relationship with compliance to GFD.

Given the controversies related to changes in anthropometric indices and body composition observed in individuals following a GFD, this problem unquestionably requires further study. It would be of extreme importance to conduct a long-term assessment of the effects produced by a GFD on body composition, beginning from childhood, when patients receive CD diagnosis until they reach adulthood. It would then be easier to eliminate small fluctuations in the components of body composition associated with age and the level of gluten cross-contamination in foods, and consequently to obtain reliable results.

5. Conclusions

The children with celiac disease differ significantly in body composition compared to healthy comparators. Participants adhering to a gluten-free diet presented a trend towards higher indices of selected body composition components. To assess the predictive and prognostic value of these findings, further prospective, longer-lasting studies, including a higher number of participants are required in this population.

Author Contributions: P.W. and B.K. conceived and designed the study; P.W., Z.C., D.B., M.D., A.M. analyzed the data; P.W., D.B., M.D., A.B., I.S. and M.B.-B wrote the paper; all authors approved the final manuscript.

Funding: The study was conducted under the grant for statutory activity (Research Potential) of the Institute of Nursing and Health Sciences, Faculty of Medicine, University of Rzeszów for 2018 and 2019 years (Resolution No. WM/21/2018/P-M).

Acknowledgments: The study was conducted as the project of the Natural and Medical Center for Innovative Research in the University of Rzeszów, and it was co-financed by the Regional Operational Program for the Podkarpackie Province for the years 2007–2013, contract number UDA-RPPK.01.03.00-18-004/12-00.

Conflicts of Interest: The authors declare no conflict of interest.

References

1. Husby, S.; Koletzko, S.; Korponay-Szabó, I.R.; Mearin, M.L.; Phillips, A.; Shamir, R.; Troncone, R.; Giersiepen, K.; Branski, D.; Catassi, C.; et al. European society for pediatric gastroenterology, hepatology, and nutrition guidelines for the diagnosis of coeliac disease. *J. Pediatr. Gastroenterol. Nutr.* **2012**, *54*, 136–160. [CrossRef] [PubMed]
2. Ivarsson, A.; Myléus, A.; Norström, F.; van der Pals, M.; Rosén, A.; Högberg, L.; Danielsson, L.; Halvarsson, B.; Hammarroth, S.; Hernell, O.; et al. Prev–alence of childhood celiac disease and changes in infant feeding. *Pediatrics* **2013**, *131*, e687–e694. [CrossRef] [PubMed]
3. Almazán, M.V.; Ortega, E.; Moreno Torres, R.; Tovar, M.; Romero, J.; López-Casado, M.Á.; Jáimez, L.; Jiménez-Jáimez, J.; Ballesteros, A.; Caballero-Villarraso, J.; et al. Diagnostic screening for subclinical celiac disease using a rapid test in children aged 2–4. *Pediatr. Res.* **2015**, *78*, 280–285. [CrossRef] [PubMed]
4. Bascuñán, K.A.; Roncoroni, L.; Branchi, F.; Doneda, L.; Scricciolo, A.; Ferretti, F.; Araya, M.; Elli, L. The 5 Ws of a gluten challenge for gluten-related disorders. *Nutr. Rev.* **2018**, *76*, 79–87. [CrossRef] [PubMed]
5. Mustalahti, K.; Catassi, C.; Reunanen, A.; Fabiani, E.; Heier, M.; McMillan, S.; Murray, L.; Metzger, M.H.; Gasparin, M.; Bravi, E.; et al. The prevalence of celiac disease in Europe: Results of a centralized, international mass screening project. *Ann. Med.* **2010**, *42*, 587–595. [CrossRef] [PubMed]
6. Obtułowicz, K.; Waga, J.; Dyga, W. Gluten-mechanisms of intolerance, symptoms and treatment possibilities of IgE-related allergy for gluten in the light of actual clinical and immunological studies. *Przegl. Lek.* **2015**, *72*, 747–753. [PubMed]
7. Fasano, A.; Catassi, C. Clinical practice. Celiac disease. *N. Engl. J. Med.* **2012**, *367*, 2419–2426. [CrossRef] [PubMed]
8. Parzanese, I.; Qehajaj, D.; Patrinicola, F.; Aralica, M.; Chiriva-Internati, M.; Stifter, S.; Elli, L.; Grizzi, F. Celiac disease: From pathophysiology to treatment. *World J. Gastrointest. Pathophysiol.* **2017**, *8*, 27–38. [CrossRef] [PubMed]
9. Pulido, O.; Zarkadas, M.; Dubois, S.; Macisaac, K.; Cantin, I.; La Vieille, S.; Godefroy, S.; Rashid, M. Clinical features and symptom recovery on a gluten-free diet in Canadian adults with celiac disease. *Can. J. Gastroenterol.* **2013**, *27*, 449–453. [CrossRef] [PubMed]
10. Alzaben, A.S.; Turner, J.; Shirton, L.; Samuel, T.M.; Persad, R.; Mager, D. Assessing nutritional quality and adherence to the gluten-free diet in children and adolescents with celiac disease. *Can. J. Diet. Pract. Res.* **2015**, *76*, 56–63. [CrossRef] [PubMed]
11. Laurikka, P.; Salmi, T.; Collin, P.; Huhtala, H.; Mäki, M.; Kaukinen, K.; Kurppa, K. Gastrointestinal symptoms in celiac disease patients on a long-term gluten-free diet. *Nutrients* **2016**, *8*, E429. [CrossRef] [PubMed]
12. Shepherd, S.J.; Gibson, P.R. Nutritional inadequacies of the gluten-free diet in both recently-diagnosed and long-term patients with coeliac disease. *J. Hum. Nutr. Diet.* **2013**, *26*, 349–358. [CrossRef] [PubMed]
13. Brambilla, P.; Picca, M.; Dilillo, D.; Meneghin, F.; Cravidi, C.; Tischer, M.C.; Vivaldo, T.; Bedogni, G.; Zuccotti, G.V. Changes of body mass index in celiac children on a gluten-free diet. *Nutr. Metab. Cardiovasc. Dis.* **2013**, *23*, 177–182. [CrossRef] [PubMed]
14. Anania, C.; Pacifico, L.; Olivero, F.; Perla, F.M.; Chiesa, C. Cardiometabolic risk factors in children with celiac disease on a gluten-free diet. *World J. Clin. Pediatr.* **2017**, *6*, 143–148. [CrossRef] [PubMed]
15. Tsiountsioura, M.; Wong, J.E.; Upton, J.; McIntyre, K.; Dimakou, D.; Buchanan, E.; Cardigan, T.; Flynn, D.; Bishop, J.; Russell, R.K.; et al. Detailed assessment of nutritional status and eating patterns in children with gastrointestinal diseases attending an outpatients clinic and contemporary healthy controls. *Eur. J. Clin. Nutr.* **2014**, *68*, 700–706. [CrossRef] [PubMed]
16. Newnham, E.D.; Shepherd, S.J.; Strauss, B.J.; Hosking, P.; Gibson, P.R. Adherence to the gluten-free diet can achieve the therapeutic goals in almost all patients with coeliac disease: A 5-year longitudinal study from diagnosis. *J. Gastroenterol. Hepatol.* **2016**, *31*, 342–349. [CrossRef] [PubMed]
17. Carbone, M.C.; Pitzalis, G.; Ferri, M.; Nenna, R.; Thanasi, E.; Andreoli, A.; De Lorenzo, A.; Bonamico, M. Body composition in coeliac disease adolescents on a gluten-free diet: A longitudinal study. *Acta Diabetol.* **2003**, *40*, S171–S173. [CrossRef] [PubMed]
18. Barera, G.; Mora, S.; Brambilla, P.; Ricotti, A.; Menni, L.; Beccio, S.; Bianchi, C. Body composition in children with celiac disease and the effects of a gluten-free diet: A prospective case-control study. *Am. J. Clin. Nutr.* **2000**, *72*, 71–75. [CrossRef] [PubMed]

19. De Lorenzo, A.; Di Campli, C.; Andreoli, A.; Sasso, G.F.; Bonamico, M.; Gasbarrini, A. Assessment of body composition by bioelectrical impedance in adolescent patients with celiac disease. *Am. J. Gastroenterol.* **1999**, *94*, 2951–2955. [CrossRef] [PubMed]
20. Xing, Y.; Morgan, S.L. Celiac disease and metabolic bone disease. *J. Clin. Densitom.* **2013**, *16*, 439–444. [CrossRef] [PubMed]
21. Więch, P.; Dąbrowski, M.; Bazaliński, D.; Sałacińska, I.; Korczowski, B.; Binkowska-Bury, M. Bioelectrical impedance phase angle as an indicator of malnutrition in hospitalized children with diagnosed inflammatory bowel diseases—A case control study. *Nutrients* **2018**, *10*, 499. [CrossRef] [PubMed]
22. Bardella, M.T.; Molteni, N.; Prampolini, L.; Giunta, A.M.; Baldassarri, A.R.; Morganti, D.; Bianchi, P.A. Need for follow up in coeliac disease. *Arch. Dis. Child.* **1994**, *70*, 211–213. [CrossRef] [PubMed]
23. Troncone, R.; Mayer, M.; Spagnuolo, F.; Maiuri, L.; Greco, L. Endomysial antibodies as unreliable markers for slight dietary transgressions in adolescents with celiac disease. *J. Pediatr. Gastroenterol. Nutr.* **1995**, *21*, 69–72. [CrossRef] [PubMed]
24. Oberhuber, G.; Granditsch, G.; Vogelsang, H. The histopathology of coeliac disease: Time for a standardized report scheme for pathologists. *Eur. J. Gastroenterol. Hepatol.* **1999**, *11*, 1185–1194. [CrossRef] [PubMed]
25. Yanovski, S.Z.; Hubbard, V.S.; Heymsfield, S.B.; Lukaski, H.C. Bioelectrical impedance analysis in body composition measurement: National institutes of health technology assessment conference statement. *Am. J. Clin. Nutr.* **1996**, *64*, 524S–532S.
26. Kyle, U.G.; Bosaeus, I.; de Lorenzo, A.D.; Deurenberg, P.; Elia, M.; Manuel Gómez, J.; Heitmann, B.L.; Kent-Smith, L.; Melchior, J.C.; Pirlich, M.; et al. Bioelectrical impedance analysis—Part II: Utilization in clinical practice. *Clin. Nutr.* **2004**, *23*, 1430–1453. [CrossRef] [PubMed]
27. Kushner, R.F. Bioelectrical impedance analysis: A review of principles and applications. *J. Am. Coll. Nutr.* **1992**, *11*, 199–209. [PubMed]
28. Barone, M.; Della, V.N.; Rosania, R.; Facciorusso, A.; Trotta, A.; Cantatore, F.P.; Falco, S.; Pignatiello, S.; Viggiani, M.T.; Amoruso, A.; et al. A comparison of the nutritional status between adult celiac patients on a long-term, strictly gluten-free diet and healthy subjects. *Eur. J. Clin. Nutr.* **2016**, *70*, 23–27. [CrossRef] [PubMed]
29. Capristo, E.; Addolorato, G.; Mingrone, G.; De Gaetano, A.; Greco, A.V.; Tataranni, P.A.; Gasbarrini, G. Changes in body composition, substrate oxidation, and resting metabolic rate in adult celiac disease patients after a 1-y gluten-free diet treatment. *Am. J. Clin. Nutr.* **2000**, *72*, 76–81. [CrossRef] [PubMed]
30. Blazina, S.; Bratanic, N.; Campa, A.S.; Blagus, R.; Orel, R. Bone mineral density and importance of strict gluten-free diet in children and adolescents with celiac disease. *Bone* **2010**, *47*, 598–603. [CrossRef] [PubMed]
31. Abenavoli, L.; Delibasic, M.; Peta, V.; Turkulov, V.; De Lorenzo, A.; Medić-Stojanoska, M. Nutritional profile of adult patients with celiac disease. *Eur. Rev. Med. Pharmacol. Sci.* **2015**, *19*, 4285–4292. [PubMed]
32. Forchielli, M.L.; Fernicola, P.; Diani, L.; Scrivo, B.; Salfi, N.C.; Pessina, A.C.; Lima, M.; Conti, V.; Pession, A. Gluten-free diet and lipid profile in children with celiac disease: Comparison with general population standards. *J. Pediatr. Gastroenterol. Nutr.* **2015**, *61*, 224–229. [CrossRef] [PubMed]
33. Sue, A.; Dehlsen, K.; Ooi, C.Y. Paediatric patients with coeliac disease on a gluten-free diet: Nutritional adequacy and macro- and micronutrient imbalances. *Curr. Gastroenterol. Rep.* **2018**, *22*, 2. [CrossRef] [PubMed]
34. Bessahraoui, M.; Bouziane, N.K.; Boudraa, G.; Touhami, M. Growth and puberty in the coeliac disease of the child. *Pediatr. Res.* **2011**, *70*, 365. [CrossRef]
35. Rodrigues, M.; Yonamine, G.H.; Fernandes Satiro, C.A. Rate and determinants of non-adherence to a gluten-free diet and nutritional status assessment in children and adolescents with celiac disease in a tertiary Brazilian referral center: A cross-sectional and retrospective study. *BMC Gastroenterol.* **2018**, *18*, 15. [CrossRef]
36. Dickey, W.; Kearney, N. Overweight in celiac disease: Prevalence, clinical characteristics, and effect of a gluten-free diet. *Am. J. Gastroenterol.* **2006**, *101*, 2356–2359. [CrossRef] [PubMed]
37. Nenna, R.; Mosca, A.; Mennini, M.; Papa, R.E.; Petrarca, L.; Mercurio, R.; Montuori, M.; Piedimonte, A.; Bavastrelli, M.; De Lucia, I.C.; et al. Coeliac disease screening among a large cohort of overweight/obese children. *J. Pediatr. Gastroenterol. Nutr.* **2015**, *60*, 405–407. [CrossRef] [PubMed]
38. Reilly, N.R.; Aguilar, K.; Hassid, B.G.; Cheng, J.; Defelice, A.R.; Kazlow, P.; Bhagat, G.; Green, P.H. Celiac disease in normal weight and overweight children: Clinical features and growth outcomes following a gluten-free diet. *J. Pediatr. Gastroenterol. Nutr.* **2011**, *53*, 528–531. [CrossRef] [PubMed]

39. Siddh, L.; Sengar, G.S.; Nagraj, N.; Shyam, R.; Garg, P. Body mass index in celiac disease and effect of a gluten-free diet on body mass index. *Int. J. Adv. Med.* **2016**, *3*, 813–815. [CrossRef]
40. Radlović, N.; Mladenović, M.; Leković, Z.; Zivanović, D.; Brdar, R.; Radlović, V.; Ristić, D.; Pavlović, M.; Stojsić, Z.; Vuletić, B.; et al. Effect of gluten-free diet on the growth and nutritional status of children with coeliac disease. *Srp. Arh. Celok. Lek.* **2009**, *137*, 632–637. [CrossRef] [PubMed]
41. Glissen Brown, J.R.; Singh, P. Coeliac disease. *Paediatr. Int. Child. Health.* **2018**, *13*, 1–9. [CrossRef] [PubMed]
42. Chauhan, J.C.; Kumar, P.; Dutta, A.K.; Basu, S.; Kumar, A. Assessmentof dietary compliance to gluten free diet and psychosocialproblems in Indian children with celiac disease. *Indian J. Pediatr.* **2010**, *77*, 649–654. [CrossRef] [PubMed]
43. Roma, E.; Roubani, A.; Kolia, E.; Panayiotou, J.; Zellos, A.; Syriopoulou, V.P. Dietarycompliance and life style of children with coeliac disease. *J. Hum. Nutr. Diet.* **2010**, *23*, 176–182. [CrossRef] [PubMed]
44. Kumar, P.J.; Walker-Smith, J.; Milla, P.; Harris, G.; Colyer, J.; Halliday, R. Theteenage coeliac: Follow up study of 102 patients. *Arch. Dis. Child.* **1988**, *63*, 916–920. [CrossRef] [PubMed]
45. White, L.E.; Bannerman, E.; Gillett, P.M. Coeliac disease and the gluten-free diet: A review of the burdens; factors associated with adherence and impact on health-related quality of life, with specific focus on adolescence. *J. Hum. Nutr. Diet.* **2016**, *29*, 593–606. [CrossRef] [PubMed]

nutrients

MDPI

Article

Celiac Disease Diagnosed through Screening Programs in At-Risk Adults Is Not Associated with Worse Adherence to the Gluten-Free Diet and Might Protect from Osteopenia/Osteoporosis

Francesco Tovoli [1,*], Giulia Negrini [1], Vito Sansone [2], Chiara Faggiano [1], Teresa Catenaro [1], Luigi Bolondi [1] and Alessandro Granito [1]

1 Unit of Internal Medicine, Department of Medical and Surgical Sciences, University of Bologna, 40136 Bologna, Italy; giu.negrini@gmail.com (G.N.); chiara.fg9@gmail.com (C.F.); teresa.catenaro@studio.unibo.it (T.C.); luigi.bolondi@unibo.it (L.B.); alessandro.granito@unibo.it (A.G.)

2 Unit of Gastroenterology, Department of Medical and Surgical Sciences, University of Bologna, 40136 Bologna, Italy; vito.sansone@studio.unibo.it

* Correspondence: francesco.tovoli2@unibo.it; Tel.: +39-051-214-2214

Received: 8 November 2018; Accepted: 3 December 2018; Published: 7 December 2018

Abstract: Screening strategies to detect celiac disease (CD) in at-risk subjects are of paramount importance to prevent the possible long-term complications of this condition. It is therefore of strategic relevance to understand whether patients diagnosed through screening follow a strict gluten-free diet (GFD), as the non-compliance to this diet can make screening efforts pointless. Currently, no studies have verified whether CD patients diagnosed in their adulthood are adhering to the GFD years after the diagnosis. We retrospectively evaluated the medical records of 750 CD patients diagnosed in our center during January 2004–December 2013 to verify differences between screening detected and clinically diagnosed patients. The groups shared a similar adherence to the GFD (91.2 versus 89.8%, $p = 0.857$). Moreover, the rates of non-responsive CD, GFD-induced metabolic alterations, and persistence in controls were also similar. Instead, screening-detected patients had a significantly lower rate of osteopenia/osteoporosis at diagnosis (31.3 versus 46%, $p < 0.001$). In conclusion, screening strategies for CD in at-risk groups should be encouraged even in the adult population. Patients diagnosed through these strategies had no additional problems compared to those diagnosed for clinical suspicion and might benefit from a protective effect against metabolic bone disease.

Keywords: celiac disease; gluten; gluten-free diet; screening; outcome; gluten sensitivity; osteoporosis

1. Introduction

Celiac disease (CD) is a chronic small intestinal immune-mediated enteropathy precipitated by exposure to dietary gluten in genetically predisposed people [1]. The prevalence of CD is about 1% of the general population [1]. However, a significant underdiagnosis issue exists, and most CD patients are still to be detected [2]. The identification of CD patients relies both on a case-finding strategy in subjects with gluten-related manifestations and on a screening strategy in subjects at high risk of disease. These high-risk populations include first-degree relatives of CD patients, patients with immune deficiencies (Immunoglobulin A deficiency, common variable immunodeficiency), autoimmune diseases (in particular, type 1 diabetes mellitus), congenital chromosomal abnormalities (Down and Turner syndromes) [3–5]. Unlike CD patients diagnosed on the basis of the presence of gluten-related symptoms, patients diagnosed through screening often have milder symptoms or no symptoms at all. The gluten-free diet (GFD) has consequently a more limited impact on their symptoms, exposing these patients to a higher theoretical risk of incorrect GFD compliance (and therefore to an increased risk of complications). Therefore, it is of capital importance to verify whether screening-diagnosed patients follow the GFD, as the lack of compliance negates any benefit of an early diagnosis. Unfortunately, until now adherence to the GFD in screening-diagnosed adults has been verified only in two studies performed in Northern Europe cohorts [6,7]. The colleagues found that the adherence of screening-detected subjects was similar to that of patients diagnosed on the basis of clinical suspicion. Other hints came from a recent survey in which 236 patients completed health, quality of life, and dietary adherence questionnaires a median of 18.5 years after childhood diagnosis. Even in this case, the authors reported comparable long-term outcomes between screening-diagnosed and clinically detected patients [8]. However, until now, no study has combined the strengths of a large cohort [7] with an extended follow-up [6], leaving this topic open. Lessons from previous studies in children, in fact, taught us that the compliance may drop after an extended follow-up [9,10], especially in screening-diagnosed subjects [10] and that patients from different geographical regions may have a very different adherence to the GFD [11]. At the same time, not all of the information can be translated from the pediatric experience, as adults may have different peculiarities. For instance, the impact deriving from a significant dietary change after decades of a gluten-containing diet and the increased risk of complicated CD (which is virtually absent in childhood) [12] are to be considered. Moreover, it is in adulthood that CD-related osteoporosis and GFD-induced metabolic alterations may reach their full clinical expression [13].

The objective of our study was to verify whether CD patients diagnosed in adulthood through screening procedures had different characteristics compared to CD patients diagnosed on the basis of the presence of symptoms. In particular, we intended to analyze clinical data at baseline, adherence, and responsiveness to the GFD and metabolic problems induced by the GFD. According to our national guidelines and government policies, every CD patient has to be evaluated six months after the beginning of the GFD and every 18–24 months after that [14]. Consequently, patients followed for a long period can be considered as adhering to the follow-up procedures rather than attention-seeking subjects, thus avoiding (or at least reducing) possible biases. For this reason, we also compared the persistence in the follow-up procedures between groups.

2. Materials and Methods

2.1. Clinical Setting

We retrospectively analyzed the medical records of patients who were consecutively diagnosed with CD in our outpatient clinic (Bologna Authority Hospital S.Orsola-Malpighi, Bologna, Italy) between January 2004 and December 2013. The final cut-off of December 2013 was chosen to grant a theoretical minimum five-year follow-up even for the most recently diagnosed patients.

2.2. Inclusion and Exclusion Criteria

A diagnosis of CD performed according to the North American Society for Pediatric Gastroenterology, Hepatology, and Nutrition [4] was regarded as the key inclusion criterion. Patients with incomplete medical records or unconfirmed diagnosis were excluded from this study. (Figure 1).

All the remaining patients were considered eligible for the following comparative analysis: Clinical presentation (symptomatic versus asymptomatic), severity of histology lesions according to the Marsh–Oberhuber classification (3a versus 3b versus 3c), prevalence of iron-deficiency anaemia, prevalence of osteopenia.

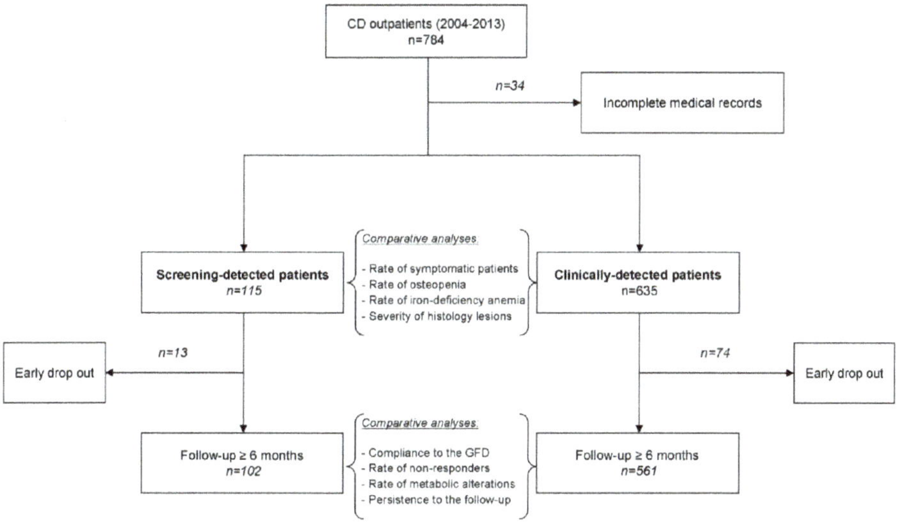

Figure 1. Patients' flow chart. CD: celiac disease

Instead, only patients who performed at least two evaluations (one of which at least six months after the beginning of the GFD) were considered to be eligible for the additional comparative analyses. These further comparisons included: Compliance to the GFD, prevalence of non-responder CD defined according to the Oslo classification [1], and prevalence of metabolic alterations (body weight increase >10 kg, total cholesterol increase >50 mg/dL, development of overt metabolic syndrome).

2.3. Clinical Evaluations

Clinical evaluations were scheduled according to the local guidelines (six months after the beginning of the GFD and every 18–24 months after that [14]). Each evaluation consisted of: (1) medical history; (2) physical examination; (3) evaluation of laboratory tests.

Medical history was examined with particular attention to reported intentional or accidental gluten ingestion, modifications of gluten-related symptoms (diarrhea, abdominal pain, bloating, dyspepsia, constipation, skin rash, myalgia, oral aftosis, etc.), onset of any new symptom, and list of current medications [14].

Physical examination included the evaluation of vital signs and body weight. Abdomen, thorax, heart, and neck examinations were also performed [14].

Laboratory tests included: Complete blood count, ferritin, calcium, glycaemia, total cholesterol, alanine and aspartate aminotransferase, thyroid-stimulating hormone, anti-thyroperoxidase and anti-thyroglobulin antibodies, anti-tissue transglutaminase immunoglobulin A, and anti-deamidated gliadin peptides immunoglobulin G antibodies. Additional tests were performed at diagnosis (other anti-organ- and non-organ-specific antibodies) or on a clinical basis (second-level metabolic and osteometabolic tests) [14].

Dual-energy X-ray absorptiometry (DXA) was performed at the diagnosis of CD.

2.4. Evaluation of Adherence to the GFD

The patients were considered to have complied to the GFD if all the following criteria were satisfied: (1) No reported intentional or accidental gluten ingestion; (2) absence of CD-related symptoms; (3) negative anti-transglutaminase IgA antibodies [4].

2.5. Ethics

This study was approved by the Institutional Review Board of the Bologna Authority Hospital S.Orsola-Malpighi (Protocol 243/2013/O/OssN) and performed according to the Declaration of Helsinki guidelines. All patients signed an informed consent.

2.6. Sample Size Considerations

The main aim of our study was to compare the rate of patients strictly following the GFD during the follow-up. On the basis of the previous reviews on the adult population [6,7], we estimated a global adherence to the GFD of 90%. To detect a decrease of 10% in one of the two study groups with an alpha error of 0.05 and a power of 90%, we estimated to enroll a minimum of 640 patients.

2.7. Statistical Analysis

Distribution of continuous variables was assessed with a Shapiro–Wilk test, which showed non-normal distributions. Consequently, continuous variables were expressed as median and interquartile range. Categorical variables were expressed as frequencies. Group comparisons were subsequently performed using the Mann–Whitney test for continuous variables and the two-tailed Fisher's test for categorical variables. Binary logistic regression was performed to assess the relationship between correct compliance with the GFD (dependent variable) and other clinical variables. Log-rank test and Cox proportional hazard models were used to evaluate the relationship between the persistence to the follow-up procedure and other clinical variables of interest. Variables for which the association in the univariate analysis was $p < 0.10$ were entered into the multivariate models. A $p < 0.05$ was considered to be the cut-off for statistical significance. All of the statistical analyses were performed with SPSS version 23.0 (SPSS Inc., Chicago, IL, USA).

3. Results

3.1. Study Population

A total of 750 CD patients were identified using the specified inclusion and exclusion criteria. Of these patients, 115 (15.3%) had been identified through screening procedures, and 635 (84.7%) because of clinical suspicion. The clinical motivations leading to the screening procedures are reported in Table 1.

Table 1. Conditions which justified the screening for celiac disease in at-risk groups.

Familiar Screening (Total)	**78 (67.8)**
Index case: brother/sister	26 (22.6)
Index case: father/mother	18 (15.7)
Index case: son/daughter	18 (15.7)
Index case: nephew/grandchild	11 (9.6)
Index case: cousin	5 (4.3)
At-Risk Associated Conditions (Total)	**37 (32.2)**
Autoimmune thyroid disease	10 (8.7)
Type-1 diabetes mellitus	6 (5.2)
Primary biliary cholangitis	3 (2.6)
IgA deficiency	3 (2.6)
Down syndrome	3 (2.6)
Vitiligo	3 (2.6)
Sjogren syndrome	1 (0.9)
Turner syndrome	1 (0.9)
Other	7 (6.1)

Data are reported as absolute frequencies (percentage).

3.2. Characteristics at Diagnosis

A comparison of the main characteristics of screening- and clinically detected patients is detailed in Table 2.

Table 2. Characteristics of screening- and clinically detected patients.

Parameter	Screening (n = 115)	Clinical Suspicion (n = 635)	p
Age (Years)	34 (22–46)	33 (22–44)	0.690
Sex (Female)	80 (69.6)	502 (79.1)	0.021
Time since Diagnosis (Years)	1.5 (0.0–5.0)	2.0 (0.0–6.50)	0.145
Symptoms	29 (25.2)	594 (93.5)	<0.001
Iron-Deficiency Anemia	25 (21.7)	324 (51.0)	<0.001
Osteopenia/Osteoporosis	36 (31.3)	292 (46.0)	0.003
Histology			
-Marsh 3a	33 (28.7)	182 (28.7)	
-Marsh 3b	43 (37.4)	180 (28.3)	0.100
-Marsh 3c	39 (33.9)	273 (42.3)	

Categorical variables are reported as absolute number (percentage), continuous variables are described as median (interquartile range).

Female sex was slightly preponderant in clinically detected patients, while the age at the diagnosis did not significantly differ between groups. As expected, the prevalence of symptomatic patients was sharply higher in clinically detected compared to screening-detected patients. In parallel, iron-deficiency anemia and osteopenia/osteoporosis were also more prevalent in the clinically detected group of patients. No differences in the severity of villous atrophy were noted.

3.3. Follow-Up

A total of 13 patients in the screening group (11.3%) and 74 clinically detected patients (11.7%) dropped out after the first evaluation in our centre (p = 1.000). The remaining patients (102 and 561, respectively) were assessed for compliance to the GFD, prevalence of non-responder CD, and metabolic alterations (Table 3).

Table 3. Comparison of the compliance to the gluten-free diet, persisting symptoms, and metabolic alterations at the follow-up evaluations between screening- and clinically detected patients.

Parameter	Screening (n = 102)	Clinical suspicion (n = 561)	p
Correct Compliance	93 (91.2)	504 (89.8)	0.857
Accidental Contaminations	2 (2.0)	25 (4.5)	0.410
Voluntary Gluten Ingestion	7 (6.9)	32 (5.7)	0.647
Gerd-like Symptoms	2 (2.0)	17 (3.0)	0.753
Ibs-like Symptoms (Total)	8 (7.8)	79 (14.1)	0.110
(a) classical ibs	4 (3.9)	43 (7.7)	0.212
(b) Diarrhea-predominant IBS	1 (1.0)	6 (1.1)	1.000
(c) Constipation-predominant IBS	3 (2.9)	30 (5.3)	0.457
Metabolic Alterations (tOtal)	15 (14.7)	96 (17.1)	0.666
(a) weight increase >10%	7 (6.9)	34 (6.1)	0.823
(b) cholesterol increase >50 mg/dL	7 (6.9)	36(6.4)	0.864
(c) metabolic syndrome	1 (1.0)	26 (4.6)	0.103

IBS: irritable bowel syndrome; GERD: gastroesophageal reflux disease. Categorical variables are reported as absolute number (percentage), continuous variables are described as median (interquartile range).

Compliance to the GFD was similar in screening- and clinically detected patients (91.2 versus 89.8%, p = 0.857). Two patients in the screening-diagnosed group and 25 patients in the clinically detected group referred possible accidental contaminations with gluten, mainly when they ate at work or at a restaurant. Instead, seven and 32 patients, in the screening- and clinically-detected groups respectively, voluntarily ingested gluten at least twice per month. At the binary logistic regression analysis, only the presence of gluten-related symptoms at baseline was marginally associated with better compliance (hazard ratio 2.110, 95% confidence interval 0.888–5.012, $p = 0.091$). On the contrary, sex ($p = 0.283$), age at the diagnosis ($p = 0.504$), and presence of a relative with CD ($p = 0.183$) did not correlate with compliance.

Overall, persistent symptoms were found in 19 (18.6%) screening-diagnosed patients and 153 (27.3%) clinically detected patients. Briefly, the aforementioned incomplete compliance to the GFD was one of the leading causes of persistent symptoms in both groups. Co-existing irritable bowel syndrome and gastroesophageal reflux disease were not significantly different across the study groups. Complicated CD was confirmed to be a rare condition. Interestingly, all seven cases of complicated CD were found in the clinically diagnosed patients and not in the screening-diagnosed group. Complications were found at diagnosis in three cases (two small bowel adenocarcinoma, one enteropathy-associated T cell lymphoma) and were diagnosed in the follow-up in the remaining five cases (three patients with type-1 refractory CD, one case of a type-2 refractory CD, and one case of hyposplenism).

Persistence in the follow-up procedures was also similar between the two groups, with a median follow up of 6.5 years (95% confidence interval 5.1–7.9) in screening-detected and 6.3 years (95% confidence interval 5.7–6.9) in clinically detected patients ($p = 0.452$) (Figure 2).

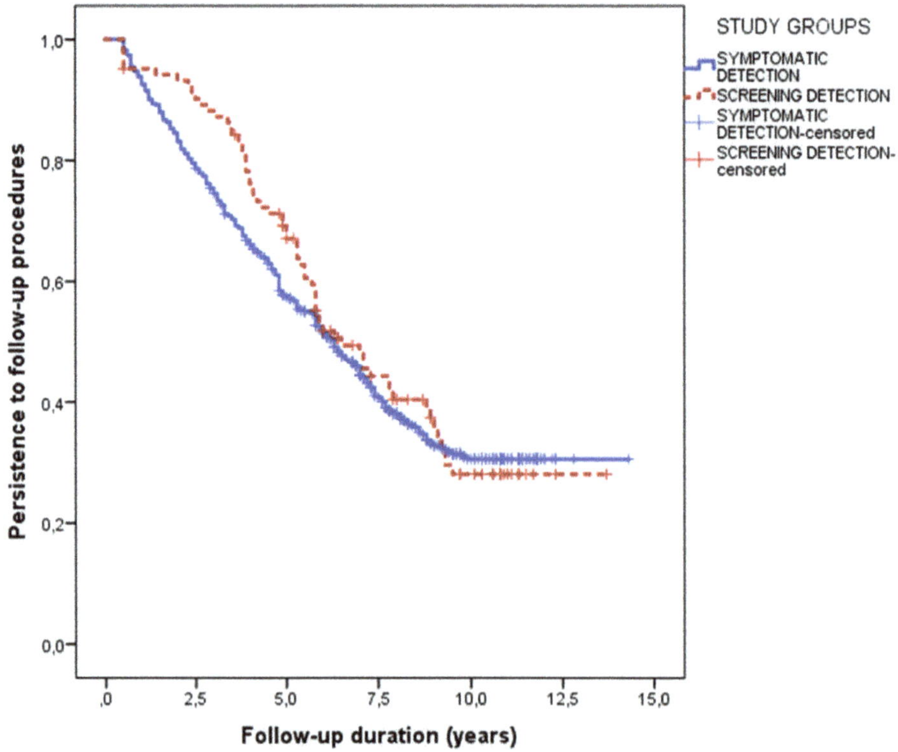

Figure 2. Persistence in the follow-up procedures in patients detected by screening and in patients diagnosed because of clinical suspicion.

Age at diagnosis was the only factor associated with persistence, with an inverse correlation (hazard ratio 0.988, 95% confidence interval 0.982–0.994, $p < 0.001$). Sex ($p = 0.325$), familiarity for

CD ($p = 0.696$), symptoms at the diagnosis ($p = 0.155$), and adherence to GFD ($p = 0.392$) were not associated with the length of the follow-up.

4. Discussion

In this paper, we assessed different clinical aspects of adult CD patients in which their condition was discovered thanks to screening programs. In particular, we explored both their baseline and their follow-up evaluations. These tasks were performed in a large cohort with a median six-year follow-up.

First, our data showed that adult CD patients diagnosed by screening had a GFD adherence which was similar to that of clinically detected patients after a six-year median follow-up. Both groups had an adherence as high as 90%. As previously stated, local policies may influence compliance. In the case of this study, it should be noted that Italy has official government policies protecting CD patients and helping them in the management of their conditions. These policies establish that diagnosed CD patients receive vouchers to buy specially produced gluten-free foods for up to 120 euro/month and call for strict respect of the local guidelines which recommend a clinical and laboratory follow-up at regular intervals. It is, therefore, possible that even patients who are diagnosed in the absence of severe symptoms are sufficiently eased in their difficult endeavors, which would favor higher compliance. The similarity in the compliance to the GFD of screening- and clinically detected CD patients had been already suggested in a series of studies on pediatric populations, mainly from North-European countries [15–17]. Data in the adult screening-detected population are more limited. Viljamaa and colleagues [6] firstly reported adherence of 82 versus 77% in 53 screening-detected and 44 clinically detected adult patients after a 14-year follow-up. In the only large study, Ukkola et al. [7] analyzed 123 screening-detected patients versus 698 patients diagnosed because of clinical suspicion. The self-reported adherence to the GFD after one year was similar between the study groups (91 versus 85%). Compared to Ukkola et al., the design of our study is different. While we lack the strengths of a prospective evaluation, we benefited from a longer follow-up and a physician-assessed adherence. Moreover, a difference in the geographical regions of enrolment should also be considered. With all these differences in mind, our results are surprisingly similar to those of Ukkola, thus validating them even in a different social context and in a more extended follow-up period. We also report novel findings based on the analysis of the persistence in the follow-up procedures, the rate of the non-responsive CD, and the metabolic alterations potentially induced by the GFD. In particular, all these factors were consistent across the study groups. It is also interesting to note that all the patients with complications belonged to the clinically detected group, even if our study was not designed nor powered enough to detect significant differences in this variable. A final word on this topic, therefore, will only come from extensive studies with decade-long follow-up.

Second, our data validated on a large scale the preliminary evidence that screening-detected patients have peculiar features during diagnosis when compared to patients recognized because of clinical suspicion. Approximately 25% of our screening-detected patients had mild gluten-related symptoms which could have led to the diagnosis, suggesting that the local screening strategies were reasonably good. This rate is, in fact, lower if compared to those previously described in adults [18] and pediatric series [15], in which at least half of the cases diagnosed by screening had symptoms. More interestingly, our screening-diagnosed patients were significantly less affected by iron-deficiency anemia and osteopenia. In a series of 19 screening-detected patients, Mustalahti and colleagues [19] firstly reported that bone mineral density (BMD) was lower than average. Following this report, Sundar et al. [20] compared the characteristics of 24 screening-detected versus 105 clinically detected CD patients, confirming a higher rate of BMD abnormalities in the latter group but also calling for further evidence from larger cohorts. We, therefore, suggest that the prevention of metabolic bone disease should strongly encourage CD screening in at-risk subjects. In fact, CD subjects are at increased risk of fractures [21,22] and benefit from GFD, which generally leads to an improvement in BMD in the first 12 months [23,24].

The strengths of our study include a large cohort of patients, the systematic clinical assessment of the compliance to the GFD, and the availability of additional information including the rate of clinical response to the GFD and its metabolic impact. We are aware that our study also comes with limitations, including its retrospective nature, the lack of systematic assessment of all features of metabolic syndrome (for instance, high-density lipoprotein cholesterol), and the lack of structured questionnaires for an even more comprehensive collection of both symptoms and dietary adherence. Finally, because of the observational nature of our study, we did not investigate the prevalence of some polymorphisms involved in iron absorption in children (DMT 1 IVS4 + 44C > A) [25] and lower bone mineral density in adults (IL1B-511T) [26], as reported in previous studies in CD patients.

5. Conclusions

Our data support the use of screening procedures for CD in the adult population. In particular, we demonstrated that an early diagnosis might protect from severe metabolic bone disease. Also, compared to clinically diagnosed patients, screening-diagnosed patients did not show an impaired adherence to the GFD nor an increased rate of GFD-related problems.

Author Contributions: Conceptualisation, A.G., L.B., and F.T.; methodology, F.T. and G.N.; formal analysis, F.T. and V.S.; investigation, G.N., C.F., and T.C.; data curation, F.T. and C.F.; writing original draft preparation, F.T. and V.S.; writing review & editing, L.B.; supervision, A.G.; funding acquisition, L.B and A.G.

Funding: All costs of the study were covered by the Oriented Finalized Research funds (R.F.O.) of the Ministry of University, Italy.

Conflicts of Interest: The authors declare no conflicts of interest.

References

1. Ludvigsson, J.L.; Leffler, D.A.; Bai, J.C.; Biagi, F.; Fasano, A.; Green, P.H.R.; Hadjivassiliou, M.; Kaukinen, K.; Kelly, C.P.; Leonard, J.N.; et al. The Oslo definitions for coeliac disease and related terms. *Gut* **2013**, *62*, 43–52. [CrossRef] [PubMed]
2. Green, P.H. Where are all those patients with Celiac disease? *Am. J. Gastroenterol.* **2007**, *102*, 1461–1463. [CrossRef] [PubMed]
3. Husby, S.; Koletzko, S.; Korponay-Szabó, I.R.; Mearin, M.L.; Phillips, A.; Shamir, R.; Troncone, R.; Giersiepen, K.; Branski, D.; Catassi, C.; et al. European Society for Pediatric Gastroenterology, Hepatology, and Nutrition guidelines for the diagnosis of coeliac disease. *J. Pediatr. Gastroenterol. Nutr.* **2012**, *54*, 136–160. [CrossRef] [PubMed]
4. Hill, I.D.; Dirks, M.H.; Liptak, G.S.; Colletti, R.B.; Fasano, A.; Guandalini, S.; Hoffenberg, E.J.; Horvath, K.; Murray, J.A.; Mitchell, P.; et al. Guideline for the diagnosis and treatment of celiac disease in children: Recommendations of the North American Society for Pediatric Gastroenterology, Hepatology and Nutrition. *J. Pediatr. Gastroenterol. Nutr.* **2005**, *40*, 1–19. [CrossRef] [PubMed]
5. Rubio-Tapia, A.; Hill, I.D.; Kelly, C.P.; Calderwood, A.H.; Murray, J.A. ACG clinical guidelines: Diagnosis and management of celiac disease. *Am. J. Gastroenterol.* **2013**, *108*, 656–676. [CrossRef] [PubMed]
6. Viljamaa, M.; Collin, P.; Huhtala, H.; Sievänen, H.; Mäki, M.; Kaukinen, K. Is coeliac disease screening in risk groups justified? A fourteen-year follow-up with special focus on compliance and quality of life. *Aliment. Pharmacol. Ther.* **2005**, *22*, 317–324. [CrossRef] [PubMed]
7. Ukkola, A.; Mäki, M.; Kurppa, K.; Collin, P.; Huhtala, H.; Kekkonen, L.; Kaukinen, K. Diet improves perception of health and well-being in symptomatic, but not asymptomatic, patients with celiac disease. *Clin. Gastroenterol. Hepatol.* **2011**, *9*, 118–123. [CrossRef] [PubMed]
8. Kivelä, L.; Popp, A.; Arvola, T.; Huhtala, H.; Kaukinen, K.; Kurppa, K. Long-term health and treatment outcomes in adult coeliac disease patients diagnosed by screening in childhood. *United Eur. Gastroenterol. J.* **2018**, *6*, 1022–1031. [CrossRef]
9. van Koppen, E.J.; Schweizer, J.J.; Csizmadia, C.G.; Krom, Y.; Hylkema, H.B.; van Geel, A.M.; Koopman, H.M.; Verloove-Vanhorick, S.P.; Mearin, M.L. Long-term health and quality-of-life consequences of mass screening for childhood celiac disease: A 10-year follow-up study. *Pediatrics* **2009**, *123*, e582-8. [CrossRef]

10. Fabiani, E.; Taccari, L.M.; Rätsch, I.M.; Di Giuseppe, S.; Coppa, G.V.; Catassi, C. Compliance with gluten-free diet in adolescents with screening-detected celiac disease: A 5-year follow-up study. *J. Pediatr.* **2000**, *136*, 841–843. [CrossRef]
11. Jadresin, O.; Misak, Z.; Sanja, K.; Sonicki, Z.; Zizić, V. Compliance with gluten-free diet in children with coeliac disease. *J. Pediatr. Gastroenterol. Nutr.* **2008**, *47*, 344–348. [CrossRef]
12. Laurikka, P.; Nurminen, S.; Kivelä, L.; Kurppa, K. Extraintestinal Manifestations of Celiac Disease: Early Detection for Better Long-Term Outcomes. *Nutrients* **2018**, *10*, 1015. [CrossRef]
13. Bathrellou, E.; Kontogianni, M.D.; Panagiotakos, D.B. Celiac disease and non-celiac gluten or wheat sensitivity and health in later life: A review. *Maturitas* **2018**, *112*, 29–33. [CrossRef]
14. Italian Guidelines for the Diagnosis and the Follow-up of Celiac Disease. 2015. Available online: http://www.celiachia.it/public/bo/upload/eventi_progetti/A.07.Booklet%20Celiachia%20-%20Impaginato.pdf (accessed on 7 November 2018).
15. Kivelä, L.; Kaukinen, K.; Huhtala, H.; Lähdeaho, M.L.; Mäki, M.; Kurppa, K. At-Risk Screened Children with Celiac Disease are Comparable in Disease Severity and Dietary Adherence to Those Found because of Clinical Suspicion: A Large Cohort Study. *J. Pediatr.* **2017**, *183*, 115–121. [CrossRef]
16. Kinos, S.; Kurppa, K.; Ukkola, A.; Collin, P.; Lähdeaho, M.L.; Huhtala, H.; Kekkonen, L.; Mäki, M.; Kaukinen, K. Burden of illness in screen-detected children with celiac disease and their families. *J. Pediatr. Gastroenterol. Nutr.* **2012**, *55*, 412–416. [CrossRef]
17. Kurppa, K.; Lauronen, O.; Collin, P.; Ukkola, A.; Laurila, K.; Huhtala, H.; Mäki, M.; Kaukinen, K. Factors associated with dietary adherence in celiac disease: A nationwide study. *Digestion* **2012**, *86*, 309–314. [CrossRef]
18. Vilppula, A.; Kaukinen, K.; Luostarinen, L.; Krekelä, I.; Patrikainen, H.; Valve, R.; Luostarinen, M.; Laurila, K.; Mäki, M.; Collin, P. Clinical benefit of gluten-free diet in screen-detected older celiac disease patients. *BMC Gastroenterol.* **2011**, *11*, 136. [CrossRef]
19. Mustalahti, K.; Collin, P.; Sievänen, H.; Salmi, J.; Mäki, M. Osteopenia in patients with clinically silent coeliac disease warrants screening. *Lancet* **1999**, *354*, 744–745. [CrossRef]
20. Sundar, N.; Crimmins, R.; Swift, G. Clinical presentation and incidence of complications in patients with coeliac disease diagnosed by relative screening. Postgrad. *Med. J.* **2007**, *83*, 273–276.
21. Heikkila, K.; Pearce, J.; Maki, M.; Kaukinen, K. Celiac disease and bone fractures: A systematic review and meta-analysis. *J. Clin. Endocrinol. Metab.* **2015**, *100*, 25–34. [CrossRef]
22. Davie, M.W.; Gaywood, I.; George, E.; Jones, P.W.; Masud, T.; Price, T.; Summers, G.D. Excess non-spine fractures in women over 50 years with celiac disease: A cross-sectional, questionnaire-based study. *Osteoporos. Int.* **2015**, *16*, 1150–1155. [CrossRef]
23. Meyer, D.; Stavropolous, S.; Diamond, B.; Shane, E.; Green, P.H. Osteoporosis in a north american adult population with celiac disease. *Am. J. Gastroenterol.* **2001**, *96*, 112–119. [CrossRef]
24. Pantaleoni, S.; Luchino, M.; Adriani, A.; Pellicano, R.; Stradella, D.; Ribaldone, D.G.; Sapone, N.; Isaia, G.C.; Stefano, M.D.; Astegiano, M. Bone mineral density at diagnosis of celiac disease and after 1 year of gluten-free diet. *Sci. World J.* **2014**, 173082. [CrossRef]
25. Tolone, C.; Bellini, G.; Punzo, F.; Papparella, A.; Miele, E.; Vitale, A.; Nobili, B.; Strisciuglio, C.; Rossi, F. The DMT1 IVS4+44C>A polymorphism and the risk of iron deficiency anemia in children with celiac disease. *PLoS ONE.* **2017**, *12*, e0185822. [CrossRef]
26. Moreno, M.L.; Crusius, J.B.; Cherñavsky, A.; Sugai, E.; Sambuelli, A.; Vazquez, H.; Mauriño, E.; Peña, A.S.; Bai, J.C. The IL-1 gene family and bone involvement in celiac disease. *Immunogenetics* **2005**, *57*, 618–620. [CrossRef]

nutrients

MDPI

Article

Exposure to Different Amounts of Dietary Gluten in Patients with Non-Celiac Gluten Sensitivity (NCGS): An Exploratory Study

Leda Roncoroni [1,2,*,†], Karla A. Bascuñán [1,3,*,†], Maurizio Vecchi [4,5], Luisa Doneda [2], Maria T. Bardella [1], Vincenza Lombardo [1], Alice Scricciolo [1], Federica Branchi [1] and Luca Elli [1]

1 Center for Prevention and Diagnosis of Celiac Disease, Gastroenterology and Endoscopy Unit, Fondazione IRCCS Ca' Granda Ospedale Maggiore Policlinico, 20135 Milan, Italy; mariateresa.bardella@yahoo.com (M.T.B.); vicky.l@hotmail.it (V.L.); scricciolo.alice@gmail.com (A.S.); federica.branchi@gmail.com (F.B.); dottorlucaelli@gmail.com (L.E.)
2 Department of Biomedical, Surgical and Dental Sciences, University of Milan, 20133 Milan, Italy; luisa.doneda@unimi.it
3 Department of Nutrition, School of Medicine, University of Chile, 8380453 Santiago, Chile
4 Department of Pathophysiology and Transplantation, University of Milan, 20122 Milan, Italy; maurizio.vecchi@policlinico.mi.it
5 Gastroenterology and Endoscopic Unit, Fondazione IRCCS Ca' Granda, Ospedale Maggiore Policlinico, 20122 Milan, Italy
* Correspondence: leda.roncoroni@unimi.it (L.R.); kbascunan@med.uchile.cl (K.A.B.); Tel.: +39-025-503-3384 (L.R.)
† These authors have contributed equally.

Received: 15 October 2018; Accepted: 7 January 2019; Published: 10 January 2019

Abstract: It is unclear whether patients with non-celiac gluten sensitivity (NCGS) can tolerate gluten. We have evaluated the changes of both gastrointestinal symptoms and quality of life for NCGS patients after the re-introduction of dietary gluten. Twenty-two NCGS patients reporting functional gastroenterological symptoms and on gluten-free diet (GFD) for the previous three weeks were exposed to incremental gluten-containing diets. Three groups were compared at baseline (immediately after 3-weeks on GFD) and immediately after the return of symptomatology: (i) a group tolerating a low-gluten diet (3.5 g gluten/day, week 1, $n = 8$), (ii) a group tolerating a mid-gluten diet (8 g gluten/day, week 2, $n = 6$), and (iii) a group tolerating a high-gluten diet (13 g gluten/day, week 3, $n = 8$). Their gastrointestinal symptoms and quality of life were assessed at baseline and post-intervention. The most common symptoms were: constipation (46%), abdominal pain (50%) and dyspepsia (38%). A decrease in several short form health survey (SF-36) sub-scores (all $p < 0.03$) after gluten re-introduction was only observed in the group tolerating the low-gluten diet; the same group showed a lower post-intervention role-emotional SF-36 score ($p = 0.01$). Most gastrointestinal symptoms remained similar after gluten re-introduction. However, a decrease in the general perception of well-being was only found after gluten re-introduction in the group tolerating a low-gluten diet ($p = 0.01$); the same was true when comparing the post-intervention general well-being perception among the three groups ($p = 0.050$). In conclusion, dissimilar responses from patients with NCGS were observed after the re-introduction of gluten, with gluten at a low dosage affecting the quality of life and general well-being of a group of patients, whereas others tolerate even higher doses of dietary gluten.

Keywords: non-celiac gluten sensitivity; gluten re-introduction; gluten-free diet; gastrointestinal symptoms

1. Introduction

Non-celiac gluten sensitivity (NCGS) is characterized by intestinal and extra-intestinal symptoms related to the ingestion of gluten-containing foods, in subjects that are not affected by either celiac disease (CD) or wheat allergy [1–3]. The symptomatology commonly found in NCGS comprises: bloating, abdominal pain, diarrhea, epigastric pain, nausea, aerophagia, lack of well-being, tiredness, headache, foggy mind, and anxiety among other symptoms [4]. Symptoms disappear after starting on a gluten-free diet (GFD) and appear again after a gluten challenge within a few hours or a couple of days [5,6]. However, this latter finding can be attributed to a placebo/nocebo effect [7,8]. Several studies have evaluated the effect of a gluten re-challenge in NCGS patients after GFD (a summary of studies is shown in Table 1). According to a recent meta-analysis, there is a wide range of patients relapsing after a gluten challenge (between 7% and 77%) and no effect of a gluten challenge was found on the risk of relapse [9]. These results are in line with another review of studies on patients with suspected NCGS, indicating that only 16% of them show clear gluten-specific symptoms [10]. These studies highlight the fact that further methodological considerations are required in studies evaluating the gluten challenge.

The current clinical consensus is that the diagnostic criteria on NCGS should include self-reported gluten intolerance, negative serology for CD (including immunoglobulin A (IgA) endomysial antibodies, IgA tissue transglutaminase antibodies, and IgG de-amidated gliadin peptide antibodies) and the absence of villous atrophy at duodenal histology (whilst on a gluten-containing diet) [1,3,11].

Similarly to CD and wheat allergy, the cornerstone of NCGS treatment is the withdrawal of gluten-containing foods. Although considered safe and effective, the lifelong elimination of gluten from the diet carries psychological and social implications. Patients with CD report about concerns related to the management of their social relationships and life routine [12]. Support and education are important to enable patients to adapt to their new diet [13]. However, given the uncertainty on the pathogenesis and trigger(s) of NCGS, it is not clear how strict such a new diet needs to be, how long its implementation and how to monitor the efficacy of the treatment other than by clinical response. Clinical experience suggests that patients affected by NCGS range from those who need to adhere to a strict GFD to those who can tolerate potential cross-contamination without any clinical consequences [14].

NCGS is a disorder treated with a GFD. There is currently discussion whether the symptoms described in NCGS are exclusively due to the ingestion of gluten proteins rather than other components included in wheat [15]. Wheat has some components that are different from gluten proteins and can be harmful to patients suffering from NCGS, including wheat germ agglutinins (WGA), amylase inhibitors/trypsin (ATI), and fermentable oligo/di/monosaccharides and polyols (FODMAP) [16–19]. ATIs are a family of structurally similar proteins, which serve as protective proteins in wheat and other cereals, by inhibiting the enzymes (trypsin and trypsin-like activities) of wheat and some parasites [20] ATIs have been described as triggers of the activation of innate immunity in intestinal cells [18]. WGAs [19], similar to ATIs, serve as protective proteins as they are resistant to heat and proteolysis. WGAs have shown to promote the production of pro-inflammatory cytokines, which affect the integrity of the intestinal epithelium [21]. Finally, FODMAP-containing foods include such components as oligosaccharides, disaccharides, monosaccharides, and sugar alcohols. They are resistant to digestion and can ferment completely or partially in the large intestine. Their efficacy in the treatment of gastrointestinal symptoms related to IBS has been described, and their function is being evaluated in various pathologies affecting the intestine [22,23].

Table 1. Summary of clinical trials evaluating a gluten re-challenge in NCGS patients.

Study (Reference)	Patients	Study Design	No. of Patients	Challenge Duration	Methods	Main Findings
Biesiekierski et al. [5]	NCGS w/IBS	DBRPCT	34 patients	up to 6 weeks	Gluten or placebo (two bread slices plus one muffin per day)	68% (13) of patients in the gluten group reported inadequate symptoms control compared with 40% (6) under placebo.
Carroccio et al. [24]	NCGS	DBRPCT		2 weeks	Capsules with wheat (20 g) vs. placebo	30% (276) of patients diagnosed as non-celiac wheat sensitivity. Wheat challenge induced >30% increase in symptoms.
Peters et al. [25]	NCGS w/IBS symptoms	DBRPCT	22 patients	3 days	Dietary challenge: gluten-free food supplemented with gluten (16 g/day), whey (16 g/day) or not supplemented (placebo)	Higher overall Spielberger State Trait Personality Inventory state depression scores compared to placebo but not whey, after gluten. Similar gastrointestinal symptoms induced after all treatments
Zanini et al. [26]	NCGS	DBRPCT	35 non-CD patients	10 days	Gluten-containing flour or gluten-free flour for 10 days, followed by a 2-week washout period	34% of patients diagnosed as having NCGS
Capannolo et al. [27]	NCGS	DBRPCT	364 patients (27 with NCGS and 337 with no specific diagnosis)	1 month	Challenge with dietary gluten vs. a GFD.	85.96% did not experience a change in symptomatology after a GFD. Low value of a gluten-containing diet for an increase in symptoms.
Rosinach et al. [28]	NCGS	DBRPCT	18 non-CD patients	6 months	11 gluten (20 g/day) and 7 placeboes	91% of patients with clinical relapse during gluten challenge (vs. 28.5% after placebo)
Picarelli et al. [29]	NCGS	DBRPCT	26 patients	1 day	Food challenge (oral provocation test) with a gluten-containing croissant (10 g of gluten per croissant) to 13 patients and a gluten-free croissant to the other 13 patients.	No difference was found between the severity of symptoms with gluten-containing croissants compared to a group of patients with gluten-free croissants.

Table 1. *Cont.*

Study (Reference)	Patients	Study Design	No. of Patients	Challenge Duration	Methods	Main Findings
Elli et al. [30]	NCGS w/functional gastrointestinal symptoms	DBRPCT	98 patients	7 days	Gluten intake (5.6 g/day) or placebo	28 patients reported symptomatic relapse with deteriorated quality of life
Skodje et al. [31]	Subjects with self-reported NCGS	DBRPCT	59 subjects	7 days	Diets containing gluten (5.7 g), fructans (2.1 g), or placebo	Overall Gastrointestinal Symptom Rating Scale for Irritable Bowel Syndrome scores increased after fructans rather than gluten.
Dale et al. [32]	Patients w/suspected NCGS	DBRPCT	20 patients	4 days	Two muffins a day (11/0 g gluten). (4 periods w/double-blinded provocation, 2 w/gluten, 2 w/placebo)	Most severe symptoms found after placebo. Only 4/20 patients correctly identified periods w/gluten.

NCGS: Non-celiac gluten sensitivity; DBRPCT: Double-blind randomized placebo-controlled trial; IBS: Irritable bowel syndrome; CD: Celiac disease; GFD: Gluten-free diet.

There is currently no data that can support any recommendations on the need for, or frequency of, repeated follow-up visits in these patients. It is considered good clinical care to study these patients at regular intervals in order to ensure they remain healthy and to involve a nutritionist to make sure they are not at risk of nutrient deficiencies. It is also advisable that the continued need for "strict" avoidance of all gluten-related products be regularly reviewed following recovery because some patients can possibly follow a less restrictive diet with no recurrence of symptoms. A lifelong strict GFD (as in CD) vs. an "on-demand" approach is the main question. Many experts recommend that patients should undergo periodic re-evaluation with the re-introduction of gluten (e.g., every 6–12 months) [8].

A GFD leads to the complete disappearance of symptoms in most patients with NCGS but in some cases the level of improvement after gluten withdrawal is only partial. However, it should be mentioned that the level of tolerance varies among individuals and there are patients with NCGS who do not tolerate even very small amounts of gluten. As it is presently unclear whether gluten sensitivity is a permanent or transient condition, the re-introduction of gluten after 1–2 years on a GFD is potentially advisable [33]. Thus, the aim of the present study was to evaluate the changes in gastrointestinal symptoms and quality of life for NCGS patients after exposure to different amounts of dietary gluten.

2. Materials and Methods

Between 2013 and 2014, patients reporting functional gastroenterological symptoms according to the Rome III criteria [34] were invited to participate in this study. All were recruited from the gastroenterological outpatient clinic at the Center for Prevention and Diagnosis of Celiac Disease, Gastroenterology and Endoscopy Unit, Fondazione IRCCS Ca' Granda Ospedale Maggiore Policlinico in Milan (Italy). The patients who agreed to participate gave their written informed consent and were enrolled in the study. The local Ethics Committee for Human Research of the City of Milan approved the study protocol. The trial was registered in ClinicalTrial.gov (NCT01864993).

The inclusion criteria were: adult age (>18 years old), being on a gluten-containing diet, with negative anti-tissue transglutaminase IgA, normal IgA dosage, negative IgE-mediated wheat allergy as verified by skin prick test and serological IgE dosage. The exclusion criteria were: diagnosis of CD, wheat allergy, inflammatory bowel disease, psychiatric disorders, major abdominal surgery (in particular, intestinal resections), diabetes mellitus, systemic autoimmune diseases, previous anaphylactic episodes, any systemic disorders, patients already following or having followed a GFD regimen in the previous six months, pregnant or breastfeeding women, and patients already on pharmacological therapy. The patients were evaluated by a gastroenterologist and a qualified nutritionist. The diagnosis of NCGS was made in accordance with the latest NCGS consensus [4]. After recruitment, patients were requested to follow a GFD plan for 3-weeks before the start of the dietary intervention (i.e., the low/mid/high-gluten diet). Their overall health, gastrointestinal symptoms, and quality of life were assessed by medical examination. Their adherence to the GFD was evaluated according to the celiac dietary adherence test (CDAT) [35]. The CDAT is a clinically relevant, easily administrated 7-item instrument which allows the standardized evaluation of GFD adherence. It is a sensitive tool developed using standard psychometric techniques. Only those patients with excellent or very good GFD adherence were included in the study. CDAT is based on a score ranging from 7 to 35 against seven questions, each on a 5-point scale, with higher scores denoting worse GFD adherence [35].

2.1. Intervention

Twenty-four patients were recruited (Figure 1). As mentioned above, all the recruited patients were instructed to follow a strict GFD for 3 weeks. After that time, the intervention period started. A qualified nutritionist designed a personalized GFD adjusted to match daily requirements for energy, macronutrients and micronutrients. A structured 3-week dietary plan was indicated and explained to every patient, to cover structured meals, foods/beverages and alternatives for food purchase.

The patients were also encouraged to immediately contact the nutritionist by phone in case of any doubt related to the diet. After the three weeks on the GFD, the intervention period started. The patients started the study with a low-gluten diet during the first week (3.5–4 g gluten/day, week 1, *n* = 24). Two patients dropped out of the study during the first week because they did not want to continue the diet. Afterwards, the patients who did not report adverse symptoms were administered a mid-gluten diet in the second week (6.7–8 g gluten/day, week 2, *n* = 14). Then, the patients who passed the second week were started on a high-gluten diet for the following week (10–13 g gluten/day, week 3, *n* = 8). Each patient had been instructed to immediately contact the research team at the end of each week should any of the previously reported symptoms at the beginning of the study return. A clinical evaluation was then arranged and the patient was to stop their gluten-containing diet and return to the GFD (i.e., for patients reporting adverse symptomatology at the end of the first week) or to the previous gluten-containing diet (i.e., for patients reporting adverse symptomatology at the end of the second and third week). In such cases, the nutritionist would also reinforce the instructions and food education on the practice of the GFD. A flow-chart of patients is shown in Figure 1. The patients with symptomatic relapse at the end of week 1 returned to the GFD (as indicated in the previous three weeks after recruitment). The patients who experienced a symptomatic relapse at the end of week 2 returned to a low-gluten diet (3.5–4 g/day) and stayed on that dietary treatment until the end of week 3. Finally, none of the patients who had undergone the high-gluten diet (*n* = 8) reported any worsening of gastrointestinal symptoms and at the end of week 3, they were instructed to return to their regular dietary pattern.

2.2. Diets

The nutritional evaluation aimed to assess anthropometrical parameters, nutritional status, and usual dietary patterns. At the beginning of the study, after clinical evaluation, a structured 7-day dietary plan was generated for each patient, adjusted to his/her daily nutritional requirements for energy, macronutrients and micronutrients. For each week, according to the low/mid/high-gluten amount contained, meals were listed (breakfast, morning snack, lunch, afternoon snack, dinner and other snacks during the day) with specific foods/beverages (see examples in Table 2). For week 1 the source of gluten was only wheat pasta (50 g, about 3.5–4 g of gluten) administered during dinner. In week 2 the sources of gluten were wheat pasta (50 g, about 3.5–4 g of gluten) during dinner and wheat bread (50 g, about 3.2–4 g gluten) during the daytime. For week 3 the sources of gluten were wheat pasta (60 g at lunch and 60 g at dinner, ~8.4–9.6 g gluten) and wheat bread (30 g during the day, 1.9–3 g gluten). The gluten content of each of the three diets was calculated referring to Schalk et al. [36]. In that study, the gluten content was determined through a comprehensive strategy to isolate gluten protein fractions and gluten protein types (GPT) from wheat, rye, barley, and oat flours. All of the isolated GPTs were fully characterized by means of analytical reversed-phase high-performance liquid chromatography (RP-HPLC), sodium dodecyl sulfate-polyacrylamide gel electrophoresis (SDS-PAGE), N-terminal sequencing, electrospray-ionization quadrupole time-of-flight mass spectrometry (LC-ESI-QTOF-MS) and untargeted LC-MS/MS of chymotryptic hydrolysates of the single GPT. Successively, all of the GPTs were reproducibly isolated in high purity from the flours and were made suitable to be used as a reference material, i.e., for calibration of liquid chromatography tandem mass spectrometry methods or enzyme-linked immunosorbent assays (ELISAs) [36].

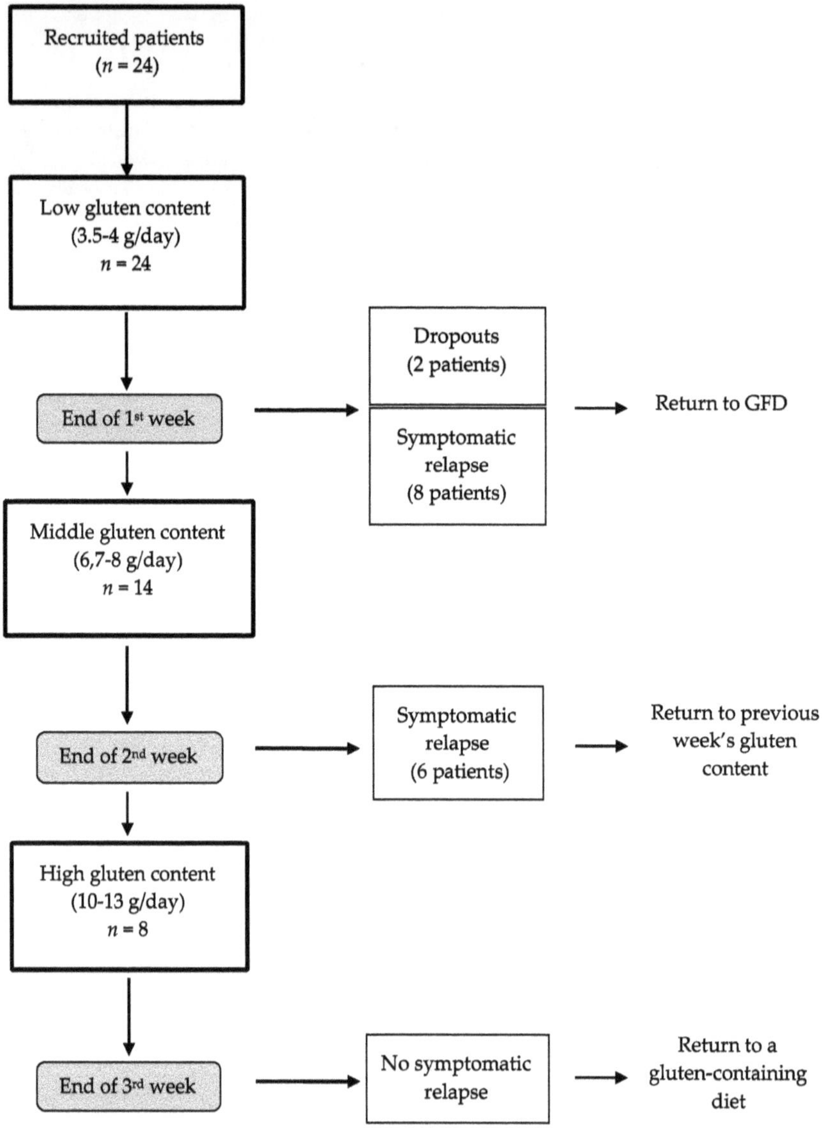

Figure 1. Flow-chart of the patients' activity in the study. Two patients (drop-outs) decided to abandon the diet during the first week of intervention; GFD: gluten-free diet.

Table 2. Example of the three dietary plans used and differing in the amount of gluten contained [1].

Meal	Low-Gluten (3.5–4 g Gluten)	Mid-Gluten (6.7–8 g Gluten)	High-Gluten (10–13 g Gluten)
Breakfast	1 small cup of coffee, 300 mL partly skimmed milk, 1 gluten-free croissant	1 small cup of coffee, 300 mL partly skimmed milk, 4 gluten-free biscuits	1 small cup of coffee, 300 mL partly skimmed milk, 4 gluten-free rusks
Morning snack	1 kiwifruit	1 apple	1 banana
Lunch	100 g gluten-free pasta, 90 g mixed vegetables, 1 portion of chard, 4 mandarins	100 g gluten-free pasta, 40 g cow ricotta cheese, 100 g potatoes, 2 bananas	60 g wheat pasta with broccoli, 2 teaspoonfuls grated Parmesan cheese, 1 portion of mixed salad, 2.5 glasses of fruit salad
Afternoon snack	1 bowl of strawberries	1 bowl of strawberries	1 pear
Dinner	50 g wheat pasta with zucchini, 100 g turkey thigh 200 g potatoes, 5 slices of pineapple	50 g wheat pasta with tomato sauce, 1 spoon of fresh peas 120 g pork, 1 portion of chard 5 mandarins	60 g wheat pasta with tomato sauce, 100 g halibut, 200 g potatoes, 2 glasses of fruit salad
During the day	40 g gluten-free bread, 6.5 teaspoonfuls virgin olive oil	50 g of white wheat bread, 3.5 teaspoonfuls virgin olive oil	30 g white wheat bread, 8 teaspoonfuls virgin olive oil

[1] Example of a typical day per week for each of the three different diets, as calculated for an average 2000 Kcal/day energy requirement.

2.3. Gastrointestinal Symptoms and Quality of Life

The gastrointestinal symptoms and quality of life of each patient were assessed at the beginning of the study and soon after the return of symptoms after administering one of the gluten-containing diets (i.e., after gluten exposure). A visual analogue scale (VAS) was used to assess the patient's gastrointestinal symptoms and general perception of well-being as previously described by our group [23]. This instrument recorded the severity of specific symptoms: abdominal pain, bloating, postprandial fullness, early satiety, epigastric pain, non-specific functional gastrointestinal symptoms, and satisfaction with stool consistency. For each question, each patient was asked to put a mark along a 10-cm long line with one end 0 meaning "absence of symptom" and the other end 10 "severe symptomatology". A further VAS evaluated the satisfaction about the current level of general well-being, with 0 meaning "completely unsatisfied" and 10 "absolutely satisfied".

The patient's quality of life was evaluated through the short form health survey (SF-36) questionnaire. This instrument comprises 36 questions that conceptually refer to eight health domains [37]. The patients were asked to answer each question and then domain-specific scores ranging between 0 and 100 were calculated, where 100 represented the best possible perception of quality of life.

2.4. Statistical Analysis

The data are provided as mean $\pm$ SEM or median (interquartile range) unless indicated otherwise. Twenty-two patients were included for analysis. Comparisons were made according to the group of patients that reported the return of symptomatology after gluten exposure, that is 3 groups:

low-gluten (patients that reported adverse symptomatology after 1 week on a gluten-containing diet, $n = 8$), mid-gluten (patients that reported adverse symptomatology after 2 weeks on a gluten-containing diet, $n = 6$), and high-gluten (patients that reported adverse symptomatology after 3 weeks on a gluten-containing diet, $n = 8$). One-way ANOVA was used to evaluate between-group differences as to age and body-mass index; Fisher's exact test was used to compare categorical variables (i.e., gender distribution and presence of gastrointestinal symptoms) between the groups. The within-group differences of SF-36 and VAS scores before (immediately after 3-weeks on a GFD) and after gluten exposure (i.e., baseline vs. the time when gastrointestinal symptoms returned after the gluten-containing diets) were assessed using a non-parametric Wilcoxon's rank sum test. The between-group differences were evaluated after gluten exposure using the non-parametric Kruskal-Wallis test. STATA® ver. 13.1 software (StataCorp, College Station, TX, USA) was used for statistics and statistical significance was set at a 5% α-level.

3. Results

3.1. Patients

All patients included in the study obtained a CDAT score from 7 to 13, thus indicating very good adherence to the GFD. As shown in Table 3, the patients were middle-aged, mainly women, and within the normal weight range. Regarding the clinical symptomatology at baseline, symptoms such as constipation, abdominal pain, and dyspepsia were the most frequently reported by the whole sample (46%, 50%, and 38%, respectively). All three groups were comparable regarding both general characteristics and present gastrointestinal symptoms at baseline (Table 3). In regards to the estimated gluten content in the foods used in the intervention diets, the gluten content was 3.5–4 g/day in the low-gluten diet, 6.7–8 g/day in the mid-gluten diet, and 10–13 g/day in the high-gluten diet.

Table 3. General characteristics of the group of patients at baseline [1].

	Low-Gluten (3.5–4 g/day, $n = 8$)	Mid-Gluten (6.7–8 g/day, $n = 6$)	High-Gluten (10–13 g/day, $n = 8$)	p-Value †
Age, years	44.6 ± 4.5	45.5 ± 3.1	44.6 ± 5.2	0.98
Gender, F/M	7/1	6/0	7/1	0.99
BMI, kg/m^2	23.0 ± 1.7	23.8 ± 1.8	21.8 ± 0.7	0.65
Diarrhea, n (%)	1 (12.5)	0 (0)	1 (12.5)	0.99
Bloating, n (%)	0 (0)	2 (33.3)	1 (12.5)	0.24
Constipation, n (%)	3 (37.5)	5 (83.3)	3 (37.5)	0.21
Abdominal pain, n (%)	5 (62.5)	4 (66.6)	3 (37.5)	0.64
Dyspepsia, n (%)	6 (75)	1 (16.6)	2 (25)	0.08

[1] Data are shown as mean ± SEM for continuous variables and frequency and/or relative number for nominal variables. † p-value for comparison between groups using one-way ANOVA or Fisher's exact test for categorical variables. F: female; M: male; BMI: body mass index.

3.2. Quality of Life

The resulting SF-36 scores are shown in Table 4. There was a significant decrease in several SF-36 sub-scores (role physical, role emotional, bodily pain, mental health, vitality and social interaction, all $p < 0.03$) after gluten exposure in the group of patients receiving the low-gluten diet but not in the groups receiving mid- and high-gluten content (Table 4). However, when comparing the change in SF-36 scores after dietary gluten exposure between the three groups, we observed a change only in the role emotional score, which was lower in the low-gluten content group. No post-intervention differences were found regarding the general health score among the three groups (Table 4).

3.3. Gastrointestinal Symptoms

The within-group comparisons showed no significant changes in most of the evaluated gastrointestinal symptoms before and after dietary intervention (Table 5). However, a decrease in the general perception of well-being was found in the low-gluten group (but not in the mid- and high-gluten groups) after intervention ($p = 0.01$). In line, when comparing the three groups after dietary gluten exposure, a further decrease of the general well-being level was found in the low-gluten group compared with the mid- and high-gluten groups ($p = 0.050$, Table 5).

Table 4. SF-36 subscales and global score for quality of life [1].

	Low-Gluten (3.5–4 g/day, $n = 8$)			Mid-Gluten (6.7–8 g/day, $n = 6$)			High-Gluten (10–13 g/day, $n = 8$)			
	Baseline	7-Day	*p*-Value †	Baseline	14-Day	*p*-Value †	Baseline	21-Day	*p*-Value †	*p*-Value ‡
Physical functioning	100.0 (5.0)	95.0 (10.0)	0.10	100.0 (20.0)	82.5 (45.0)	0.17	100.0 (2.5)	100.0 (2.5)	0.94	0.13
Role physical	100.0 (25.0)	50.0 (37.5)	0.03	87.5 (25.0)	100.0 (50.0)	0.72	87.5 (37.5)	87.5 (62.5)	0.65	0.19
Role emotional	79.0 (26.0)	41.0 (31.0)	0.004	79.0 (26.0)	62.5 (32.0)	0.92	84.0 (27.5)	67.5 (40.5)	0.83	0.01
Bodily pain	76.0 (22.5)	53.5 (47.5)	0.008	76.0 (22.5)	64.0 (11.0)	0.87	66.5 (50.0)	69.5 (44.0)	0.30	0.15
Mental health	65.0 (20)	47.5 (17.5)	0.12	65.0 (20.0)	55.0 (20.0)	0.74	72.5 (15.0)	57.5 (37.5)	0.79	0.48
Vitality	87.0 (12.5)	56.0 (18.5)	0.02	87.0 (12.5)	62.5 (38.0)	0.50	100.0 (31.5)	68.5 (44.0)	0.34	0.67
Social interaction	100.0 (17.0)	33.0 (33.0)	0.007	100.0 (67.0)	100.0 (34.0)	0.10	100.0 (33.5)	100.0 (17.0)	0.39	0.30
General health	82.0 (18.0)	62.0 (34.0)	0.15	76.0 (20.0)	72.0 (16.0)	0.46	78.0 (10.0)	72.0 (24.0)	0.99	0.49

[1] Data are shown as median values (interquartile range); † *p*-value for comparison within each group (low-, mid- and high-gluten) using a non-parametric Wilcoxon's rank sum test; ‡ *p*-value for between-groups comparison (low-, mid-, and high-gluten) post diet using the Kruskal-Wallis test.

Table 5. Visual analogue scale scores for gastrointestinal symptoms [1].

	Low-Gluten (3.5–4 g/day, $n = 8$)			Mid-Gluten (6.7–8 g/day, $n = 6$)			High-Gluten (10–13 g/day, $n = 8$)			
	Baseline	7-Day	*p*-Value †	Baseline	14-Day	*p*-Value †	Baseline	21-Day	*p*-Value †	*p*-Value ‡
Abdominal pain	0 (1.3)	2.6 (6.1)	0.16	5.3 (4.5)	4.9 (3.6)	0.87	0 (0.4)	0.5 (7.8)	0.22	0.66
Stool satisfaction	3.8 (9.1)	0 (3.4)	0.16	7.0 (9.8)	3.2 (5.4)	0.25	7.6 (8.8)	4.1 (8.8)	0.99	0.21
Abdominal bloating	0 (3.9)	3.0 (8.4)	0.19	5.4 (5.5)	5.2 (6.0)	0.87	0 (2.2)	3.5 (8.8)	0.19	0.68
Postprandial fullness	0 (4.4)	4.3 (7.4)	0.12	0 (6.7)	0 (2.9)	0.84	0 (0.0)	2.5 (6.6)	0.29	0.37
Early satiety feeling	0.2 (1.8)	3.5 (5.2)	0.13	0 (1.0)	0 (1.4)	0.84	0 (0.0)	1.3 (6.4)	0.09	0.36
Epigastric burn	0 (0.9)	2.0 (8.2)	0.07	0 (2.0)	0 (4.4)	0.85	0 (1.9)	0.7 (5.8)	0.41	0.42
General well-being	9.1 (2.9)	2.1 (2.9)	0.01	7.9 (3.1)	5.9 (4.5)	0.14	8.5 (1.9)	5.1 (4.3)	0.21	0.05

[1] Data are shown as median values (interquartile range); † *p*-value for comparison within each group (low-, mid- and high-gluten) using a non-parametric Wilcoxon's rank sum test. ‡ *p*-value for between-groups comparison (low-, mid- and high-gluten) post diet using the Kruskal-Wallis test.

4. Discussion

This study evaluated the effects of a short-term re-introduction of gluten on individuals diagnosed with NCGS. Our results show that a level of tolerance is present in patients without showing any adverse signs or gastrointestinal symptoms when consuming gluten. There was a different response among individuals with NCGS when exposed to different amounts of dietary gluten. A subgroup of patients had an immediate response with some worsening of their quality of life and general well-being at a low-gluten dosage, whereas other patients were able to tolerate medium and high doses of gluten, indicating that these latter groups can be administered some gluten without adverse health effects.

At present, it is well known that a GFD is the treatment of choice for patients suffering from NGCS. Several randomized controlled trials (RCTs) [10] have been carried out to identify gluten as the trigger of symptoms (Table 1). Those reports have shown variable results and are not conclusive regarding the cause-effect relationship of gluten and gastrointestinal symptoms [30,32]. We have previously suggested that gluten can be a major trigger of gastrointestinal symptoms in line with other [5,38,39]. Although the data to date suggest a benefit from a GFD for a selected group of patients, it is possible that the improvement in symptoms might not be due to gluten itself. Other components in wheat may trigger the reported symptoms in these patients, suggesting the clinical feature of non-celiac wheat sensitivity. This last entity has not completely been clarified as it is not clear whether patients are suffering from gluten-related symptoms or another component of wheat (such as fructans) [40]. Regardless of the nomenclature, Carroccio et al. [41] provided a clinically useful approach confirming non-celiac wheat sensitivity as a unique clinical condition. Their results suggest the existence of two different groups of patients with this condition: one with characteristics similar to CD and the other with characteristics resembling food allergy [41]. The current nomenclature of gluten sensitivity [1], NCGS [5] and gluten-related disorders does not resolve this problem and may confuse clinicians as to which component in wheat might be triggering patients' symptomatology. Expert recommendations have proposed a periodic evaluation with re-introduction of gluten for NCGS patients on consideration of the economic costs and quality of life that a lifelong GFD entails [8].

Regarding the quality-of-life perception, previous data of our group from a cross-over study has shown that patients with NCGS treated with a GFD enjoy an improvement in the majority of the SF-36 scores after 7 days [30]. In our study, we observed that the group who tolerated only a low amount of dietary gluten was the only group showing a decrease in several SF-36 sub-scores. On the other hand, it is important to point out that the groups on a mid- and high-gluten diet did not show any significant change in their quality of life. This finding is intriguing because it would suggest that a greater gluten intake by patients with NCGS would not necessarily further affect their quality of life, thus reinforcing the idea of inter-individual variability against gluten in this group.

After the re-introduction of gluten, the gastrointestinal symptomatology showed no main changes against our dietary intervention. Moreover, no differences were found after gluten exposure among the three groups (i.e., at the end of the intervention period). However, we did find a change in the perception of general well-being, which was significantly affected in the group receiving a low level of gluten; such a result is in line with what we found on the patients' quality of life. Overall, these findings suggest that with regard to quality of life and general well-being the changes observed in the group on a low-gluten diet would be related to a systemic response to gluten consumption rather than only gastrointestinal symptomatology or, at least, a combination of both. Even if our results are interesting per se they require further confirmation in larger samples and with different populations of patients suffering from NCGS.

This was an exploratory study that worked on a small sample of patients to evaluate the re-introduction of gluten through dietary modifications in a homogeneous group of patients correctly diagnosed with NCGS. As to limitations, we would like to point out that all the patients did not receive all their gluten doses in a balanced cross-over design. This was mainly due to ethical considerations since, at the time the clinical picture began to worsen, the patients stopped the administered diet and returned to their established treatment with GFD.

To summarize, we have shown a dissimilar response after the reintroduction of gluten in patients with NCGS who were on GFD for the last 3-weeks. We have also shown that for a group of them the re-introduction of gluten at low dosage affected their quality of life and general well-being, whereas other patients could tolerate higher doses of dietary gluten. Further studies are needed to establish whether NCGS patients require a dietary regimen free of gluten or just a gluten-restricted diet. Therefore, a controlled re-introduction of gluten potentially helps the improvement of selected patients that are able to tolerate gluten intake by developing a personalized diet containing gluten without the reappearance of symptoms. Further research is needed to assess the long-term clinical response of the increase in the dietary gluten content as concerns symptomatology and quality of life for patients with NCGS.

Author Contributions: Conceptualization, L.R., K.A.B. and L.E.; Methodology, L.R., K.A.B., L.D. and L.E.; Investigation, L.R., V.L., A.S., F.B. and L.E.; Data Curation, L.R. and K.A.B.; Formal analysis, K.A.B.; Writing-Original Draft Preparation, K.A.B., L.R. and L.E.; Writing Review & Editing, L.R., K.A.B., L.D. and M.T.B.; M.V. and L.E.; Funding Acquisition, L.E.

Funding: This research was funded by Fondazione IRCCS Ca' Granda and through grants from the Italian Ministry of Health and Lombardy's Regional Government Authority (Ministero della Salute and Regione Lombardia, call No. 2011-02348234), and the APC was funded by Fondazione IRCCS Ca' Granda Ospedale Maggiore Policlinico and Università degli Studi di Milano, Milan, Italy.

Conflicts of Interest: The authors declare no conflict of interest. The funders had no role in the design of the study; in the collection, analysis, or interpretation of data; in the writing of the manuscript, or in the decision to publish the results.

References

1. Sapone, A.; Bai, J.C.; Ciacci, C.; Dolinsek, J.; Green, P.H.R.; Hadjivassiliou, M.; Kaukinen, K.; Rostami, K.; Sanders, D.S.; Schumann, M.; et al. Spectrum of gluten-related disorders: Consensus on new nomenclature and classification. *BMC Med.* **2012**, *10*, 13. [CrossRef] [PubMed]
2. Bascuñán, K.A.; Roncoroni, L.; Branchi, F.; Doneda, L.; Scricciolo, A.; Ferretti, F.; Aray, M.; Elli, L. The 5 Ws of a gluten challenge for gluten-related disorders. *Nutr. Rev.* **2018**, *76*, 79–87. [CrossRef] [PubMed]
3. Catassi, C.; Bai, J.C.; Bonaz, B.; Bouma, G.; Calabrò, A.; Carroccio, A.; Castillejo, G.; Ciacci, C.; Cristofori, F.; Dolinsek, J.; et al. Non-celiac gluten sensitivity: The new frontier of gluten related disorders. *Nutrients* **2013**, *5*, 3839–3853. [CrossRef]
4. Catassi, C.; Elli, L.; Bonaz, B.; Bouma, G.; Carroccio, A.; Castillejo, G.; Cellier, C.; Cristofori, F.; de Magistris, L.; Dolinsek, J.; et al. Diagnosis of non-celiac gluten sensitivity (NCGS): The salerno experts' criteria. *Nutrients* **2015**, *7*, 4966–4977. [CrossRef]
5. Biesiekierski, J.R.; Newnham, E.D.; Irving, P.M.; Barrett, J.S.; Haines, M.; Doecke, J.D.; Shepherd, S.J.; Muir, J.G.; Gibson, P.R. Gluten Causes Gastrointestinal Symptoms in Subjects Without Celiac Disease: A Double-Blind Randomized Placebo-Controlled Trial. *Am. J. Gastroenterol.* **2011**, *106*, 508. [CrossRef] [PubMed]
6. Volta, U.; Bardella, M.T.; Calabrò, A.; Troncone, R.; Corazza, G.R.; Bagnato, C.; Belcari, C.; Bellantoni, A.; Caio, G.; Calella, F.; et al. An Italian prospective multicenter survey on patients suspected of having non-celiac gluten sensitivity. *BMC Med.* **2014**, *12*, 85. [CrossRef] [PubMed]
7. Parrish, C.R. Non-Celiac Gluten Sensitivity; Where are we now in 2015? *Pract. Gastroenterol.* **2015**, *142*, 40–48.
8. Fasano, A.; Sapone, A.; Zevallos, V.; Schuppan, D. Nonceliac gluten sensitivity. *Gastroenterology* **2015**, *148*, 1195–1204. [CrossRef]
9. Lionetti, E.; Pulvirenti, A.; Vallorani, M.; Catassi, G.; Verma, A.K.; Gatti, S.; Catassi, C. Re-challenge Studies in Non-celiac Gluten Sensitivity: A Systematic Review and Meta-Analysis. *Front. Physiol.* **2017**, *8*, 621. [CrossRef]
10. Molina-Infante, J.; Carroccio, A. Suspected Nonceliac Gluten Sensitivity Confirmed in Few Patients After Gluten Challenge in Double-Blind, Placebo-Controlled Trials. *Clin. Gastroenterol. Hepatol.* **2017**, *15*, 339–348. [CrossRef]
11. Rubio-Tapia, A.; Hill, I.D.; Kelly, C.P.; Calderwood, A.H.; Murray, J.A. ACG clinical guidelines: Diagnosis and management of celiac disease. *Am. J. Gastroenterol.* **2013**, *108*, 656–676, quiz 677. [CrossRef] [PubMed]

12. Sverker, A.; Hensing, G.; Hallert, C. "Controlled by food"—Lived experiences of coeliac disease. *J. Hum. Nutr. Diet.* **2005**, *18*, 171–180. [CrossRef] [PubMed]
13. Bascuñán, K.A.; Vespa, M.C.; Araya, M. Celiac disease: Understanding the gluten-free diet. *Eur. J. Nutr.* **2017**, *56*, 449–459. [CrossRef] [PubMed]
14. Hill, I.D.; Fasano, A.; Guandalini, S.; Hoffenberg, E.; Levy, J.; Reilly, N.; Verma, R. NASPGHAN clinical report on the diagnosis and treatment of gluten-related disorders. *J. Pediatr. Gastroenterol. Nutr.* **2016**, *63*, 156–165. [CrossRef] [PubMed]
15. Catassi, C.; Alaedini, A.; Bojarski, C.; Bonaz, B.; Bouma, G.; Carroccio, A.; Castillejo, G.; De Magistris, L.; Dieterich, W.; Di Liberto, D.; et al. The overlapping area of non-celiac gluten sensitivity (NCGS) and wheat-sensitive irritable bowel syndrome (IBS): An update. *Nutrients* **2017**, *9*, 1268. [CrossRef] [PubMed]
16. Uhde, M.; Ajamian, M.; Caio, G.; De Giorgio, R.; Indart, A.; Green, P.H.; Verna, E.C.; Volta, U.; Alaedini, A. Intestinal cell damage and systemic immune activation in individuals reporting sensitivity to wheat in the absence of coeliac disease. *Gut* **2016**, *65*, 1930–1937. [CrossRef] [PubMed]
17. Pinto-Sánchez, M.I.; Verdú, E.F. Non-coeliac gluten sensitivity: Are we closer to separating the wheat from the chaff? *Gut* **2016**. [CrossRef]
18. Junker, Y.; Zeissig, S.; Kim, S.-J.; Barisani, D.; Wieser, H.; Leffler, D.A.; Zevallos, V.; Libermann, T.A.; Dillon, S.; Freitag, T.L.; et al. Wheat amylase trypsin inhibitors drive intestinal inflammation via activation of toll-like receptor 4. *J. Exp. Med.* **2012**, *209*, 2395–2408. [CrossRef]
19. de Punder, K.; Pruimboom, L. The dietary intake of wheat and other cereal grains and their role in inflammation. *Nutrients* **2013**, *5*, 771–787. [CrossRef]
20. Tatham, A.S.; Shewry, P.R. Allergens to wheat and related cereals. *Clin. Exp. Allergy* **2008**, *38*, 1712–1726.
21. Pellegrina, C.D.; Perbellini, O.; Scupoli, M.T.; Tomelleri, C.; Zanetti, C.; Zoccatelli, G.; Fusi, M.; Peruffo, A.; Rizzi, C.; Chignola, R. Effects of wheat germ agglutinin on human gastrointestinal epithelium: Insights from an experimental model of immune/epithelial cell interaction. *Toxicol. Appl. Pharmacol.* **2009**, *237*, 146–153. [CrossRef] [PubMed]
22. Manning, L.P.; Biesiekierski, J.R. Use of dietary interventions for functional gastrointestinal disorders. *Curr. Opin. Pharmacol.* **2018**, *43*, 132–138. [CrossRef] [PubMed]
23. Roncoroni, L.; Bascuñán, K.A.; Doneda, L.; Scricciolo, A.; Lombardo, V.; Branchi, F.; Ferretti, F.; Dell'osso, B.; Montanari, V.; Bardella, M.T.; et al. A low FODMAP gluten-free diet improves functional gastrointestinal disorders and overall mental health of celiac disease patients: A randomized controlled trial. *Nutrients* **2018**, *10*, 8. [CrossRef]
24. Carroccio, A.; Mansueto, P.; Iacono, G.; Soresi, M.; D'Alcamo, A.; Cavataio, F.; Brusca, I.; Florena, A.M.; Ambrosiano, G.; Seidita, A.; et al. Non-celiac wheat sensitivity diagnosed by double-blind placebo-controlled challenge: Exploring a new clinical entity. *Am. J. Gastroenterol.* **2012**, *107*, 1898–1906, quiz 1907. [CrossRef] [PubMed]
25. Peters, S.L.; Biesiekierski, J.R.; Yelland, G.W.; Muir, J.G.; Gibson, P.R. Randomised clinical trial: Gluten may cause depression in subjects with non-coeliac gluten sensitivity—An exploratory clinical study. *Aliment. Pharmacol. Ther.* **2014**, *39*, 1104–1112. [CrossRef] [PubMed]
26. Zanini, B.; Basché, R.; Ferraresi, A.; Ricci, C.; Lanzarotto, F.; Marullo, M.; Villanacci, V.; Hidalgo, A.; Lanzini, A. Randomised clinical study: Gluten challenge induces symptom recurrence in only a minority of patients who meet clinical criteria for non-coeliac gluten sensitivity. *Aliment. Pharmacol. Ther.* **2015**, *42*, 968–976. [CrossRef]
27. Capannolo, A.; Viscido, A.; Barkad, M.A.; Valerii, G.; Ciccone, F.; Melideo, D.; Frieri, G.; Latella, G. Non-Celiac Gluten Sensitivity among Patients Perceiving Gluten-Related Symptoms. *Digestion* **2015**, *92*, 8–13. [CrossRef] [PubMed]
28. Rosinach, M.; Fernández-Bañares, F.; Carrasco, A.; Ibarra, M.; Temiño, R.; Salas, A.; Esteve, M. Double-Blind Randomized Clinical Trial: Gluten versus Placebo Rechallenge in Patients with Lymphocytic Enteritis and Suspected Celiac Disease. *PLoS ONE* **2016**, *11*, e0157879. [CrossRef] [PubMed]
29. Picarelli, A.; Borghini, R.; Di Tola, M.; Marino, M.; Urciuoli, C.; Isonne, C.; Puzzono, M.; Porowska, B.; Rumi, G.; Lonardi, S.; et al. Intestinal, systemic, and oral gluten-related alterations in patients with nonceliac gluten sensitivity. *J. Clin. Gastroenterol.* **2016**, *50*, 849–858. [CrossRef]

30. Elli, L.; Tomba, C.; Branchi, F.; Roncoroni, L.; Lombardo, V.; Bardella, M.T.; Ferretti, F.; Conte, D.; Valiante, F.; Fini, L.; et al. Evidence for the presence of non-celiac gluten sensitivity in patients with functional gastrointestinal symptoms: Results from a multicenter randomized double-blind placebo-controlled gluten challenge. *Nutrients* **2016**, *8*, 84. [CrossRef] [PubMed]
31. Skodje, G.I.; Sarna, V.K.; Minelle, I.H.; Rolfsen, K.L.; Muir, J.G.; Gibson, P.R.; Veierød, M.B.; Henriksen, C.; Lundin, K.E.A. Fructan, Rather Than Gluten, Induces Symptoms in Patients With Self-Reported Non-Celiac Gluten Sensitivity. *Gastroenterology* **2018**, *154*, 529–539.e2. [CrossRef] [PubMed]
32. Dale, H.F.; Hatlebakk, J.G.; Hovdenak, N.; Ystad, S.O.; Lied, G.A. The effect of a controlled gluten challenge in a group of patients with suspected non-coeliac gluten sensitivity: A randomized, double-blind placebo-controlled challenge. *Neurogastroenterol. Motil.* **2018**, e13332. [CrossRef] [PubMed]
33. Volta, U.; Caio, G.; Tovoli, F.; De Giorgio, R. Non-celiac gluten sensitivity: Questions still to be answered despite increasing awareness. *Cell. Mol. Immunol.* **2013**, *10*, 383. [CrossRef] [PubMed]
34. Drossman, D.A.; Dumitrascu, D.L. Rome III: New standard for functional gastrointestinal disorders. *J. Gastrointest. Liver Dis.* **2006**, *15*, 237–241.
35. Leffler, D.A.; Dennis, M.; Edwards George, J.B.; Jamma, S.; Magge, S.; Cook, E.F.; Schuppan, D.; Kelly, C.P. A Simple Validated Gluten-Free Diet Adherence Survey for Adults With Celiac Disease. *Clin. Gastroenterol. Hepatol.* **2009**, *7*, 530–536.e2. [CrossRef]
36. Schalk, K.; Lexhaller, B.; Koehler, P.; Scherf, K.A. Isolation and characterization of gluten protein types from wheat, rye, barley and oats for use as reference materials. *PLoS ONE* **2017**, *12*, e0172819. [CrossRef]
37. Ware, J.E.; Sherbourne, C.D. The MOS 36-item short-form health survey (SF-36). I. Conceptual framework and item selection. *Med. Care* **1992**, 473–483. [CrossRef]
38. Di Sabatino, A.; Volta, U.; Salvatore, C.; Biancheri, P.; Caio, G.; De Giorgio, R.; Di Stefano, M.; Corazza, G.R. Small Amounts of Gluten in Subjects With Suspected Nonceliac Gluten Sensitivity: A Randomized, Double-Blind, Placebo-Controlled, Cross-Over Trial. *Clin. Gastroenterol. Hepatol.* **2015**, *13*, 1604–1612.e3. [CrossRef]
39. Shahbazkhani, B.; Sadeghi, A.; Malekzadeh, R.; Khatavi, F.; Etemadi, M.; Kalantri, E.; Rostami-Nejad, M.; Rostami, K. Non-Celiac Gluten Sensitivity Has Narrowed the Spectrum of Irritable Bowel Syndrome: A Double-Blind Randomized Placebo-Controlled Trial. *Nutrients* **2015**, *7*, 4542–4554. [CrossRef]
40. Sanders, D.S.; Aziz, I. Editorial: Non-celiac wheat sensitivity: Separating the wheat from the chat! *Am. J. Gastroenterol.* **2012**, *107*, 1908–1912. [CrossRef]
41. Carroccio, A.; Rini, G.; Mansueto, P. Non-celiac wheat sensitivity is a more appropriate label than non-celiac gluten sensitivity. *Gastroenterology* **2014**, *146*, 320–321. [CrossRef] [PubMed]

nutrients

Article

Celiac Immunogenic Potential of α-Gliadin Epitope Variants from *Triticum* and *Aegilops* Species

Ángela Ruiz-Carnicer [1], Isabel Comino [1], Verónica Segura [1], Carmen V. Ozuna [2], María de Lourdes Moreno [1], Miguel Ángel López-Casado [3], María Isabel Torres [4], Francisco Barro [2] and Carolina Sousa [1,*]

1 Departamento de Microbiología y Parasitología, Facultad de Farmacia, Universidad de Sevilla, 41012 Sevilla, Spain; acarnicer@us.es (Á.R.-C.); icomino@us.es (I.C.); vsegura@us.es (V.S.); lmoreno@us.es (M.d.L.M.)
2 Departamento de Mejora Genética Vegetal, Instituto de Agricultura Sostenible (IAS-CSIC), 14004 Córdoba, Spain; carmen.ozuna@eez.csic.es (C.V.O.); fbarro@ias.csic.es (F.B.)
3 Departamento de Gastronterología pediátrica, Hospital Virgen de las Nieves, 18014 Granada, Spain; drlopezcasado@digestivointegral.es
4 Departamento de Biología Experimental, Campus Universitario Las Lagunillas, 23071 Jaén, Spain; mitorres@ujaen.es
* Correspondence: csoumar@us.es; Tel.: +34-954-556-452

Received: 28 December 2018; Accepted: 17 January 2019; Published: 22 January 2019

Abstract: The high global demand of wheat and its subsequent consumption arise from the physicochemical properties of bread dough and its contribution to the protein intake in the human diet. Gluten is the main structural complex of wheat proteins and subjects affected by celiac disease (CD) cannot tolerate gluten protein. Within gluten proteins, α-gliadins constitute the most immunogenic fraction since they contain the main T-cell stimulating epitopes (DQ2.5-glia-α1, DQ2.5-glia-α2, and DQ2.5-glia-α3). In this work, the celiac immunotoxic potential of α-gliadins was studied within Triticeae: diploid, tetraploid, and hexaploid species. The abundance and immunostimulatory capacity of CD canonical epitopes and variants (with one or two mismatches) in all α-gliadin sequences were determined. The results showed that the canonical epitopes DQ2.5-glia-α1 and DQ2.5-glia-α3 were more frequent than DQ2.5-glia-α2. A higher abundance of canonical DQ2.5-glia-α1 epitope was found to be associated with genomes of the BBAADD, AA, and DD types; however, the abundance of DQ2.5-glia-α3 epitope variants was very high in BBAADD and BBAA wheat despite their low abundance in the canonical epitope. The most abundant substitution was that of proline to serine, which was disposed mainly on the three canonical DQ2.5 domains on position 8. Interestingly, our results demonstrated that the natural introduction of Q to H at any position eliminates the toxicity of the three T-cell epitopes in the α-gliadins. The results provided a rational approach for the introduction of natural amino acid substitutions to eliminate the toxicity of three T-cell epitopes, while maintaining the technological properties of commercial wheats.

Keywords: celiac disease; α-gliadin; 33-mer; DQ2.5-glia-α1; DQ2.5-glia-α2; DQ2.5-glia-α3 epitopes; wheat species

1. Introduction

Wheat is one of the most widely cultivated cereals in the world and constitutes a major source of energy, protein, and fiber in the diet. Increasing global demand for wheat and its subsequent consumption, with an annual production of about 750 million tons, is due to its unique viscoelastic properties for its inclusion in food products and to industrialization and westernization [1–3]. The wheat group has evolved through allopolyploidization, that is, through hybridization between species from the genera *Aegilops* and *Triticum* followed by genome doubling [4]. Genetic studies have provided valuable information regarding which wild cereal species are the relatives of modern domesticated cereals, and which geographical wild plant produced the domesticated forms that are used in food production today [5]. The diploid wild wheat that was first domesticated is thought to have been *Triticum monococcum* (A^mA^m), which is still growing in some parts of the world both for animal feed and human consumption. Wheats with more than one genome are known as polyploid wheats. The AA genome of the tetraploid wheats is closely similar to that of *T. urartu*, and the BB genome is related to *Aegilops speltoides* (BB). The wild tetraploid, formed after the hybridization, was designated as *Triticum turgidum* ssp. *dicoccoides* (wild emmer; BBAA), and the first domesticated tetraploid was *T. turgidum* ssp. *dicoccum* (cultivated emmer; BBAA), from which, the cultivated *T. turgidum* ssp. *durum* has evolved. The hexaploid wheat, *Triticum aestivum* ssp. *aestivum* (BBAADD), consists of three genomes designated A, B, and D. The A and B genomes of hexaploid wheats come from the A and B genomes of tetraploid wheat. The hexaploid wheats resulted from the hybridization of cultivated emmer and a wild grass species identified as *Aegilops tauschii* (DD), followed by polyploid formation which gave rise to a new species that has three genomes designated BBAADD [6,7]. The main wheat species grown throughout the world is the hexaploid *T. aestivum*, usually called "common" or "bread" wheat. In terms of total production, the next variety in importance is the tetraploid durum or macaroni wheat (*T. turgidum* L. subsp. *durum* Desf.). This is adapted to hot dry climates and is widely used for the production of pasta. Common wheat species account for nearly 94% of the total production, with durum wheat representing 5%, and other wheat forms about 1% [6,8].

Although wheat has always been recognized as a fundamental food, this cereal cannot be tolerated by certain individuals since it is responsible for significant pathologies, called gluten-related disorders, such as celiac disease (CD), wheat allergy, non-celiac gluten sensitivity, gluten ataxia, and dermatitis herpetiformis [9]. CD is an immune-mediated systemic disorder elicited by the ingestion of gluten in genetically susceptible individuals. It affects around 1% of the global population and is based on a variable combination of intestinal and extra-intestinal signs and symptoms, celiac specific antibodies, HLA-DQ2/8 haplotypes, and enteropathy [9–11]. Gluten proteins are rich in proline and glutamine residues, which make them resistant to being fully digested in the gastrointestinal track. Partial digestion of gluten generates small peptides that provoke autoimmune disorders in celiac people. The most accepted model for explaining CD immunopathogenesis is the two-signal model [12] characterized by a first innate immune response followed by a secondary antigen-specific adaptive response. According to this model, certain peptides, such as the 19-mer gliadin peptide, trigger an innate immune response [13] mainly characterized by the production of interleukin 15 (IL-15) by epithelial cells. The result is the disruption of the epithelial barrier by increasing the permeability and inducing enterocyte apoptosis [14]. As a consequence, the immune-adaptive peptides, like the 33-mer, can now reach the lamina propria where they are deaminated by the tissue transglutaminase (tTG2). Such deamidation provides a negative charge to gliadin peptides and hence enhances their affinity to bind within the HLA-DQ2/8 bound, which is also the 'susceptibility gene' in CD, expressed on the surface of dendritic cells (DCs) [15–17]. DCs are therefore central in CD pathogenesis since they present a gluten antigen to T cells, [18] thereby driving progression of the pro-inflammatory antigen-specific adaptive immune response, which will turn into the symptomatology of the disease.

Gluten is a complex mixture of storage proteins of cereals such as wheat, rye, barley, oats, and their hybrid derivatives. Gluten proteins have been classified according to their solubility [19]. In wheat, these proteins are defined as gliadins (soluble in 60–70% ethanol) and glutenins (only soluble under stronger conditions, i.e. acids, reducing agents and detergents, urea, etc.) [20]. According to their electrophoretic mobilities, gliadins are divided into three groups: α- and β-gliadins, γ-gliadins, and ω-gliadins [19], while the glutenins are divided into the high molecular weight (HMW) and the low molecular weight (LMW) glutenin subunits (GSs) [21,22]. Among the gliadins, the α-gliadins have the strongest immunogenicity [23], and four T-cell stimulatory epitopes have been identified as being responsible for eliciting the immunogenicity of α-gliadin. Two of these are the major epitopes and they are present in the 33-mer peptide, which is the main contributor to the immunogenicity of the gluten [24] and contains six copies of these two overlapping T-cell epitopes: three copies of the DQ2.5-glia-α1 and three copies of the DQ2.5-glia-α2. The other two T-cell stimulatory epitopes are minor epitopes: DQ2.5-glia-α3 and DQ8-glia-α1 [24–27]. However, natural substitutions of these canonical epitopes could also contribute to the toxicity of wheat [28], and it could suggest that the total CD immunogenicity of gluten protein is a result of the canonical epitopes and their variants, some of which are more abundant than the canonical epitopes themselves. Gluten can have different immunogenic potential sequences whose proportions in each species are also variable. For this reason, it is important to study the amino acid substitutions in the variants of these epitopes; interestingly, these variants could increase, reduce, or suppress the CD response.

In earlier work, next-generation sequencing and Sanger sequencing of α-gliadins from diploid and polyploid wheats provided six types of α-gliadins with major differences in their frequencies. The canonical CD epitopes and their variants were identified in the different types of α-gliadins [29]. In the present study, we used the sequence data with one or two mismatches and canonical epitopes obtained in Ozuna et al. [29], and we have built upon the previous research by exploring the abundance of different DQ2.5-glia-α1, DQ2.5-glia-α2, and DQ2.5-glia-α3 epitope variants per species in diploid and polyploid wheats. Moreover, the immunogenic potential of these epitope variants in wheat species was studied by testing their binding capacity to anti-33-mer monoclonal antibodies (moAbs) [30,31] and to induce T-cell proliferation. The anti-33-mer antibodies were able to detect the presence of gliadin 33-mer related epitopes in prolamins from wheat, barley, rye, and various oats varieties as well as in food samples and human samples to monitor gluten free diet (GFD) compliance and transgressions [32]. Our study showed that the canonical epitopes DQ2.5-glia-α1 and DQ2.5-glia-α3 were more frequent than DQ2.5-glia-α2. The most abundant natural modification was found in the DQ2.5-glia-α3 domain in all the sequences studied. However, this variant decreased its immunogenicity with respect to the canonical epitope. On the other hand, one of the most representative variants of DQ2.5-glia-α2 (40%) showed an immunogenicity equivalent to the canonical epitope. Our results provide a rational approach for the introduction or selection of natural amino acid substitutions to eliminate the toxicity of three α-gliadin T-cell epitopes, while keeping the technological properties of the commercial wheats.

2. Materials and Methods

2.1. Catalogue and Abundance of CD Epitopes from Diploid, Tetraploid, and Hexaploid Wheat Varieties

Canonical epitopes DQ2.5-glia-α1 (PF/YPQPQLPY), DQ2.5-glia-α2 (PQPQLPYPQ), and DQ2.5-glia-α3 (FRPQQPYPQ) and variants with one or two mismatches provided by Ozuna et al. [29] were obtained from diploid, tetraploid, and hexaploid wheats (Figure 1).

The frequency/abundance of each peptide in the sequences of the different wheats was studied *in silico*. The abundance of each epitope was calculated by multiplying the total number of epitopes found in a given gene by the frequency of that gene in the genome.

These canonical CD epitopes and their most representative variants with one or two mismatches were synthesized as deaminated and non-deaminated 9-mer peptides. The peptides were supplied by Biomedal S.L. (Seville, Spain).

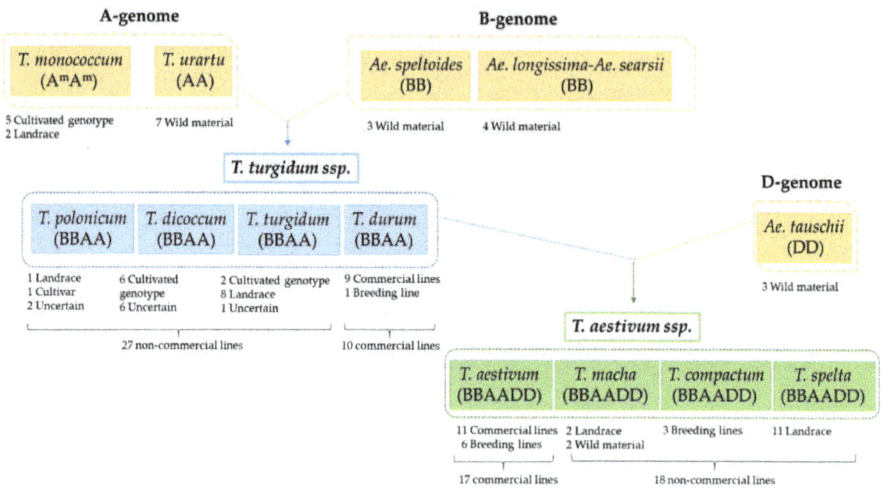

Figure 1. Schematic representation of 96 accessions from *Triticum* and *Aegilops* sp. showing their origin and breeding status. In total, there are thirty-five accessions of hexaploid wheats, thirty-seven accessions of tetraploid wheats, and twenty-four accessions of diploid wheats. AA, BB, and DD: diploids; BBAA: tetraploids; BBAADD: hexaploids (partially adapted from Ozuna and Barro) [3].

2.2. Enzyme-Linked Immunosorbent Assay (ELISA)

Maxisorp microtitre plates (Nunc, Roskilde, Denmark) were coated with gliadin solution (Sigma, St Louis, MO, USA) and incubated overnight at 4 °C. The plates were washed with phosphate-buffered saline (PBS) containing 0.05% Tween 20 and blocked with PBS-bovine serum albumin (BSA) 3% for 1 h at room temperature (RT), and 33-mer peptide was used as standard. Serial dilutions of peptides were made, to each of which horseradish peroxidase (HRP)-conjugate with anti-33-mer antibody (moAb) was added [32]. The samples were pre-incubated at RT for 1 h and then added to the wells. After 1 h of incubation at RT, the plates were washed and substrate solution (TMB, Sigma) was added. The reaction was stopped at 15 min with 1 M sulfuric acid and the absorbance at 450 nm was measured (microplate reader UVM340; Asys Hitech GmbH, Eugendorf, Austria). Two separate assays were performed, each with two repetitions.

2.3. Peripheral Blood Mononuclear Cells (PBMCs) and Cell Cultures

Peripheral blood mononuclear cells from 18 child patients with active CD on a gluten-containing diet were isolated from 6 mL of heparinized blood by Histopaque gradient centrifugation and cultured at a density of 1×10^6 cells per milliliter in 96-multiwell culture plates in RPMI-1640 culture medium (Sigma-Aldrich) supplemented with 10% fetal bovine serum (GIBCO-Invitrogen Ltd), 1% penicillin-streptomycin, and 0.1% gentamicin (Sigma-Aldrich). After 48 h, PBMCs were incubated with different peptides (50 μg/mL). After 48 h of stimulation, the free supernatants were collected and stored at −80 °C until the interferon gamma (IFN-γ) analyses were carried out.

2.4. Cell Proliferation Analysis

T-cell proliferation was determined after 48 h of incubation using the ELISA 5-bromo-2-deoxyuridine (BrdU) cell proliferation test (Millipore Chemicon, Temecula, California, USA). The stimulation index (SI) value was calculated by dividing the mean absorbance at 450 nm after stimulation by the mean absorbance of T cells exposed to the culture medium alone (negative control).

2.5. IFN-γ Production

Supernatants from the PBMC culture were collected after 48 h and stored at 80 °C for IFN- γ determination using a commercial ELISA kit in accordance with the manufacturer's instructions (Thermo Scientific, Madrid, Spain). Standards were run on each plate. The sensitivity of the assay was <2 pg/mL.

2.6. Statistical Analysis of T Cells and IFN-γ Assays

Each experiment was carried out in duplicate on separate days. The data is expressed as mean and *SD*. All statistical analyses were performed with the STATGRAPHICS Centurion XVI program. The analysis of variance (ANOVA), followed by the Tukey test for mean multiple comparison, was used. In this study, p values lower than 0.05 ($p < 0.05$) were considered significant.

3. Results and Discussion

3.1. Relative Abundance of DQ2.5-Glia-α1, DQ2.5-Glia-α2, and DQ2.5-Glia-α3 Domains and Their Variants in Triticum and Aegilops Species

The complete repertoire of peptides involved in the pathogenesis of CD remains a daunting task due to the great heterogeneity of gluten proteins [23,26]. Several studies have demonstrated that peptides derived from α-gliadins induce the strongest T-cell responses in the vast majority of patients [23,33–35]. The α-gliadins can have different sequences and their proportions in each species are also variable. In the present study, we have explored the abundance of different DQ2.5-glia-α1, DQ2.5-glia-α2, and DQ2.5-glia-α3 variants in 96 genotypes from diploid and polyploid wheats. Among these genotypes, 27 accessions were commercial lines and 69 were non-commercial lines (Figure 1).

The DQ2.5-glia-α epitopes are located in the 33-mer region of α-gliadins (Figure 2a). Although seventy-eight variants were found for these three canonical epitopes across the Triticeae species [29], only the most representative variants (covered by >80 reads), encompassing one or two mismatches, were used for this study; of which 9 variants were from DQ2.5-glia-α1, 10 from DQ2.5-glia-α2, and 14 from DQ2.5-glia-α3 (Figure 2b).

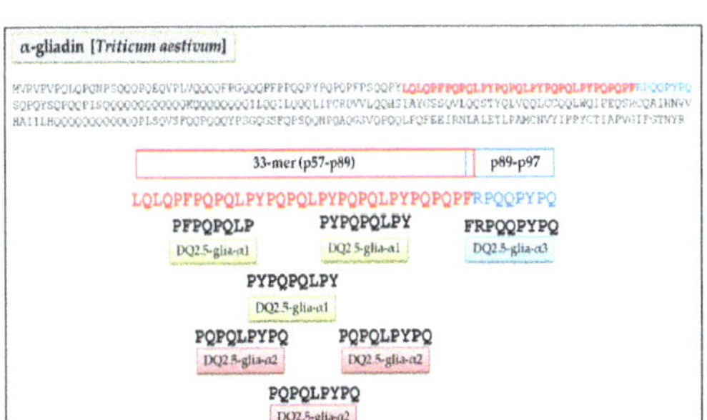

(a)

Canonical epitope	DQ2.5-glia-α1	DQ2.5-glia-α2	DQ2.5-glia-α3
	PFPQPQLPY Y	PQPQLPYPQ	FRPQQPYPQ
Mismatch	**CD epitope variants**		
One mismatch	PFPQLQLPY	PQPQLPYSQ	FPPQQPYPQ
	PFLQPQLPY	PQPHLPYPQ	FSPQQPYPQ
	PFPQPQLSY	PQLQLPYPQ	FRPQQSYPQ
	PFSQPQLPY	PQPQLPYPH	FLPQQPYPQ
	PYPQPHLPY	PQPQLPYLQ	FQPQQPYPQ
	PYPHPQLPY	PQPQLLYPQ	FRPQQPQPQ
	PYPQPQLLY		FRPQQPYLQ
			FRQQQPYPQ
Two mismatches	PFPQLQQPY	PQPQPQYPQ	FLPQLPYPQ
	PYPQPQLFP	LQPQLPYSQ	FPPQQSYPQ
		SQPQLPYSQ	FPPQLPYPQ
		PQPQLPHSQ	FPSQQPYPQ
			FPAQQPYPQ
			FPPQQPYPH

(b)

Figure 2. Celiac disease (CD) epitopes and variants derived from α-gliadin. (**a**) Location of canonical epitopes DQ-2.5-glia-α1, DQ-2.5-glia-α2, and DQ-2.5-glia-α3 into α-gliadin protein. (**b**) Variants of the canonical CD epitopes with one or two mismatches selected with more than 80 reads found in *Triticum* and *Aegilops* ssp. The mismatches are indicated in red.

In view of the total abundance of the different canonical epitopes, DQ2.5-glia-α1 and DQ2.5-glia-α3 were more abundant than DQ2.5-glia-α2 ($p < 0.05$, Figure 3). There were no significant differences between the abundance of DQ2.5-glia-α1 and DQ2.5-glia-α3, however, we found higher variability of the DQ2.5-glia-α1 canonical epitope in hexaploid wheats, since its abundance fluctuated widely depending on the different hexaploid species, while it remained evenly distributed in the DQ2.5-glia-α3 canonical epitope (p = 0.02, Figure 3).

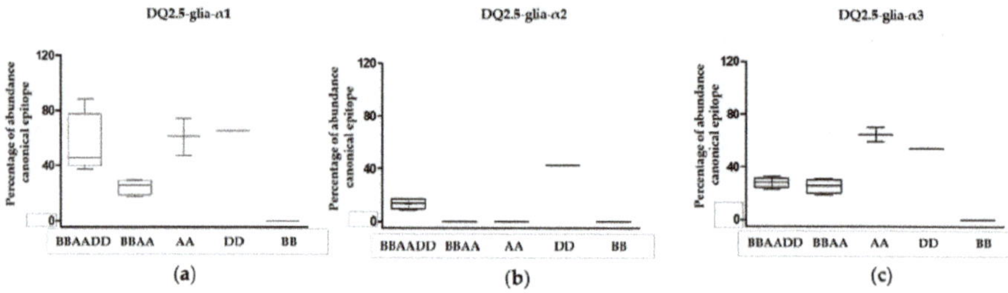

Figure 3. Abundance of CD canonical epitope and variants per wheat genome type. (**a**) Abundance of the canonical epitope DQ2.5-glia-α1 and variants, (**b**) abundance of the canonical DQ2.5-glia-α2 epitope and variants, and (**c**) abundance of the canonical DQ2.5-glia-α3 epitope and variants. BBAADD: hexaploid genome; BBAA: tetraploid genome; AA, DD, and BB: diploid genomes.

Figure 4 shows the abundance of CD canonical epitopes and variants per species. The percentage of DQ2.5-glia-α1 canonical epitope with respect to variants was 80%. This epitope was present in all wheat genomes with the exception of BB diploids. The highest abundance was found in *T. compactum*, *T. monococcum*, and *Ae. tauschii*. The most abundant variant (range from 0.1% to 20%) was $P_1Y_2P_3Q_4P_5Q_6L_7\underline{\mathbf{F_8P_9}}$ with two mismatches (P to F at p8 and Y to P at p9). This variant was present in all wheat genomes with the exception of BB and DD diploids. The next most abundant variant was the substitution of P to L at p5, but this variant was present in only BBAA and BB genomes (Figure 5).

The percentage of DQ2.5-glia-α2 canonical epitope with respect to the different variants of this epitope was 14%, and this epitope was only present in hexaploids BBAADD and DD diploids. This finding may indicate that this epitope came from *Ae. tauschii*, the donor of the D genome to bread wheat. The DQ2.5-glia-α2 variants $P_1Q_2P_3Q_4L_5P_6Y_7\underline{\mathbf{S_8}}Q_9$ and $P_1Q_2P_3Q_4\underline{\mathbf{P_5Q_6}}Y_7P_8Q_9$ were the most frequent (80%). The highest abundance score (range from 46% to 74%) of $P_1Q_2P_3Q_4L_5P_6Y_7\underline{\mathbf{S_8}}Q_9$ (P to S substitution at p8) occurred in AA diploids and was absent from DD and BB diploid genomes. In contrast, $P_1Q_2P_3Q_4\underline{\mathbf{P_5Q_6}}Y_7P_8Q_9$ (L to P at p5 and P to Q at p6), with two mismatches, presented high abundance in all genomes, with the exception of *T. monococcum* (A^mA^m diploid) (Figures 4 and 5).

Regarding the DQ2.5-glia-α3, the epitope variant $F_1\underline{\mathbf{P_2}}P_3Q_4Q_5P_6Y_7P_8Q_9$ (with R to P substitution at p2) was the most frequent, with an abundance greater than 75% across all species, except in *Triticum polonicum* (BBAA) and *Triticum urartu* (A^uA^u), with abundances of 67.9% and 42.2%, respectively. The second and third most frequent variants, $F_1\underline{\mathbf{L_2}}P_3Q_4\underline{\mathbf{L_5}}P_6Y_7P_8Q_9$ (R to L at p2 and Q to L at p5) and $F_1\underline{\mathbf{P_2}}P_3Q_4Q_5\underline{\mathbf{S_6}}Y_7P_8Q_9$ (R to P at p2 and P to S at p6), had two mismatches and were absent in AA and DD diploid genomes, which could indicate that the BB genome is the origin of this variant in the polyploid varieties; in fact, the abundance of this epitope variant in the remaining genomes was very similar (≈20%) (Figures 4 and 5).

The process of hybridization between *Ae. tauschii* and *T. dicoccum* provided the DD genome, and new gluten gene combinations, to hexaploid wheats, thereby considerably improving their bread baking properties compared to that of tetraploid wheats, particularly the HMW-glutenin subunits [36]. However, the DD genome also encodes for gliadins that have been reported as highly immunogenic, as the DD genome has the highest number of potential immunogenic α-gliadin peptides [37], while those from the BB genome contribute the least [38,39]. We found that the three canonical epitopes are present in the DD genome, with a representation ranging from 43% to 65%. In hexaploids (BBAADD), all canonical epitopes are also present, but in a smaller proportion (<40%) than the DD genome. In contrast, in the AA genome, only DQ2.5-glia-α1 and DQ2.5-glia-α3 are present, and the BB genome is not represented by any of the canonical epitopes.

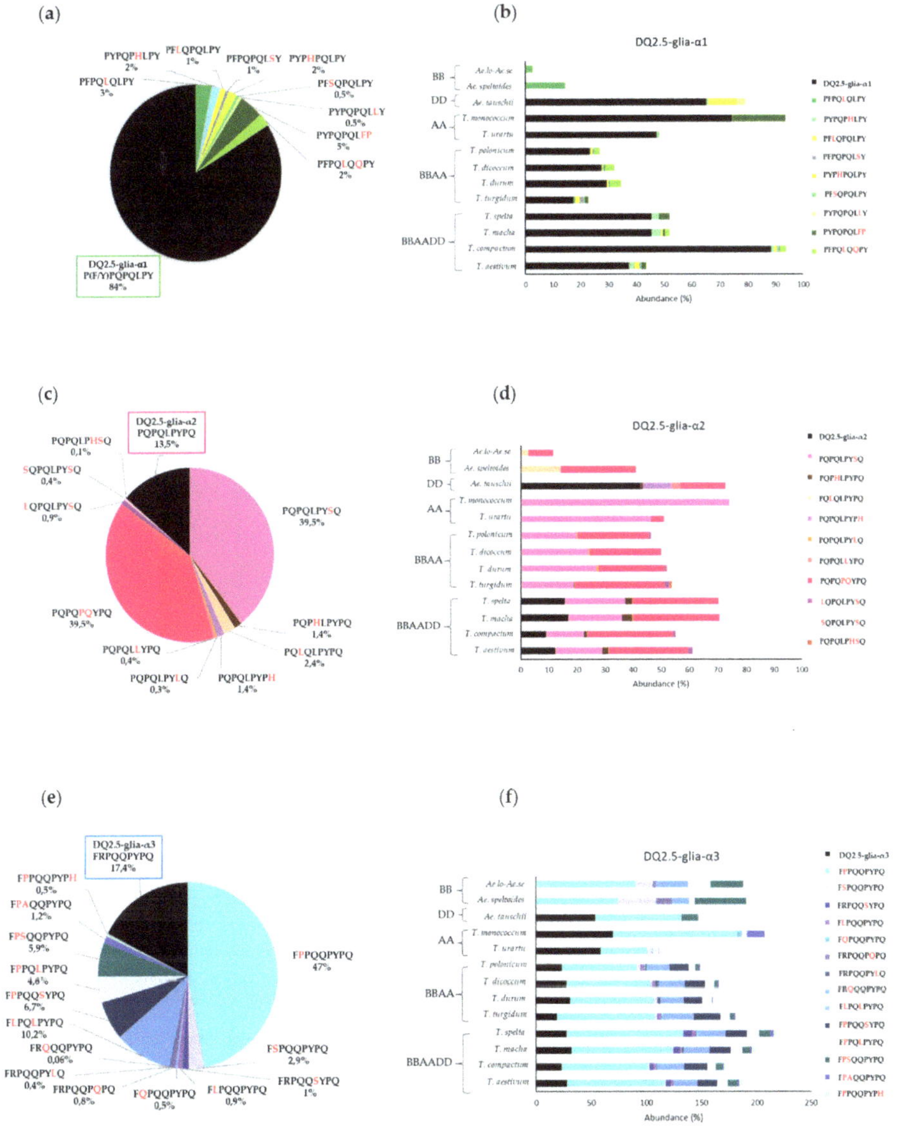

Figure 4. Abundance of CD canonical epitopes and variants per wheat species. (**a**) Abundance in the DQ2.5-glia-α1 epitope variants, (**b**) abundance in DQ2.5-glia-α1 epitope variants by species, (**c**) abundance in DQ2.5-glia-α2 epitope variants, (**d**) abundance in DQ2.5-glia-α2 epitope variants by species, (**e**) abundance in DQ2.5-glia-α3 epitope variants, and (**f**) abundance in DQ2.5-glia-α2 epitope variants by species.

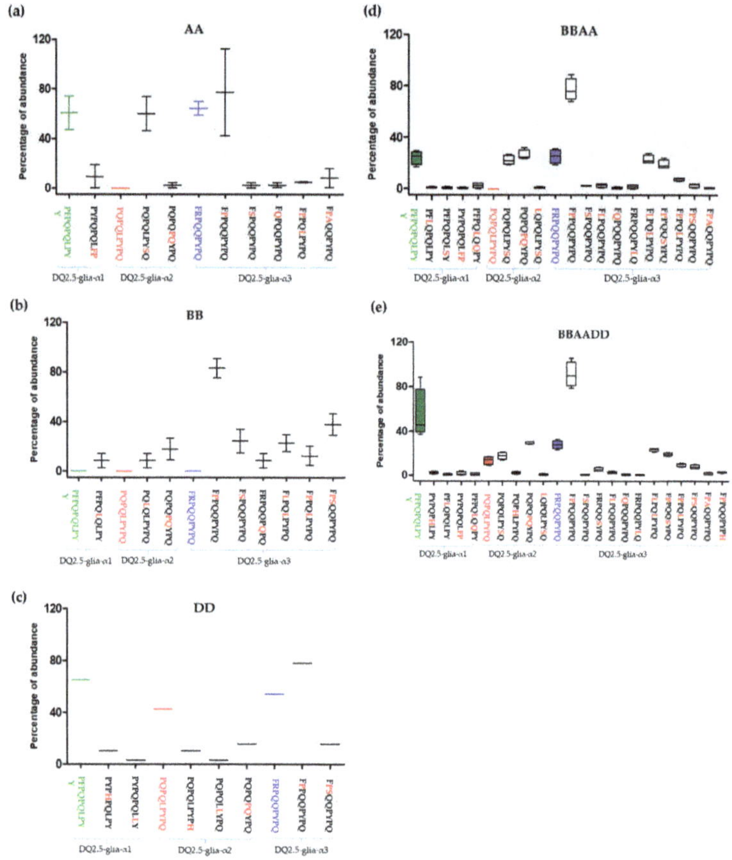

Figure 5. Abundance of epitope variants according to wheat genome type. The epitopes represented showed more than 1% of abundance in each gliadin domain. (**a**) AA genome, (**b**) BB genome, (**c**) DD genome, (**d**) BBAA genome, and (**e**) BBAADD genome. DQ2.5-glia-α1 epitope: green; DQ2.5-glia-α2 epitope: red; DQ2.5-glia-α3 epitope: blue.

3.2. Anti-33-mer MoAb Binding Capacity and T-cell Stimulatory of DQ2.5-α-Gliadin-Derived Peptides

Several of the amino acid variants that we found in the α-gliadin epitope sequences had never been described previously, while a number had been described but had never been tested for their immunogenic and stimulatory capacities. In order to determine which variants are capable of inducing a CD stimulatory response, the variants from DQ2.5-glia-α epitopes were synthesized as native and deaminated peptides and tested for their capacity to bind to anti-33-mer monoclonal antibodies (moAbs) and to induce T-cell proliferation, respectively (Figure 6). The latter was confirmed with gamma interferon assays (IFN-γ). The positioning of deamidated glutamine residues is strongly related to the positioning of proline residues, which is particularly strict in the case of DQ2.5 epitopes (but not DQ8 epitopes), as DQ2.5 only accepts proline at a certain position in the peptide binding groove [26,40]. The capacity of DQ2.5-glia-α epitopes to trigger proliferation of T cells was tested in deaminated peptides, deamidation of glutamine (Q) at p6 in DQ2.5-glia-α1 domain, p4 in DQ2.5-glia-α2 domain, and p4 in DQ2.5-glia-α3 domain.

The DQ2.5-glia-α1 and DQ2.5-glia-α2 epitopes were regarded as major CD epitopes, as they are recognized by most of CD patients [41]. The anti-33-mer moAbs reacted strongly with the canonical DQ2.5-glia-α1 epitope $P_1\{F/Y\}_2P_3Q_4P_5Q_6L_7P_8Y_9$. In comparison with the canonical CD epitope, the variants $P_1F_2\underline{\mathbf{L_3}}Q_4P_5Q_6L_7P_8Y_9$ (proline (P) to leucine (L) substitution at p3) and $P_1F_2\underline{\mathbf{S_3}}Q_4P_5Q_6L_7P_8Y_9$ (P to serine (S) substitution at p3) showed a cross-reactivity (CR) of 37.7% and 55.4%, respectively. With regard to studies of PBMCs in DQ2.5-glia-α1 variants, the single substitution P to S at p3 maintained similar stimulation capacity to that of the canonical epitope, although it was not abundant (0.2% to 0.8%) in wheat species. Similarly, the variant with P to L substitution at p3 was very low in abundance (0.1% to 1.6%) and was found in all the polyploid species except for *T. spelta,* while in diploids it was only found in species with the AA genome. However, substitutions of Q to histidine (H) at p4 and p6, respectively, abolished the stimulatory capacity of this epitope, probably because it provides a positive charge or via its influence in the deamidation at p6, as previously observed by Schumann et al. [42]. Moreover, P to L at p8, or two substitutions, also abolished the stimulatory capacity and showed no affinity for the moAbs (Figure 6a).

As indicated in Figure 6b, the variant $P_1Q_2P_3Q_4L_5P_6Y_7\underline{\mathbf{S_8}}Q_9$ (P to S substitution at p8) showed an anti-33-mer binding capacity and PBMC stimulation similar to that of the DQ2.5-glia-α2 canonical CD epitope. This common variant was found in polyploid and diploid species with AA genome, but was not found in BB and DD genomes. Those peptides with two mismatches, such as $P_1Q_2P_3Q_4\underline{\mathbf{P_5Q_6}}Y_7P_8Q_9$ (substitutions L to P at p5 and P to Q at p6), $\underline{\mathbf{L_1}}Q_2P_3Q_4L_5P_6Y_7\underline{\mathbf{S_8}}Q_9$ (substitutions P to L at p1 and P to S at p8), $\underline{\mathbf{S_1}}Q_2P_3Q_4L_5P_6Y_7\underline{\mathbf{S_8}}Q_9$ (substitutions P to S at p1 and p8), and $P_1Q_2P_3Q_4L_5P_6\underline{\mathbf{H_7S_8}}Q_9$ (substitutions tyrosine (Y) to H at p7, and P to S at p8) showed a CR of 30–40% with respect to the canonical CD epitope and a stimulation index (SI) from 13 to 23 for PBMC stimulation. In contrast, the replacement of P to L at p3, p6, or p8 showed no reactivity with the moAbs. Among all of these variants, $P_1Q_2P_3Q_4L_5P_6Y_7\underline{\mathbf{S_8}}Q_9$ and $P_1Q_2P_3Q_4\underline{\mathbf{P_5Q_6}}Y_7P_8Q_9$ were the most frequent variants of the DQ2.5-glia-α2. The modification of P to S at p8 showed high stimulation with the moAbs and PBMCs, however, two mismatches of L to P at p5 and P to Q at p6 in the same sequence caused a threefold decrease in the immunogenicity of the DQ2.5-glia-α2 canonical epitope. This change is abundant in the BBAA genome, especially in the *T. turgidum* species.

Proliferation assays for PBMC with the canonical DQ2.5-glia-α3 epitope $F_1R_2P_3E_4Q_5P_6Y_7P_8Q_9$ were tested with E on p4 by tTG2-deamidation of the original Q. Several peptides released an increased stimulatory effect on T cells, such as the DQ2.5-glia-α3 variant $F_1\underline{\mathbf{L_2}}P_3Q_4\underline{\mathbf{L_5}}P_6Y_7P_8Q_9$ with two mismatches. However, other variants for this epitope, with several amino acid substitutions, had no stimulatory effect on T cells, including P to S substitution at p6, Y to Q at p7, P to Q at p3, and two substitutions of arginine (R) to P at p2 and Q to H at p9 and R to P at p2 and P to A at p3 (Figure 6c). The replacement of R to L at p2 and Q to L at p5 in the variant $F_1\underline{\mathbf{L_2}}P_3Q_4\underline{\mathbf{L_5}}P_6Y_7P_8Q_9$ gave it greater stimulation capacity, given that this variant was highly abundant for the DQ2.5-glia-α3 epitope, it was found in all the polyploid species and in the BB diploid genome. However, the non-abundant variant $F_1\underline{\mathbf{P_2}}P_3Q_4\underline{\mathbf{L_5}}P_6Y_7P_8Q_9$ with the change of R to P at p2 and Q to L at p5 increased both the binding of the moAbs and stimulation with T cells. The variant $F_1R_2P_3Q_4L_5P_6Y_7\underline{\mathbf{L_8}}Q_9$ with one mismatch (P to L at p8) showed T-cell stimulatory capacity and moAb binding, but was low in abundance (0.6% to 2.5%). Nevertheless, one of the most abundant variants, $F_1\underline{\mathbf{S_2}}P_3Q_4Q_5P_6Y_7P_8Q_9$, showed no T-cell stimulatory capacity and binding of the moAb and was found in the BB diploid genome.

According to the model of HLA-DQ2, the key amino acid residues for DQ2 binding lie at positions 1, 7, and 9, with preferential residues at positions 4 and 6 [43,44]. On the other hand, Elli et al. [45] found that substitutions at positions 2, 3, 5, and 8 also profoundly affected T-cell stimulation, indicating that these residues may all interact with the T-cell receptor (TCR). Our findings showed that the change at position 2 affected T-cell stimulation in the domain DQ2.5-glia-α1, at p8 in the DQ2.5-glia-α2 domain. In addition, the changes at positions 2, 5, and 8 in the DQ2.5-glia-α3 domain profoundly affected T-cell stimulation. Our results now provide new insights into an alternative approach, since we have showed that, by introducing specific amino acid substitutions, such as Q to H, at any position, the toxicity of the three T-cell α-gliadin epitopes could be eliminated. As such, the high level of variation influencing the immunogenicity of the major CD epitopes may offer possibilities to generate new wheat lines with reduced CD-immunogenicity, which may be potentially used as starting points for the breeding of safe wheats.

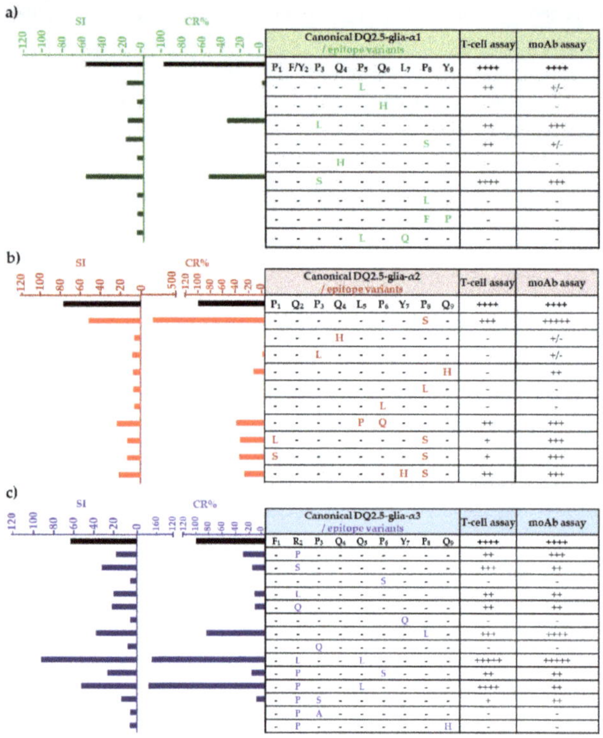

Figure 6. T-cell proliferation and anti-33-mer binding capacity of DQ2.5-glia-α1, DQ2.5-glia-α2, and DQ2.5-glia-α3 epitope variants and canonical epitope. (**a**) DQ-2.5-glia-α1 epitope and variants, (**b**) DQ-2.5-glia-α2 epitope and variants, and (**c**) DQ-2.5-glia-α3 epitope and variants. Variants and the canonical epitope were synthesized as deaminated 9-mer peptides to peripheral blood mononuclear cell (PBMC) assay. Proliferative responses of T cells were defined as a stimulation index (SI), which means the specific proliferation of a sample divided by the background proliferation ([PBMC + peptide]/[PBMC]). Glutamate residues (E) that would be formed by TG2-mediated deamination, which are important for recognition by T cells, are shown in italics. For the T-cell assay, the responses are represented relative to the maximum response given by the CD canonical epitope indicated by ++++. Therefore, - corresponds with 15%; + corresponds with 15–25%; ++ corresponds with 25–50%; +++ corresponds with 50–75%; ++++ corresponds with 75–100%; and +++++ corresponds with >100%. For the monoclonal antibody (moAb) assay, the amount of antigen detected is represented relative to the maximum amount (mol/L) detected in a given assay by the CD canonical epitope indicated by ++++. Therefore, - corresponds with 0%; +/- corresponds with < 5%; + corresponds with 5–10%; ++ corresponds with 10–30%; +++ corresponds to 30–60%; ++++ corresponds to 60–100%; and +++++corresponds to > 100%. CR; cross-reactivity, was calculated as follows: (IC50 of the antigen for which the moAb was raised/IC50 of each antigen assayed) × 100. The IC50 is defined as the concentration of the line that reduces the peak absorbance by 50% in the assay. Each of the letters represents the amino acid substitution of the variants.

4. Conclusions

The results presented here about CD DQ2.5 epitopes provide the basis for the introduction and/or selection of natural amino acid substitutions to eliminate the toxicity of the α-gliadin T-cell epitopes. Our findings show that the most abundant epitope in the DQ2.5-glia-α1 domain is the CD canonical epitope. Considering the DQ2.5-glia-α2 domain, the variants $P_1Q_2P_3Q_4L_5P_6Y_7\underline{\mathbf{S_8}}Q_9$ and $P_1Q_2P_3Q_4\underline{\mathbf{P_5Q_6}}Y_7P_8Q_9$ are the most abundant in this domain, while $F_1\underline{\mathbf{P_2}}P_3Q_4Q_5P_6Y_7P_8Q_9$ is the most abundant in the DQ2.5-glia-α3 domain. Moreover, the $F_1\underline{\mathbf{P_2}}P_3Q_4Q_5P_6Y_7P_8Q_9$ variant was also the most frequent of all the sequences studied. Our data indicate that the changes of P to S and R to P may be the most representative changes and the natural introduction of Q to H at any position eliminates the toxicity of the three T-cell epitopes. These results may offer possibilities to generate wheat varieties with a reduced CD-immunogenicity. Such varieties would help to reduce the presence of immunogenic CD epitopes in wheat flour and, while not safe for consumption by patients, might help to prevent the onset of CD in people that carry genetic risk factors. Overall, the more the scientific community knows about immunogenicity of the gliadins, the closer an alternative therapy besides GFDwill be achieved.

Author Contributions: Conceptualization, Á.R.-C., F.B., and C.S.; Data curation, Á.R.-C., C.V.O., and M.I.T.; Formal analysis, Á.R.-C., C.V.O., and M.I.T.; Investigation, Á.R.-C., I.C., V.S., M.d.L.M., C.V.O., M.Á.L.-C., M.I.T., F.B., and C.S.; Methodology, Á.R.-C., C.V.O., M.I.T., F.B., and C.S.; Resources, C.V.O., F.B., and C.S.; Writing—original draft, Á.R.-C., I.C., V.S., M.d.L.M., C.V.O., M.Á.L.-C., M.I.T., F.B., and C.S.; Writing—review & editing, Á.R.-C., I.C., V.S., M.d.L.M., C.V.O., M.Á.L.-C., M.I.T., F.B., and C.S.

Funding: The Spanish Ministry of Economy and Competitiveness (project AGL2013-48946-C) supported this work.

Acknowledgments: The Spanish Ministry of Economy and Competitiveness supported this work.

Conflicts of Interest: The authors declare no conflict of interest. None of the authors has any conflict of interest that could affect the performance of the work or the interpretation of the data.

References

1. Shewry, P.R.; Hey, S.J. The contribution of wheat to human diet and health. *Food Energy Secur.* **2015**, *4*, 178–202. [CrossRef] [PubMed]
2. Food and Agriculture Organization of the United Nations. Available online: http://faostat3.fao.org (accessed on 15 October 2018).
3. Ozuna, C.V.; Barro, F. Characterization of gluten proteins and celiac disease-related immunogenic epitopes in the Triticeae: Cereal domestication and breeding contributed to decrease the content of gliadins and gluten. *Mol. Breed.* **2018**, *38*, 22. [CrossRef]
4. Feldman, M.; Levy, A.A. Genome evolution due to allopolyploidization in wheat. *Genetics* **2012**, *192*, 763–774. [CrossRef] [PubMed]
5. López-Merino, L.; Leroy, S.A.G.; Haldorsen, S.; Heun, M.; Reynolds, A. Can *Triticum urartu* (Poaceae) be identified by pollen analysis? Implications for detecting the ancestor of the extinct two-grained einkorn-like wheat. *Bot. J. Linn. Soc.* **2015**, *177*, 278–289. [CrossRef] [PubMed]
6. Petersen, G.; Seberg, O.; Yde, M.; Berthelsen, K. Phylogenetic relationships of Triticum and Aegilops and evidence for the origin of the A, B, and D genomes of common wheat (*Triticum aestivum*). *Mol. Phylogenet. Evol.* **2006**, *39*, 70–82. [CrossRef]
7. Kasarda, D.D. Can an increase in celiac disease be attributed to an increase in the gluten content of wheat as a consequence of wheat breeding? *J. Agric. Food Chem.* **2013**, *61*, 1155–1159. [CrossRef] [PubMed]
8. Arzani, A.; Ashraf, M. Cultivated Ancient Wheats (*Triticum* spp.): A Potential Source of Health-Beneficial Food Products. *Compr. Rev. Food Sci. Food Saf.* **2017**, *16*, 477–488. [CrossRef]
9. Ludvigsson, J.F.; Leffler, D.A.; Bai, J.C.; Biagi, F.; Fasano, A.; Green, P.H.R.; Hadjivassiliou, M.; Kaukinen, K.; Kelly, C.P.; Leonard, J.N.; et al. The Oslo definitions for coeliac disease and related terms. *Gut* **2013**, *62*, 43–52. [CrossRef]
10. Fasano, A.; Sapone, A.; Zevallos, V.; Schuppan, D. Nonceliac gluten and wheat sensitivity. *Gastroenterology* **2015**, *148*, 1195–1204. [CrossRef]

11. Herrera, M.J.; Hermoso, M.A.; Quera, R. An update on the pathogenesis of celiac disease. *Revista Medica de Chile* **2009**, *137*, 1617–1626.
12. Brandtzaeg, P. The changing immunological paradigm in coeliac disease. *Immunol. Lett* **2006**, *105*, 127–139. [CrossRef] [PubMed]
13. Maiuri, L.; Ciacci, C.; Ricciardelli, I.; Vacca, L.; Raia, V.; Auricchio, S.; Picard, J.; Osman, M.; Quaratino, S.; Londei, M. Association between innate response to gliadin and activation of pathogenic T cells in coeliac disease. *Lancet* **2003**, *362*, 30–37. [CrossRef]
14. Maiuri, L.; Ciacci, C.; Auricchio, S.; Brown, V.; Quaratino, S.; Londei, M. Interleukin 15 mediates epithelial changes in celiac disease. *Gastroenterology* **2000**, *119*, 996–1006. [CrossRef] [PubMed]
15. Qiao, S.W.; Bergseng, E.; Molberg, O.; Xia, J.; Fleckenstein, B.; Khosla, C.; Sollid, L.M. Antigen Presentation to Celiac Lesion-Derived T Cells of a 33-Mer Gliadin Peptide Naturally Formed by Gastrointestinal Digestion. *J. Immunol* **2004**, *173*, 1757–1762. [CrossRef] [PubMed]
16. Ráki, M.; Tollefsen, S.; Molberg, Ø.; Lundin, K.E.A.; Sollid, L.M.; Jahnsen, F.L. A Unique Dendritic Cell Subset Accumulates in the Celiac Lesion and Efficiently Activates Gluten-Reactive T Cells. *Gastroenterology* **2006**, *131*, 428–438. [CrossRef] [PubMed]
17. Tollefsen, S.; Arentz-Hansen, H.; Fleckenstein, B.; Molberg, Ø.; Ráki, M.; Kwok, W.W.; Jung, G.; Lundin, K.E.A.; Sollid, L.M. HLA-DQ2 and -DQ8 signatures of gluten T cell epitopes in celiac disease. *J. Clin. Investig.* **2006**, *116*, 2226–2236. [CrossRef] [PubMed]
18. Bernardo, D. Human intestinal dendritic cells as controllers of mucosal immunity. *Rev. Esp. Enferm. Dig.* **2013**, *105*, 279–290. [CrossRef] [PubMed]
19. Martínez-Esteso, M.J.; Nørgaard, J.; Brohée, M.; Haraszi, R.; Maquet, A.; O'Connor, G. Defining the wheat gluten peptide fingerprint via a discovery and targeted proteomics approach. *J. Proteom.* **2016**, *147*, 156–168. [CrossRef]
20. Allred, L.K.; Ritter, B.W. Recognition of gliadin and glutenin fractions in four commercial gluten assays. *J. AOAC Int.* **2010**, *93*, 190–196.
21. Shewry, P.R.; Halford, N.G. Cereal seed storage proteins: Structures, properties and role in grain utilization. *J. Exp. Bot.* **2002**, *53*, 947–958. [CrossRef]
22. Mena, M.C.; Sousa, C.; Mena, M.C.; Sousa, C. CHAPTER 16. Analytical Tools for Gluten Detection: Policies and Regulation. *OmniaSci. Monogr.* **2015**, 527–564. [CrossRef]
23. Camarca, A.; Anderson, R.P.; Mamone, G.; Fierro, O.; Facchiano, A.; Costantini, S.; Zanzi, D.; Sidney, J.; Auricchio, S.; Sette, A.; et al. Intestinal T Cell Responses to Gluten Peptides Are Largely Heterogeneous: Implications for a Peptide-Based Therapy in Celiac Disease. *J. Immunol.* **2009**, *182*, 4158–4166. [CrossRef] [PubMed]
24. Shan, L.; Molberg, Ø.; Parrot, I.; Hausch, F.; Filiz, F.; Gray, G.M.; Sollid, L.M.; Khosla, C. Structural basis for gluten intolerance in Celiac Sprue. *Science* **2002**, *297*, 2275–2279. [CrossRef] [PubMed]
25. Molberg, Ø.; Uhlen, A.K.; Jensen, T.; Flæte, N.S.; Fleckenstein, B.; Arentz-Hansen, H.; Raki, M.; Lundin, K.E.A.; Sollid, L.M. Mapping of gluten T-cell epitopes in the bread wheat ancestors: Implications for celiac disease. *Gastroenterology* **2005**, *128*, 393–401. [CrossRef] [PubMed]
26. Sollid, L.M.; Qiao, S.W.; Anderson, R.P.; Gianfrani, C.; Koning, F. Nomenclature and listing of celiac disease relevant gluten T-cell epitopes restricted by HLA-DQ molecules. *Immunogenetics* **2012**, *64*, 455–460. [CrossRef] [PubMed]
27. Escarnot, E.; Gofflot, S.; Sinnaeve, G.; Dubois, B.; Bertin, P.; Mingeot, D. Reactivity of gluten proteins from spelt and bread wheat accessions towards A1 and G12 antibodies in the framework of celiac disease. *Food Chem.* **2018**, *268*, 522–532. [CrossRef] [PubMed]
28. Dubois, B.; Bertin, P.; Muhovski, Y.; Escarnot, E.; Mingeot, D. Development of TaqMan probes targeting the four major celiac disease epitopes found in α-gliadin sequences of spelt (*Triticum aestivum* ssp. spelta) and bread wheat (*Triticum aestivum* ssp. aestivum). *Plant Methods* **2017**, *13*, 1–14. [CrossRef]
29. Ozuna, C.V.; Iehisa, J.C.M.; Giménez, M.J.; Alvarez, J.B.; Sousa, C.; Barro, F. Diversification of the celiac disease α-gliadin complex in wheat: A 33-mer peptide with six overlapping epitopes, evolved following polyploidization. *Plant J.* **2015**, *82*, 794–805. [CrossRef]
30. Moron, B.; Cebolla, A.; Manyani, H.; Alvarez-Maqueda, M.; Megias, M.; Thomas, M.D.C.; Lopez, M.C.; Sousa, C. Sensitive detection of cereal fractions that are toxic to celiac disease patients by using monoclonal antibodies to a main immunogenic wheat peptide. *Am. J. Clin. Nutr.* **2008**, *87*, 405–414. [CrossRef]

31. Morón, B.; Bethune, M.T.; Comino, I.; Manyani, H.; Ferragud, M.; López, M.C.; Cebolla, Á.; Khosla, C.; Sousa, C. Toward the assessment of food toxicity for celiac patients: Characterization of monoclonal antibodies to a main immunogenic gluten peptide. *PLoS ONE* **2008**, *3*, 1–13. [CrossRef]
32. Comino, I.; Real, A.; Vivas, S.; Síglez, M.Á.; Caminero, A.; Nistal, E.; Casqueiro, J.; Rodríguez-Herrera, A.; Cebolla, Á.; Sousa, C. Monitoring of gluten-free diet compliance in celiac patients by assessment of gliadin 33-mer equivalent epitopes in feces. *Am. J. Clin. Nutr.* **2012**, *95*, 670–677. [CrossRef] [PubMed]
33. ArentzHansen, H.; McAdam, S.N.; Molberg, Ø.; Fleckenstein, B.; Lundin, K.E.A.; Jørgensen, T.J.D.; Jung, G.; Roepstorff, P.; Sollid, L.M. Celiac lesion T cells recognize epitopes that cluster in regions of gliadins rich in proline residues. *Gastroenterology* **2002**, *123*, 803–809. [CrossRef]
34. Vader, W.; Stepniak, D.; Kooy, Y.; Mearin, L.; Thompson, A.; van Rood, J.J.; Spaenij, L.; Koning, F. The HLA-DQ2 gene dose effect in celiac disease is directly related to the magnitude and breadth of gluten-specific T cell responses. *Proc. Natl. Acad. Sci. USA* **2003**, *100*, 12390–12395. [CrossRef] [PubMed]
35. Ciccocioppo, R.; Di Sabatino, A.; Corazza, G.R. The immune recognition of gluten in coeliac disease. *Clin. Exp. Immunol.* **2005**, *140*, 408–416. [CrossRef] [PubMed]
36. Payne, P.I.; Jackson, E.A.; Holt, L.M. The association between γ-gliadin 45 and gluten strength in durum wheat varieties: A direct causal effect or the result of genetic linkage? *J. Cereal Sci.* **1984**, *2*, 73–81. [CrossRef]
37. Jouanin, A.; Gilissen, L.J.W.J.; Boyd, L.A.; Cockram, J.; Leigh, F.J.; Wallington, E.J.; van den Broeck, H.C.; van der Meer, I.M.; Schaart, J.G.; Visser, R.G.F.; et al. Food processing and breeding strategies for coeliac-safe and healthy wheat products. *Food Res. Int.* **2018**, *110*, 11–21. [CrossRef]
38. Van Herpen, T.W.J.M.; Goryunova, S.V.; van der Schoot, J.; Mitreva, M.; Salentijn, E.; Vorst, O.; Schenk, M.F.; van Veelen, P.A.; Koning, F.; van Soest, L.J.M.; et al. Alpha-gliadin genes from the A, B, and D genomes of wheat contain different sets of celiac disease epitopes. *BMC Genom.* **2006**, *7*, 1–13. [CrossRef]
39. Salentijn, E.M.; Goryunova, S.V.; Bas, N.; van der Meer, I.M.; van den Broeck, H.C.; Bastien, T.; Gilissen, L.J.W.J.; Smulders, M.J.M. Tetraploid and hexaploid wheat varieties reveal large differences in expression of alpha-gliadins from homoeologous Gli-2 loci. *BMC Genom.* **2009**, *10*, 48. [CrossRef]
40. Kim, C.Y.; Quarsten, H.; Bergseng, E.; Khosla, C.; Sollid, L.M. Structural basis for HLA-DQ2-mediated presentation of gluten epitopes in celiac disease. *Proc. Natl. Acad. Sci. USA* **2004**, *101*, 4175–4179. [CrossRef]
41. Tye-Din, J.A.; Stewart, J.A.; Dromey, J.A.; Beissbarth, T.; Van Heel, D.A.; Tatham, A.; Henderson, K.; Mannering, S.I.; Gianfrani, C.; Jewell, D.P.; et al. Comprehensive, quantitative mapping of T cell epitopes in gluten in celiac disease. *Sci. Transl. Med.* **2010**, *2*. [CrossRef]
42. Schumann, M.; Siegmund, B.; Schulzke, J.D.; Fromm, M. Celiac Disease: Role of the Epithelial Barrier. *Cell. Mol. Gastroenterol. Hepatol.* **2017**, *3*, 150–162. [CrossRef] [PubMed]
43. Vartdal, F.; Johansen, B.H.; Friede, T.; Thorpe, C.J.; Stevanović, S.; Eriksen, J.E.; Sletten, K.; Thorsby, E.; Rammensee, H.G.; Sollid, L.M. The peptide binding motif of the disease associated HLA-DQ (α 1(*) 0501, β 1(*) 0201) molecule. *Eur. J. Immunol.* **1996**, *26*, 2764–2772. [CrossRef] [PubMed]
44. Arentz-Hansen, H.; Korner, R.; Molberg, O.; Quarsten, H.; Vader, W.; Kooy, Y.M.C.; Lundin, K.E.A.; Koning, F.; Roepstorff, P.; Sollid, L.M.; et al. The intestinal T cell response to a-gliadin in adult celiac disesae is focused on a single deamidated glutamine targeted by tissue transglutaminase. *J. Exp. Med.* **2000**, *191*, 603–612. [CrossRef]
45. Ellis, H.J.; Pollock, E.L.; Engel, W.; Fraser, J.S.; Rosen-Bronson, S.; Wieser, H.; Ciclitira, P.J. Investigation of the putative immunodominant T cell epitopes in coeliac disease. *Gut* **2003**, *52*, 212–217. [CrossRef] [PubMed]

MDPI
St. Alban-Anlage 66
4052 Basel
Switzerland
Tel. +41 61 683 77 34
Fax +41 61 302 89 18
www.mdpi.com

Nutrients Editorial Office
E-mail: nutrients@mdpi.com
www.mdpi.com/journal/nutrients

www.ingramcontent.com/pod-product-compliance
Lightning Source LLC
Chambersburg PA
CBHW041752220926
51847CB00014B/177
9783038977360